DATE

Substance Abuse

Alan David Kaye • Nalini Vadivelu
Richard D. Urman

Editors

Substance Abuse

Inpatient and Outpatient Management
for Every Clinician

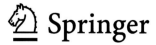 Springer

Editors
Alan David Kaye
Departments of Anesthesiology
  and Pharmacology
Louisiana State University Health
  Sciences Center, Louisiana State
  University Interim Hospital,
  and Ochsner Kenner Hospital
New Orleans, LA, USA

Nalini Vadivelu
Department of Anesthesiology
Yale University School of Medicine
  and Yale-New Haven Hospital
New Haven, CT, USA

Richard D. Urman
Department of Anesthesiology,
  Perioperative and Pain Medicine
Brigham and Women's Hospital
  Harvard Medical School
Boston, MA, USA

ISBN 978-1-4939-1950-5   ISBN 978-1-4939-1951-2 (eBook)
DOI 10.1007/978-1-4939-1951-2
Springer New York Heidelberg Dordrecht London

Library of Congress Control Number: 2014954439

Printed on acid-free paper

Springer is part of Springer Science+Business Media (www.springer.com)

To my wife, Dr. Kim Kaye, and my children, Aaron and Rachel Kaye, for being the best family a man could ask for in his life.

To my mother, Florence Feldman, who, while enduring a lifetime of pain and suffering with seven back surgeries, taught me to accomplish tasks and to reach my dreams and goals.

To Daniel Garcia, my nephew, and his entire family including: Sheree Kaye Garcia, my sister; Andrew Garcia, my nephew; Debra Garcia, my niece; and Amanda Garcia, my niece.

To all my teachers and colleagues at the University of Arizona in Tucson, Ochsner Clinic in New Orleans, Massachusetts General Hospital/Harvard School of Medicine in Boston, Tulane School of Medicine in New Orleans, Texas Tech Health Sciences Center in Lubbock, and LSU School of Medicine in New Orleans.

Alan David Kaye, MD, PhD

To my parents, Major General C. Vadivelu and Mrs. Gnanambigai Vadivelu, for their absolute trust in me always. To my husband, Thangamuthu Kodumudi, for his constant support. To my sons, Gopal Kodumudi and Vijay Kodumudi, who, with the highest standards of propriety, inspire me to reach out to perfection. To my siblings and their families for their friendship always, and to my colleagues and innumerable friends everywhere for countless helpful things.

Nalini Vadivelu, MD

To my patients, who inspired me to write this book to help other practitioners improve their care.
To my mentors for their encouragement and support.
To my students and trainees so that they can use this guide to better understand the needs of these patients.
To my family: my wife, Dr. Zina Matlyuk-Urman, M.D.; my daughters, Abigail and Isabelle, who make it all possible and worth it, every day.
And finally, to my parents, Tanya and Dennis Urman.

Richard D. Urman, MD, MBA

Foreword

Substance Abuse: Inpatient and Outpatient Management for Every Clinician will certainly be a welcomed and very well-timed new text addition to the libraries of practitioners who not only treat patients with substance abuse, but who also care for patients who experience chronic pain and require medication with analgesics and adjuvants with abuse potentials. The timing of this new text coincides with several recently publicized public health trends including the worldwide epidemic of prescription drug abuse and "drugged" driving, the identification of validated risk factors for substance abuse, and a paradigm shift in the management and prevention of substance abuse [1].

Schools of Medicine and Public Health,
Louisiana State University
New Orleans, LA, USA

James H. Diaz, MD, MPH,
DrPH, FACMT

Reference

1. Smith RM. Anesthesia for infants and children. St. Louis (MI): C.V. Mosby; 1959.

Preface

Virtually every family and every community will have to deal with substance abuse in one way or another, as there are epidemic rates of affliction in the United States and worldwide. For most people with a substance abuse issue, there are remarkably familiar stages, problematic consequences, and numerous brain chemistry changes that have been better appreciated in recent years.

Society portrays someone with substance abuse issues as a homeless, uneducated, lower socioeconomic individual offering little understanding or compassion. This is most naïve, as a person with a substance abuse disorder can be anyone, a grandmother, a teenager from an affluent family, or a prominent successful person admired for his or her talents in athletics, arts, sciences, or business. How much is related to genetics versus the environment has been a long-standing debate. Many of the common molecular mechanisms and general themes related to substance abuse are better understood today, even though the prevalence of addiction and abuse have never been higher, particularly alcohol abuse, tobacco use, opioid medication abuse, and eating disorders.

The editors of this book have not been immune to the consequences of substance abuse. We have witnessed star quarterbacks die related to acute alcohol binge in high school, family members brought to emergency rooms and rehabilitation facilities for prescription and heroin abuse, pleasant appearing patients, including grandmothers and clergy, fail urine toxicology screens at our pain clinics, and reasonable and compliant patients shot and killed in their homes related to dealing with the same drugs they were prescribed for appropriate spinal cord pathologies or pain syndromes. Over and above these terrible stories, the suffering of loving family members cannot be understated. As examples, anyone who grew up in a home with an alcoholic parent or an overeating child knows that substance abuse, though with many appearances and nuances, is a problem all of us share. Data indicate lack of success for many of these substance abuse issues. This failure is tragic with our ever-evolving technology and robust pharmaceutical industry. On a positive note, science is constantly developing new medications with an ever-evolving and better-understood subtype receptor target or enzyme to combat physical and mental processes prominent with substance abuse-mediated sequelae.

As editors of *Substance Abuse: Inpatient and Outpatient Management for Every Clinician* we have recruited outstanding scientists and clinicians to better outline the current understanding of substance abuse, discuss cutting-edge research, and to summarize treatment options. We hope this book is utilized by health care professionals and non-health care professionals for many years to come. We thank the authors that have contributed outstanding chapters to make our book easy to read yet in depth and pertinent to the reader. Finally, we all need to appreciate that each person we help in life should be thought of as a family member. With this in mind, we can all make decisions to help others and give of ourselves, when those around us have critical and difficult moments. The world is made for comebacks and there is no greater gift than your time, patience, and love for others.

New Orleans, LA, USA   Alan David Kaye, MD, PhD
New Haven, CT, USA   Nalini Vadivelu, MD, DNB
Boston, MA, USA   Richard D. Urman, MD, MBA

Contents

Contributors

Mohammed Jamil Abu-Asi, M.B.B.S., M.R.C.P. Department of Anesthetics, Epsom and St. Helier University Hospitals NHS, Surrey, UK

Magdalena Anitescu, M.D., Ph.D. Department of Anesthesia and Critical Care, University of Chicago Medical Center, Chicago, IL, USA

Danie Babypaul, M.B.B.S., D.A., M.D. Department of Anesthetics, Royal Glamorgan Hospital, LlantrisantRhondda Cynon Taf, UK

Debasish Basu, M.D., Ph.D. Department of Psychiatry, Postgraduate Institute of Medical Education and Research, Drug De-Addiction and Treatment Center, Chandigarh, India

Peter A. Blume, D.P.M. Department of Podiatric Medicine and Surgery, Yale New Haven Hospital/VA Healthcare System, New Haven, CT, USA

Department of Surgery, Anesthesia and Orthopedics and Rehabilitation Medicine Yale University School of Medicine, Yale New Haven Hospital, New Haven, CT, USA

Michael N. Brown, M.D., D.C. Seattle, WA, USA

Ethan O. Bryson, M.D. Department of Anesthesiology and Psychiatry, Icahn School of Medicine at Mount Sinai, New York, NY, USA

Sara Bustamante, F.F.P.M.R.C.A., F.R.C.A. Department of Anesthetics and Pain Management, Epsom, St. Helier University Hospitals NHS Trust, Carshalton, Surrey, UK

Ryan Chadha, M.D. Department of Anesthesiology, Yale University School of Medicine, Yale-New Haven Hospital, New Haven, CT, USA

Sumit Chatterji, M.A., M.B., B.Chir., F.R.C.P. Respiratory Department, Peterborough & Stamford Hospitals, Cambridge, UK

Grace Chen, M.D. Department of Anesthesiology and Perioperative Medicine, Oregon Health and Sciences University, Portland, OR, USA

Michal Czernicki, F.R.C.A. F.F.P.M.R.C.A., M.D. Department of Anesthesia and Pain Management, Nottingham University Hospital in United Kingdom, Nottingham, Nottinghamshire, UK

Yashwin Agnelo D'Costa, M.B.B.S., M.D. Department of Anesthetics, St. Helier Hospital, Carshalton, Surrey, UK

Susan Dabu-Bondoc, M.D. Department of Anesthesiology, Yale New Haven Hospital, Yale School of Medicine, New Haven, CT, USA

Xiaoli Dai, M.D. Department of Anesthesiology, University of Mississippi Medical Center, Jackson, MS, USA

Anjuli Desai, M.D. Department of Pain Medicine, Temple University Hospital, Philadelphia, PA, USA

Ranjit Deshpande, M.B.B.S. Department of Anesthesiology, Yale University School of Medicine, New Haven, CT, USA

Gulshan Doulatram, M.D. Department of Anesthesiology, University of Texas Medical Branch, Galveston, TX, USA

Philip R. Effraim, M.D., Ph.D. Department of Anesthesiology, Yale New Haven Hospital, New Haven, CT, USA

Chioma N. Odukwe Enu, D.P.M. Department of Podiatric Medicine and Surgery, Yale New Haven Hospital/VA Healthcare System, New Haven, CT, USA

Ike Eriator, M.D., M.P.H. Department of Anesthesiology, University of Mississippi Medical Center, Jackson, MS, USA

Frank John English Falco, M.D. Mid Atlantic Spine and Pain Physicians, Newark, DE, USA

American Society of Interventional Pain Physicians, Paducah, KY, USA

Temple University Medical School, Philadelphia, PA, USA

Pain Medicine Fellowship Program, Temple University Hospital, Newark, DE, USA

Michael Alan Fishman, M.D., M.B.A. Department of Anesthesiology, Yale University School of Medicine, New Haven, CT, USA

Cynthia French, M.S., B.S.N., C.R.N.A.

Larissa Galante, M.S.N., B.S.N., C.R.N.A.

Gabriel V. Gambardella, D.P.M. Department of Pediatric Medicine and Surgery, Yale New Haven Hospital, New Haven, CT, USA

Kingsuk Ganguly, M.D. Department of Anesthesiology, Perioperative and Pain Medicine, Stanford University School of Medicine, Redwood City, CA, USA

Clifford Gevirtz, M.D., M.P.H. LSU New Orleans Health Sciences Center, Harrison, NY, USA

Jhaodi Gong, M.D. Department of Anesthesiology, Yale University School of Medicine, New Haven, CT, USA

Ranganathan Govindaraj, M.D., F.R.C.A. Department of Anesthesiology, University of Texas Medical Branch, Galveston, TX, USA

Kirsten B. Grace, M.S.N., B.S.N., F.N.P-C., A.P.R.N.

Karina Gritsenko, M.D. Department of Anesthesiology, Montefiore Medical Center—Albert Einstein College of Medicine, Bronx, NY, USA

Maria Teresa Gudin, M.D., F.R.C.A., F.F.P.M.R.C.A. Department of Anesthesiology, Getafe University Hospital, Madrid, Spain

Sumit Gulati, M.D. Department of Pain Medicine, The Walton Centre NHS Foundation Trust, Liverpool, UK

Ala Haddadin, M.D. Department of Anesthesiology, Yale University School of Medicine, New Haven, CT, USA

Hans C. Hansen, M.D. The Pain Relief Center, Conover, NC, USA

Kareem Hubbard, M.D. Redwood Medical Center, Pleasanton, CA, USA

Chrystina Jeter, M.D. Department of Anesthesiology, Perioperative and Pain Medicine, University School of Medicine, Redwood City, CA, USA

Jatin Joshi, M.D. Memorial Sloan Kettering Cancer Center, Hospital for Special Surgery, Weill Cornell Medical College, New York, NY, USA

Emily Kahn, M.D. Department of Anesthesiology, Yale-New Haven Hospital, New Haven, CT, USA

Alan David Kaye, M.D., Ph.D., D.A.B.A., D.A.B.P.M., D.A.B.I.P.P. Departments of Anesthesiology and Pharmacology, Louisiana State University Health Sciences Center, Louisiana State University Interim Hospital, and Ochsner Kenner Hospital, New Orleans, LA, USA

Adam Marc Kaye, Pharm.D., F.A.S.C.P., F.C.Ph.A. Department of Pharmacy Practice, Thomas J. Long School of Pharmacy and Health Sciences, University of the Pacific, Stockton, CA, USA

Ameana Khan, M.B.B.S. Department of Anaesthetics, Milton Keynes Hospital, Rickmansworth, Hertfordshire, UK

Song Kim, B.S. Tulane University School of Medicine, New Orleans, LA, USA

Martin D. Knolle, M.A., M.B., B.Chir., Ph.D., M.R.C.P. Addenbrooke's Hospital, Cambridge University Hospital NHS Foundation Trust, Cambridge, UK

Daniel Krashin, M.D. Department of Psychiatry and Pain and Anesthesia, Harborview Medical Center, University of Washington, Seattle, WA, USA

Sreekumar Kunnumpurath, M.B.B.S., M.D., F.F.P.M.R.C.A., F.R.C.A., F.C.A.R.C.S.I. Department of Anesthetics and Pain Management, Epsom and St. Helier University Hospitals NHS Trust, Carshalton, UK

Steven Michael Lampert, M.D. Department of Anesthesiology, Perioperative and Pain Medicine, Brigham & Women's Hospital, Harvard Medical School, Boston, MA, USA

Sahra Lantz-Dretnik, M.B.B.S., B.Sc. (Hon.) St George's Hospital, London, UK

Janet Lucas, L.C.S.W. Family Medicine Residency Program, Glendale Adventist Medical Center, Glendale, CA, USA

Bobby Ray Malbrough, Esq., B.A., J.D. Attorney at Law, New Orleans, LA, USA

Adnan Khan Malik, M.D. Department of Anesthesiology, Yale-New Haven Hospital, New Haven, CT, USA

Laxmaiah Manchikanti, M.D. Anesthesiology and Perioperative Medicine, University of Louisville, Paducah, KY, USA

Steve Martino, Ph.D. Psychology Service, VA Connecticut Healthcare System, West Haven, CT, USA

Yale University School of Medicine, Department of Psychiatry, New Haven, CT, USA

Kim Mauer, M.D. Department of Anesthesiology, Oregon Health & Sciences University, Portland, OR, USA

Bill Mejia, L.C.S.W. Department of Palliative Care, Social Work, and Spiritual Care, Huntington Memorial Hospital, Pasadena, CA, USA

Ann Marie Melookaran, M.D. Department of Anesthesiology, Yale-New Haven Hospital, New Haven, CT, USA

Suresh Menon, M.D., F.R.C.A. Department of Anaesthetics, Milton Keynes, UK

Hosni Mikhael, M.D. Department of Anesthesiology, Yale-New Haven Hospital, New Haven, CT, USA

Sukanya Mitra, M.D., Ph.D. Department of Anesthesia and Intensive Care, Government Medical College and Hospital, Chandigarh, India

Natalia Murinova, M.D., M.H.A. Department of Neurology, University of Washington, Seattle, WA, USA

Iyabo Muse, M.D. Department of Anesthesiology, Montefiore Medical Center—Albert Einstein College of Medicine, Bronx, NY, USA

Narendren Narayanasamy, M.D. Department of Anesthesiology, Washington University School of Medicine, St. Louis, MO, USA

Jordan L. Newmark, M.D. Department of Anesthesiology, Perioperative and Pain Medicine, Stanford University School of Medicine, Redwood City, CA, USA

Elizabeth Ngo, D.O. Department of Physical Medicine and Rehabilitation, University of California, Irvine, Costa Mesa, CA, USA

Efosa Ogiamien, B.S. University of Mississippi School of Medicine, Jackson, MS, USA

Jasmina Perinpanayagam, M.B.B.S., B.Sc. (Hons.) Department of Anesthetics, Epsom and St. Helier University Hospitals NHS, Carshalton, Surrey, UK

David Pilkey, Ph.D. Psychology Service, VA Connecticut Healthcare System, West Haven, CT, USA

Yale University School of Medicine, Department of Psychiatry, New Haven, CT, USA

Thomas B. Pulimood, FRCP, FHEA. West Suffolk Hospital, A University of Cambridge Teaching Hospital, Edmunds, UK

Vinay Puttanniah, M.D. Department of Anesthesiology and Critical Care Mediline, Memorial Sloan Kettering Cancer Center, New York, NY, USA

Tilak D. Raj, M.D., M.R.C.P., F.R.C.A. Department of Anesthesiology, Oklahoma University Health Sciences Center/OU Medical Center, Oklahoma City, OK, USA

Rahul Rastogi, M.D. Department of Anesthesiology, Washington University School of Medicine, St. Louis, MO, USA

Anne Riffenburgh, L.C.S.W. The Huntington Cancer Center, Palliative Care, Huntington Memorial Hospital, Pasadena, CA, USA

Matthew Verne Satterly, M.D. Department of Anesthesiology, Center for Advanced Medicine, Pain Management Center, Washington University School of Medicine, St. Louis, MO, USA

Brian M. Schmidt, D.P.M. Department of Podiatric Medicine and Surgery, Yale New Haven Hospital/VA Healthcare System, New Haven, CT, USA

Andrei D. Sdrulla, M.D., Ph.D. Department of Anesthesiology and Perioperative Medicine, Oregon Health and Sciences University, Portland, OR, USA

Amit A. Shah, M.D. Department of Anesthesiology, Yale New Haven Hospital, New Haven, CT, USA

Shalini Shah, M.D. Department of Anesthesiology and Peri-operative Care, University of California, Irvine, Orange, CA, USA

Debra Short, Pharm.D. Stockton, CA, USA

Sanford M. Silverman, M.D. Comprehensive Pain Medicine, Florida Society of Interventional Pain Physicians (FSIPP), Pompano Beach, FL, USA

Gnana S. Simon, M.D., M.B.A. Department of Anesthesiology, Yale-New Haven Hospital, New Haven, CT, USA

Paul Sraow, M.D., M.S. Spine & Sports Rehabilitation Institute, Tempe, AZ, USA

Howard Steinberg, Ph.D. Psychology Service, VA Connecticut Healthcare System, West Haven, CT, USA

Yale University School of Medicine, Department of Psychiatry, New Haven, CT, USA

Natacha Telusca, M.D. Department of Anesthesiology, Perioperative and Pain Medicine, Stanford University School of Medicine, Redwood City, CA, USA

Donna-Ann M. Thomas, M.D. Department of Anesthesiology, Yale University School of Medicine, New Haven, CT, USA

Andrea Trescot, M.D. Pain and Headache Center, Wasilla, AK, USA

Richard D. Urman, M.D., M.B.A., C.P.E. Department of Anesthesiology, Perioperative and Pain Medicine, Brigham and Women's Hospital, Harvard Medical School, Boston, MA, USA

Nalini Vadivelu, M.D. Department of Anesthesiology, Yale University, New Haven, CT, USA

Amaresh Vydyanathan, M.B.B.S., M.S. Assistant Professor of Anesthesiology Fellowship Co-Director Regional Anesthesia and Acute Pain Medicine Montefiore Medical Center, Bronx, NY, USA

Shu-Ming Wang, M.D. Department of Anesthesiology, St. Francis Hospital, Hartford, CT, USA

Lara Zador, M.D. Department of Anesthesia, Yale New Haven Hospital, New Haven, CT, USA

Qingbing Zhu, M.D., Ph.D. Department of Anesthesiology, Yale University, School of Medicine, New Haven, CT, USA

Chapter 1
Definition and Demographics of Addiction

Andrei D. Sdrulla, Grace Chen, and Kim Mauer

Key Points

- Introduction/background
- Definition of addiction/demographics
- Alcohol-related disorders
- Amphetamine and amphetamine-like related disorders
- Caffeine-related disorders
- Nicotine-related disorders
- Opioid-related disorders
- Hallucinogen-related disorders
- Sedative-, hypnotic-, or anxiolytic-related disorders

Introduction

Addiction in the context of psychiatry has historically meant dysfunctional use of a substance that leads to psychosocial pathology. Over time, the concept of the object that leads to dysfunction has widened from illicit drugs to everyday necessities such as food, sex, and even technology such as the Internet. Dysfunction may be measured by a validated questionnaire such as the SF-12 [1]. The DSM IV subclassifies substance dependence and abuse pathologies as: alcohol-related, amphetamine or amphetamine-like, caffeine-related, cannabis-related, cocaine, hallucinogen, inhalant-related, nicotine, opioid, phencyclidine (PCP), sedative/hypnotic or anxiolytic, polysubstance and unknown, "other" substance disorders.

A.D. Sdrulla, M.D., Ph.D. (✉) • G. Chen, M.D. • K. Mauer, M.D.
Department of Anesthesiology and Perioperative Medicine, Oregon Health & Sciences University, 3181 SW Sam Jackson Park Road, Portland, OR 97239, USA
e-mail: Sdrulla@ohsu.edu; Cheng@ohsu.edu; Mauer@ohsu.edu

© Springer Science+Business Media New York 2015
A.D. Kaye et al. (eds.), *Substance Abuse*, DOI 10.1007/978-1-4939-1951-2_1

The DSM IV defines addiction as abuse and dependence. "Abuse" refers to use that impairs the individual's ability to function in one or more important areas. "Dependence" includes physical withdrawal if abstaining, and a lifestyle centered on obtaining and using the drug. Interestingly, most patients with substance abuse problems do not develop dependence [2]. Indeed, the risk of developing dependence from abuse is 26.6 % of individuals with alcohol abuse, 9.4 % with cannabis abuse, and 15.6 % with cocaine abuse.

The compulsive use of illicit or legal substances is thought to reflect dysregulation of neurotransmitters in the brain. For example, stimulants such as amphetamine and cocaine promote dopamine release, opioids act like endogenous endorphins, and similar to benzodiazepines, are GABA agonists. More broadly there are "dirty" drugs, such as alcohol that affect several types of neurotransmitter receptors including dopamine, serotonin, opiate, GABA, glutamate, acetylcholine, and endocanabinoid receptors.

According to the National Survey on Drug Use and Health (NSDUH), in 2010 55 % of American adults consumed at least some alcohol, while marijuana was the most commonly used illicit drug (41 %), and enough opioids were prescribed in 2012 to medicate every American every 4 h [3]. As noted above, tobacco, not surprisingly, causes the most preventable deaths [4]. Thus, addiction is a profound medical and sociological problem in the USA and around the world.

Definition of Addiction

There are two principal, widely used definitions associated with addiction, from the DSM and ASAM. The DSM IV definition uses the words of "abuse" and "dependence" to describe the clinical consequences of addiction (Table 1.1). Rather than being one psychopathology, the DSM IV classifies abuse and dependence according to the particular object of pursuit. For example, the DSM IV defines alcohol abuse and dependence as maladaptive patterns of consumption leading to clinically significant impairment or distress [5].

The most recent version of the DSM IV avoided the word "addiction" and instead used "abuse and dependence" primarily because addiction has pejorative connotations and might place an unnecessary burden on patients. However, this choice of wording created some confusion. Clinicians generally consider "dependence" as physical dependence, not necessarily including the compulsive seeking behavior that is at the core of addiction-based dysfunction. With this confusion between compulsive dysfunctional behavior and physiologic process, patients and clinicians alike often have difficulty distinguishing between psychiatric pathology and physiologic sequelae. For example, patients who had been exposed to opioid medication for pain may have withdrawal symptoms such as piloerection, anxiety, tearing and yawning. This is evidence of physiologic dependence; whether or not the patient has dysfunctional behavior in response to the physiologic dependence is what determines psychiatric pathology.

Table 1.1 Criteria for substance abuse and substance dependence

Criteria for substance abuse	Criteria for substance dependence
A pattern of substance use leading to significant impairment or distress, as manifested by one or more of the following during in the past 12-month period:	Dependence or significant impairment or distress, as manifested by 3 or more of the following during a 12-month period:
1. Failure to fulfill major role obligations at work, school, home such as repeated absences or poor work performance related to substance use; substance-related absences, suspensions, or expulsions from school; neglect of children or household	1. Tolerance or markedly increased amounts of the substance to achieve intoxication or desired effect or markedly diminished effect with continued use of the same amount of substance
2. Frequent use of substances in situation in which it is physically hazardous (e.g., driving an automobile or operating a machine when impaired by substance use)	2. Withdrawal symptoms or the use of certain substances to avoid withdrawal symptoms
3. Frequent legal problems (e.g., arrests, disorderly conduct) for substance abuse	3. Use of a substance in larger amounts or over a longer period than was intended
4. Continued use despite having persistent or recurrent social or interpersonal problems (e.g., arguments with spouse about consequences of intoxication, physical fights)	4. Persistent desire or unsuccessful efforts to cut down or control substance use
	5. Involvement in chronic behavior to obtain the substance, use the substance, or recover from its effects
	6. Reduction or abandonment of social, occupational or recreational activities because of substance use
	7. Use of substances even though there is a persistent or recurrent physical or psychological problem that is likely to have been caused or exacerbated by the substance

According to the newest definition proposed by the ASAM, addiction is not only behavioral but also a chronic brain disease. Addiction encompasses (a) inability to consistently abstain; (b) impairment in behavioral control; (c) craving or increased "hunger" for drugs or rewarding experiences; (d) diminished recognition of significant problems with one's behavior and interpersonal relationships; and (e) a dysfunctional emotional response [6]. This new definition by ASAM contrasts with the DSM IV definition in many ways. First, as mentioned above, DSM IV does not use the word "addiction" but rather "dependence and abuse." Second, the DSM IV does not aim to attribute a cause as the dysfunction is described in terms of clinically significant impairment or distress. Third, the DSM IV elucidates individual impairments instead of a unifying disease. An overview of DSM IV Drug Use Disorders (2001–2002) is presented below (Table 1.2) [7].

Table 1.2 Twelve-month and lifetime prevalence of specific DSM IV drug use disorders

Drug use disorders	Prevalence, % (SE)	
	12-Month	Lifetime
Any drug use disorder	2.0 (0.1)	10.3 (0.3)
• Any drug abuse	1.4 (0.1)	7.7 (0.2)
• Any drug dependence	0.6 (0.1)	2.6 (0.1)
Sedative use disorder	0.2 (0.02)	1.1 (0.1)
• Sedative abuse	0.1 (0.02)	0.8 (0.1)
• Sedative dependence	0.1 (0.02)	0.3 (0.03)
Tranquilizer use disorder	0.1 (0.02)	1.0 (0.1)
• Tranquilizer abuse	0.1 (0.02)	0.8 (0.1)
• Tranquilizer dependence	0.1 (0.02)	0.2 (0.03)
Opioid use disorder	0.4 (0.1)	1.4 (0.1)
• Opioid abuse	0.2 (0.04)	1.1 (0.1)
• Opioid dependence	0.1 (0.02)	0.3 (0.04)
Amphetamine use disorder	0.2 (0.03)	2.0 (0.1)
• Amphetamine abuse	0.1 (0.02)	1.4 (0.1)
• Amphetamine dependence	0.1 (0.02)	0.6 (0.1)
Hallucinogen use disorder	0.1 (0.02)	1.7 (0.1)
• Hallucinogen abuse	0.1 (0.02)	1.5 (0.1)
• Hallucinogen dependence	0.02 (0.01)	0.2 (0.03)
Cannabis use disorder	1.5 (0.1)	8.5 (0.3)
• Cannabis abuse	1.1 (0.1)	7.2 (0.2)
• Cannabis dependence	0.3 (0.04)	1.3 (0.1)
Cocaine use disorder	0.3 (0.03)	2.8 (0.1)
• Cocaine abuse	0.1 (0.02)	1.8 (0.1)
• Cocaine dependence	1.1 (0.02)	1.0 (0.1)
Solvent/inhalant abuse[a]	0.02 (0.01)	0.3 (0.04)

[a]The base rate for solvent/inhalant dependence was 0.00 %; DSM IV (Diagnostic and Statistical Manual of Mental Disorders, Fourth Edition) Diagnostic and Statistical Manual of Mental Disorders, Fourth Edition. American Psychiatric Association [42]

Demographics

According to the 2012 NSDUH, an annual survey sponsored by the Substance Abuse and Mental Health Services Administration (SAMHSA) of non-institutionalized civilians who are 12 years or older, an estimated 23.9 million were current (past month) illicit drug users. This striking number represents a staggering 9.2 % of the population. Illicit drugs include marijuana/hashish, cocaine (including crack), heroin, hallucinogens, inhalants, or prescription-type psychotherapeutics (pain relievers, tranquilizers, stimulants, and sedatives) [8]. Each of these is discussed in the following sections.

Alcohol-Related Disorders

Alcohol is the oldest substance of abuse. In 1994, 14 million Americans had alcohol-related disorders [9]. A study from 2012 documented that drinking starts at age 12 and included 2.2 % of 12 year olds, drinking peaks in adults age 21–26 at 60 % and includes binge or heavy drinking, then drinking steadily declines after age 65 to 10 % (Fig. 1.1) [8].

In the USA, alcohol-related disorders cost an estimated $166 billion every year [10]. This cost is manifested in motor vehicle crashes, lost work place productivity, neuropsychological impairment, and other psychiatric comorbidities. Hasin et al. conducted in-person interviews with 43,093 US adults to gather epidemiologic data about alcohol use disorders.

They found that the prevalence of lifetime and 12-month alcohol *abuse* was 17.8 and 4.7 % while the prevalence of lifetime and 12-month alcohol *dependence* was 12.5 and 3.8 %.

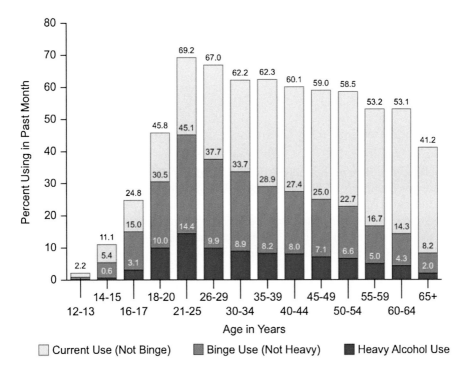

Fig. 1.1 A study from 2012 documented that drinking starts at age 12 and included 2.2 % of 12 year olds, drinking peaks in adults age 21–26 at 60 % and includes binge or heavy drinking, then drinking steadily declines after age 65 to 10 %

Similar to previous epidemiological studies, alcohol dependence was significantly more prevalent among men, whites, Native Americans, younger and unmarried adults, and those in lower income brackets [11].

Psychiatric disorders tend to cluster and this is relevant to substance abuse. According to the 1996 comorbidity survey, patients with alcohol dependence/abuse are 3.9 times more likely to be depressed, 6.3 times more likely to be bipolar, and 4.6 times more likely to have generalized anxiety disorder [12]. In the 2007 analysis of comorbid conditions to alcoholism, drug dependence is almost 20 times more prevalent in patients who suffer from alcohol use disorder when the study population is controlled for sociodemographics. Interestingly, Hasin et al. observed that alcohol dependence together with other substance disorders appears to be due in part to unique factors underlying etiology for each pair of disorders studied, while comorbidity of alcohol dependence with mood, anxiety, and personality disorders appears more attributable to factors shared among these other disorders. Americans who are between the ages of 30–67 are most at risk for lifelong alcohol abuse. The relatively lower prevalence of alcohol abuse in the Asian population is attributed to genetic polymorphisms that affect alcohol metabolism [13]. Alcohol abuse is also lower among African Americans, but the cause for this reduced prevalence is not yet known.

In a 2013 study of more than 7,000 patients, the highest proportion of individuals with alcohol abuse was persons 45 years of age or older, male, white, married or living with someone, employed, US-born, and living in urban areas, with at least some college education, and an individual income of less than $20,000 per year (some of these are contrary to one or more statements above) [2].

Amphetamine and Amphetamine-Like Related Disorders

Amphetamines have become a very prominent drug of abuse, and as a class include the psychostimulants amphetamine, dextroamphetamine, and methamphetamine. Amphetamines are chirals, dextro-, and levo-amphetamine with levo-amphetamine being more potent. Amphetamines are indirect sympathomimetics that stimulate release and inhibit reuptake of monoamines such as serotonin and dopamine. Methylphenidate and amphetamine are Schedule II controlled medications that have medical uses for narcolepsy, obesity, and attention deficit/hyperactivity disorder [14]. Amphetamine was first synthesized in the 1870s and was subsequently popularized to treat obesity and narcolepsy, and was used widely during World War II to keep soldiers alert. Abuse of methamphetamines became prevalent in the 1960s and 1970s when addicts discovered that IV use produces more rapid and profound euphoria than oral doses. Remarkably, amphetamine is one of the most abused illicit drugs in the world, more than heroin and cocaine combined [15]. The widespread abuse of amphetamine has a profound impact on social order and prosperity. The US Department of Justice reported that identity theft in 2007 significantly increased specifically to fund the purchase of amphetamines [16]. In the USA in 2005, an estimated $4.2 billion was spent on criminal justice costs associated with methamphetamine [17]. For the individual patient, amphetamine abuse is frequently associated with profound depressions and significantly increased chances of aortic dissection [18] and Parkinson's Disease [19] and the health risks vary according to gender and ethnicity. Overall, as a consequence of methamphetamine abuse, back/neck injuries (27 %), severe dental problems (26 %), gunshot/knife injury (25 %), and sexually transmitted diseases (STDs) (24 %) were commonly reported. Racial/ethnic differences were observed for conditions including gunshot/knife injuries, hearing loss; learning disabilities disproportionately affect Latino populations, while asthma and STDs disproportionately affect African Americans [20].

Gruenewald et al. studied the spread of amphetamine abuse in California from 1995 to 2008 and found a 13-fold increase, or about a 17 % increase per year [21]. The growth is mostly in non-dense urban areas with large white and Hispanic populations. Amphetamines are relatively cheap to produce and readily available and this may be one of the major causes underlying the dramatic increase in use and abuse worldwide.

Caffeine-Related Disorders

Caffeine is legal and the most commonly used drug in the world, but is not considered an abused substance by the DSM IV. Caffeine is an adenosine receptor antagonist that produces similar psychomotor activation as cocaine or amphetamines and is pervasive in fast paced societies where mild stimulants are socially acceptable [22]. Most psychiatrists recognize that caffeine abstinence causes withdrawal symptoms such as headache and fatigue. Within the context of the DSM IV, however, psychiatrists disagree about the severity even though 73 % believe that caffeine withdrawal can have clinical importance [23]. Indeed, more than half of those did not want caffeine use disorder to be included in the DSM IV because of fears that psychiatry is perceived as being concerned with the banal. When students are interviewed about their high rates of caffeine use for cognitive enhancement and their low rates of illicit drug use, they cited medical, ethical, and legal reasons why caffeine was the preferred drug [24]. Caffeine use is not generally considered a profound sociological or medical problem.

Cannabis-Related [25] Disorders

Cannabis is a widely used drug and, notably, CB1 receptors are the most highly expressed receptors in the brain. Currently, cannabis legalization fuels heated political debates. Proponents argue that cannabis use is safe and that it is a legitimate treatment for conditions such as glaucoma, pain, and anxiety, but cannabis use has been implicated in myocardial infarctions [26], anxiety, depression, and psychosis [27]. In an attempt to dissuade people from the use of alcohol or cannabis it is frequently stressed that use of these substances correlates with a poorer quality of life. However, Swain et al. studied the relationship between quality of life and alcohol or cannabis use in young adults and found that quality of life correlated with circumstantial life events and not substance use [28].

Perhaps the most significant point for a clinician who encounters a patient with cannabis use disorder is to not miss a possible psychiatric disorder, as cannabis users frequently have comorbid mood disorders such as depression, anxiety, and schizophrenia [25]. Social anxiety disorders are more likely to be related to cannabis dependence than abuse [29]. Also, cannabis use may have a genetic component as shown by an Australian twins study published in 2012. In a separate study of 3,824 young adults born between 1972 and 1979 cannabis use was very common with 75.2 % of males and 64.7 % of females reporting some use in their lifetimes, and 24.5 % of males and 11.8 % of females meeting criteria for DSM IV cannabis abuse or dependence. Rates of other drug use disorders and common psychiatric conditions were highly correlated with the extent of cannabis involvement and there was consistent evidence of heritable influences across a range of cannabis phenotypes including early ($\leq$15 years) opportunity to use, early ($\leq$16 years) onset use, and DSM abuse/dependence. Early age of onset of cannabis use was strongly associated with increased rates of subsequent use of other illicit drugs and with illicit drug abuse/dependence [30]. Thus, cannabis use is both popular and poses very real psychosocial challenges.

Nicotine-Related Disorders

Tobacco use is responsible for the most preventable deaths in America, and amounts to a staggering $200 billion each year in health costs [4]. Approximately 70 % of smokers want to quit but only 3–7 % succeed [31]. In 2012, an estimated 69.5 million Americans aged 12 or older were current users of tobacco products, representing ~26 % of the population. Nicotine is thought to achieve its highly addictive property through stimulating phasic dopamine release and the consequent feeling of reward [32]. Nicotine use had been associated with a variety of health problems beyond cancer, including non-unions in orthopedic surgeries, extensive aortoiliac atherosclerosis [33], and wound dehiscence in soft tissue surgeries [34].

Interestingly, many longitudinal studies found associations between childhood inattention/hyperactivity and defiant behavior disorders with parental nicotine abuse. In one 15-year longitudinal study of young patients who suffer from substance abuse, 37 % had a nicotine use disorder [35]. This population is at increased risk for health concerns at much earlier ages. For example, in study of young stroke patients, half of those between 18 and 55 were smokers at the time of their stroke [36].

Tobacco abuse has a clear correlation with education. According to the CDC, in the USA, the smoking rate among people with post-graduate degrees is 5 % as compared to 45 % for those people with GEDs. There are also ethnic factors as 31.5 % of American Indians/Alaska Natives (non-Hispanic), 9.9 % of Asians (non-Hispanic; excludes Native Hawaiians and Pacific Islanders), 19.4 % of blacks (non-Hispanic), 12.9 % of Hispanics, and 20.6 % of whites (non-Hispanic) are smokers. In terms of gender, women are less likely to be smokers than are men [37], and geographically, smoking is highest in the midwest and southeast regions of the country.

While smoking rates in the USA are high, there are other places with much higher smoking rates. The World Health Organization (WHO) reports that Guinea, Argentina, and Lebanon have adult smoking rates approaching 50 % [38].

Opioid-Related Disorders

The use of opioids to treat patients with chronic pain has increased dramatically over the last two decades [39–41]. This has been accompanied by escalating prescription drug abuse, particularly for the opioid analgesics and opioid abuse is now epidemic in our society. With more patients being prescribed opioids, there are now greater numbers of patients with physical dependence and/or addiction. In this case, it is particularly important to understand the difference between dependence and addiction before adding the label, and its consequences, to your patient's record.

Addiction is a chronic neurobiological brain disease that occurs with exposure to reward-producing drugs such as opioids. It is thought that certain patients may be more biologically and psychosocially susceptible to addiction than others. Addiction can be evidenced by specific behaviors, such as poor control over drug use and continued use of the drug despite physical, mental, and/or social harm. Although most chronic pain patients who take opioids on a long-term basis will become physically dependent on them, very few will ever become addicted to them.

A cross-sectional study showed that, among patients on opioids at a tertiary pain center, the prevalence of addiction was 14 % when the International Statistical Classification of Diseases and Related Health Problems (ICD), [a medical classification list by the WHO] ICD-10 criteria were used [42]. There are well-established risk factors for developing addiction during pain treatment with opioids. These include genetic predisposition, personal or family history of addiction, psychiatric disorders such as depression and anxiety, younger age, high opioid doses, use of short-acting opioids, high pain level, multiple pain complaints, self-reported craving, and concurrent use of tobacco, alcohol, and benzodiazepines [42–44].

In addition to dependence, long-term use of opioids may cause "classic" opioid-induced adverse effects (constipation, nausea, dizziness, cognitive deficits), as well as more serious consequences such as cognitive disorders, opioid-induced hyperalgesia, and immune and endocrine system suppression [45–47]. Indeed it is often difficult to distinguish between opioid-induced hyperalgesia and tolerance.

Which drugs become popular on the street, and why? One factor is clearly their availability. In 2011, oxycodone was the most diverted prescription drug and the opioid most patients were taking when entering drug treatment programs [48]. OxyContin, the long-acting formulation of oxycodone, has also been widely diverted and abused, and is believed to be a major driver of the prescription opioid abuse epidemic over the past 15 years [48]. After several years in clinical development and then in the FDA approval processes, Purdue Pharma released a new formulation of OxyContin in August 2010, replacing the original formulation. The new formulation of OxyContin is tamper-resistant, using a physical barrier designed to resist crushing and other manipulation, in order to deter abuse. Indeed, the tamper-resistant formulation appears to have dramatically decreased the diversion of OxyContin [49].

There is clearly a gender distinction as women are more likely than men to have opioid medication addiction issues. Consequently the rates of toxic reactions among women have tripled since 1999, and opioid poisoning related hospitalizations have increased for women but not for men. Factors related to poisoning include over-prescription, overuse by the patient, adverse effects, or toxic reactions related to drug–drug interactions. A study of unintentional pharmaceutical overdose fatalities reported that prescribed opioids were present in 44 % of women [50]

Women are also at greater risk for misuse/abuse. Women who take opioids long-term are twice as likely to abuse their opioids than to abuse alcohol [51], while men who take opioids have a greater incidence of alcohol abuse. For men, they are twice as likely to have opioid misuse rather than alcohol abuse. In contrast depression and anxiety predispose to opioid misuse independent of gender [52–54]. Opioid use and abuse are likely to continue to be serious medical and sociological problems.

Hallucinogen-Related Disorders

Hallucinogenic compounds are usually alkaloids extracted from plants or mushrooms that mimic endogenous neurotransmitters. Perhaps the most famous hallucinogen is the synthetic compound, LSD (D-lysergic acid diethylamide) but also popular are peyote, an extract from a spineless cactus that includes mescaline, psilocybin produced by certain species of mushrooms, as well as the synthetic compound PCP (aka Angel Dust). Hallucinogen use became prominent in the 1960s. Use declined in the 1970s and 1980s and increased again in the 1990s, particularly among teenagers. The 1997 National Household Survey conducted by SAMHSA. SAMSHA showed that 20.7 million of the 216 million persons represented in the 1997 NHSDA survey (10 %) had used hallucinogens in their lifetime [55].

PCP is an NMDA receptor antagonist that can cause schizophrenia-like symptoms in healthy individuals. PCP was developed in the 1950s as an anesthetic but was never approved for human use because of adverse psychological effects. Prenatal administration of PCP causes apoptotic neurodegeneration particularly in the frontal cortex [56]. Interestingly, PCP abuse varies geographically. In 2010, there were no reports of PCP among primary treatment admissions for the 28-county

Los Angeles Area but PCP was one of the three most common substances that caused traffic related deaths in Washington DC. In fact, in 2009, 6.4 % of the drug items seized in Washington, DC, tested positive for PCP, making it the fourth most frequently found drug there, after marijuana, cocaine, and heroin [57]. Thus, while hallucinogen use has seen a revival in recent years, PCP use stands out as a particularly prominent example with associated medical and psychosocial components.

Sedative-, Hypnotic-, or Anxiolytic-Related Disorders

Assessments from the National Addictions Vigilance Intervention and Prevention Program (NAVIPPRO) (10/01/2009 through 03/31/2012) of the past 30-day non-medical use of prescription stimulants (1.29 %) showed that their use was significantly lower than that of prescription opioids (19.79 %) or sedatives (10.62 %) [58]. Those who reported nonmedical use of sedative and hypnotic drugs tend to have previous histories of drug abuse and personality traits including impulsivity and hopelessness [59].

Heavy use of sedatives was positively associated with diagnoses for sedative use disorder and prescription opioid use disorder, a higher number of motives for sedative use, and reporting "sedative use in ways other than as prescribed" [60]. In terms of gender, women abuse sedatives along with opioids for pain conditions more frequently than do men, while men use sedatives more frequently along with alcohol [61].

A cross-sectional survey conducted between 2002 and 2004 on 92,020 respondents over the age of 18, revealed nonmedical use of sedatives and tranquilizers was ~2.3 %. This study also revealed correlations with panic symptoms and elevated serious mental illness, female sex, white/hispanic/other ethnicity, criminal arrest, being uninsured and/or unemployed, alcohol abuse or dependence, cigarette use, illicit drug use, younger age of initiating illicit substance use, and a history of IV drug use. Those who demonstrated abuse/dependence to sedatives tend to be agoraphobic, older, unmarried, have a low education level and have been arrested [62].

Propofol is an intravenous hypnotic anesthetic that is not currently listed as a controlled medication by the FDA. Nevertheless, its abuse potential has been of widespread interest since the Michael Jackson case in which he was given propofol as a sleep aid, and was ultimately fatal. Reviews of the albeit scarce literature on propofol as an abused medication revealed multiple reports describing tolerance, dependence, withdrawal phenomena, abuse, and death from recreational use [63].

Conclusion

Substance abuse and dependence are costly diseases for the patient and for society. Hopefully, defining addiction as a neurobiological disease instead of a behavioral problem will engender more empathy for the patient and more research for effective treatments. The demographics of addiction point to increased education and social advancement as meaningful preventative measures to reign in the ramifications of this prevalent and growing biological disease.

Summary

- Addiction implies biological disease that is manifested as behavioral dysfunction.
- To avoid additional burden for patients who struggle with this dysfunction, the DSM IV does not use the word "addiction" but instead uses the terms "abuse" and "dependence."
- Abuse is the compulsive seeking of a substance, and dependence is the biological withdrawal from abstaining.
- Abuse does not necessarily lead to dependence and, conversely, biological dependence does not necessarily engender abuse.
- While substance dependence and abuse rates remain high (~22 %), they have not changed in the past 10 years.
- There are several substances that account for the vast majority of dependence and abuse. In particular alcohol abuse is highest in male patients between ages 21 and 25 and approaches 25 %.
- Also prominent, despite aggressive education and taxation is tobacco. According to a recent survey, there has been a drop in the number of people who started using tobacco from 7 % in 2002 to 5 % in 2012. The seriousness of tobacco use is highlighted by the fact that tobacco use is the number one cause of preventable death in the USA. Most smokers are in lower socioeconomic ranks and are less well educated.
- Marijuana is another prevalent drug and the percentage of people who have tried marijuana in the USA is approximately 37 % of the population, according to a recent Gallop Poll.

References

1. Gandek B, Ware JE, Aaronson NK, Alonso J, Apolone G, Bjorner J, Bazier J, Bullinger M, Fukuhara S, Kaasa S, Lepllege A, Sullivan M. Tests of data quality, scaling assumptions, and reliability of the SF-36 in eleven countries: results from the IQOLA Project. International Quality of Life Assessment. J Clin Epidemiol. 1998;51(11):1149–58.
2. Flórez-Salamanca L, et al. Probability and predictors of transition from abuse to dependence on alcohol, cannabis, and cocaine: results from the national epidemiologic survey on alcohol and related conditions. Am J Drug Alcohol Abuse. 2013;39(3):168–79.
3. 2010 National Survey on Drug Use and Health (NSDUH) sponsored by the U.S. Department of Health and Human Services, SubstanceAbuse and Mental Health Services Administration (SAMHSA), Office of Applied Studies (OAS).

4. CDC. Smoking-attributable mortality, years of potential life lost, and productivity losses—United States, 2000–2004. MMWR Morb Mortal Wkly Rep. 2008;59:1135–40.
5. American Psychiatric Association. Diagnostic and statistical manual of mental disorders. 4th ed. Washington, DC: American Psychiatric Association; 1994.
6. American Society of Addiction Medicine (ASAM). Public Policy Statement: Definition of addiction. 2011. Available from http://www.asam.org/advocacy/find-a-policy-statement/view-policy-statement/public-policy-statements/2011/12/15/the-definition-of-addiction
7. Compton WM, et al. Prevalence, correlates, disability, and comorbidity of DSM-IV drug abuse and dependence in the United States: results from the national epidemiologic survey on alcohol and related conditions. Arch Gen Psychiatry. 2007;64(5):566.
8. Substance Abuse and Mental Health Services Administration. Results from the 2012 National Survey on Drug Use and Health: summary of national findings. NSDUH series H-46, HHS publication no. (SMA) 13-4795. Rockville, MD: Substance Abuse and Mental Health Services Administration; 2013.
9. Grant BF, et al. Prevalence of DSM-IV alcohol abuse and dependence: United States, 1992. Alcohol Health Res World. 1994;18(3):243–8.
10. Harwood H, et al. The economic costs of alcohol and drug abuse in the United States, 1992. Rockville, MD: National Institute on Drug Abuse; 1998.
11. Hasin DS, Stinson FS, Ogburn E, Grant BF. Prevalence, correlates, disability, and comorbidity of DSM-IV alcohol abuse and dependence in the United States: results from the national epidemiologic survey on alcohol and related conditions. Arch Gen Psychiatry. 2007;64(7):830–42.
12. Kessler RC, Nelson CB, Mcgonagle KA, et al. Epidemiology of co-occurring addictive and mental disorders: implications for prevention and service utilization. Am J Orthopsychiatry. 1996;66(1):17–31.
13. Cook TA, Luczak SE, Shea SH, Ehlers CL, Carr LG, Wall TL. Associations of ALDH2 and ADH1B genotypes with response to alcohol in Asian Americans. J Stud Alcohol. 2005;66(2):196–204.
14. National Drug Intelligence Center. Prescription drug abuse and youth. In Carson-DeWitt R, editor. Information brief. 2002. Available from http://www.usdoj.gov/ndic/pubs1/1765/index.htm; MEDLINEplus. Accessed 13 October 2006.
15. EMCDDA European Monitoring Centre for Drugs and Drug Addiction. Annual report: the state of the drugs problem in Europe. 2008. Available from http://www.emcdda.europa.eu/publications/annual-report/2008
16. U.S. Department of Justice. Methamphetamine-related identity theft. (No. 2007-L0424-003). Washington, DC: U.S. Department of Justice; 2007.
17. Nicosia N, Pacula RL, Kilmer B, Lundberg R, Chiesa J. The economic cost of methamphetamine use in the United States, 2005 (No. MG-829-MPF/NIDA). Santa Monica, CA: The RAND Corporation; 2009.
18. Westover AN, Nakonezny PA. Aortic dissection in young adults who abuse amphetamines. Am Heart J. 2010;160(2):315–21.
19. Callaghan RC, et al. Increased risk of Parkinson's disease in individuals hospitalized with conditions related to the use of methamphetamine or other amphetamine-type drugs. Drug Alcohol Depend. 2012;120(1):35–40.
20. Herbeck DM, Brecht M-L, Pham AZ. Racial/ethnic differences in health status and morbidity among adults who use methamphetamine. Psychol Health Med. 2013;18(3):262–74.
21. Gruenewald PJ, et al. Mapping the spread of methamphetamine abuse in California from 1995 to 2008. Am J Public Health. 2013;103(7):1262–70.
22. Ferré S. Caffeine and substance use disorders. J Caffeine Res. 2013;3(2):57–8.
23. Budney AJ, et al. Caffeine withdrawal and dependence: a convenience survey among addiction professionals. J Caffeine Res. 2013;3(2):67–71.
24. Franke AG, Lieb K, Hildt E. What users think about the differences between caffeine and illicit/prescription stimulants for cognitive enhancement. PLoS One. 2012;7(6):e40047.

25. Mesias B, et al. Abuse or dependence on cannabis and other psychiatric disorders. Madrid study on dual pathology prevalence. Actas Esp Psiquiatr. 2013;41(2):122–9.
26. Caldicott DG, Holmes J, Roberts-Thomson KC, Mahar L. Keep off the grass: marijuana use and acute cardiovascular events. Eur J Emerg Med. 2005;12:236–44.
27. Hall W, Degenhardt L. Adverse health effects of non-medical cannabis use. Lancet. 2009; 374:1383–91.
28. Swain NR, et al. Alcohol and cannabis abuse/dependence symptoms and life satisfaction in young adulthood. Drug Alcohol Rev. 2012;31(3):327–33.
29. Buckner JD, et al. The relationship between cannabis use disorders and social anxiety disorder in the National Epidemiological Study of Alcohol and Related Conditions (NESARC). Drug Alcohol Depend. 2012;124(1):128–34.
30. Lynskey MT, et al. An Australian twin study of cannabis and other illicit drug use and misuse, and other psychopathology. Twin Res Hum Genet. 2012;1(1):1–11.
31. Benowitz NL. Nicotine addiction. N Engl J Med. 2010;362:2295–303.
32. Wanat MJ, Willuhn I, Clark JJ, Phillips PE. Phasic dopamine release in appetitive behaviors and drug addiction. Curr Drug Abuse Rev. 2009;2:195–213.
33. Sixt S, et al. Endovascular treatment for extensive aortoiliac artery reconstruction: a single-center experience based on 1712 interventions. J Endovasc Ther. 2013;20(1):64–73.
34. Ozimek A, Clavien PA, Antonio N. Wound dehiscence. In: Totally implantable venous access devices. Milan: Springer; 2012. p. 157–60.
35. Pingault JB, et al. Childhood trajectories of inattention, hyperactivity and oppositional behaviors and prediction of substance abuse/dependence: a 15-year longitudinal population-based study. Mol Psychiatry. 2012;18(7):806–12.
36. de los Ríos F. Trends in substance abuse preceding stroke among young adults a population-based study. Stroke. 2012;43(12):3179–83.
37. Centers for Disease Control and Prevention. Current cigarette smoking among adults—United States, 2011. Morb Mortal Wkly Rep. 2012;61(44):889–94.
38. Degenhardt L, et al. Toward a global view of alcohol, tobacco, cannabis, and cocaine use: findings from the WHO World Mental Health Surveys. PLoS Med. 2008;5(7):e141.
39. Eriksen J, Jensen MK, Sjogren P, Ekholm O, Rasmussen NK. Epidemiology of chronic non-malignant pain in Denmark. Pain. 2003;106:221–8.
40. Toblin RI, Mack KA, Perveen G, Paulozzi LJ. A population-based survey of chronic pain and its treatment with prescription drugs. Pain. 2011;152:1249–55.
41. Kurita GP, Sjogren P, Juel K, Hojsted J, Ekholm O. The burden of chronic pain: a cross-sectional survey focusing on diseases, immigration, and opioid use. Pain. 2012;153:2332–8.
42. Hojsted J, Nielsen PR, Guldstrand SK, Frich L, Sjogren P. Classification and identification of opioid addiction in chronic pain patients. Eur J Pain. 2010;14:1014–20.
43. Hojsted J, Sjogren P. Addiction to opioids in chronic pain patients: a literature review. Eur J Pain. 2007;11:490–518.
44. Hurley RW, Adams MC. Sex, gender, and pain: an overview of a complex field. Anesth Analg. 2008;107:309–17.
45. Hojseted J, Sjogren P. An update on the role of opioids in the management of chronic pain of non-malignant origin. Curr Opin Anaesthesiol. 2007;20:451–5.
46. Katz N, Mazer NA. The impact of opioids on the endocrine system. Clin J Pain. 2009;25:170–5.
47. Lennon FE, Moss J, Singleton PA. The mu-opioid receptor in cancer progression: is there a direct effect? Anesthesiology. 2012;116:940–5.
48. Cicero TJ, Ellis MS, Surratt HL, Kurtz SP. Factors influencing the selection of hydrocodone and oxycodone as primary opioids in substance abusers seeking treatment in the United States. Pain. 2013;154(12):2693–2648.
49. Cicero TJ, Ellis MS, Surratt HL. Effect of abuse-deterrent formulation of OxyContin. New England Journal of Medicine. 2012;367(2):187–189.

50. Hall AJ, Logan JE, Toblin RL, et al. Patterns of abuse among unintentional pharmaceutical overdose fatalities. JAMA. 2008;300(22):2613–20.
51. Cicero TJ, Wong G, Tian Y, Lynskey M, Todorov A, Isenberg K. Co-morbidity and utilization of medical services by pain patients receiving opioid medications: data from an insurance claims database. Pain. 2009;144(1-2):20–7.
52. Edlund MJ, Steffick D, Hudson T, Harris KM, Sullivan M. Risk factors for clinically recognized opioid abuse and dependence among veterans using opioids for chronic non-cancer pain. Pain. 2007;129(3):355–62.
53. Ives TJ, Chelminski PR, Hammett-Stabler CA, et al. Predictors of opioid misuse in patients with chronic pain: a prospective cohort study. BMC Health Serv Res. 2006;6:46.
54. Wasan AD, Butler SF, Budman SH, Benoit C, Fernandez K, Jamison RN. Psychiatric history and psychologic adjustment as risk factors for aberrant drug-related behavior among patients with chronic pain. Clin J Pain. 2007;23(4):307–15.
55. SAMHSA, National Household Survey on Drug Abuse. 1997. Available from http://www.samhsa.gov/data/nhsda/1997main/nhsda1997mfWeb-43.htm#P8904_188945
56. Wang C, et al. Long-term behavioral and neurodegenerative effects of perinatal phencyclidine administration: implications for schizophrenia. Neuroscience. 2001;107(4):535–50.
57. Brecht M-L. Patterns and trends in drug abuse in Los Angeles County, California: 2010. Proceedings of the Community Epidemiology Work Group, June 2011. Available from http://www.drugabuse.gov/sites/default/files/cewgjune2011_vol_ii_508.pdf.
58. Cassidy TA, McNaughton EC, Varughese S, Russo L, Zulueta M, Butler SF. Nonmedical use of prescription ADHD stimulant medications among adults in a substance abuse treatment population: Early findings from the NAVIPPRO surveillance system. Journal of Attention Disorders. 2013 July 30.
59. McLarnon ME, et al. Drug misuse and diversion in adults prescribed anxiolytics and sedatives. Pharmacotherapy. 2011;31(3):262–72.
60. Nattala P, et al. Heavy use versus less heavy use of sedatives among non-medical sedative users: characteristics and correlates. Addict Behav. 2011;36(1):103–9.
61. Saunders KW, et al. Concurrent use of alcohol and sedatives among persons prescribed chronic opioid therapy: prevalence and risk factors. J Pain. 2012;13(3):266–75.
62. Becker WC, Fiellin DA, Desai RA. Non-medical use, abuse and dependence on sedatives and tranquilizers among US adults: psychiatric and socio-demographic correlates. Drug Alcohol Depend. 2007;90(2):280–7.
63. Wilson C, Canning P, Martin Caravati E. The abuse potential of propofol. Clin Toxicol. 2010;48(3):165–70.

Chapter 2
Legal Issues

Bobby Ray Malbrough

Key Points

- Drug addiction and crime
- Pain management rules
- Pain management clinics
- Legislative strategies
- Medical license revocation
- Laws regulating controlled substances

Drug Addiction and Crime

Drug abuse and addiction have placed a drain on society, law enforcement, and the court system, not to mention the toll it has taken on countless human lives. The most recent incident that comes to mind is the death of Michael Jackson and his apparent addiction to Propofol. The role Jackson's physician played resulted in a criminal conviction as determined by a jury. Perhaps the role involved the physician being placed in a compromised position that resulted in the exercise of poor judgment and substandard medical management. Regardless, the problem of drug addiction is mounting and every segment of society need take notice—including physicians.

The statistics involving drugs and crime in the United States are staggering—and somewhat surprising. For example, the prison population in America reveals that 1 in 100 US citizens is now confined in jail or prison and 80 % of the offenders abuse alcohol or other drugs; 50 % of jailed or prison inmates are clinically addicted,

B.R. Malbrough, Esq., B.A., J.D. (✉)
Attorney at Law, New Orleans, LA, USA
e-mail: brm@ocblaw.com

© Springer Science+Business Media New York 2015
A.D. Kaye et al. (eds.), *Substance Abuse*, DOI 10.1007/978-1-4939-1951-2_2

and 60 % of individuals arrested for most types of crimes test positive for illegal drugs at arrest. Perhaps not surprising is that 60–80 % of drug abusers commit a new crime (typically a drug-driven crime) after release from prison, and approximately 95 % return to drug abuse after release from prison [1]. Drug courts have been established in most jurisdictions in an attempt to stem the tide of prison over-population, and in response to the fact that imprisonment has little effect on drug abuse. Drug courts seek to strike a balance between the need to protect community safety and the need to improve public health and well-being. It is in conjunction with this approach that the physician can best attend to the needs of patients addicted to drugs while recognizing the enormous problems that face all of society.

Pain Management Rules

Pain management physicians who deal daily with patients afflicted with chronic pain issues know all-too-well the fine line between medical management of pain and addiction. The enactment of Pain Management Rules establishes specific guide-lines for physicians to follow, such as an appropriate physical exam and a subjective reasonable belief on the part of the physician prescribing narcotic medication that the patient is truly in pain as opposed to having an addiction. Other factors such as behavioral indicators, implicit and explicit patient admissions, and evidence of doc-tor shopping are all factors the physician must weigh and evaluate. While the guide-lines are clear and succinct, following them has proven to be a problem for the hundreds and even thousands of physicians who find themselves with suspended or revoked licenses, and worse yet facing federal or state criminal prosecution.

Pain Management Clinics

The quantity of prescription painkillers sold to pharmacies, hospitals, and doctors' offices was four times greater in 2010 than in 1999. Enough prescription painkillers were prescribed in 2010 to medicate every American adult around-the-clock for 1 month. Nearly nine out of every ten poisoning deaths are caused by drugs. Every day in the United States 105 people die as a result of drug overdose, and another 6,748 are treated in emergency departments for the misuse or abuse of drugs [2]. As a result of this epidemic, and the emergence of "pill mills," pain clinic regulations have been adopted in every state in the union, primarily designed to prevent facili-ties from prescribing controlled substances indiscriminately or inappropriately [3].

It is no secret that Pain Management Clinics have heretofore been a haven for doctor-shopping and pill-dispensing factories. Typically, drug addiction in society results in increased crime and increased violent crime. However, surprisingly the association between drugs and criminal behavior is not solely due to people com-mitting crimes to further their drug habit. Drug use is actually a factor in many crimes that have nothing to do with obtaining money for drugs. Drug use is implicated in 50 % of violent crimes, 50 % of instances of domestic violence, and 80 % of child abuse and neglect cases [4]. The burdens placed on society, law enforcement, and the court system are a matter of daily news. The financial burdens placed on Medicare, Medicaid, and public health hospitals amount to billions of dollars annually. It is the obligation of the physician by not only his/her oath to prevent addiction, but to reverse it—but certainly not to contribute to it.

Legislative Strategies

Physicians need to be aware of the seven types of legislative strategies that have been implemented and have the potential to impact prescription drug misuse, abuse, and overdose. These seven types of "laws" are as follows:

1. Laws requiring examination before prescribing.
2. Laws requiring tamper-resistant prescription forms.
3. Laws regulating pain clinics.
4. Laws setting prescription drug limits.
5. Laws prohibiting "doctor shopping"/fraud.
6. Laws requiring patient identification before dispensing.
7. Laws providing immunity from prosecution/mitigation at sentencing for individuals seeking assistance during an overdose.

Each state has its own set of laws and it behooves the physician to become intimately familiar with the laws of the state wherein the physician practices to assure full compliance.

While the right to practice medicine is deemed a fundamental right, the protection of public health is a duty of the State in its exercise of inherent police powers, and thus it is universally held that it is the duty of the State to regulate and control the practice of medicine. This regulation and control of the practice of medicine is vested in the various state legislatures and involves legislative control over which the federal government lacks jurisdiction. There exists federal legislation that provides grants for training and fellowships which contain guidelines under federal legislation, but the general control of the practice of medicine vests with the individual state legislatures. This does not mean to imply that the federal government cannot enact laws regarding illegal narcotic use and distribution. However, all-in-all, the primary method of regulating the practice of medicine is state legislation requiring physicians and other healthcare professionals (dentists, nurses, chiropractors, physician assistants, nurse practitioners, etc.) to do or refrain from specified activity, or controlling and regulating the manner and circumstances in which certain phases of the practice of medicine shall be performed. Near the top of the list are regulations controlling the administration of anesthetics and narcotics. The most important method of regulating the practice of medicine, and other healthcare professionals, is through licensing and the revocation of licenses for specified causes or misconduct.

The issuance of a license to practice medicine does not translate into a contract, and therefore the holder of the license has no right to continue the practice of medicine in the future unrestricted. Any license can be revoked for good cause shown. It is axiomatic that with the power to issue a license comes the power of revocation when the "license" has been improperly issued or when the holder of the license is guilty of improper or unlawful conduct. To be certain, there can be no ambiguity in the law regarding right and wrong conduct. As long as the law enacted by the legislature proscribes reasonable regulations declared with specificity and definiteness, allowing the practitioner to accurately gauge their meaning without confusion, a license can be revoked for causes enumerated in the legislation. Therefore, it is imperative that the physician familiarizes himself/herself with the laws of the state involved, and to seek legal assistance in the interpretation of any areas of the law that may appear ambiguous.

License Revocation

As noted, one of the primary causes of license revocation is the inappropriate, wrongful, or excessive prescription of anesthetic or narcotic medications. Typically these instances involve one or more of the following: (1) the prescription of drugs without a physical examination or an indication of therapeutic necessity; (2) the prescription of drugs to known narcotics addicts or habitual users, and (3) permitting unauthorized persons to obtain or prescribe drugs in the name of the authorized practitioner [5].

Laws Regulating Controlled Substances

In addition to license revocation for practitioners who violate proscribed rules and regulations, the practitioner can also face state and federal criminal liability. The United States Congress has passed a plethora of laws regulating controlled substances. The Food and Drugs Act of 1906 was the beginning of over 200 laws concerning public health and consumer protection. Other laws such as the Federal Food, Drug, and Cosmetic Act (1938) and Kefauver Harris Amendment of 1962 were passed. In 1969 President Richard M. Nixon announced a comprehensive new program to more effectively deal with the narcotic and dangerous drug problems at the federal level, combining all existing federal laws into a single, comprehensive statute. The result was the Federal Controlled Substances Act (CSA), 21 U.S.C. § 801, passed by the 91st Congress as Title II of the Comprehensive Drug Abuse Prevention and Control Act of 1970. The CSA is the federal US drug policy regulating the manufacture, importation, possession, use and distribution of certain substances. This Act created the five Schedules (classifications) of drugs.

Enforcement of the Act is relegated to the Drug Enforcement Administration (DEA) established in 1973. An investigation by the DEA can be begun at any time based upon information received from laboratories, state or local law enforcement and regulatory agencies, or any other source of information. Federal or state prosecution can result from violation of the CSA—such prosecution typically leads to license revocation or suspension, depending on the severity of the violation. There can be no substitute to being familiar with the applicable laws, both federal and state.

In addition to the criminal consequence and license revocation or suspension associated with the illegal administration/distribution of narcotics, there is the civil side of the equation. Typically a civil suit will be stayed pending the outcome of the criminal investigation and trial. A guilty verdict or a guilty plea in a criminal proceeding is normally admissible in a civil proceeding, making the end-result of a civil proceeding, which typically requires evidence by preponderance much easier. Any judgment or settlement against a healthcare provider in a civil proceeding requires notification to the National Data Bank. Any judgment paid would normally be paid by the healthcare provider's professional liability insurer, with the exception in some cases being in euthanasia deaths. However, an argument can and has been made that the illegal dispensing of a scheduled narcotic is outside the stated coverage of the professional liability insurance agreement when the physician has been determined to dispense the medication for monetary reasons as opposed to reasons for treatment purposes only. Awards for the inappropriate administration/prescribing of narcotics and other scheduled substances vary from state-to-state, and range across the board from as little as a few thousand dollars to millions of dollars.

Summary

Physicians and other healthcare providers must walk a fine line when it comes to treating patients with substance abuse problems or potential substance abuse problems. The role of the physician is to treat the whole patient—whether the ailment is a physical issue or a substance abuse issue. It is essential for the physician to become intimately familiar with all of the applicable federal laws and the laws applicable to the state of practice, and to develop a systematic record-keeping process in order to manage effectively the treatment protocol. There is little to no margin for error by the physician in treating those addicted to narcotics—but there is the potential to change the lives of such persons—hopefully, forever.

What really is the physician's role in treating drug abuse and the crisis of prescription abuse? Simply stated, it is the responsibility of the physician to obtain advance training in prescribing controlled substances to avoid causing or contributing to the problem. Medical schools have not met the need adequately, and it is the physician's responsibility in recognizing and managing addictive disease to attend workshops and seminars to become more knowledgeable in treating the disease. Inadequate education in medical school and residency training about addiction and abuse has resulted in physicians wittingly or unwittingly contributing to the prescription drug epidemic because physicians lack the skill, knowledge and training to diagnose and treat addictive disease. This lack of skill, knowledge and training can lead to licensing issues, including revocation or suspension, and criminal and civil legal issues. Typically, a criminal case revolves around violation of a state or federal statute. A civil case, on the other hand, revolves around the applicable standard of care, or whether the physician possessed the requisite skill, knowledge or training in a given field of medicine.

Thus, there are myriad pitfalls and potential traps for the physician who ventures into this very challenging field. Lest there be need for a reminder of The Hippocratic Oath: "If I fulfill this oath and do not violate it, may it be granted to me to enjoy life and art, being honored with fame among all men for all time to come; if I transgress it and swear falsely, may the opposite of all this be my lot."

References

1. National Association of Drug Court Professionals. http://www.nadcp.org/learn/drug-courts-work/drugs-and-crime-America
2. Substance Abuse and Mental health Services Administration. Highlights of the 2011 Drug Abuse Warning Network (DAWN) findings on drug-related emergency department visits. The DAWN Report. Rockville: US Department of Health and Human Services, Substance Abuse and Mental Health Administration; 2013. http://www/samhsa/gov/data/2k13/DAWN127/sr127-DAWN-highlights.htm
3. Centers for Disease Control and Prevention. http://www.cdc.gov/homeandrecreationalsafety/Poisoning/laws/pain_clinic.html
4. Commentary: Drug Courts' positive effects on families and society. http://www/drugfree.org/join-together/addiction/commentary-drug-courts-positive-effects. Accessed 17 May 2013.
5. Medical Licensure Com'n of Alabama v. Herrera, 918 So.2d 918, 19 A.L.R. 6th (Ala. Civ. App. 2005); Elai v. Arizona State Bd. Of Dental Examiners, 168 Ariz, 221, 812 P.2d 1039 (Ct. App. Div. 1 1990); Fisher v. La. St. Bd. Of Med. Examiners, 353 So.2d 729 (La.App. 4 Cir. 1977); Glover v. Bd. Of Med. Quality Assur., 231 Cal. App. 3d 203, 282 Cal. Rptr. 137 (1st Dist. 1991); Pannone v. N.Y, St. Ed. Dept., 54 A.D.2d 1014, 338 N.Y.S.2d 174 (3Dep't 1976); Gallo v. St. Bd. Of Med. Exam., 257 So.2d 97 (Fla. Dist. Ct. App 3d Dist. 1972); Arkansas St. Med. Bd. V. Grimmett, 250 Ark. 1, 463S.W.2d 662 (1971).

Chapter 3
Signs and Symptoms of Substance Abuse

Elizabeth Ngo and Shalini Shah

Key Points
- Taking a history
- Physical examination
- Research trials

Introduction

Substance abuse has become a growing problem for many practicing clinicians [1–3]. The signs and symptoms are often subtle and being able to make a diagnosis requires the clinician to take a detailed look into the patient's history, speaking to family members and co-workers, as well as utilization of screening tools. The challenging issues that clinicians often come across are: being able to detect and make a diagnosis of the substance abuse problem, addressing the problem with the patient, and also assessing the patients who are at high risk for developing problems with dependence or abuse in order to prevent occurrence or relapse.

In particular, many clinicians find the practice of prescribing opiates to be one of the most challenging. Studies have shown that opiate dependence/abuse has historically been underdiagnosed even though the incidence of prescription opioid abuse

E. Ngo, D.O. (✉)
Department of Physical Medicine and Rehabilitation, University of California, Irvine,
1112 Dennis Dr., Costa Mesa, CA 92626, USA
e-mail: engo324@gmail.com

S. Shah, M.D.
Department of Anesthesiology and Peri-operative Care, University of California, Irvine,
101 The City Drive, Building 53, Orange, CA 92868, USA
e-mail: ssshah1@uci.edu

© Springer Science+Business Media New York 2015
A.D. Kaye et al. (eds.), *Substance Abuse*, DOI 10.1007/978-1-4939-1951-2_3

has increased by 400 % from 628,000 to 2.7 million between the years 1990 and 2000, with this trend continuing to be on the rise [3]. In fact, in the last decade there has been a marked increased use of opioids for chronic non-cancer pain as well as an increase in opioid dependence/abuse and accidental overdose [4]. Between 1992 and 2002, there has been a 350 % increase in the number of yearly admissions for primary prescription opioid abuse in the United States [3].

These findings raise an important question: if opiate dependence/abuse is an ever-increasing problem in this country, then why is it still consistently being under-diagnosed and undertreated? It would make sense that for such a pervasive problem that we would have improved methods to increase sensitivity in screening for this problem in our patients. There are multiple factors involved and identification of these barriers will help clinicians gain a better understanding of the problem and, in turn, improve treatment for their patients.

To start with, being able to identify the signs and symptoms of opiate depen-dence/abuse may depend on the clinician being sensitive and vigilant for any changes in the individual's behavior or social interactions, or any difficulties with maintaining responsibilities at home or work. This process can be time-consuming, especially for practitioners today who face time-constraints on how much time they can spend with each patient and are judged by the clock in terms of their productiv-ity. In order to gain a more complete assessment, clinicians may need to gather information from family members and employers in addition to reports from the individual, which require the clinician to spend even more time to establish a diagnosis.

There are other barriers that prevent those with opioid dependence or abuse to be diagnosed and treated. Unlike other illicit street drugs such as heroin, cocaine, or methamphetamine, prescription drugs are often not viewed with the same kind of stigma and disapproval by the community. In fact, many of the abusers of narcotics come from affluent, upper-class backgrounds [5]. These individuals can afford the more costly purchases of prescription drugs, as compared to street drugs. Moreover, they do not fit into the "drug-seeker" prototype, which makes it difficult to identify if they have a problem with drug dependence or abuse. In addition, there are sub-groups of people such as healthcare professionals who have access to prescription drugs and are aware of the euphoric effects of these drugs, which put them at increased risk of developing dependence to these drugs [5]. Unfortunately, health-care professionals are also known to have one of the lowest rates for following-up and seeking medical treatment. Being able to detect an issue with drug dependence in this group of patients can be problematic.

Many individuals, including some practitioners, do not regard drug addiction as a medical illness but rather a condition that is self-induced and a weakness in will power so that efforts to treat it will inevitably fail [2]. Also worthwhile to mention is the social implications and fear many clinicians associate with opiate prescribing in general [1]. The phenomenon of "opiophobia" refers to the fear of opioid pre-scribing with an inherent prejudice against these types of drugs regardless of their appropriate utility [1].

Healthcare workers often have the fear of patients abusing or becoming addicted to the pain medications [1]. They also have a fear of being perceived as contributing to the increasing rates of abuse or addiction in patients [1]. And finally, many clinicians are concerned with potential regulatory investigation [1, 2]. Due to these underlying fears, it is not uncommon for pain patients to be undertreated and develop a type of pseudo-addiction. Many clinicians will mistakenly diagnose the patient with dependence/abuse and decrease their pain medication when, in fact, the patient actually needs an increased dosage to achieve therapeutic levels and obtain adequate analgesic effects.

Diagnosing and screening patients for substance dependence/abuse is often a challenging task due to the time-consuming nature and need for awareness and hypervigilance among clinicians and medical personnel. To achieve better outcomes with detecting issues of drug dependence/abuse will require improved training of all healthcare professionals: e.g. physicians from multidisciplines, physician assistants, psychologists, social workers, nursing staff, and medical students [2]. Having a multidisciplinary team can increase the success with identification of the early signs and symptoms of drug dependence/abuse and help with treatment plan once the problem is identified.

Taking a History

Many patients have risk factors that can be identified before starting them on any opioid medications [6]. For example, if the patient has had a personal history of substance dependence/abuse such as with opioids, alcohol, or illicit drugs they are at increased risk of developing dependence/abuse for other medications such as opioids [1, 2, 6]. In fact, it is not uncommon for patients to have a history of poly-substance dependence. The TROUP studies found that the effects of substance use disorders on predicting increased risk of opioid dependence/abuse were especially strong [4]. These patients are also at increased risk for relapse even after they are treated. Long-term administration of addictive drugs produces alterations in the brain that increase vulnerability to relapse and facilitate craving even months or years after successful detoxification [7].

Another trait that positively correlates with increased risk of substance abuse/dependence is a history of mental disorders [1, 4, 6]. Although mental disorders are not as strongly correlated compared to a history of substance abuse disorder, mental disorders have been shown to be more common [4]. Patients who abuse or misuse pain medication are extremely likely to have other psychosocial issues (such as personality disorders, clinical depression, and anxiety disorders) that need to be concurrently treated along with the pain condition itself for which the medication is being prescribed [1].

The patient's environment is also an important consideration when assessing for substance dependence or abuse. Patients who report living close to a parent, sibling, or spouse who has a history of a drug dependence or abuse are at increased risk for developing the problem later in life [2]. Patients who are a part of a detoxification clinic are also obviously at increased risk due to their high vulnerability and tendency to experiment with all drugs, including opioids [5]. Inquiring about life events that can lead to self-titration of medication and escalation of drug dosages such as the death of a loved one, recent divorce, or loss of a job can be helpful to gain insight into any emotional issues the patient is dealing with.

There is some evidence that genetics can also influence a person's predisposition to developing substance dependence/abuse [2, 6, 7]. The metabolism of drugs determined by genetic factors also has been shown to increase the risk for addiction. For example, the more known allele that encodes for the isoenzyme aldehyde dehydrogenase is involved in the metabolism of acetaldehyde (which is responsible for the aversive effects of alcohol) is less active in certain individuals and ethnic groups making them less prone to develop alcohol abuse [7]. On the contrary, some individuals have reduced sensitivity to alcohol and increased chances for developing alcohol dependence or abuse. And yet another minor (A1) allele of the TaqIA D2 dopamine receptor gene has been linked to severe alcoholism, polysubstance and psychostimulant abuse, and opioid and nicotine dependence [7].

Age is a non-modifiable risk factor that has been correlated with risk of opioid dependence or abuse [1, 4]. In the TROUP study, younger individuals were much more likely to have abuse/dependence with odds ratio especially large for individuals 50 years or younger [4]. Age was found to be highly protective from abuse of opioid dependence or other abuse [4]. The American Geriatrics Society in 2009 recommended that opioids generally be used in geriatric populations before NSAIDs and Cox-II inhibitors with acetaminophen recommended as first-line agent.

There are some red flags that should alert the clinician that there could be a problem with opioid dependence or abuse (see Table 3.1) [6]. There are also certain questions about the medication history that the clinician should inquire when suspecting a problem (see Table 3.2) [8]. As mentioned previously, detecting substance dependence or abuse can require the clinician to take a very detailed history, asking specific questions about the individual's home and work environment in addition to obtaining details about their medication history (Table 3.3).

The clinician should raise concerns when the patient begins to have problems functioning at work or fulfilling responsibilities at home. Patients who have issues with substance dependence/abuse may have difficulty keeping a job. Unemployment is associated with worse outcome compared to patients who are opioid dependent but who can still maintain a job [2]. Therefore, encouraging the patient to maintain some form of job, even if it is not the same job they previously had, may be worthwhile. Behavioral changes or mood disorders such as anxiety or depression can start to become more apparent. As a consequence, the patient may start to withdraw and encounter difficulties in their personal and professional relationships.

Table 3.1 Portenoy's predictive factors for problematic drug use

More predictive:

- Selling prescription drugs
- Forging prescriptions
- Stealing drugs
- Injecting oral formulations
- Obtaining prescription drugs from nonmedical sources
- Concurrently abusing alcohol or illicit drugs
- Escalating doses on multiple occasions or otherwise failing to comply with prescribed regimen despite warnings
- Repeatedly seeking prescriptions from other physicians or emergency rooms without informing the original physician
- Multiple episodes of prescription "loss"
- Evidence of deterioration in the ability to function at work, in the family, or in social settings, that appears to be related to drug use
- Repeated resistance to changes in therapy despite clear evidence of adverse physical or psychological effects from the drug

Less predictive:

- Aggressive complaining about the need for more drug
- Drug hoarding during periods of reduced symptoms
- Unsanctioned dose escalation or other noncompliance with therapy on one or two occasions
- Unapproved use of the drug to treat other symptoms
- Resistance to a change in therapy, with expressions of anxiety related to the return of severe symptoms

Adapted and modified from: Portenoy RK. Opioid therapy for chronic nonmalignant pain: a review of the critical issues. Journal of Pain and Symptom Management. 1996;(11):203-17. Copyright 1996 by the US Cancer Pain Relief Committee

Table 3.2 Medication history

- What was the prescribed medication, dosage form, dose, and frequency?
- What was the actual frequency at which the medication was taken?
- How long did the patient take the medication?
- Over what period of time did the patient take the medication?
- When was the patient on the medication?
- Was the medication self-administered or administered by others?
- Were there any side effects that were unreported to the referring physician? Why were the side effects not reported?
- Why was the medication stopped?

Adapted from: Sees KL, Clark HW. Opioid use in the treatment of chronic pain: assessment of addiction. Journal of pain and symptom management. 1993;8(5):257-64. Epub 1993/07/01

Table 3.3 Useful questions for probing addiction in chronic pain patients

1. Drug-taking reliability
• Does the patient take opioids or other psychoactive medications as prescribed?
• Frequency? Dose?
2. Loss of control of drug use
• Does the patient have partially used bottles of medications at home?
• Will the patient bring them in for verification?
3. Indications of drug-seeking behavior
• Frequently reports losing medications?
• Demands drugs of high street value?
• Has prescriptions from multiple doctors?
• Has prescriptions filled at multiple pharmacies?
4. Abuse of drugs other than those prescribed
• Alcohol? Cocaine? Marijuana? Heroin? Amphetamines?
• Opioids? Benzodiazepines?
5. Contact with the street-drug culture
• Friends or family members who are street-drug users?
• Does the patient buy street drugs for any purpose?
6. Adverse life consequences not due to chronic pain, but due to the effects of opioids or other drugs
• Inability to work?
• Loss of friends or alienation of family?
• Decreased interest in recreational activities?
• Adverse health consequences?
7. Cooperation with full treatment plan and alternative pain management techniques
• Avoiding situations that induce pain?
• Using nonnarcotic medications?
• Using physical therapy?
• Using TENS units if indicated?
• Meditation or biofeedback?

Adapted and modified from Sees KL, Clark HW. Opioid use in the treatment of chronic pain: assessment of addiction. Journal of pain and symptom management. 1993;8(5):257-64. Epub 1993/07/01

Physical Examination

The physical examination is also important for assessing problems with substance dependence/abuse. The encounter gives the clinician a chance to interact with the patient and gather more objective findings through their observations. During the physical examination, the clinician should look for general mood and affect (e.g. does the patient look depressed or anxious?). These initial encounters can allow the clinician to understand any mental/emotional difficulties the patient may have and be able to refer the patient to appropriate support groups if needed.

Table 3.4 Signs and symptoms of opioid and cocaine/amphetamines intoxication versus withdrawal

Opioid intoxication	Opioid withdrawal	Cocaine intoxication	Cocaine withdrawal
• Miosis (pinpoint pupils)	• Mydriasis (pupil dilation)	• Agitation	• Hypersomnolence
• Decreased mental status or coma	• Agitation	• Mydriasis (pupil dilation)	• Hyperphagia
• Hypoventilation	• Diaphoresis (heavy perspiration)	• Diaphoresis	• Anhedonia
• Bradycardia	• Tachypnea	• Hypertension	• Boredom
• Hypotension	• Piloerection (hair erection)	• Tachycardia	• Anxiety
• Hypothermia	• Hypertension	• Hyperthermia	• Generalized malaise
• Decreased bowel motility	• Muscle cramps	• Increased energy	• Difficulty with memory and concentration
	• Diarrhea	• Decreased fatigue	• Suicidal ideation
	• Yawning	• Paranoia	
	• Vomiting	• Decreased appetite	
	• Diarrhea		

The clinician can look for physical signs of maladaptive drug use. Venous puncture marks may show up in hidden areas on the body such as on the abdomen, the neck, the genitals, or in between the fingers or toes. There have been reports from hospitals located in socioeconomically disadvantaged areas of patients who show up with repeated skin abscesses in various parts of their body due to "skin popping" (subcutaneous administration of drugs under the skin). Mucosa damage in the nasal passageway may be seen due to usage of that route for administering drugs. In addition, there are different signs and symptoms of opiate and amphetamine/cocaine intoxication versus withdrawal (see Table 3.4). Being familiar with these signs will aid the clinician to establish a correct diagnosis.

Research Trials

Screening tools and urine toxicology testing designed to detect opioid misuse are used clinically but scant evidence currently exists to allow the formulation of an algorithm for judicious use of these tools [1]. An evidence-based algorithmic approach to risk mitigation that can be applied in a cost-effective manner to guide therapy is urgently needed [1]. There have been some good clinical trials that have shown pertinent correlations between various risk factors for opioid dependence or abuse.

The TROUP (Trends and Risks of Opioid Use for Pain) study is the largest study to date of risk factors for opioid and non-opioid substance dependence/abuse among patients with chronic non-cancer pain on chronic opioid therapy [4]. There were several findings from the results of the study. In support of what has been found in current literature, the study concluded that age is an important risk factor in assessing for opioid dependence/abuse. Therefore, the results suggest that clinicians should be especially cautious in balancing the risks and benefits of chronic opioid therapy in younger individuals. Mental health disorders and a history of prior substance dependence/abuse were both positively correlated with high post-index opioid and non-opioid substance dependence/abuse. Mental health disorders can be successfully treated and may decrease the risk of development of opioid dependence/abuse in chronic opioid therapy. Individuals on greater than 120 mg morphine equivalent also had significantly increased diagnoses of post-index opioid and non-opioid dependence/abuse, making them a high-risk group. Individuals on daily rather than intermittent dosage and those on multiple opioid types are also at increased risk for abuse. Patients who used only Schedule III or IV opioids had lower rates of post-index opioid dependence/abuse compared to those in the opioid type categories that included Schedule II opioids. Of note, policy changes aimed at decreasing the incidence and prevalence of opioid dependence need to include both Schedule II opioids as well as Schedule III and IV opioids [4].

There is still controversy over how to strategically minimize the risk of drug addiction when prescribing opioids. There is a general preference for long-acting opioids such as OxyContin or MS Contin because the longer duration of drug effect offers baseline coverage of pain control while the low frequency in daily dosing provides "delayed reinforcement". The behavioral effects of taking multiple doses of opioids throughout the day can be habit-forming with short-term opioids but is not a phenomenon seen with long-term opioids. However, the RADARS (Researched Abuse, Diversion and Addiction-Related Surveillance) system that was initiated by Purdue Pharma showed that even though there was modest growth in drug abuse seen with all analgesics, one of the most pronounced was that seen with OxyContin [5]. Results showed that OxyContin abuse was prevalent in all areas of the country, but unevenly concentrated in the eastern and southeastern part of the United States. OxyContin was rarely the sole prescription drug abused and most frequently associated with polysubstance abuse. Notably, nearly all of the OxyContin abusers (>87 %) had extensive current and past histories of substance abuse. Few legitimate, drug-naïve patients become addicted as a result of the intended use of OxyContin as an analgesic [5].

Conclusion

Substance dependence and abuse is clearly a growing problem in the country. Therefore, better screening tools need to be developed and undergo clinical trials to assess their efficacy. More importantly, an evidence-based algorithmic approach to risk mitigation that can be applied in a cost-effective manner to guide therapy is urgently needed. There also needs to be a movement to educate and improve awareness of the problem among clinicians from multidisciplines and all healthcare providers. Identification of the barriers that prevent patients from getting treatment for substance dependence/abuse is also essential in this movement. Finally, there needs to be a cultural shift in the medical community from opioid fear and disapproval to one of acceptance and understanding of opiate dependence/abuse as a medical illness just like any other disease process that needs to be treated [9].

References

1. Hartrick CT, Gatchel RJ, Conroy S. Identification and management of pain medication abuse and misuse: current state and future directions. Expert Rev Neurother. 2012;12(5): 601–10. Epub 2012/05/04.
2. National Consensus Development Panel on Effective Medical Treatment of Opiate Addiction. Effective medical treatment of opiate addiction. JAMA. 1998;280(22):1936–43. Epub 1998/12/16.
3. Sigmon SC. Characterizing the emerging population of prescription opioid abusers. Am J Addict. 2006;15(3):208–12. Epub 2006/08/23.
4. Edlund MJ, Martin BC, Fan MY, Devries A, Braden JB, Sullivan MD. Risks for opioid abuse and dependence among recipients of chronic opioid therapy: results from the TROUP study. Drug Alcohol Depend. 2010;112(1–2):90–8. Epub 2010/07/17.
5. Cicero TJ, Inciardi JA, Munoz A. Trends in abuse of Oxycontin and other opioid analgesics in the United States: 2002-2004. J Pain. 2005;6(10):662–72. Epub 2005/10/06.
6. Robinson RC, Gatchel RJ, Polatin P, Deschner M, Noe C, Gajraj N. Screening for problematic prescription opioid use. Clin J Pain. 2001;17(3):220–8. Epub 2001/10/06.
7. Cami J, Farre M. Drug addiction. N Engl J Med. 2003;349(10):975–86. Epub 2003/09/05.
8. Sees KL, Clark HW. Opioid use in the treatment of chronic pain: assessment of addiction. J Pain Symptom Manage. 1993;8(5):257–64. Epub 1993/07/01.
9. Krantz MJ, Mehler PS. Treating opioid dependence. Growing implications for primary care. Arch Intern Med. 2004;164(3):277–88. Epub 2004/02/11.

Chapter 4
Speaking with Your Patient about the Problem

Shalini Shah

Key Points

- Mindset to approach
- Use of language and stigmatization: terminology
- Guide to asking about drug use
- DOs and DONT'S when asking about drug and/or alcohol use
- Terminology and words that work
- Motivational interviewing

Introduction

Anyone who aspires to help another will quickly learn how difficult it is to change people, or readiness to wish to change. Those involved in preventing, treating, and supporting recovery for substance abuse have learned that language and words can be powerful motivators when used appropriately to clarify, encourage, and enlighten. On the other hand, improper language can often discourage, stigmatize, isolate, and totally undermine one's efforts to begin recovery from substance abuse.

Based on trials that brief alcohol and drug counselling reduces consumption, adverse, health consequences, healthcare expenditures, and morbidity and mortality in patients who consume above recommended limits, the US Preventative Services Task Force recommends routine alcohol and drug screening followed by brief counselling with patients who screen positive [1]. Effective and informative counselling includes an upfront discussion about the problem, discussion of risks

S. Shah, M.D. (✉)
Department of Anesthesiology and Perioperative Care, University of California, Irvine,
101 The City Drive, Building 53, Orange, CA 92868, USA
e-mail: ssshah1@uci.edu

© Springer Science+Business Media New York 2015
A.D. Kaye et al. (eds.), *Substance Abuse*, DOI 10.1007/978-1-4939-1951-2_4

associated with this problem, and strategies to curb use, along with feedback in a patient-focused manner.

While providers generally understand the importance of an upfront and open discussion into the problem as a clinical responsibility, the rates of counselling are low [2], and efforts have generally not yet been successful [3, 4]. Some of the barriers providers report include an unwillingness or "unreadiness" by the patient to make steps toward change, unwillingness of patients to even address a substance abuse issue, fear from the provider that the patient may physically act upon the provider and his/her family, fear from the provider that the patient may take legal or administrative action against the providers' medical license, and a general indifference perceived by the provider that the patient does not care about his/her own health. These issues, coupled with a general skepticism about effectiveness of counselling, lack of time, and stigmatization of substance abuse are the major themes identified in qualitative and exploratory studies on how providers discuss substance abuse with their patients.

In this chapter we will explore various mindsets to approach substance abuse discussions with one's patients, use of language, and stigmatization, examples of approaches and themes learned through various video and audio-taping studies exploring appropriateness of how to discuss the issue effectively with patients. Finally, we will explore the idea of Motivational Interviewing, a tactic which was first coined in the early 1980s, and its efficacy with prescription adherence, immediacy of effect, and long-term adherence for recovery. We understand that we may not be able to change the ways of all of our patients with substance abuse issues, however, we hope that we can educate the reader in using the most appropriate and effective strategies when you believe a patient is ready and willing and motivated for recovery.

Mindset to Approach

Drugs and alcohol are often regarded negatively by society and associated with forms of judgment. By asking open-ended questions and removing any assumptions and bias from the interview, providers are more likely to gather honest information on drug and alcohol use from the patient [5]. As stated earlier, words can be powerful when used to inform, clarify, encourage, support, enlighten, and unify. On the other hand, stigmatizing words often discourage, isolate, misinform, shame, and embarrass. Recognizing the power of words, this chapter will help raise awareness of the providers' own language and own personal mindset about substance abuse discussions, that we may be inadvertently biased and pass that on to the patient. That is to say, attention to language is a critical step toward the reduction of stigma, but it is only one step. Reducing stigma involves not only changes in language, but also a significant change in providers' perceptions, attitudes, and policies. These developments are essential to creating a society that supports prevention, treatment, and recovery for substance abuse patients.

Use of Language and Stigmatization: Terminology

Specific competencies are expected out of providers in order to perform a discussion with patients. They include:

1. Describe the importance of talking about alcohol and drugs with ALL patients
2. Address drug and substance abuse with ALL patients
3. Take a complete substance abuse history

   (a) Ask patients questions in a nonjudgmental manner
   (b) Demonstrate comfort in talking about the subject of substance abuse
   (c) Use an effective screening tool for abuse i.e. CAGE questionnaire

4. Reflect on own biases involved with drugs and alcohol use

Phrasing

How one phrases the question is important. Example: *You haven't felt the need to cut down on the amount of alcohol you drink, have you?*

The way this question is worded is too leading and does not provide the patient the opportunity to provide sincere and honest answers. The question contains implicit bias and judgment. Actually if the patient HAS felt like cutting down, it becomes harder for him to answer this question truthfully. Instead: Ask: *Have you ever felt the need to cut down on the amount of alcohol you drink?* This open-ended question allows the patient to answer "Yes–No".

Setting

Consider the setting of the interview. Is this a primary care visit or is this a psychiatry visit or a drug rehabilitation program? When one asks questions, make sure they are tailored to the individual person and situation.

Denial

Consider the continuum of denial. Denial is often a component of addictive illness and it is imperative for the provider to be aware the patient may still be in denial of their active state of abuse or misuse. Do not take everything the patient states as the truth. Reviewing a patient's record make reveal discrepancies in terms of substances used, last use date, and frequency of use, and often times the record may provide a more accurate history of substance use.

Stages of Addiction

Consider the stages of addiction. Recognize that there are stages of addiction and recovery and that your questions have to be tailored to the current state of that patient. Relapse is also very common during recovery, and remind yourself as the provider of this fact so that you remove bias when a patient reveals he has had multiple relapses.

Guide to Asking About Drug Use

One can start the conversation simply by asking:
Do you use any recreational drugs? If they answer YES, you may want to ask:

- What type of drugs?
- When did you start?
- Frequency?
- Method of Administration
- Have you ever been in trouble because of your use?
- Who do you use with?
- Have you ever tried to stop using?
- How you pay for the drugs?
- How do they make you feel?

If the patient answers NO, then confirm he has understood your question and what exactly you define as drugs. Ask if he has ever used drugs in the past. *Do you use any prescription or nonprescription drugs other than as directed by a doctor*? It may be helpful to ask these questions as separate questions since some individuals do not consider taking prescription medication in the same category as recreational drugs, whether or not they were the ones being prescribed in the medications or not.

DOs and DONT'S When Asking about Drug and/or Alcohol Use

DO:

- Ask open-ended questions
- Quantify the drug or alcohol use
- Be empathetic
- Be alert, suspicious, and circumspect
- Be willing to be inquisitive

DON'T:

- Ask leading questions
- Ask questions in a judgmental way
- Judge a patient or his response
- Assume he is answering truthfully
- Settle for vague answers such as "sometimes," "not very often"

Terminology and Words That Work

The following terms are considered effective in advancing people's understanding of substance use disorders as a health issue. These are only a selected discussion of terminology, however, these terms are key in ANY discussion with patients about substance abuse.

Addiction

Why it works: This widely understood term describes "uncontrollable, compulsive drug seeking and use, even in the face of negative health and social consequences" [6]. There is a distinction between *addiction* and *dependence*, although many use the words interchangeably. *Addiction* conveys both social and health problems, whereas *dependence* only encompasses the latter.

Caveats: Clinically speaking, both the DSM criteria and the ICD codes use the term "dependence," not addiction. Addiction cannot be used as an umbrella term for substance use disorders, because not all substance use reaches the level of addiction. Also, addiction as a stand-alone term could potentially encompass any addictive behavior i.e. gambling, shopping, sexual disorders, as well as alcohol and drugs.

Dependence

Why it works: Dependence is useful as a term because it represents a clinical entity as a diagnosis without including stigmatizing terminology. Physical dependence is a "state of adaption that often includes tolerance and is manifested with withdrawal syndrome that can be produced by cessation or drug dose reduction, and/or an administration of an antagonist" [7].

Caveats: The reader should note it is possible to be physically dependent on a drug without being addicted (i.e. the use of regulated opioid medication), and it is also possible to be addicted (i.e. gambling) without being physically dependent [8].

Disease Management

Why it works: Disease management is "the management of severe behavioral health disorders in ways that enhance clinical outcomes and reduce social costs" [9]. It relates to the process of suppressing symptoms/cravings while providing service intervention. Disease management's focus is on *service and cost efficiency*, as distinct from "recovery management" whose focus is on the *individual*.

Intervention

Why it works: Intervention is a broad term used to describe an interruption of progress of an illness or potential illness. It is used in clinical scenarios to describe the process in which a concerned group executes a formally prepared plan to encourage a person to get help for a substance use disorder. The following descriptors are quoted from the *Substance Abuse and Mental Health Services Administration (SAMHSA) 2003, Dept. of Health and Human Services* [10].

Universal Preventative Intervention

Targeted to the general public or a whole population that has not been identified on the basis of individual risk.

Selective Preventative Intervention

Targeted to individuals or a sub-group of the population whose risk of developing a mental or substance use disorder is significantly higher than average.

Indicated Preventive Intervention

Targeted to high-risk individuals who are identified as having minimal but detectable signs of symptoms foreshadowing a mental or substance use disorder, or biological markers indicating a predisposition for a disorder, but who do not meet accepted clinical diagnostic criteria at the time.

Treatment Intervention

Therapeutic services designed to reduce the length of time a disorder exists, halt its progression of severity, or if not possible, increase the length of time between acute episodes.

Maintenance Intervention

Services, generally supportive, educational, and/or pharmacological in nature, provided on a long-term basis to individuals who have met DSM-IV diagnostic criteria, are considered in remission, and whose underlying illness continues.

Patient

Why it works: this word accurately refers the person to be suffering from an illness. It re-enforces the notion that substance abuse disorders constitute a health issue.

Recovery

Why it works: SAMHSA 2003 defines recovery as "abstinence plus a full return to biological, psychological, and social functioning" [11]. It is a way of elevating the concept of recovery to resiliency.

Caveats: There is no formal consensus on the precise definition of recovery, or the boundary of what recovery constitutes. Unless the context is clear, a modifier is needed (recovery of alcohol, partial recovery from drug use, etc.).

Relapse

Why it works: It is a recognized term to describe the recurrence of symptoms and behaviors of substance use disorders following a period of remission.

Caveats: The term has negative connotations for it often has projected a tone of morality. Some recommend the term "recurrence" for its alignment with the nature of other chronic illnesses.

Treatment

Why it works: According to the American Society of Addiction Medicine (ASAM), "treatment is the use of any planned, intentional intervention in the health, behavior, personal, and/or family life of an individual suffering from alcoholism or from another drug dependency designed to enable the affected individual to achieve and maintain sobriety, physical and mental health, and a maximum functional ability" [12]. It effectively denotes a health intervention.

Caveats: Treatment does not denote the entire recovery process has completed, nor is professional treatment the only path to recovery.

Motivational Interviewing

What is the most effective way to communicate with your patient about substance abuse once the problem has been identified? The evidence for "motivational interviewing" is strong in the areas of addictive health behavior, and appears to improve outcomes when added to other treatment approaches. Motivational interviewing (MI) is "a client centered, directive therapeutic style to enhance readiness for change by helping clients explore and resolve ambivalence" [13]. In short, MI elicits the client's own motivation for change—help patients with the readiness to change.

Motivational interviewing (MI) was concretely developed in 1983, although the theory behind its tactics has been used informally since the late 1950s. It was developed as a way to help patients work through ambivalence and commit themselves to change—the success of the "change" is work for the cognitive behavioral therapists, but the readiness for change is the basis of MI. MI combines a support and empathy with a directive method for resolving ambivalence in the direction of change. Drawing on Bem's self-perception theory that people tend to become more committed to that which they hear themselves defend, MI explores the client's own arguments for change [14]. The provider or interviewer seeks to evoke this "change talk"—expressions of the client's desire, ability, reasons, and need for change—and responds with reflective listening. The net effect of evoking change talk in an empathetic and supportive manner is to strengthen the client's commitment to change [13]. MI is therefore differentiated into two phases: the first is focused on increasing motivation for change, and the second on consolidating commitment [15].

MI is normally provided in only one–two sessions and like other psychotherapies, is a complex skill method that is learned over time. It does not operate from a deficiency model which seeks to instill knowledge or insight or correct thinking. Rather, the clinician seeks to evoke confidence in the human desire and capacity to grow in positive direction i.e. "You have what you need to succeed". Proper training focuses on recognition of time to change, which can be met with significant client resistance. It is not the job of the clinician to fight this resistance, but instead to strategize a way to roll with the resistance, calling attention to the ambivalence and redirecting the emphasis toward change.

Research indicates that MI is particularly useful with clients who are less motivated or ready for change, and who are more angry or oppositional [16]. The treatment outcome literature for MI is growing rapidly and to this date, seems to be the most evidence-based method to initiate the conversation about change with one's substance abuse patient. In observational studies across sites that employ MI, it was noted the wide variability in effect sizes across studies. For example, in PROJECT MATCH, a nine-site outcome-based study of MI, the observed effect sizes have varied between 0 and 3 standard deviations [17]. This means that in using the same method (MI), across sites and populations, very different effect sizes were noted despite clinician efforts to standardize training and treatment procedures. Thus, it appears that variation in the delivery of MI can have substantial impact on its outcome.

A second broad observation is that the effect of MI tends to be immediate and to last up to a year of follow-up. This is found in studies in which clients were randomized to receive or not receive MI and follow-up period is between 0 and 12 months. In this case, the effect of MI in improving outcome is maintained or increased over time, hovering around 6 months [13].

Conclusion

In its origins, MI was not derived from theory, but rather it arose from specification of principles underlying intuitive clinical practice [18]. The client-centered perspective of Dr Carl Rogers in 1959 was the guiding spirit of MI, in the hopes that patients would follow through with their commitment to change, particularly relating to improved outcomes in treating alcohol problems [19, 20] and decreasing frequency of drinking after treatment. Thus, if a practitioner's goal is to maintain prescription adherence and also combine with immediacy of effect, motivational interviewing techniques have been documented to be the ideal vehicle to begin the discussion on talking to your patient

References

1. Kinsey A, McCormick BA, Cochran NE, Back A, Merrill JO, Williams EC, Bradley KA. How primary care providers talk to patients about alcohol. A qualitative study. J Gen Intern Med. 2006;21:955–72.
2. Rush IL, Ellis K, Crowe T, Powell L. How general practitioners view alcohol use: clearing up the confusion. Can Fam Physician. 1994;40:1570–8.
3. Babor TE, Higgins-Biddle J, Dauser D, Elggins P, Berleson JA. Alcohol screening and brief intervention in primary care settings: implementation models and predictors. J Stud Alcohol. 2005;66:361–8.
4. Funk M, Wutzke S, Kaner E, et al. A multi-center controlled trial of strategies to promote dissemination and implementation of brief alcohol intervention in primary health care: findings of a World Health Organization collaborative study. J Stud Alcohol. 2005;66:379–88.
5. Sanchez L. Talking with patients about Alcohol and Drugs; Medical Interviewing and the Doctor-Patient Relationship. Tufts School of Medicine Lecture Notes. 2011.
6. Lescher A. The essence of drug addiction. www.jointogether.org. Accessed 21 March 2001.
7. American Academy of Pain Medicine, American Pain Society, American Society of Addiction Medicine. Consensus document: definitions related to the use of opioids for the treatment of pain. 2001. www.asam.org/ppol/paindef.htm
8. Allen D. Drugs and society: addiction defined. New Orleans, LA: University of New Orleans, Department of Sociology.
9. White W, Boyle M, Loveland D. A model to transcend the limitations of addiction treatment. Behav Health Manag. 2003;3:38–44.
10. Substance Abuse and Mental Health Services Administration. Request for applications No TI 03-009: Cooperative agreements for screening, brief intervention, referral and treatment. Washington, D.C.: Department of Health and Human Services; 2003.

11. Gorski TT, Kelly JM, Havens L, Peters RH. Relapse prevention and the substance-abusing criminal offender, Technical assistance publication series 8. Rockville: Department of Health and Human Services Press; 1993. p. 9.
12. American Society of Addiction Medicine. ASAM public policy statement: treatment for alcoholism and other drug dependencies. 2001.
13. Hettema J, Steele J, Miller WR. Motivational interviewing. Annu Rev Clin Psychol. 2005; 1:91–111.
14. Bem DJ. Self-perception theory. In: Berkowitz L, editor. Advances in experimental social psychology, vol. 6. New York: Academic; 1972. p. 1–62.
15. Miller WR, Rollnick S. Motivational interviewing: preparing people for change, vol. 2. New York: Guilford; 2002.
16. Prochaska JO, DiClemente CC. The trans-theoretical approach: crossing traditional boundaries of therapy. Homewood: Dow/Jones Irwin; 1984.
17. MATCH Project Res Group. Therapist effects in three treatments for alcohol problems. Psychother Res. 1988;8:455–74.
18. Miller WR. Motivational interviewing with problem drinkers. Behav Psychother. 1983; 11:147–72.
19. Miller WR, Baca LM. Two year followup of bibliotherapy and therapist-directed controlled drinking training for problem drinkers. Behav Ther. 1983;14:441–8.
20. Valle SK. Interpersonal functioning of alcoholism counselors and treatment outcome. J Stud Alcohol. 1981;42:783–90.

Chapter 5
Screening and Assessment for Substance Abuse

Elizabeth Ngo and Shalini Shah

Key Points

- Definitions
- Pathobiochemical process
- Risk factors
- Undertreatment of pain
- Screening tools
- Questionnaires
- The cold pressor test
- Urine drug screening
- Random pill counts
- Opioid withdrawal challenge
- Database check

Introduction

Substance abuse has become a rising public health problem in the United States [1]. Notably, the incidence of opioid abuse as well as accidental opioid-related overdose has dramatically increased in the past decade [2–5]. Despite overall healthcare workers' efforts to limit the amount of opioids prescribed and unnecessary

E. Ngo, D.O.
Department of Physical Medicine and Rehabilitation, University of California, Irvine,
1112 Dennis Dr., Costa Mesa, CA 92626, USA
e-mail: engo324@gmail.com

S. Shah, M.D. (✉)
Department of Anesthesiology and Peri-operative Care, University of California, Irvine,
101 The City Drive, Building 53, Orange, CA 92868, USA
e-mail: ssshah1@uci.edu

© Springer Science+Business Media New York 2015
A.D. Kaye et al. (eds.), *Substance Abuse*, DOI 10.1007/978-1-4939-1951-2_5

escalation of dosages, opioid abuse continues to be a concern in the medical community. To begin with, there are a number of challenges when assessing patients for opioid abuse. Chronic pain patients are a special group of patients due to the complexity of their condition. The underlying pathophysiology is a combination of factors that include neurobiochemical processes as well as psychosocial, environmental, and genetic variability.

The current tools that we have for screening patients for opioid abuse include self-reports, questionnaires, state-level databanks, the physical examination, and laboratory testing. However, there are limitations of each of these screening tools. For example, self-reports of medication use and dosages can be unreliable. On the other hand, physical examination and laboratory tests cannot measure the level of pain or pain relief that is experienced by the patient. Databank searches are commonly used in the clinical setting as part of the assessment for opioid dependence or abuse, but there is still low evidence to support its efficacy as a screening tool [2]. More research is needed to establish an evidence-based algorithm to screening for opioid abuse.

Definitions

Clear and distinct definitions need to be established to provide an accurate assessment of the patient's diagnosis. Table 5.1 provides definitions that are important for the clinician to understand when assessing a patient for opioid dependence or abuse [6–11]. A distinction worth mentioning is that opioid tolerance is an expected physiological response for chronic opioid patients but this does not necessarily lead to maladaptive patterns of addiction [7–9]. Moreover, physical dependence and tolerance alone do not equate with addiction [9]. Opioid tolerance, however, can lead to higher opioid dosages, which is associated with opioid dependence.

Table 5.1 Definitions that are important for the clinician to understand when assessing a patient for opioid dependence or abuse

Opioid: A compound or drug that binds to receptors in the brain involved in the control of pain and other functions (e.g., morphine, heroin, hydrocodone, oxycodone)
Polysubstance Abuse: The abuse of two or more drugs at the same time, such as CNS depressants and alcohol
Prescription Drug Abuse: The use of a medication without a prescription in a way other than as prescribed or for the experience or feeling elicited. This term is used interchangeably with "nonmedical" use
Substance Abuse: maladaptive pattern of substance use manifested by recurrent and significant adverse consequences related to the repeated use of substances. There may be repeated failure to fulfill major role obligations, repeated use in situations in which it is physically hazardous, multiple legal problems, and recurrent social and interpersonal problems [4, 6]

(continued)

Table 5.1 (continued)

Substance dependence: a cluster of cognitive, behavioral, and physiological symptoms indicating that a person is continuing to use a substance despite having clinically significant substance-related problems. For substance dependence to be diagnosed, at least three of the following must be present: symptoms of tolerance; symptoms of withdrawal; the use of a substance in larger amounts or for longer periods than intended; persistent desire or unsuccessful attempts to reduce or control use; the spending of considerable time in efforts to obtain the substance; a reduction in important social, occupational, or recreational activities because of drug use; and continued use of a substance despite attendant health, social, or economic problems [5, 7]
Addiction: a psychological and behavioral syndrome characterized by an intense desire for the drug and overwhelming concerns about continued availability; evidence of compulsive drug use (characterized, for example, by unsanctioned dose escalation, continued dosing despite significant side effects, use of the drug to treat symptoms not targeted by therapy, or unapproved use during periods of no symptoms; and evidence of one or more of a group of associated behaviors, including manipulation of the treating physician or medical system for the purposes of obtaining additional drug (altering prescriptions, for example), acquisition of drugs from other medical sources or from a nonmedical source, drug hoarding or sales, or unapproved use of other drugs (particularly alcohol or other sedative/hypotics) [7, 11]
Physical Dependence: An adaptive physiological state that occurs with regular drug use and results in a withdrawal syndrome when drug use is stopped; often occurs with tolerance. Physical dependence can happen with chronic and even appropriate use of many medications, and by itself does not constitute addiction
Tolerance: A condition in which higher doses of a drug are required to produce the same effect achieved during initial use; often associated with physical dependence
Withdrawal: Symptoms that occur after chronic use of a drug is reduced abruptly or stopped
Detoxification: A process in which the body rids itself of a drug or its metabolites. This is often the first step in drug abuse treatment. During this period, withdrawal symptoms can emerge that may require medical treatment

Pathobiochemical Process

There is considerable individual variability and differences in the physiologic make-up of each person. Variation in sensitivity to drug effect, drug metabolism, and adaptation to the effects of chronic exposure to a drug may also contribute to the susceptibility for opioid abuse [2, 8]. Interindividual differences in response to opioid therapy and downregulation in receptor numbers or sensitivity can lead to the need for dose escalation in some patients. The mesolimbic system is involved in modulation of the reward experience through both positive reinforcement (euphoria) and negative reinforcement (avoidance of withdrawal symptoms), and can also present with interindividual variability [8]. Altered behavior of dopaminergic neurons in the ventral tegmental area associated with reward mechanisms can transition from regulated to compulsive drug use [2]. Vulnerability to relapse is thought to be mediated by neuroplasticity in cortical glutaminergic pathways projecting to the nucleus accumbens [2].

Risk Factors

Consideration of risk factors is essential when assessing for problems with opioid dependence or abuse. Having a personal history of prior substance abuse or mental health disorder increases a patient's risk of opioid abuse [7]. In addition, younger age, smoking, and having certain genetic subtypes can also predispose to increased risk for opioid abuse [5, 8, 12]. Interestingly, patients with a close relative such as a parent, sibling, or a spouse with a history of substance abuse are also at higher risk for opioid abuse [3, 7, 13].

Undertreatment of Pain

An important topic that is often overlooked is the undertreatment of pain. Patients who have pain that is not adequately treated can develop "pseudoaddiction" [2, 7]. This term refers to behaviors that may be described as drug seeking, e.g. taking larger amounts of medications than prescribed, running out of medications prematurely, anger and escalating demands for increased pain medication. However, the cause of the problem is the gross undertreatment of pain and when adequate pain relief is given, the symptoms are eliminated [10].

Screening Tools

Questionnaires [2, 14, 15]

Beck Depression Inventory (BDI-II)

This is a 21-item multiple-choice self-report inventory. It was originally developed to provide a quantitative assessment of the intensity of depression. The questionnaire is composed of items related to symptoms of depression such as hopelessness, anhedonia, inability to concentrate, guilt, lack of appetite, and fatigue. Since then, the BDI has been revised and is now known as the BDI-II. The cutoffs used for the BDI-II differ from the original. Each question is still graded on a scale from 0 to 3 and the scoring is as follows: 0–13: minimal depression; 14–19: mild depression; 20–28: moderate depression; and 29–63: severe depression. Higher total scores indicate more severe depressive symptoms. This scale can be useful for monitoring treatment response.

CAGE

An acronym representing the four questions commonly used to assess for substance abuse and dependence. The questions are not sensitive for detecting the full spectrum of unhealthy drug use but two affirmative responses have shown in some studies to have high sensitivity and specificity for alcohol abuse and dependence. The four questions that are asked to patients are: (1) Have you ever felt you needed to **C**ut down on your drinking? (2) Have people **A**nnoyed you by criticizing your drinking? (3) Have you ever felt **G**uilty about drinking? (4) Have you ever felt you needed a drink first thing in the morning (**E**ye-opener) to steady your nerves or to get rid of a hangover?

Visual Pain Analogue (VPA)

This scale measures pain on a level from 0 to 10. Patients are asked to make an "X" mark on a 10-cm horizontal line, hashed at two-point intervals with higher numbers reflecting greater pain. A pain score is determined by rounding up to the next whole number subsequent to the marking made by the patient.

Oswestry Pain Disability Questionnaire (OSW)

This is a self-rating scale that evaluates the degree of functional impairment caused by pain in activities of daily living such as in personal care, mobility, employment, and social life.

Patient Health Questionnaire (PHQ-9)

This is a self-administered questionnaire comprising of nine questions that incorporates the DSM-IV criteria for major depression and an additional item that assesses for psychosocial impairment. Each item is scored on a four-point Likert scale from "0" (not at all) to "3" (nearly every day) and total scores range from 0 to 27, with 0 to 4 indicates no depression; 5 to 9 mild depression; 10 to 14 moderate depression; 15 to 19 moderately severe depression; and 20 to 27 indicates severe depression.

Pain Medication Questionnaire (PMQ)

This 26-item self-report inventory prompts patients to select the description that best matches their experiences, thoughts, and needs related to their pain medication. Grading is on a five-point Likert scale from 0 (disagree) to 4 (agree) and is used to assess risk of opioid medication misuse specifically in chronic pain patients and to measure progress in those patients already taking opioids. High PMQ scores are associated with history of substance abuse, higher levels of psychosocial distress, and poorer functioning.

Patient Information Form

This is a clinic-specific form that elicits pertinent information such as patient demographics, level of education, employment status, details and date of prior injuries, involvement in worker's compensation or other litigation, medication and dosages, history of substance abuse or mental health disorder, prior surgeries, and chronic health problems.

The Dallas Pain Questionnaire

This is 16-item self-report questionnaire containing items related to pain and disability as it affects activities of daily living, mood, work, interpersonal relationships, and social life. Patients mark an "X" along a 0 to 100 % scale anchored with descriptors. Higher total scores represent greater levels of disability with (0–39) mildly-disabling pain; (40–84) moderately disabling pain; and (85+) severely disability pain.

Opioid Risk Tool (ORT)

This brief, simple-scoring inventory contains five items that screen for deviant behaviors associated with substance abuse in pain patients. The five items that contribute to increased risk for substance abuse are as follows: personal or family history of substance abuse with a separate check box for alcohol, illegal drugs, and prescription drugs; age (between 16 and 45); history of preadolescent sexual abuse, and psychological disease and/or depression. There is a distinction between males and females for each item scored with total score (0–3) low risk; (4–7) moderate risk; and (>8) high risk.

Screener and Opioid Assessment for Patients with Pain (SOAPP-R)

This self-administered 24-item questionnaire, administered to pain patients and contains items that inquire about prior experience with pain medication, changes in interpersonal relationships, mood, and past history of substance abuse. It is used to predict possible opioid abuse in chronic pain patients.

Minnesota Multiphasic Personality Inventory (MMPI-2)

This 567-item self-report questionnaire comprises of true or false statements related to psychiatric symptoms and personality organizations. It is a widely used test and has numerous uses in counseling, therapy, employment in high-risk public-safety positions, and to assist clinicians with the diagnosis of mental disorders and design of effective treatment strategies, including in chronic pain management.

The Cold Pressor Test

The apparatus is a temperature-controlled water bath of 1.0 degree Celsius that is continuously stirred by a pump. Patients are asked to place their nondominant hand in the cold pressor test bath with fingers wide apart and asked to maintain their hand in the cold water for as long as they could tolerate. They are then asked to report the exact point in time when the cold sensation begins to elicit pain. Immediately after hand withdrawal, patients are asked to mark their maximal pain intensity on a visual analogue scale (VAS) from 0 to 100 with 100 representing "the worst pain one can imagine" [16]. The time until the pain was first perceived is defined as the latency to pain onset. Some studies have shown that this latency is expected to be shorter for patients prone to opioid addiction compared to control group [16].

Urine Drug Screening

Urine toxicology testing is one of the most commonly used screening tools and sometimes thought of as the "gold standard" for deducing a problem with substance abuse [2]. There are two main types of UDS available, which are the immunoassay drug testing and the laboratory-based specific drug identification.

The immunoassay drug testing offers rapid results, is relatively inexpensive, and can be used readily in the outpatient setting. The test is based on the principle of competitive binding; antibodies bind to antigens when exposed to a drug or its metabolite. The ability of the immunoassay to detect a drug or its metabolite is based on a predetermined cut off concentration, depends on the concentration of the substance in the urine, and results are usually reported as positive or negative. Drawbacks include both false-positive and false-negative results, which can represent significant pitfalls for clinicians.

Liquid or gas chromatography combined with mass spectrometry can determine the presence and quantity of drugs present in a urine sample. These can serve as a confirmatory tool following initial immunoassay testing. The advantages of these laboratory-based drug identification processes include identification of specific drugs and their metabolites and quantitative measures of each drug compound.

Many pain clinics utilize the UDS before initiation of treatment with chronic opioids and often randomly throughout the course of treatment. However, there are cases of false-positive testing due to production of drug metabolites that show up on the urine toxicology testing from certain medications, so results must be interpreted with caution. For example, hydromorphone is a metabolite of hydrocodone and both can show up positive on the UDS. Morphine sulfate can test positive on a UDS in a patient taking codeine. Also an initial true positive UDS may not necessarily predict future aberrant behaviors after initiation of treatment [2]. Conversely, an initial negative screening does not definitely exclude the possibility of future misuse of opioids or aberrant drug behaviors [2].

Random Pill Counts

Some clinicians ask patients to participate in random pill counts during scheduled office visits in order to verify that the patient is taking their opioids as prescribed and not self-titrating dosages or selling them to others.

Opioid Withdrawal Challenge

Evidence to support opioid dependence can be obtained with a naloxone hydrochloride (Narcan) challenge test to induce symptoms of withdrawal [3]. However, this is not as commonly done due to concern for patient safety and ethical principles of benevolence to avoid inducing more harm to the patient.

Database Check

Statewide databases can aid in verifying medication dosages and dates of refills. They are also used to identify the providers who are prescribing opioid medications for the patient, encourage the patient to have one provider manage these medications, and to avoid obtaining opioid prescriptions from multiple sources which increases risk for opioid abuse. There is still unclear evidence as to whether these databases are effective in reducing opioid abuse [2]. Still, they are widely used by clinicians and often combined with an opioid agreement between the provider and the patient that documents in writing the expectations for adherence, goals, and treatment plan for the patient.

Conclusion

Opioid abuse is a growing problem and continues to be a threat to healthcare. Availability of effective screening tools to help clinicians identify problems with opioid abuse is an essential part of the equation. But perhaps more urgently needed is an evidence-based algorithm to guide clinicians with the following goals: identifying risk factors and high-risk populations; implementing appropriate screening tools; recognizing the signs and symptoms of aberrant drug behaviors related to opioid abuse; and addressing the issue of opioid abuse with the patient if it arises. The screening tools that presently exist to detect opioid abuse still have limited sensitivities. Therefore, these limitations underscore the fact that we still need to rely largely on clinicians' instincts to help identify patients who are at risk for opioid abuse.

References

1. Santora PB, Hutton HE. Longitudinal trends in hospital admissions with co-occurring alcohol/drug diagnoses, 1994-2002. J Subst Abuse Treat. 2008;35(1):1–12. Epub 2007/10/16.
2. Hartrick CT, Gatchel RJ, Conroy S. Identification and management of pain medication abuse and misuse: current state and future directions. Expert Rev Neurother. 2012;12(5):601–10. Epub 2012/05/04.
3. National Consensus Development Panel on Effective Medical Treatment of Opiate Addiction. Effective medical treatment of opiate addiction. JAMA. 1998;280(22):1936–43. Epub 1998/12/16.
4. Sigmon SC. Characterizing the emerging population of prescription opioid abusers. Am J Addict. 2006;15(3):208–12. Epub 2006/08/23.
5. Edlund MJ, Martin BC, Fan MY, Devries A, Braden JB, Sullivan MD. Risks for opioid abuse and dependence among recipients of chronic opioid therapy: results from the TROUP study. Drug Alcohol Depend. 2010;112(1–2):90–8. Epub 2010/07/17.
6. Cicero TJ, Inciardi JA, Munoz A. Trends in abuse of Oxycontin and other opioid analgesics in the United States: 2002-2004. J Pain. 2005;6(10):662–72. Epub 2005/10/06.
7. Robinson RC, Gatchel RJ, Polatin P, Deschner M, Noe C, Gajraj N. Screening for problematic prescription opioid use. Clin J Pain. 2001;17(3):220–8. Epub 2001/10/06.
8. Cami J, Farre M. Drug addiction. N Engl J Med. 2003;349(10):975–86. Epub 2003/09/05.
9. Sees KL, Clark HW. Opioid use in the treatment of chronic pain: assessment of addiction. J Pain Symptom Manage. 1993;8(5):257–64. Epub 1993/07/01.
10. Krantz MJ, Mehler PS. Treating opioid dependence. Growing implications for primary care. Arch Intern Med. 2004;164(3):277–88. Epub 2004/02/11.
11. Portenoy RK. Chronic opioid therapy in nonmalignant pain. J Pain Symptom Manage. 1990;5(1 Suppl):S46–62. Epub 1990/02/01.
12. Bruner AB, Fishman M. Adolescents and illicit drug use. JAMA. 1998;280(7):597–8. Epub 1998/08/26.
13. McCabe SE, Cranford JA, Boyd CJ, Teter CJ. Motives, diversion and routes of administration associated with nonmedical use of prescription opioids. Addict Behav. 2007;32(3):562–75. Epub 2006/07/18.

14. Adams LL, Gatchel RJ, Robinson RC, Polatin P, Gajraj N, Deschner M, et al. Development of a self-report screening instrument for assessing potential opioid medication misuse in chronic pain patients. J Pain Symptom Manage. 2004;27(5):440–59. Epub 2004/05/04.
15. Brown J, Setnik B, Lee K, Wase L, Roland CL, Cleveland JM, et al. Assessment, stratification, and monitoring of the risk for prescription opioid misuse and abuse in the primary care setting. J Opioid Manag. 2011;7(6):467–83. Epub 2012/02/11.
16. Pud D, Cohen D, Lawental E, Eisenberg E. Opioids and abnormal pain perception: new evidence from a study of chronic opioid addicts and healthy subjects. Drug Alcohol Depend. 2006;82(3):218–23. Epub 2005/10/19.

Chapter 6
Assessment of Pain

Jatin Joshi and Vinay Puttanniah

Key Points

- Assessment
- Pain history
- Physical examination
- Diagnostic tests
- Pain assessment tools
- Perioperative pain assessment

Pain is an unpleasant sensory and emotional experience associated with actual or potential tissue damage [1]. It is also a subjective phenomenon that is modulated by emotional and past experiences, personal beliefs, and social norms. Consequently, the assessment of pain cannot be as objective and as well defined as, for example, blood pressure monitoring or the calculation of serum creatinine.

Pain assessment should begin prior to a patient's presentation for surgery, through the intraoperative and postoperative period, and continue to the post-discharge visit. Assessment should be performed on a repeated basis and take into account the patient's ability to effectively communicate, mental status, preferences, comorbid conditions, type of surgical procedure, length of stay, and preoperative pain state (i.e., history of chronic pain, complex regional pain syndrome, opioid tolerance).

J. Joshi, M.D.
Memorial Sloan Kettering Cancer Center, Hospital for Special Surgery,
Weill Cornell Medical College, New York, NY, USA
e-mail: Jatin.joshi@gmail.com

V. Puttanniah, M.D. (✉)
Department of Anesthesiology and Critical Care Mediline, Memorial Sloan Kettering
Cancer Center, 1275 York Avenue, New York, NY 100675, USA
e-mail: puttannv@mskcc.org

© Springer Science+Business Media New York 2015
A.D. Kaye et al. (eds.), *Substance Abuse*, DOI 10.1007/978-1-4939-1951-2_6

A systematic method of pain assessment is an essential component of perioperative care. Poorly controlled pain can lead to poor medical outcomes and psychologically distressful experiences for patients. Inaccurate assessment may lead to inappropriate or ineffective therapeutic management of pain [2].

Assessment

Accurate pain assessment and appropriate management in the pre-, intra-, and postoperative periods is contingent on obtaining a detailed pain history, performing a thorough physical examination, and reviewing or obtaining relevant diagnostic tests.

Pain History

The collection of pain history begins with obtaining a comprehensive medical history, with particular attention on pathological sources of pain, their frequency, location intensity, and duration. Comorbid conditions will affect the choice of pain management strategy. For example, a patient with pancreatitis with chronic abdominal pain presenting for repair of a tibial fracture will have a complicated presentation of pain. In addition to the acute pain of a fracture, the patient's chronic pain of pancreatitis and possible opioid tolerance are factors that may complicate the pain presentation making accurate assessment imperative. A detailed pain history should address all of the following components as listed in Table 6.1.

Physical Examination

The assessment of pain in the perioperative setting requires a complete physical examination with specific focus on the region of pain and area of recent surgical procedure. In addition to the expected pain of the perioperative setting, such as

Table 6.1 Components of pain history

Onset of pain	Exacerbating or provoking factors
Temporal pattern of pain	Ameliorating factors
Location	Prior history of similar pain
Intensity	Response to analgesics and interventions
Radiation of pain	Referred vs. localized pain
Quality of pain	Patient's attitude toward pain and management

incision related discomfort, pain incited by unanticipated complications should be excluded. For example, a patient with recent repair of an extremity fracture may be experiencing pain from expanding hematoma causing a compartment syndrome.

The physical exam should include neurologic, musculoskeletal and mental status assessment. A through neurologic exam can help elucidate subtle physical exam findings and also identify neuropathic components of pain [3–5]. Provocative maneuvers, such as palpation, are helpful in understanding the etiology and nature of pain. Elicitation of pain may further exacerbate symptoms, and one should be prepared to treat pain resulting from physical examination [6]. Additionally, psychogenic pain or secondary gain should be excluded.

Diagnostic Tests

Although history and physical examination are often all that is necessary to determine the nature and severity of a patient's pain, diagnostic testing is sometimes necessary [4]. X-ray, computerized tomography, bone scans and MRI can be used to evaluate abnormalities in bone, soft tissue, organs and neural structures. Diagnostic percutaneous nerve blocks can also help differentiate between somatic, visceral, and neuropathic pain.

Diagnostic imaging and laboratory tests in the perioperative period can be critical in excluding pathological conditions causing pain. For example chest X-ray and cardiac markers can help rule out pneumonia or myocardial infarction as causes of chest pain.

Pain Assessment Tools

Multiple studies suggest that the formal measurement of pain leads to improved management of pain [3]. Pain assessment in the perioperative period should be simplified for ease of patient participation. The major component of assessment and determinant of method of treatment is "intensity of pain." The tool used for pain assessment should be appropriate for the patient's age, physical and mental status, and preference. For example, a patient who is delirious or intubated cannot participate in pain assessment that requires significant self-assessment [2]. Pain assessment in pediatrics and the cognitively impaired should be proactive and developmentally appropriate. There are several pain intensity measures used in clinical practice, including unidimensional self-report scales, multidimension instruments, and pain diaries (Figs. 6.1 and 6.2 and Tables 6.2 and 6.3) [4, 7–9].

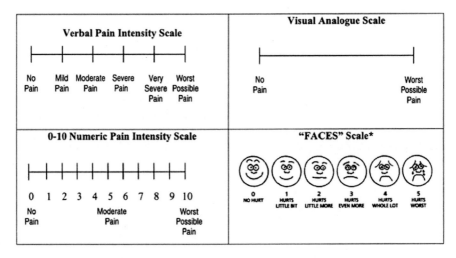

Fig. 6.1 Pain intensity scales [7]

Perioperative Pain Assessment

Preoperative Pain Assessment

Ideally, assessment of pain begins during preoperative patient evaluation and planning. During this time, a proactive plan for postoperative pain management can be formulated. Assessment and planning involves consideration of [10]:

1. Type of surgery
2. Expected severity of postoperative pain
3. Underlying medical conditions
4. Current pain state and medication regimen
5. Risks–benefits of available pain management techniques
6. Patient preferences
7. Prior experiences with perioperative pain

   Pain inventory in the preoperative assessment is used to guide perioperative pain management and improves accuracy of pain assessment postoperatively.

Intraoperative Pain Assessment

Intraoperative assessment of pain during general anesthesia requires monitoring of physiological and behavioral responses to pain [11]. While patients face intense pain of surgical stimulus, they are unable to communicate distress because of the use of intravenous and inhalational anesthetics, paralytics, and mechanical

---

Brief Pain Inventory

Name   Date   Time

1. Throughout our lives, most of us have had pain from time to time (such as minor headaches, sprains, toothaches). Have you had pain other than these everyday types of pain today?

   1. Yes   2. No

2. On the diagram, shade in the areas where you feel pain. Put an X on the area that hurts the most.

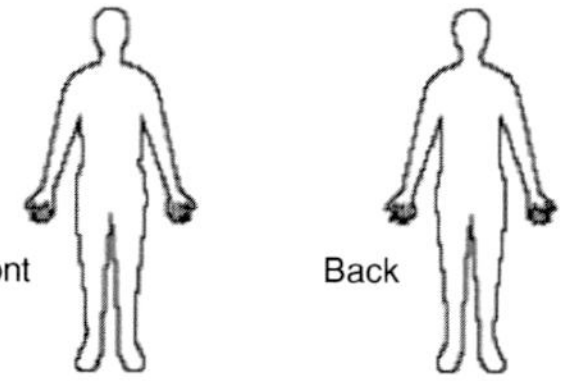

   Front   Back

3. Please rate your pain by circling the one number that best describes your pain at its worst in the past 24 hours.

   0   1   2   3   4   5   6   7   8   9   10
   No pain   Pain as bad as
                                        you can imagine

4. Please rate your pain by circling the one number that best describes your pain at its least in the last 24 hours.

   0   1   2   3   4   5   6   7   8   9   10
   No pain   Pain as bad as
                                        you can imagine

5. Please rate your pain by circling the one number that best describes your pain on average.

   0   1   2   3   4   5   6   7   8   9   10
   No pain   Pain as bad as
                                        you can imagine

6. Please rate your pain by circling the one number that best how much pain you have right now.

   0   1   2   3   4   5   6   7   8   9   10
   No pain   Pain as bad as
                                        you can imagine

7. What treatment or medication are you receiving for the pain?

   _____

   _____

   _____

   _____

   _____

8. In the past 24 hours, how much relif have pain treatments or medication provided? Please circle the one percentage that most shows how much relief you have received.

   0% 10 20 30 40 50 60 70 80 90 100%
   No relief   Complete
                                          relief

9. Circle the one number that describes how, during the past 24 hours, pain has interfered with your:

   A. General activity
   0   1   2   3   4   5   6   7   8   9   10
   Does not   Completely
   Interfere   interferes

   B. Mood
   0   1   2   3   4   5   6   7   8   9   10
   Does not   Completely
   Interfere   interferes

   C. Walking ability
   0   1   2   3   4   5   6   7   8   9   10
   Does not   Completely
   Interfere   interferes

   D. Normal work (includes both work outside the home and housework)
   0   1   2   3   4   5   6   7   8   9   10
   Does not   Completely
   Interfere   interferes

   E. Relations with other people
   0   1   2   3   4   5   6   7   8   9   10
   Does not   Completely
   Interfere   interferes

   F. Sleep
   0   1   2   3   4   5   6   7   8   9   10
   Does not   Completely
   Interfere   interferes

   G. Enjoyment of life
   0   1   2   3   4   5   6   7   8   9   10
   Does not   Completely
   Interfere   interferes

   H. Ability to concentrate
   0   1   2   3   4   5   6   7   8   9   10
   Does not   Completely
   Interfere   interferes

   I. Appetite
   0   1   2   3   4   5   6   7   8   9   10
   Does not   Completely
   Interfere   interferes

Fig. 6.2 Brief pain inventory

Table 6.2 Unidimensional self-report scales [8]

Assessment scale	Description	Advantages/disadvantages
Verbal Descriptor Scale	The patient chooses from a list of adjectives that reflect gradations of pain intensity using a 5-word scale (mild, discomforting, horrible, excruciating)	Advantages • Can indicate trends over time or after interventions • Easy to score and easily understood Disadvantages • Assumes fluency in given language • Provides a limited selection of descriptors • Patients tend to select moderate descriptors
Numerical Rating Scale	The patient assigns a number on a numeric scale (usually 0–10, with 0 being no pain and 10 being the worst pain) to grade the severity of their pain	Advantages • Reproducibility • Easily understood • Sensitive to small changes in pain • Most frequently used Disadvantages • Not validated as a screening test
FACES Pain Rating Scale	The patient selects one of six sketches of facial features ranging from happy, smiling face to a sad teary face. Each sketch is assigned a numeric value	Advantages • Children as young as 3 may reliably use this scale • May be beneficial for mentally impaired patients • Shows adequate test–retest reliability Disadvantages • Limited number of data points
Visual Analog Scale (VAS)	The patient marks the severity of his pain on a 100 mm line with no gradations. The mark is then measured from the end of the line and the score given in mm over 100. For example, if the patient's mark is measured at 67 mm his score would be 67/100	Advantages • Infinite response options • Valid for research purposes • Supported as a sensitive measure of pain and change in pain Disadvantages • Requires abstract thinking • More time consuming to administer • The distance constituting a clinically significant change has not been reliably established • Consistency of response has been low for the chronic pain population

Table 6.3 Multidimensional pain assessment scales [8]

Assessment scale	Description	Advantage/disadvantage
McGill Pain Assessment Scales (MPQ)	Measures 3 dimensions of pain (sensory, affective, and evaluative) using descriptive words	**Advantages** • Reliable for clinical research • Good to capture the whole pain experience **Disadvantages** • Time consuming (5–15 min)
Brief Pain Inventory (BPI)	Patients rate the severity of the pain at its "worst", "least", and "average" within the past 24 h at the time the rating is made. Pain can be represented on a schematic body diagram	**Advantages** • Addressed pain and impact of pain on activity and function • Cross-cultural • Validated in cancer and arthritis research **Disadvantages** • Time consuming
Pain Diary	Evaluates impact of pain on activities, mood, and functionality	**Advantages** • Accurate for day-to-day impacts of pain • Can use electronic pain diaries **Disadvantages** • Not a good study tool
Pain Assessment in Advanced Dementia (PAINAD)	Uses the assessment of key pain behaviors such as respiratory pattern, facial expressions, consolability, and body language	**Advantages** • Easy to use and understand • Can be used in non-communicative patient (dementia, intubated patients, etc.) **Disadvantages** • Relies on proper patient observation by caregiver

ventilation. For example, a typical physiologic response to pain and inappropriate depth of general anesthesia is sympathetic stimulation, which may cause tachycardia, increased respiratory rate, and hypertension.

Signs indicative of insufficient pain control, despite adequate depth of general anesthesia, are identified in Table 6.4 [12].

Typically, the intensity of physiologic responses is proportional to the stimulus. However, intraindividual physiological variation, comorbid disease, preoperative and intraoperative medications (i.e., anesthetics, beta blockers, vasopressors), and surgical events may alter the anticipated response to nociception.

An anesthesiologist's preoperative pain and medical assessment is used to individualize and optimize pain management in the intraoperative setting. Strategies employed by anesthesiologists to appropriately manage pain include: preemptive

Table 6.4 Responses to pain during general anesthesia [12]

Organ System	Response
Cardiovascular	Increased heart rate
	Increased blood pressure
Respiratory	Changes in respiratory rate and tidal volume
Mucocutaneous	Moist/sticky skin
Ocular	Lacrimation

analgesics (i.e., local anesthetic infiltration at incision sites), intraoperative narcotic and anesthetic choice and dosing, and regional anesthesia.

Assessment of pain in patients who have had regional anesthesia must incorporate the appropriate choice of regional anesthesia for type of surgery and the level of blockade required to anesthetize surgical incision. Unfortunately, regional anesthetics do not always provide an "all encompassing" control of perioperative pain. There can be variability in the quality of pain control and the anatomic "coverage" derived from regional anesthesia. For example, a patient who has received an epidural or femoral nerve block for knee surgery may not achieve sufficient pain control for surgical incision and postoperative pain.

The success of regional anesthesia in managing pain is dependent on several factors, including: type of regional anesthesia; adequacy of placement; choice, concentration, volume and rate of infusion of local anesthetic or opiate; duration of blockade, physiological side effect (i.e., hypotension and bradycardia) and preexisting neuromuscular disorders. All these factors must be taken into account in the assessment of pain in perioperative patients receiving regional anesthesia. Additionally, even with successful regional anesthesia, there may be neuromuscular and vascular complications or quality of pain control may wear off over time, necessitating routine reassessment.

Postoperative Pain Assessment

Immediately postoperatively, assessment includes evaluating behavioral responses to pain including splinting, grimacing, moaning, grunting, distorted posture, and reluctance to move [2]. Though these responses are not a prerequisite to experiencing pain, they are especially helpful markers in the nonverbal or cognitively impaired patient.

Postoperative pain assessment should incorporate:

1. Type of surgical procedure and expected pain response
2. Intraoperative and postoperative complications (i.e., conversion from laparoscopic to open incision, development of hematoma, compartment syndrome, myocardial ischemia, unanticipated nerve injury)
3. Anticipated length of stay
4. Preoperative pain state and treatment

The documentation of pain assessment at standard intervals is absolutely essential in communication of pain state amongst clinicians and to guide therapeutic management. In fact, pain is often referred to as the fifth vital sign given its importance in postoperative recovery and physiologic function [2]. Assessment of pain in the immediate postoperative period can be as simple as asking "How bad is your pain?" However, formalized tools, as described above, should be used when possible for standardized and reproducible assessment. VAS scores are widely used in the immediate postoperative period. Discomfort should also be assessed in terms of nausea, patient position, and medication side effects.

Assessment of pain should be an ongoing effort throughout the hospital stay and through postoperative office visits. The purpose of reassessment is to evaluate the current therapeutic pain regimen and to guide further management. Pain should be reassessed after any intervention or change to help continue to optimize the patient's pain relief and recovery.

Additionally, reassessment serves to evaluate development of "breakthrough" pain, pain that persists despite a basal level of analgesia [13]. Patients with breakthrough pain [14] are identified informally and by tools such as the Breakthrough Pain Questionnaire [15], which also determines the nature of pain ([16], Box 3-1).

Conclusion

Every healthcare institution should have a systematic and formalized method of pain assessment in the perioperative setting. A multidisciplinary approach incorporating all clinical care personnel is absolutely essential in identifying, managing, and preventing pain and its sequelae. A comprehensive pain assessment program involves:

1. Early patient evaluation in the preoperative setting that individualizes a pain management plan
2. Vigilant intraoperative monitoring and multifactorial pain management techniques
3. Formalized postoperative pain assessment and reassessment through the post-discharge period

References

1. Bonica JJ. The need of a taxonomy. Pain. 1979;6(3):247–8.
2. Wells N, Pasero C, McCaffery M. Improving the quality of care through pain assessment and management. In: Hughes RG, editor. Patient safety and quality: an evidence-based handbook for nurses, Chapter 17. Rockville: Agency for Healthcare Research and Quality; 2008.
3. Cleeland CS, Ryan KM. Pain assessment: global use of the brief pain inventory. Ann Acad Med. 1994;23:129–35.

4. LeBel A. Assessment of pain. In: Ballantyne JC, editor. The Massachusetts general hospital handbook of pain management. 3rd ed. Philadelphia: Lippincott Williams and Wilkins; 2006. p. 58–75.

5. Bennett M. The LANSS pain scale: the leeds assessment of neuropathic symptoms and signs. Pain. 2001;92(1–2):147–57.

6. Hagen NA. Reproducing a cancer patient's pain on physical examination: bedside provocative maneuvers. J Pain Symptom Manage. 1999;18(6):406–11.

7. Turk DC, Burwinkle TM. Assessment of chronic pain in rehabilitation: outcomes measures in clinical trials and clinical practice. Rehabil Psychol. 2005;50(1):56–64.

8. Urman V. Assessment of pain: patient evaluation. Pocket pain medicine. Philadelphia: Lippincott Williams and Wilkins; 2011.

9. Perry G. Medical care of older persons in residential aged care facilities. 4th ed. East Melbourne: The Royal Australian College of General Practitioners; 2006.

10. American Society of Anesthesiologists Task Force on Acute Pain Management. Practice guidelines for acute pain management in the perioperative setting: an updated report by the American Society of Anesthesiologists Task Force on Acute Pain Management. Anesthesiology. 2012;116(2):248–73.

11. Carr DR, Jacox AK, Chapman CR, et al. Acute pain management: operative or medical procedures and trauma, No 1. U.S. Dept. of Health and Human Services: Rockville; 1992. AHCPR Pub No 92-0032; Public Health Service.

12. Stomberg MW, Sjöström B, Haljamäe H. Routine intra-operative assessment of pain and/or depth of anaesthesia by nurse anaesthetists in clinical practice. J Clin Nurs. 2001;10(4): 429–36.

13. Portenoy PK, et al. Breakthrough pain and impact in patients with cancer pain. Pain. 1999; 81:129–34.

14. Caraceni, et al. Pain measurement tools and methods in clinical research in palliative care: Recommendations of an Expert Working Group of the European Association of Palliative Care. J Pain Symptom Manage. 2002;23(3):239–55.

15. Portenoy, et al. Prevalence and characteristics of breakthrough pain in opioid-treated patients with chronic noncancer. J Pain Med. 2006;7:583–91.

16. Ruth, Denise, The diagnosis and treatment of breakthrough pain. Chapter 3—Assessment box 3.1. In: Perry G, editor. Fine. Oxford: Oxford American Pain Library; 2008.

Chapter 7
Food and Abuse

Ike Eriator, Efosa Ogiamien, and Xiaoli Dai

Key Points

- Food and substance abuse: pathophysiological links
- Clinical therapy
- Translating science into policy

Introduction

The dictionary meaning of food is any material, usually of plant or animal origin, that contains or consists of essential body nutrients, such as carbohydrates, fats, proteins, vitamins, or minerals, and is ingested and assimilated by an organism to produce energy, stimulate growth, and maintain life. To abuse is to use wrongly or improperly, to use to bad effect or for a bad purpose. Food is thus essential for life, health, and procreativity. Yet, excessive consumption of certain foods is detrimental to health. Many of the foods that are most dangerous are also very pleasurable to consume. Consistently consuming too much food can result in major health consequences. Obesity is a medical condition in which excess body fat accumulates to the extent that it may have an adverse effect on health, leading to increased health problems and reduced life expectancy. Obesity is defined by a body-mass index (BMI) greater than 30 kg/m^2. Overweight individuals are those with a BMI of $25–29.9 \text{ kg/m}^2$.

I. Eriator, M.D., M.P.H. (✉) • X. Dai, M.D.
Department of Anesthesiology, University of Mississippi Medical Center,
2500 North State Street, Jackson, MS 39216, USA
e-mail: ieriator@umc.edu; xdai@umc.edu

E. Ogiamien, B.S.
University of Mississippi School of Medicine, 2500 North State Street,
Jackson, MS 39216, USA
e-mail: eogiamien@umc.edu

© Springer Science+Business Media New York 2015
A.D. Kaye et al. (eds.), *Substance Abuse*, DOI 10.1007/978-1-4939-1951-2_7

Obesity constitutes one of the greatest public health challenges of the 21st century and the most serious public health problem facing the USA. Next to tobacco, it is the leading behavioral cause of death in the USA, and it is poised to become the most important determinant of health in the future. Many western or first world societies are currently faced with the twin evils of increasing numbers of people consuming more food than needed for energy balance, as well as poorly adhering to low-calorie prescriptions despite the known adverse effects of obesity. About half of the people on weight-loss programs are likely to weigh more, 4 years after their diet compared to their weight before they started the diet [1]. No nation has been successful in controlling or reversing the obesity epidemic. Efforts made towards addressing this epidemic at the level of basic science, clinical practice, and social policy have had limited success. There are significant associated health, economic, and social effects on the individual and society. It costs about $1,400 more annually to treat an obese patient when compared with a healthy weight individual. Healthcare costs of obesity in the USA were estimated at $147 billion in 2008, up from $78.5 billion in 1998 [2]. The subclinical problems may be more substantial, considering the proportion of adults and children who over eat enough to compromise their health. Reports of emotional eating, strong food cravings, binge eating, difficulties with controlling high-calorie food consumption despite known consequences are widespread, with annual healthcare costs associated with being obese or overweight in the USA projected to exceed $850 billion by 2030 [3].

Until a few centuries ago, obesity was a sign of wealth or health and was much more prevalent in the rich. This still holds true in many poor countries. In fact, tens of thousands of children still die each day from starvation. However, in the developed countries, the problem is the magnification of abundance, and the pace at which the incidence of obesity has been rising in the developed countries in the last 50 years is probably too rapid to be explained by genomic changes. Rather, apart from very rare genetic mutations, it is enabled mostly by an "obesigenic" food environment [4]. The era of foraging for food in groups and using primitive tools with no technology for transportation and handling mostly small food items, with personal access often based on social hierarchy, have been replaced by an efficiently run mass-produced, highly processed, hyperpalatable food available at low cost. In most mammals, including human, sweet receptors evolved in ancestral environments poor in sugars and are not adapted to high concentrations of sugar-rich diets widely available in modern societies [5], much like coca leaves being processed into cocaine. The supranormal stimulation of these receptors generates supranormal reward with the potential to override self-control mechanisms. For instance, a sucrose solution on a pacifier is known to provide sufficient soothing for performing neonatal circumcision [6].

Approximately 200 million men and 300 million women are currently obese worldwide. About two thirds of the USA population is overweight and a third of the population is obese. Severe obesity (a BMI of 40 and above) among adults in the USA quadrupled between 1986 and 2000. An estimated 1 in 3 adolescents in the USA are overweight, a figure that has tripled in the past 20 years. About 80 % of this group is expected to become obese adults. Obesity rates among preschool children have also increased, leading to unexpected rates of diabetes, hypertension, and even heart attacks. No clear program for reversing this trend has yet emerged. The World Health Organization has classified obesity as one of the top ten global health problems.

The phenotype of obesity is heterogenous. Not all individuals who are overweight are addicted to food. The etiology of the current epidemic of obesity is complex and multifactorial, and contributing factors include metabolic processes, genotype, sedentary lifestyle, and increased availability of high-energy, palatable food as part of the current food environment. There is an agreement that a key root cause of the epidemic is hyperphagia, which may be defined as overeating or eating beyond one's energy needs on a chronic basis [7].

Obesity rates have also been rising rapidly throughout the world. Although there are many contributing factors, the changing food environment deserves special attention. Evidence from epidemiological studies also indicates that the rise in obesity rates is linked to the rise in the per capita consumption of proposed addictive foods such as refined carbohydrates [8]. The rate of rise in countries such as France and United Kingdom has been significantly correlated with the availability of highly processed food and fast-food chains [9, 10]. Obesity has increased as there has been an increase in the availability and in the average portion size. In the past two decades, the daily caloric intake, mostly from increases in carbohydrate and refined sugar, has increased by 650 calories per person. Meat, once consumed as wild game, is now genetically engineered, with fat content as much as 50 %. Ice cream is no longer an expensive item. There has also been a disintegration of structured meal. People eat nowadays while watching televisions, while on the computer, while at sporting events, and in all kinds of social gatherings. Most gas stations sell food or snacks. Every car is now equipped with places for food or drinks. Some fast-food delivery places operate all day and all night.

Current brain, behavioral and genetic findings point to shared vulnerabilities underlying the pathological pursuit of substance and non-substance rewards [11]. Eating, in general, stimulates reward pathways. So does music, humor, attractive faces, being in love, winning a prize, and other "pleasant" stimuli. Dopamine is the "pleasure" or "anti-stress" molecule. Lack of dopamine reportedly leads to multiple pleasure-seeking behavior including glucose binges, gambling, sex addiction, and substance abuse. Dopamine is released in the nucleus accumbens and ventral tegmentum area following the administration of most substances of abuse, in a similar way to the ingestion of food. Such release of dopamine is a direct function of the palatability of the food.

There are deep commonalities between overconsumption of sugars and drug addictions. Alcohol and sugar are biochemically congruent substances, since ethanol is the fermented by-product of fructose. Both hijack the natural reward pathway by stimulating dopamine signaling in the ventral striatum in the brain, generate cross tolerance and cross dependence, and administration of naloxone can precipitate withdrawal. In addition, neuroadaptations in the brains of obese individuals mimic those of individuals addicted to drugs [5, 12]. Just as some individuals can drink alcohol responsibly and others cannot, there are individual differences in reactions to food (due to genetic predisposition or to prior experience) and some people can consume food in moderation more easily than others [13].

Excessive and compulsive eating often shares some of the same processes and behavioral phenotypes with substance abuse and dependence. Tolerance, withdrawal, using larger amounts, persistent desire/unsuccessful attempts to cut down use, spending a large amount of time acquiring the substance, using it, or recovering from it, sacrificing occupational, social or recreational activities because of the substance and continued substance use despite recurrent physical and/or psychological problems, all apply to obesity.

Although modern neurobiology of feeding is still conceptualized on the classic principle of homeostasis, it is obvious that the reward system can be hijacked by hyperpalatable food, overwhelming the intrinsic homeostatic mechanisms. Food made hyperpalatable by significant increase in their content of fat, sugar, salt flavor, and additives appear to surpass the rewarding properties of traditional foods. These extremely potent reinforcers can be hard to resist, and can lead to non-homeostatic eating and obesity [11].

Food and Substance Abuse: Pathophysiological Links

Sweet taste perception is an innate capacity that depends on G-protein coupled receptor subunits located on the tongue. The stimulation of these receptors by sweet tasting food generates a sensation that most humans find intensely rewarding [5]. Such sweet sensations generated by sugar-sweetened foods and drinks are probably one of the most frequent and intense pleasures of modern humans. The sight or smell of food is biologically programmed to grasp the attention. The effectiveness of the food in stimulating the brain's reward system influences the likelihood of the future intake of the food. Obese individuals show significantly greater brain activation during activated and actual consumption of food in the primary gustatory cortex, somatosensory cortex and anterior cingulate cortex when compared to lean individuals [14]. Human studies confirm that during ingestion, high-calorie foods selectively activate the dorsal striatum in addition to other areas like the anterior insula, the hippocampus and parietal lobe in obese women when compared to normal weight individuals. High-calorie foods elicited greater activation in the brain areas mediating motivational and emotional responses to food in the obese individuals when compared to normal weight individuals. Such hyperactive areas are also hyperactive to drug cues in addiction [15, 16]. In functional studies of the reward network, increased connectivity between the orbitofrontal cortex and nucleus accumbens has been demonstrated in obese individuals compared to lean individuals, consistent with findings in substance addiction. This may contribute to a stronger salience value of the agent [17, 18].

Animals given intermittent access to sugar exhibit features of withdrawal and tolerance as well as cross sensitization to drugs of abuse. Rats fed diets high in sugar and fat manifest reward dysfunction associated with drug addiction, compulsive eating, continued consumption despite receipt of shocks, and also had downregulation of striatal dopamine receptors [19].

Normal food intake is regulated by homeostatic processes and is influenced by the same reward and motivational processes that control drug seeking [11]. Human and animal studies have demonstrated that the reinforcing effects of psychostimulant drugs are related to increased brain dopamine levels and the subjective perception of pleasure positively correlates with the amount of dopamine released [20]. In addition, the individual differences in the reinforcing effects of such drugs are predicted by the levels of dopamine D2 receptors. Low D2 receptor levels are associated with greater reinforcing effects of the drug. When healthy food-deprived individuals are presented with favorite foods, dopamine is similarly released during the presentation of food-related cues as well as after consumption of the meal. The amount of dopamine released in the dorsal striatum correlates with the pleasantness of the meal. Increased regional cerebral blood flow occurs in the dorsal striatum and this correlates positively with the pleasantness ratings during ingestion of chocolate [21].

Aside from obesity, the overlaps between food intake and addiction have relevance to the study of eating disorders, such as anorexia nervosa and binge eating disorder. Both over- and undereating can affect the brain reward systems in a way that promotes the intake of drugs of abuse. Anorexia nervosa, which is characterized by severe undernutrition, may result in some features of addiction. Such patients manifest behavioral repertoire of weight loss, restricted food intake, and excessive exercise such that these behaviors interfere with other activities in much the same way that substance abuse does. Binge eating disorder has stood out as having particular relevance to "food addiction." Binge eating is characterized by discrete episodes of rapid and excessive food consumption not necessarily driven by hunger or metabolic need. It is a consistent self-reported trait among overweight and obese patients. Common binge foods are usually energy dense, highly palatable foods rich in sugar and/or fat. Binge eating disorder shares many characteristics with addictive behaviors including diminished control overuse of the food and continued use despite negative consequences [11].

Craving is a characteristic feature of both obesity and addiction. It may underlie overeating and drug abuse, and interfere with maintenance of abstinence. Chocolate is the most frequently craved food, especially by women. Other foods including starches, fats, and sweets are also craved. Energy-dilute beverages whether sweetened or not, are sometimes mentioned as objects of food cravings, unlike vegetables and fruits which are almost never mentioned. Using brain imaging studies, many of the areas of the brain activated in food craving seem to overlap with those that are active in craving related to drugs of abuse. This has been demonstrated for the anterior cingulate gyrus, hippocampus, insula, striatum, and the prefrontal cortex. Food cravings are associated with dysphoria and negative moods including depression, boredom, listlessness, stress, and fatigue—all of which are minimized by the ingestion of the craved substances. Just as withdrawal is not necessary to produce drug cravings, nutritional deprivation is not necessary to produce food cravings [13]. Environmental cues are effective triggers for food craving as well; the sight or smell of food or even food imagery may serve as triggers.

Tolerance occurs when larger quantity of the agent is required to produce the same effect. Tolerance is at least partially due to the downregulation of central dopamine signaling as a result of repeated exposure to substances that activate this pathway. Such attenuated dopamine signaling has been shown in individuals who are addicted to drugs. With regards to food consumption, several studies have shown that depletions in dopamine signaling are present in animals and humans that are hyperphagic. This association may mean that obesity results in increased intake because the effect of the rewarding properties of these foods has decreased. In a double-blind, randomized study of overweight women, a reduction in the intensity of mitigating negative emotions over repeated consumption of the same quantity of the carbohydrate-rich meal was reported [22].

While the dopamine system play a key role in reward processing, other systems are also important. The endocannabinoid system directly modulates reward and drug seeking. The endogenous opioid system is also involved in reward processing. Dietary obesity may also be linked to defects in systems apart from the reward circuits that may work synergistically or independently to induce hyperphagia. Some obese persons may apparently eat more because of specific defects in satiation or hunger, such as the high prevalence of melanocortin-4 receptor mutations leading to lack of satiation. Polymorphisms in leptin, leptin receptor, or CCK gene can lead to changes in snacking frequency or meal size. Some obese people have altered sensory thresholds for sweetness and may regulate reward by increasing intake in order to arrive at the same total reward. Such a taste defect could work synergistically with reward deficits. So alterations in reward per se are not the cause of all obesity, but they may be sufficient in the majority of the population [7].

The preponderance of the evidence from animal and human literature suggests that common dietary obesity satisfies all the Diagnostic and Statistical Manual of mental disorders (DSM) criteria for an addictive disorder. While there are obese people who can gain weight because of defects in satiety and genetic predisposition, this group do not represent the vast majority of obese people in modern societies. The average rate of hyperphagia in most obese people is sufficient to induce significant weight gain. Only a moderate increase in daily caloric intake would be required for such an effect over time. The addictive potential in obesity is most likely mediated by the blunting of the CNS response to palatable food through the midbrain dopamine pathways, which induces an increase in food intake to compensate [7].

Clinical Therapy

Obesity is often one of the most difficult and frustrating problems for patients and physicians. A lot of effort is spent with little benefit. Americans spend billions of dollars annually for weight loss through dieting and exercising. But most diet plans have very low success rates and most dieters have regained the weight within 3–5 years. Weight-loss diets, for example, even in the best treatment centers, result in an average 8 % reduction in body weight. This lack of clinical success has created a never-ending demand for new weight-loss treatments. Approximately 45 % of women and 25 % of men are "dieting" at any one time, spending billions of dollars each year on diet books, diet meals, weight-loss classes, diet drugs, exercise programs, "fat farms," and other weight-loss aids [23].

In a 2-year study, 322 moderately obese subjects (mean age, 52 years; mean body-mass index of 31) were randomly assigned to one of three diets: low-fat, restricted-calorie; Mediterranean, restricted-calorie; or low-carbohydrate, nonrestricted-calorie. The rate of adherence to a study diet was 95.4 % at 1 year and 84.6 % at 2 years. The mean weight loss was 2.9 kg for the low-fat group, 4.4 kg for the Mediterranean-diet group, and 4.7 kg for the low-carbohydrate group ($p < 0.001$). Of the 272 participants who completed the intervention, the mean weight losses were 3.3, 4.6, and 5.5 kg, respectively. The relative reduction in the ratio of total cholesterol to high-density lipoprotein cholesterol was 20 % in the low-carbohydrate group and 12 % in the low-fat group ($p = 0.01$). Among the 36 subjects with diabetes, changes in fasting plasma glucose and insulin levels were more favorable among those assigned to the Mediterranean diet than among those assigned to the low-fat diet [24].

Sustained weight loss requires long-term changes in eating and exercise behavior. Patients must learn specific skills to facilitate decreased calorie intake and increased energy expenditure. Behavioral therapy helps patients to identify cues that trigger inappropriate eating and learn new responses to them. Behavior therapy, combined with diet and exercise, forms the core of the most standard "lifestyle modification" approaches to weight management. Behavior therapy can be implemented in groups or as individual therapy. Trained psychologists and dieticians commonly lead such efforts, but office-based clinicians can often learn to use many of the same techniques. Intensity of interaction appears to be one of the predictors of success [23]. Healthcare providers can use the SBIRT approach, which stands for screening, Brief Intervention and Referral to Treatment. This involves asking every patient about substance use, determining significant problem use, implementing an intervention or referral. Providers need continued education units on chemical dependency in food.

Standard behavior therapy relies on specific techniques to teach the skills needed to change problematic behaviors. The major issue with applying this treatment to inappropriate food consumption is that the problem being extinguished is much more reinforcing in the short term, compared to the behavior being encouraged. Behavioral techniques include: [A] Goal-setting. Patients are taught to set specific quantifiable, realistic goals at the outset of behavior therapy and during each week of therapy. Succeeding at meeting realistic goals create a sense of self-efficacy and can reinforce further change. [B] Self-monitoring. Patients are taught to monitor both food and beverage intake and physical activity. Specific attention is directed at teaching patients how to estimate portion sizes since patients may underestimate intake by 50 %. The context, degree of hunger, and emotional state of each time of eating is also recorded. This may allow eating-related factors to be targeted for modification. Patients are also instructed to record all programmed physical activity. [C] Stimulus control. Patients are instructed to identify stimuli that increase the likelihood of both desired and undesired behaviors. Particular emphasis is placed on attempting to modify nonfood cues that are associated with eating. Other simple techniques include keeping certain problem foods out of the house, using smaller diameter plates and glasses. [D] Cognitive skills. Patients are taught skills for problem solving and cognitive restructuring. Patients are asked to identify problems, consider potential solutions, list the advantages and disadvantages of each, select a feasible solution, and evaluate the results. Cognitive restructuring involves identification of dysfunctional thoughts that interfere with goals and replacing such thoughts with more rational ones. Formal cognitive behavioral therapy can also be used as part of weight management. CBT places more emphasis on cognitive change, rather than behavioral change, as the primary focus of treatment [23].

Cue Exposure with Response Prevention (CERP) is a behavioral strategy adopted from drug abuse therapy and is geared towards extinguishing the association between conditioned food stimuli (like the sight or smell of food) and the unconditioned stimuli which serve as positive reinforcement (eating). This has shown success in small-scale studies with binge eaters [25].

A systematic review and meta-analysis of 61 studies to identify which behavioral change techniques were associated with increased self-efficacy and physical activity in obese adults found an overall small effect of the interventions on self-efficacy ($d=0.23$, 95 % confidence interval (CI): 0.16–0.29, $p<0.001$) and a medium sized effect on physical activity behavior ($d=0.50$, 95 % CI 0.38–0.63, $p<0.001$). The 4 behavioral change techniques that were significantly associated with positive changes in self-efficacy were "action planning", "time management", "prompt self-monitoring of behavioral outcome" and "plan social support/social change". These latter two behavioral change techniques were also associated with positive changes in physical activity [26]. Social support is an additional essential component for any successful weight-loss program. Most successful programs use peer group support. Diet partnerships are effective for some patients. Involvement of family members is also important. A comprehensive review of published results of weight-loss programs strongly suggests that close provider–patient contact is a better predictor of success than the particular weight-loss intervention [23].

Overeaters Anonymous (OA) was founded in 1960 and is a 12-step program for people with problems related to food. The only requirement for membership is the desire to stop eating compulsively. Like other 12-step programs, OA views compulsive eating as having a physical, mental, and spiritual dimension. The first step begins with the admission of the powerlessness over food, and the next 11 steps are tailored to bring healing. Several groups have split from OA to focus more on recovery from food addiction. Such groups include Food Addicts Anonymous (FAA), Food Addicts in Recovery Anonymous (FA), Recovering Food Addicts Anonymous (RFA), and Grey Sheeters Anonymous (GSA).

Phentermine is a sympathomimetic amine that promotes anorexia. It is the most commonly used drug for treatment of obesity currently. Average weight loss is about 3.6 kg over 24 weeks. It is only approved for short-term therapy, but is commonly used off label beyond the approved 12 weeks. Orlistat binds to lipases in the intestinal tract and inhibits the hydrolysis of fat and thus its absorption. Average weight decrease is about 2.75 kg over 52 weeks. It also limits the absorption of fat-soluble vitamins. Sibutramine is a centrally acting serotonin–norepinephrine reuptake inhibitor structurally related to amphetamines, though it had a distinct mechanism of action. It was withdrawn from the US market in 2010 due to side effects. Rimonabant was the first selective cannabinoid1 receptor blocker to be approved for use anywhere in the world, but was withdrawn from the market due to side effects. A notable historical exception to the lack of results with anti-obesity drugs is the controlled substance, d-amphetamine, which was used over the counter as a weight-loss medicine until the early seventie. Interestingly, amphetamine is a dopaminergic drug that induces massive dopamine release in the brain. In the case of binge eating disorder and anorexia, preliminary results indicate that drugs like baclofen and topiramate are effective in reducing binge eating, craving, and weight gain [7].

Considering the similarities between food and drug cravings, it would make sense to co-opt lessons from drug addiction in the fight against obesity. Mu opioid receptor antagonists block rewards from drugs such as heroin and morphine, and they blunt the reward from hyperpalatable foods [27]. Naltrexone, an opioid antagonist has potential in the treatment of obesity. Naltrexone in combination with bupropion for the treatment of obesity is in phase III clinical trial. Baclofen has shown clinical promise in substance addiction as well as the consumption of highly palatable foods [28].

Bariatric surgery is for many morbidly obese patients the viable means for initiating a successful anti-obesity program and is currently the only therapy that produces long-term weight loss of 15 % or more of the initial weight. It is recommended for those with a body-mass index of 40 kg/m^2 or higher (or those with 35 kg/m^2 or higher that have associated comorbidities) following failure of conservative therapy. Surgery type may be of the restrictive type (for instance the Laparoscopic Adjustable Gastric Banding, vertical sleeve gastrectomy), or the malabsorptive type (for instance biliopancreatic Diversion with Duodenal Switch) or a combination of the two (for instance the Roux-en Y Gastric Bypass). Bariatric surgery on the average leads to a 10–15 kg/m^2 reduction in the BMI and a weight loss of about 30–50 kg. Maximum weight loss is achieved in about 12–18 months after the procedure, though some patients will regain some of the weight several years later.

Translating Science into Policy

Initial approaches to obesity as a disease and the related metabolic conditions have focused primarily on individual risk factors like genetics, personal responsibilities, and individual behavioral changes, with a paucity of attention to the possible interaction with the "unhealthy food environment" based on the engineering and deceptive marketing of hyperpalatable foods. An explanation dating back to the early part of the last century enunciated a diet built on a logic that blamed lack of will power, bad food choices, and unhealthy life styles for the problem.

Ingredients for potentially addictive food, for instance, corn sugar, remain inexpensive because of substantial governmental subsidies. Hyperpalatable foods are the most frequently marketed products specifically targeting children and adolescents [29, 30]. Food with greater abuse potential (high sugar and high fat) are more widely available, and cost less than food with higher nutritional value. Based on lessons from alcohol regulations, it would be expected that reducing the availability of such hyperpalatable foods, in favor of those with more nutritional value would help to decrease food related problems.

Meal or portion sizes are also important. They are not under strong biological control. People tend to eat all what they are served. Plate sizes can have significant effects. Portions in the USA have doubled in the last two decades [4], driven by a free market economy. It costs very little more to serve a large compared to a small portion or meal. Restaurant patrons feel they are getting more for their money when they buy from vendors with the largest portion size. To maintain market share, competing food providers often engage in a battle of escalating portion sizes. Although such large portion sizes are known to fuel obesity, the corporate defense is that consumers have the choice to eat only a part of what they are served. However, people ordinarily may not be able to exercise such dietary restrains [4] because of the evolutionary biological programming. Even in settings of a fixed price for all you can eat, taking large portions will be the norm, since the likelihood of taking a large portion to conform with everyone else is high. Of course, the food industry is catering to consumers' demand! The cost efficiencies in industrial scale food production are gigantic, and it will be unrealistic to expect that many consumers will soon return to the fresh fruits, vegetables, and meat from the local grower.

Hyperpalatable foods usually include multiple ingredients, and research into which specific component may be addictive is still in the early stages. Fast foods also have several other attributes that may increase its salience. The majority of fast-food meals are accompanied by a soda, which increases the sugar content about 10-fold. Caffeine is a "model" substance of dependence and coffeinated drinks are driving the recent increase in fast-food sales. High fat and salt content of fast food may increase the addictive potential. Obese individuals eat more fast food than those who are normal weight. Obesity is characterized by resistance to insulin, leptin, and other hormonal signals that would normally control appetite and limit reward. Stress and dieting may sensitize an individual to reward. Fast-food advertisements, restaurants, and menus all provide environmental cues that may trigger addictive overeating. The Food and Drug Administration (FDA) requires that food additives be generally regarded as safe. But addictive effects on the brain have not been considered in this area of safety.

Policy actions that have been suggested include education and information interventions, advertising and marketing measures, changing the image of healthy foods, ensuring access to and availability of healthier food, school and worksite initiatives to create a supportive environment, economic subsidies that facilitate healthier food choices, heavy taxation on unhealthy foods, reduction of fat or added sugars and salt in manufactured products, and strict nutrition labeling regulations. Marketing works. Clear parameters of what constitutes healthy food must continue to be disseminated.

Governments have a role in creating or maintaining an environment that fosters good health. However, the checks and balances of the political system in the USA, especially the fierce partisan fights of an evenly divided congress, will make any major reform difficult. The politics of obesity is the latest version of the modern form of public health politics, focusing on private behavior that gets bogged down in a legislative stalemate despite a clear warning about current and future crisis. Litigation is therefore replacing legislation as the ticket to corporate accountability. In addition, "Big Food" is a lucrative and efficient industry, global in scope and has significant political sway, just like "Big Tobacco". These industries rely on similar tactics to redirect blame, such as emphasizing personal responsibility, spreading misinformation and doubt, and employing lobbyists, lawyers, and trade organizations to resist state regulations [31]. Policy changes often have arch enemies in those who benefit from the current system and only receive lukewarm support from those who will benefit from the new system.

Estimates are that obesity will soon overtake tobacco use as the leading cause of death in the USA, likely because the public largely does not perceive it as a significant threat and there is low public support for policies aimed at curbing obesity—like reducing television watching and taxing sugar-sweetened beverages. In addition, there is skepticism owing to the stigmatization of obesity as a personal weakness or moral failure, and the rate of adults receiving primary obesity prevention is only about 2.6 % [32].

On the positive side, the American Medical Association has recognized obesity as a disease that requires medical intervention. Under the Affordable Care Act, screening and counseling can be covered by most insurance companies with no patient cost sharing as part of the preventive services benefits. Updated nutrition guidelines for school lunch have gone into effect. And beginning with 2014–2015 school year, candy bars, high-fat chips, full-calorie soft drinks, chocolate sandwich cookies will no longer be sold during the school day in the school vending machines or a la carte lines. United States Department of Agriculture (USDA) Smart Snacks in Schools nutrition standards set down limits for calories, fat, sugar, and sodium. Several cities have proposed ordinances banning the sale of sugared beverages in municipal buildings.

The food industry has a long history of reformulating products in response to market conditions. In 2011, San Francisco promulgated a Health Food Incentive ordinance which banned toy giveaways with children's meals at fast-food restaurants unless the meal met San Francisco's strict nutritional standards. The ban targeted the Happy Meal-style toys, claiming that the inclusion of an incentive item unfairly targeted marketing at children who are unable to make healthy decisions for themselves. But instead of changing the content of Happy Meals or eliminating the toys, McDonald complied by charging ten cents for the addition of a toy and the proceeds went to the benefit of the Ronald McDonald House Charity.

There is a significant and consistent body of research that have documented similar structural and functional changes in important areas that underlie behavioral regulation, reward, executive function, and decision making in obesity and addiction. Like drugs of abuse, obesity is a disease of modern civilization. Intersecting clinical approaches and strategies for treatment and prevention are needed. Modern food environment is so immoderate that it should be obvious that physiological manipulations designed to restrain excessive eating will have little hope of succeeding on its own. Physiological controls can be effective only under conditions that enable them to be operative. Until these conditions come together, the translation of research into improved public health and clinical care will remain marginal.

Conclusion

The overwhelming interest in modern society in eating beyond that which is required for energy balance suggest that it is no longer only for survival. Alternative approaches are needed to combat this expensive, deadly personal, and public health disease. Reframing the obesity issue from the addiction perspective may encourage the development of novel human and animal laboratory paradigms, which would provide mechanistic insight into how individuals can become dependent on food.

Public health approaches, environmental modifications, global initiatives, corporate and individual responsibilities must come together in a joint effort to address these food and diet diseases of modern times [19]. Exclusive focus on personal responsibilities to the exclusion of corporate responsibilities in the case of tobacco probably accounted for decades of delayed policy changes and drug related interventions. Taxations, limits on access and marketing and legal actions by the state attorney generals in the USA are public health imperatives that helped curb the burden of tobacco health concerns in the USA. Such policies focused on changing the availability, costs, and the attributes of tobacco products have resulted in significant public health gains and perhaps the greatest public health victory of the 20th century. Similar evidence-based policy interventions will help to curb the epidemic of food related disorders—one of the greatest public health challenges of the current times. But the most important consequence of such changes will be the changes that individuals undertake in their behavior and choices. At this epoch of medical development, much of the incremental improvement in our quality of life and life span is likely to come from behavioral changes. Food abuse and obesity are prime targets for change.

References

1. Mann T, Tomiyama J, Westling E, Lew AM, et al. Medicare's search for effective obesity treatments: diets are not the answer. Am Psychologist. 2007;62:220–33.
2. Finkelstein EA, Trogdon JG, Cohen JW, Dietz W. Annual medical spending attributable to obesity: payer-and service-specific estimates. Health Aff. 2009;28:w822–31.
3. Wang Y, Beydoun MA, Liang L, et al. Will all Americans become overweight or obese? Estimating the progression and cost of the US obesity epidemic. Obesity. 2008;16:519–30.

4. Rowland NE. Order and disorder: temporal organization of eating. Behav Brain Res. 2012; 231:272–8.
5. Lenoir M, Serre F, Cantin L, Ahmed SH. Intense sweetness surpasses cocaine reward. PLoS One. 2007;2(8):e698 (1–10).
6. Herschel M, Khoshnood B, Ellman C, Maydew N, Mittendorf R. Neonatal circumcision. Randomized trial of a sucrose pacifier for pain control. Arch Pediatr Adolesc Med. 1998;152: 279–84.
7. Allen PJ, Batra P, Geiger BM, Wommack T, et al. Rationale and consequences of reclassifying obesity as an addictive disorder: Neurobiology, food environment and social policy perspectives. Physiol Behav. 2012;107:126–37.
8. Putnam JJ, Allshouse JE. Food consumption, prices, and expenditures, 1970-97. Statistical Bulletin [No. (SB-965)]. Washington, DC: USDA; 1999.
9. Fantasia R. Fast food in France. Theory Soc. 1995;24:201–43.
10. Debres K. Burgers for Britain: a cultural geography of McDonald's UK. J Cult Geogr. 2005; 22:115–39.
11. Frascella J, Potenza MN, Brown LL, Chidress AR. Shared brain vulnerabilities open the way for nonsubstance addictions: carving addiction at a new joint? Ann N Y Acad Sci. 2010; 1187:294–315.
12. Wang GJ, Volkow ND, Thanos PK, Fowler JS. Similarity between obesity and drug addiction as assessed by neurofunctional imaging: a concept review. J Addict Dis. 2004;23:39–53.
13. Pelchat ML. Food addiction in humans. J Nutr. 2009;139:620–2.
14. Stice E, Spoor S, Bohon C, Veldhuizen MG, Small DM. Relation of reward from food intake and anticipated food intake to obesity: a functional magnetic resonance imaging study. J Abnorm Psychol. 2008;117:924–35.
15. Rothemund Y, Preuschhof C, Bohner G, et al. Differential activation of the dorsal striatum by high calorie visual food stimuli in obese individuals. Neuroimage. 2007;37:410–21.
16. Stoeckel LE, Weller RE, Cook 3rd EW, Twieg DB, et al. Widespread reward system activation in obese women in response to pictures of high calorie foods. Neuroimage. 2008;41:636–47.
17. Stoeckel LE, Kim J, Weller RE, Cox JE, et al. Effective connectivity of a reward network in obese women. Brain Res Bull. 2009;79:388–95.
18. Ma N, Liu Y, Li N, Wang CX, et al. Addiction related alteration in resting state brain connectivity. Neuroimage. 2010;49:738–44.
19. Gearhardt AN, Grilo CM, Dileone RJ, et al. Can food be addictive? Public health and policy implications. Addiction. 2011;106:1208–12.
20. Volkow ND, Wang GJ, Fowler JS, Logan J, et al. Reinforcing effects of psychostimulants in human are associated with increases in brain dopamine and occupancy of D2 receptors. J Pharmacol Exp Ther. 1999;291:409–15.
21. Small DM, Zatorre RJ, Dagher A, Evans AC, Jones-Gotman M. Changes in brain activity related to eating chocolate: from pleasure to aversion. Brain. 2001;124:1720–33.
22. Spring B, Schneider K, Smith M, Kendzor D, Appelhans B, Hedeker D, et al. Abuse potential of carbohydrates for overweight carbohydrate cravers. Psychopharmacology (Berl). 2008;197: 637–47.
23. Baron R. Obesity, Chapter 19. In: Feldman MD, Christensen JF, editors. Behavioral medicine: a guide for clinical practice. 3rd ed. Maidenhead: McGraw Hill; 2008. p. 171–8.
24. Shai I, Schwarzfuchs D, Henkin Y, Shahar D, et al. Weight loss with a low-carbohydrate, mediterranean, or low-fat diet. N Engl J Med. 2008;359:229–41.
25. Umberg EN, Shader RI, Hsu LKG, Greenblatt DJ. From disordered eating to addiction; the "food drug" in bulimia nervosa. J Clin Psychopharmacol. 2012;32:376–89.
26. Olander EK, Fletcher H, Williams S, Atkinson L, et al. What are the most effective techniques in changing obese individuals' physical activity self-efficacy and behavior: a systematic review and meta-analysis. Int J Behav Nutr Phys Act. 2013;10:29. doi:10.1186/1479-5868-10-29. Accessed 15 Sept 2013.
27. Gosnell BA, Levine AS. Reward systems and food intake: role of opioids. Int J Obes (London). 2009;33 Suppl 2:S54–8.

28. Corwin RL, Wojnicki FH. Baclofen, raclopride, and naltrexone differentially affect intake of fat and sucrose under limited access conditions. Behav Pharmacol. 2009;20:537–48.
29. Powell LM, Sczypka G, Chaloupka FJ, Braunschweig CL. Nutritional content of television food advertisements seen by children and adolescents in the United States. Pediatrics. 2007; 120:576–83.
30. Harris JL, Pomeranz JL, Lobstein T, Brownell KD. A crisis in the marketplace: how food marketing contributes to childhood obesity and what can be done. Annu Rev Public Health. 2009;30:211–25.
31. Chopra M, Darnton-Hill I. Tobacco and obesity epidemics: not so different after all? BMJ. 2004;328:1558–60.
32. Lutfiyya MN, Nika B, Ng L, Tragos C, Won R, Lipsky MS. Primary prevention of overweight and obesity: an analysis of national survey data. J Gen Intern Med. 2008;23:821–3.

Chapter 8
Alcohol Dependence Syndrome

Ameana Khan, Suresh Menon, and Sreekumar Kunnumpurath

Key Points

- Pathophysiology
- Causes
- Screening for alcohol dependency
- Signs and symptoms of withdrawal
- Signs and symptoms of delirium
- Signs and symptoms of chronic alcohol abuse
- Investigations
- Acute treatment/management
- Long-term management

A. Khan, M.B.B.S. (✉)
Department of Anaesthetics, Milton Keynes Hospital,
328 Watford Road, Croxley Green, Rickmansworth, Hertfordshire WD3 3DE, UK
e-mail: ameana2011@gmail.com

S. Menon, M.D., F.R.C.A.
Department of Anaesthetics, Milton Keynes NHS foundation trust, Standing Way,
Eaglestone, Milton Keynes MK6 5LD, UK
e-mail: drsureshmenon27@googlemail.com

S. Kunnumpurath, M.B.B.S., M.D., F.F.P.M.R.C.A., F.R.C.A., F.C.A.R.C.S.I.
Department of Anaesthetics and Pain Management, Epsom and St Helier
University Hospitals NHS Trust, Wryth Lane, Carshalton SM5 1AA, UK
e-mail: skunnumpurath@gmail.com

© Springer Science+Business Media New York 2015   77
A.D. Kaye et al. (eds.), *Substance Abuse*, DOI 10.1007/978-1-4939-1951-2_8

Introduction

The Word Health Organisation [1, 2] (WHO) estimates that 140 million people are suffering from a degree of alcohol dependency. Alcohol is the world's third largest risk factor for disease and disability, 4 % of all deaths and 4.6 % of disability-adjusted life-years are attributed to alcohol.

Alcohol dependency has direct and indirect effects, which include alcohol related diseases. Internationally 20–30 % of all liver diseases, cancers (oesophageal, colon, breast) and epilepsy are a result of alcohol abuse. Conversely, indirect effects of alcohol dependency include road traffic accidents, homicides, and other injuries. Alcohol dependence is increasingly affecting the younger generations (15–29 years), annually 320,000 are direct results of alcohol use [3].

In the United States alcohol dependency is the third preventable cause of death including 50 % of all liver cirrhosis cases, which is the 12th leading cause of death. The US national longitudinal alcohol epidemiology study has shown alcohol dependence syndrome is prevalent in 20 % of all inpatients in hospital. It is estimated that 1 in 6 patients have a problem [4, 5].

Economically, the burden of alcohol abuse has negatively impacted on the justice and law enforcement sector due to increased incidents of crime and violence. Furthermore, health sector resources have been drained as a result of dealing with alcohol related health problems. In developed countries such as the United States, the total economic cost of alcohol in 1998 was $234854, which amounts to $837 per person. On further examination of these figures, 72.7 % of the total cost was for indirect effects relating to alcohol, including the loss of productivity, followed by direct health cost of 12.7 %, law enforcement costs 3.4 % and other direct costs 3.4 %. Rehm estimated the global impact of alcohol abuse and found the costs ranged from 1.3 % to 3.3 % of gross domestic product (GDP). Essentially, this highlights the severity of alcohol abuse, with its direct and indirect effects not only crippling to the economy and burden on the taxpayers [6].

Alcohol dependence syndrome, or more commonly known as *Alcoholism*, is an uncontrolled compulsion to consume excessive amounts of alcohol. Physical signs of the addiction include withdrawal symptoms and tolerance. For an addict the urge to drink alcohol overrides any physical or mental health problems and any social responsibilities [3].

Alcohol abuse: is an uncontrolled compulsion for alcohol leading to problems (psychological or social) without any physical addiction [7].

The Diagnostic and Statistical Manual of Mental Disorders, (DSM-IV-TR), defines alcohol dependency as a drinking behavior which leads to a significant amount of distress and impairment. Three of the following are required over a period of 12 months to make a diagnosis: [8]

- The presence of tolerance to alcohol.
- Abstinence from alcohol results in withdrawal symptoms.
- Alcohol is taken in larger volume or over longer periods of time than intended.

Table 8.1 Guidance on alcohol consumption for males

Country/grams per drink	Units per day	Grams per day	Units per week	Grams per week
USA/14 g	1–2	14–28 g	14	196 g
UK/8 g	>4	>32 g	> 21	>168 g

Table 8.2 Guidance on alcohol consumption for females

Country/grams per drink	Units per day	Grams per day	Units per week	Grams per week
USA/14 g	1	14 g	7	98 g
UK/8 g	>3	24 g	>14	112 g

- Impaired control where there is an overwhelming desire for alcohol or an individual is unable to reduce or control alcohol consumption.
- Time spent in alcohol related activities to obtain alcohol and recovering from effects.
- The individual neglects daily activities and gives priority to activities to obtain alcohol.
- Consumption of alcohol is continued despite knowledge of physical or psychological problems, which are likely to be caused or exacerbated by alcohol use.

Recommendations of safe alcohol consumption vary slightly according to country (Tables 8.1 and 8.2) [9].

Pathophysiology

Alcohol interferes with the brains neurotransmitters, including stimulating dopamine, γ-Aminobutyric acid (GABA), glutamate, and endorphines. Dopamine affects the mesolimbic system and the nucleus accumbens, which is commonly referred to as the reward pathway. Stimulation of this pathway leads to reward seeking behavior which can result in alcohol intoxication. Opioids have a similar effect on the reward pathway and lead to a feeling of euphoria [10].

GABA has an inhibitory effect; it acts via 2 receptors $GABA_A$ $GABA_B$ which can be found in the brain including the amygdala which regulates emotional state. Chronic alcohol exposure can cause both decreased and increased release of GABA in different areas of the brain. The increased release leads to a relaxed sedated effect. When alcohol is withdrawn it creates hyperexcitability within the brain which results in anxiety and possible seizures.

Glutamate is a major excitatory neurotransmitter which binds to N-methyl-D-aspartate receptor (NMDA) in the regions of the brain including nucleus accumbens, central nucleus, and amygdala. Alcohol exposure leads to inhibition of glutamate in the brain. Chronic inhibition of glutamate, secondary to alcohol use, results in the brain maintaining normal physiological function by increasing the release of glutamate activity and sensitivity of NMDA receptors. Thus, when alcohol is withdrawn it will cause hyperexcitability of the central nervous system, leading to excitatory neurotoxicity. This state leads to brain cell death, cerebellar degeneration, and physical dependence.

Causes

Genetics: Alcoholism is a multifactorial condition with complex genetic and environmental components. The Human genome project has made way for more recent genetic studies. Research in alcohol dependency has shown polymorphism in DNA sequence for genes encoding for alcohol dehydrogenase 1B (ALDH1B gene), aldehyde dehydrogenase 2 (ALDH2 gene), and various other alcohol metabolising enzymes which predispose individuals to alcohol dependency. Moreover, more recent research by Villafuerte et al. have shown GABA2 plays a role in impulsiveness through variation of insula activity responses. Research has indicated that alcohol use at an early age by individuals who already have genetic predisposition increases risk of alcohol abuse [11, 12].

Studies on twins have shown identical twins have a higher incidence than noidentical twins of alcohol dependency. Additionally, the study showed that high alcohol consumption by the father increases the risk of alcohol dependency in the offspring [13].

Psychiatric disorders: Higher rates of alcohol dependency has been seen in individuals with comorbid mood, anxiety disorders, depression, antisocial, and other personality disorders and schizophrenia [14].

Sex: Alcoholism is more common in males compared to females. The incidence of alcoholism is increasing in females and more frequent in older age. Globally, out of all deaths 6.2 % of male and 1.1 % of female deaths are attributed to alcohol abuse.

Developed countries: The world's highest alcohol consumption is in developed countries such as Europe and United Sates. Alcohol abuse is seen in more lower socioeconomic regions [15].

Stress: The impact of alcohol use depends on the severity and duration of stress experienced. The types of stresses which predispose individuals to alcohol dependency consist of general, catastrophic events (e.g. natural disasters), childhood maltreatment and child abuse.

Environmental: Individuals brought up in an environment of heavy drinking and exposed to other risk factors including psychological disorders such as depression, are more vulnerable to alcohol dependency. Social pressure particularly from peers can lead to increased misuse and eventual alcohol dependency.

Screening for Alcohol Dependency

Using a screening tool such as the CAGE questionnaire, can aid clinicians in the history taking process to make a diagnosis of alcohol dependency. With a score of 2 or more the patient is likely to have an alcohol dependency (see Table 8.3). Though this could easily be applied in clinical practice, research has shown the CAGE questionnaire is less sensitive with females and the elderly, it does not screen for binge drinking and should ideally be done face to face [16, 17].

WHO has created a screening tool called AUDIT (Alcohol Use Disorders Identification Test) [18] which has been designed to address gender, age, and cultural differences (see Table 8.4). A score of ≥8 is an indication for hazardous and potential harmful use of alcohol with a possible dependency. A lower cut off of 7 is used for all females and men older than 65 years. This screening tool is significantly more advantageous as it identifies binge drinking, focuses on recent alcohol use, and can be given as a paper questionnaire. However, one disadvantage is that it is specifically designed for primary care.

Table 8.3 CAGE questionnaire

1	Have you ever felt the need to Cut down on your drinking?
2	Have people Annoyed you by criticizing your drinking?
3	Have you ever felt bad or Guilty about your drinking?
4	Have you ever had an Eye-opener in the morning to steady your nerves or get rid of a hangover?

Table 8.4 Alcohol Use Disorders Identification Test (each question is 0–4 points depending on the frequency of alcohol use)

1	How often do you have a drink containing alcohol?
2	How many drinks containing alcohol do you have on a typical day when you are drinking?
3	How often do you have 6 or more drinks on one occasion?
4	How often during the past year have you found that you were not able to stop drinking once you had started?
5	How often during the past year have you failed to do what was normally expected of you because of drinking?
6	How often during the past year have you needed a first drink in the morning to get yourself going after a heavy drinking session?
7	How often during the past year have you had a feeling of guilt or remorse after drinking?
8	How often during the past year have you been unable to remember what happened the night before because you had been drinking?
9	Have you or has someone else been injured as a result of your drinking?
10	Has a relative or friend or a doctor been concerned about your drinking or suggested you cut down?

Table 8.5 Paddington Alcohol Test

1	Do you drink alcohol?
2	What is the most you drink in one day?
3	How often do you drink this much?
4	Do you feel your attendance is related to alcohol?
5	We would like to offer you advice about your alcohol consumption; would you be willing to see our alcohol nurse specialist?

Paddington Alcohol Test (PAT see Table 8.5) is designed to be used in the Emergency department setting if the patient presents any of the following [19]:

- Presentation: Fall/Collapse/Head injury/Assault/Accident /unwell/non-specific gastrointestinal/cardiac/psychiatric/repeat attender
- Clinical Signs of alcohol use
- Blood Alcohol Concentration >80 mgs/100 ml

In the PAT test if a patient drinks more than recommend units per day, week or are attending emergency department due to alcohol related problems, they are PAT test positive.

Presentation

Withdrawal symptoms occur when alcohol is withdrawn. There is generalised hyperexcitability of the central nervous system which is dominated by the autonomic system, leading to a risk of delirium tremors and seizures which can be life threatening. The possibility of seizures or tremors is most likely to occur within the first 48 h, whilst delirium usually occurs within the first 72 h of abstinence from alcohol. The acute withdrawal phase can last 1–3 weeks. Following the initial physical withdrawal a feeling of heightened anxiety, low mood/depression, lethargy, and insomnia are commonly present in individuals up to 3–6 weeks. There have been a small number of cases where it has lasted up to 2 years [20].

Repeated abstinence from alcohol can lead to more severe physical withdrawal symptoms leading to an increased risk of delirium tremors and seizures. This process is referred to as the sedative-hypnotic withdrawal or Kindling effect [21].

Signs and Symptoms of Withdrawal

- Agitation and anxiety
- Nausea and vomiting
- Diaphoresis
- Headache
- Tremor

- Seizures
- Hallucination (visual and hallucinations) but are orientated

Signs and Symptoms of Delirium

- Delirium
- Hypertension
- Raised temperature

Chronic alcohol abuse does affect the majority of organs in the body, such as the liver, causing alcoholic hepatitis which is the inflammation of hepatocytes. Inflammatory cytokines can induce cell apoptosis and necrosis. Recurrent inflammation of the liver can lead to liver fibrosis. Damage to the liver results in liver dysfunction and could affect clotting, carbohydrate metabolism, and cholesterol synthesis. Liver loses its ability to degrade waste products such as bilirubin and ammonia. A fatty liver results from increased production of aldehyde dehydrogenase which increases the fatty acid synthesis. The liver's inability to breakdown oestrogen results in **hyper oestrogenization causing signs such as** spider naevi, palmer erythema, Caput medusa and in males can lead to features such gynaecomastia and as testicular atrophy.

Signs and Symptoms of Chronic Alcohol Abuse

- Jaundice
- Ascites
- Spider naevi >5
- Palmar erythema
- Caput medusa
- Splenomegaly
- Hepatomegaly
- Bruising
- Xanthelasma
- Gynaecomastia
- Testicular atrophy
- Dupuytren's contractures
- Asterixis (liver flap)

Wernicke-Korsakoff syndrome/Alcoholic encephalopathy results from a severe acute thiamine (vitamin B1) deficiency, which is usually described as triad of the following:

- Confusion
- Ataxia
- Opthamoplegia (nystagmus, VI nerve palsy)

Wernicke psychosis:

- Amnesia (both anterograde and retrograde)
- Confabulations
- Withdrawal symptoms

Social Problems

Alcohol abuse is associated with individuals partaking in high-risk activities including unprotected sex and socially disruptive behaviors and criminal activities. Marital problems, including domestic violence are more commonly related to alcohol abuse and it is usually underestimated as women are reluctant to report the incidence. There is also a higher risk of child neglect, abuse, isolation and insecurity in families of alcohol abusers in addition to financial problems. Children of alcohol abusers are more likely to perform badly in school, eventually becoming drop-outs. The productivity and career declines in heavy drinkers as they have more sick-leave days than other employees.

Investigations

Acute intoxication (direct testing):

- Alcohol blood level
- Alcohol breath test
- Ethyl glucuronide (EtG)

    Chronic intoxication (indirect testing):

- Elevated gamma glutamyltransferase (GGT), aspartate aminotransferase (AST), alanine aminotransferase (ALT),
- Macrocytosis (elevated mean corpuscular volume (MCV))
- Elevated carbohydrate-deficient transferrin (CDT)

Acute Treatment/Management [22]

Alcohol withdrawal:

- Patient should be nursed in a well-lit room to help prevent disorientation.
- Keep external stimuli, especially noise, to a minimum
- Rehydration intravenous (IV) access for fluids e.g. crystalloids (to be cautious in patient with chronic liver disease as it can make ascites worse), and monitor fluid balance.

Table 8.6 Vitamin supplements

Indication	Regime	How frequently on 24 h	No. of days
Suspicion/known alcohol abuse	Pabrinex 2–3 pairs of ampules IV	TDS	5 days
	Thiamine 100 mg PO	BD	7 days
	Vitamin B tablets 2 tablets (compound strong) PO	TDS	7 days
	Vitamin C 50 mg PO	BD	7 days
Severe hypophosphataemia <0.6 mM	phosphate IV (polyfusor phosphate)	STAT	Until corrected

Key: IV intravenous, PO by mouth, TDS three times a day. BD twice a day, STAT straight away, mg milligrams

Table 8.7 Chordiazepoxide example of standard regime

Day	Morning (mg)	Midday (mg)	Afternoon (mg)	Night (mg)	Total (mg)
1	30	30	30	30	120
2	30	20	20	30	100
3	20	20	20	20	80
4	15	15	15	15	60
5	10	10	10	10	40
6	10			10	20
7				10	10

- Check electrolytes and correct any abnormality. Monitor blood sugar for hypoglycaemia and treat if required.
- Septic screen and relevant diagnostic tests to rule out other causes for symptoms.

Vitamin supplements:

Thiamine replacement e.g. Pabrinex is given to prevent treatment of Wernicke's encephalopathy (see Table 8.6).

Sedation: Long acting benzodiazepines such as chlordiazepoxide (Librium) and diazepam (Valium) are commonly used; if the patient has liver impairment Lorazepam is suitable. In extreme circumstances where the patient is severely agitated treat with regular doses of haloperidol 5mgs PO/IM (by mouth/intramuscularly).

It is important to undertake regular set of observations including ECG (Electrocardiography), blood pressure, pulse oximetry, respiratory rate and temperature. The initial dose of chlordiazepoxide should be determined by the severity of alcohol withdrawal.

The dose of chlordiazepoxide may be increased and it is advisable to add additional doses of this on an as-required basis. A variable dose of chordiazepoxide 5–20 mg QDS (four times a day) can be used for the initial 24 h, then a standard regime can be followed (see Table 8.7). It is important that the patient is monitored closely and on a regular basis.

Withdrawal seizures: Including epileptic forms of seizures, normally grand mal, which usually occurs in the first 24–48 h, are commonly seen in chronic alcoholics. Prophylactic treatment for seizures in patients with a past medical history of withdrawal seizures should be managed with diazepam 20 mg or Chlordiazepoxide, followed by a further 2 doses at 1 h intervals. If status epilepticus occurs it should be managed with IV Diazepam 2 mg/min. A maximum dose of 10–20 mg or IV Lorazepam 2 mg/min to a maximum 4–8 mg. Computed tomography (CT) of the head and lumbar puncture would be indicated in recurrent or prolonged seizures or status epilepticus to rule out any possible structural or infectious pathology.

Long-Term Management

Transtheoretical Approach developed by Prochaska is a technique used to aid clinicians in understanding the stages patients go through in reaching a state of alcohol abstinence. These stages consist of precontemplation, contemplation, preparation, action and maintenance (see Fig. 8.1). Within this cycle the individual can move backwards and forwards [23].

Support groups like Alcoholic Anonymous (AA) use a 12-step approach e.g. step 1: acknowledgment of having alcohol addiction. Help change the behavior of

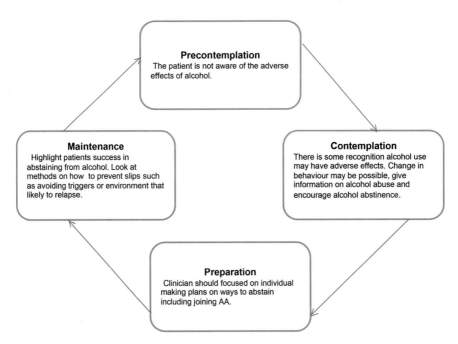

Fig. 8.1 Centre for substance abuse treatment in the United States, 4 stage process in alcohol abstinence

alcohol-dependent individuals by using positive reinforcement, creating a support network, and role models. Each individual upon joining is assigned a sponsor who is also a recovering alcoholic who is in a position to supervise and provide support to the new member. These groups provided long-term support for a recovering alcoholic. There are similar groups such as LifeRing Secular Recovery, Women for society. Involving individual's family in the rehabilitation process will help improve patients' chance of alcohol abstinence.

Summary

Alcohol abuse is a growing problem globally and is not a necessary obvious clinical illness to diagnosis, majority of people with alcohol dependency are usually in denial about alcohol use. As clinicians using simple screening tool can aid diagnosis of alcohol dependence. Each individual have different reasons for starting to drink heavily and have varying degrees of health problems attributed alcohol abuse. For example a patient with alcoholic hepatitis and malnutrition suffering from depression as result of loss of parents at a young age will require input from various professionals. A medical clinician will be required to manage patient's hepatitis A dietician input for malnutrition. A psychiatrist review would be appropriate to assess patient depression who may suggest counselling and antidepressants. The patient may require a social worker if there are problems with housing, unemployment, and family. It is important to use a holistic approach to manage patients with alcohol dependency as when they present to you will only be seeing the tip of the iceberg of the problem [24].

References

1. Klingemann H. Alcohol and its social consequences—the forgotten dimension. World Health Organisation Regional Office for Europe: Copenhagen; 2001.
2. Jellinek M. Management of substance abuse. Lexicon of alcohol and drug terms published by the World Health Organization. Geneva: WHO; 2013.
3. Agrawal A, Sartor C, et al. Evidence for an interaction between age at 1st drink and genetic influences on DSM-IV alcohol dependence symptoms. Alcohol Clin Exp Res. 2009;33(12): 2047–56.
4. Heron M. Deaths: leading causes for 2009. National Vital Statistics Reports, volume 61, no. 7. North Charleston: CreateSpace Independent Publishing Platform; 2012.
5. Heron P, Hoyert L, Murphy L, et al. Deaths: final data for 2006. National Vital Statistics Reports. Hyattsville. 2009;57(14):1–136.
6. Rehm M. Global burden of disease and injury and economic cost attribution to alcohol use and alcohol-use disorders. Lancet. 2009;373:2223–33.
7. A.D.A.M. Medical Encyclopedia. Alcoholism and alcohol abuse. Pubmed Health; 2011. http://www.ncbi.nlm.nih.gov/pubmedhealth/PMH0001940

8. Adapted from American Psychiatric Association (APA). Diagnostic and statistical manual of mental disorders. 4th ed. Washington, DC: APA; 2000.
9. International Centre for Alcohol Policies. 'Internal Drinking Guidelines'. International Centre for Alcohol Polices Analysis, Balance, Partnership; 2010. www.icap.org/table/Internationaldrinkingguidelines
10. Glipin N, Koob G. Neurobiology of alcohol dependence. Focus on motivational mechanism, volume 31, no. 3. Bethesda: National Institute on Alcohol Abuse and Alcoholism; 2008.
11. Villafuerte S, Heitzeg M, et al. Impulsiveness and insula activation during reward anticipation are associated with genetic variants in GABRA2 in a family sample enriched for alcoholism. Mol Psychiatry. 2012;17(5):511–9.
12. Niemlea O. Biomarkers in alcoholism. Clin Chim Acta. 2007;377(1–2):39–49.
13. Hicks B, Krueger R, et al. Family transmission and heritability of externalizing disorders: a twin-family study. Arch Gen Psychiatry. 2004;61(9):922–8.
14. Nery F, Stanley J, et al. Bipolar disorder comorbid with alcoholism: A (1)H magnetic resonance spectroscopy study. J Psychiatr Res. 2010;44(5):278–85.
15. Elia M. Alcohol, nutrition. Kumar and Clark clinical medicine. 6th ed. Philadelphia: Saunders Ltd.; 2005. p. 262–3.
16. Dhalla S, Kopec J. The CAGE questionnaire for alcohol misuse: a review of reliability and validity studies. Clin Invest Med. 2007;30(1):33–41.
17. Ewing J. Detecting alcoholism. The CAGE questionnaire. JAMA. 1984;252(14):1905–7.
18. Babor T, Higgins-Biddle J, et al. AUDIT, the alcohol use disorders identification test guidelines for primary care second edition. Geneva: World Health Organization, Department of mental health and substance dependence; 2001. http://www.talkingalcohol.com/files/pdfs/WHO_audit.pdf
19. Touqute R, Brown A. Paddington alcohol test 2011. Alcohol learning centre; 2011. www.alcohollearningcentre.org.uk/Topics/Browse/Hospitals/EmergencyMedicine/?parent=5168&child=5169
20. Heilig M, Egli M, et al. Acute withdrawal, protracted abstinence and negative affect in alcoholism: are they linked? Addict Biol. 2010;15(2):169–84.
21. Ramrakha P, Moore K. Acute alcohol withdrawal, neurological emergencies. Oxford handbook of acute medicine. 2nd ed. Oxford: Oxford University Press; 2004. p. 500–1.
22. Centre for Substance Abuse Treatment. Treatment improvement protocol (tip) series, no. 35. Rockville: Substance Abuse and Mental Health Services Administration (US); 1999. p. 99–3354.
23. Prochaska J, DiClemente C. The transtheoretical approach: crossing traditional boundaries of therapy, vol. 40. Homewood: Dow Jones-Irwin; 1984. p. 519–28.
24. Wood V. Guidelines for the management of alcohol issues in the acute general hospital setting. Doncanster and Bassetlaw Hospital NHS Foundation Trust; 2006. www.alcohollearningcentre.org.uk/_library/17__Doncaster_Guidelines_For_The_Management_Of_Patients_with_Alcohol_Misuse_In_The_Acute_General_Hospital_Setting.pdf

Chapter 9
Tobacco

Debasish Basu, Sukanya Mitra, and Nalini Vadivelu

Key Points

- Facts regarding tobacco dependence
- Tobacco cessation and guidelines
- Behavioral support and counseling
- Brief intervention
- Minimal intervention
- Intensive counseling
- Relapse prevention
- Modern use of technology
- Pharmacotherapy
- Nicotine replacement therapy (NRT)
- Non-nicotine pharmacotherapy
- Nicotine partial receptor agonists

Tobacco use, a human-created epidemic, kills one third of the people who use it. Across the world, smoking is the most common form of tobacco use. In several countries, both smoking as well as smokeless tobacco is used among all age groups.

D. Basu, M.D., Ph.D. (✉)
Department of Psychiatry, Postgraduate Institute of Medical Education and Research,
Drug De-Addiction and Treatment Center, Chandigarh, India
e-mail: db_sm2002@yahoo.com

S. Mitra, M.D., Ph.D.
Department of Anesthesia and Intensive Care, Government Medical College and Hospital,
Chandigarh, India
e-mail: drsmitra12@yahoo.com

N. Vadivelu, M.D.
Department of Anesthesiology, Yale University, New Haven, CT, USA
e-mail: nalinivg@gmail.com

© Springer Science+Business Media New York 2015
A.D. Kaye et al. (eds.), *Substance Abuse*, DOI 10.1007/978-1-4939-1951-2_9

In 2002, 50 % of the people killed from tobacco use were from developing countries. In the next two decades, unless urgent action is taken, the number might double and 70 % of deaths are likely be from developing countries. Tobacco-related deaths will be more than eight million in 2030 which is more than the total number of deaths from malaria, maternal and major childhood conditions, and tuberculosis combined [1].

In USA, despite less use than in the 1950s and 1960s, tobacco remains the leading cause of preventable and premature death, killing an estimated 443,000 people each year. Cigarette smoking costs the nation $96 billion in direct medical costs and $97 on in lost productivity annually [2].

There is an abundant and established scientific literature showing the myriads of harms caused by tobacco use on virtually every body organs and systems. The US Surgeon General Report on health effects of smoking clearly documents this [3]. The hazardous effects of involuntary smoking ("passive smoking," "environmental tobacco smoke") are also very well documented [4].

Facts Regarding Tobacco Dependence

Tobacco dependence is a chronic relapsing medical disorder like ulcerative colitis or diabetes, with a very high rate of relapse. Tobacco dependence is characterized by craving, tolerance, and withdrawal as well as continued use despite harm. Other features of dependence like salience, significant socio-occupational dysfunction, etc. are not prominent. The severity of tobacco dependence (physical) can be assessed by enquiring about the number of cigarette smoke/pouch of smokeless tobacco per day, and how early one needs to use tobacco after wake up. Fagerstrom Test for Nicotine dependence (FTND) [5] is a simple and useful six-item scale to assess the severity of smoking. This scale is also modified for use in smokeless tobacco [6].

Tobacco Cessation and Guidelines

Aggressive tobacco control has been associated with substantial benefit. It has been estimated that if adult consumption were to decrease by 50 % by the year 2020, approximately 180 million tobacco-related deaths could be avoided [7]. Cessation of tobacco use at any time in life has been found beneficial. Control of the tobacco epidemic and tobacco cessation needs multiple approaches including taxation, regulation, and prevention of tobacco use as well as the physician's offer for help. Studies from the USA have shown that the combined approach of tax increase, increase in smoke-free areas along with the physician's help for cessation have led to a reduction in tobacco use [8].

Many countries have produced national guidelines for tobacco, though many have not, even from those countries which are signatory to the WHO Framework Convention on Tobacco Control (FCTC) [9]. In a recent survey of 121 countries, all of which are signatories to FCTC, only 53 countries (44 %) had guidelines, ranging from 75 % among high-income countries to 11 % among low-income countries. Nearly all guidelines recommended brief advice (93 %), intensive specialist support (93 %) and medications (96 %), while 66 % recommended quitlines [10].

Behavioral Support and Counseling

Counseling is the simplest form of intervention for tobacco cessation. This helps in increasing the motivation to quit and enhances the ability to handle the urge to use tobacco.

Various counseling strategies ranging from brief intervention to more in-depth counseling have been developed for physicians and such resources applicable in developing countries are now available [11].

Brief Intervention

Brief Intervention has been found effective in the practice of smoking cessation. This intervention does not need much expertise and can be delivered by any health professional, preferably the treating doctor irrespective of the settings. As the name suggests, the intervention is brief and simple.

The important steps of intervention are:

(a) Advise all current tobacco users to quit
    All physicians should advise their clients to quit tobacco. Simple advice to quit by the physician has been shown to increase the quit rate (OR 1.3 95 % CI 1.1–1.6) compared to placebo or no intervention [12]. The advice should be strong, relevant, and personalized. It has been seen that specific advice linked to the patient's clinical condition works best.
(b) Educate about the addiction
    It is important to understand that addiction is a brain disease and having craving, withdrawal symptoms are part of this illness.
(c) Provide Brief Counseling
    Making sure that help is available in case of any difficulty increases person's confidence. This also consists of fixing a quit date, making environmental manipulations, tackling withdrawal symptoms, and handling relapses.

(d) Offering Medications
   Evidence is accumulating that providing medications improve the outcome
   even in the person who is not contemplating for complete quitting.
(e) Follow up:
   It is important to have a regular contact with the person.

Minimal Intervention is also Helpful

In case of tobacco intervention, a minimal intervention lasting less than 3 min
increases overall abstinence rates. At the same time more intensive intervention
(more time spent) is likely to provide increase in abstinence rates. Four or more sessions are associated with better outcome as per the meta-analysis [12].

Intensive Counseling

The psychiatrist or clinical psychologist is well placed to provide intensive and
multiple sessions counseling for tobacco cessation compared to the brief counseling that is offered by physicians. This involves comprehensively addressing
various psychosocial issues, multiple visits for a longer duration, and involvement of other mental health professionals, i.e., psychologist or psychiatric social
worker. Intensive interventions produce higher success rates than do less intensive interventions and there is a strong dose–response relation between counseling intensity and quitting success. In addition, the tobacco dependence
interventions offered by specialists represent an important treatment resource for
patients even if they have already received tobacco dependence treatment from
their own physician [12].

The major components of intensive counseling are increase in duration of each
session and multiple sessions that include detailed assessment and counseling
(Table 9.1).

Motivational Interviewing

The main component of motivational interviewing (MI) is tilting the balance
towards quitting tobacco. This can be achieved by discussing the issues with respect
to advantages/ disadvantages of using and stopping tobacco. Developing discrepancy, eliciting motivational statements i.e., why should you quit? Expressing

Table 9.1 Enhancing motivation: a practical approach [13]

Stage of motivation	What will help	What therapist can do
Pre-contemplation	Providing information about tobacco use and the benefit of quitting (Educational booklet)	Avoid confrontation
Person does not want to stop using tobacco	Helping the person to speak about tobacco use and also its impact to the people around including himself	Educate about tobacco and other substances (in case he is abusing)
		Focus on rapport building
		Encourage and appreciate any expression of the desire to quit tobacco (even in future)
Contemplation		
Acknowledges that there is a problem	Assessment of the client's feelings and thoughts about his/her tobacco use behavior	Facilitate (also provide further inputs) the analysis of pros and cons
Is considering costs and benefits of tobacco use		Help in realistic appraisal of the good and bad things about continued use of tobacco
Determination/preparation		
Making decision to quit tobacco and feels the need to do something to it	Choosing to give up tobacco and committing to specific goals	Reaffirm person's ability to make the change (self-efficacy)
Action		
Takes action to stop using tobacco	Achieving the goals by taking concrete steps	Help him/her lay a definite plan of action

empathy, avoiding argumentation, and supporting self-efficacy are important steps in MIs. This needs multiple sessions of counseling. The aim is to motivate the person for complete quitting or decrease the tobacco use. It is useful to provide educational booklet and keeping a future appointment for the tobacco users who are not currently willing to quit (Table 9.1) [13].

Relapse Prevention

Relapse is very common in tobacco use disorders. Hence relapse prevention is an integral part of psychosocial counseling. It is a state where an individual returns back to the previous pattern of tobacco use. There are multiple factors that can trigger relapses. Some of the common factors are mood (positive or negative), peer pressure, cues (internal and external), craving, etc. (Table 9.2) [12, 14].

Table 9.2 Components of relapse prevention and intensive psychosocial counseling [12, 14]

Techniques	Examples
Identify the high-risk relapse situations	Mood state, peer i.e., being around other tobacco users, drinking alcohol
Craving management	Identify the craving, using distraction, deep breathing, drinking glass of water, use chewing gum or cinnamon, urge surfing, etc. to handle
Increase in problem solving ability and coping skills	Learning cognitive strategies and behavioral interventions to reduce the cues
	Anticipate the negative or trigger situations and work accordingly
Life style changes	Time management to reduce stress, improve quality of life
	Keeping oneself busy
	Staying in nonsmoking locations
Cognitive	Increase self-efficacy i.e., I can do it
	Encourage self visualization as a nontobacco user
	Communicate care and concern
	Instill confidence and explain the addictive nature of tobacco use disorders
	Encourage to take credit and feel good for not using tobacco

Table 9.3 The comparison of efficacy of non-pharmacological interventions [8, 12, 15]

Type of intervention	Risk ratio (95 % CI) (Placebo or no treatment: 1)	No. of trials
Smoking cessation counseling		
Individual	1.39 (1.24–1.57)	22
Group	1.98 (1.60–2.46)	13
Telephone quit line	1.37 (1.26–1.50)	9
Physician intervention		
Brief advice to quit	1.66 (1.42–1.94)	17
Brief counseling	1.84 (1.60–2.13)	11

Comparison of efficacy of some of the non-pharmacological interventions is shown in Table 9.3 [12, 15].

Use of Modern Technology

Telephone-based intervention for tobacco cessation has been found to be effective. This can be a "quitline" or a proactive counseling process. Telephone-based counseling has the advantage of easy accessibility, assured privacy, and convenience.

Proactive counseling, i.e., the counselor should initiate the call as well as fix the timing, make a planning as well as reminding the client is more effective than providing only self help material [16] or a quitline [17]. The positive part of this approach is that proactive telephonic counseling increases the abstinence rates both in passive or in actively recruited smokers [18].

Internet-based counseling is emerging as a treatment option in developed countries. Most of the internet-based counseling also includes an offer NRT if required. Also, there is a component of telephone counseling incorporated in this. There is heterogeneity in different methods and studies in this area. To be effective, the counseling has to be tailored for the client and frequent automated contact is to be ensured [19].

Pharmacotherapy

Pharmacotherapy aims to reduce the intensity and quantity of tobacco use. The most effective drug is that which significantly reduces the craving, particularly in situations where tobacco is accessible. The literature regarding the efficacy of pharmacological agents has been mostly from cigarette smokers. There are a few emerging studies on smokeless tobacco particularly from *snus* users from Europe and USA. There is paucity of treatment studies on chewing tobacco. However, experience of tobacco cessation clinics in India in the last 10 years on over 30,000 patients (predominantly smokeless users) suggests that adding pharmacotherapy improves the likelihood of tobacco cessation [20].

Pharmacotherapy for nicotine dependence can be broadly divided into two classes: nicotine replacement therapy (NRT) and non-nicotine medications. These are detailed below.

Nicotine Replacement Therapy

NRT delivers nicotine which is safe and nontoxic. There are three predominant mechanisms by which NRT works, i.e., it reduces withdrawal symptoms, partially reduces the reinforcing effects of tobacco-delivered nicotine, and may provide some effects for which the patient previously relied on tobacco, such as sustaining desirable mood and attention states, making it easier to handle stressful or boring situations, and managing hunger and body weight [21]. NRT comes in five forms: gum, patch, lozenge, inhaler, and spray (Table 9.4) [22–24]. Nicotine patch has to be used once a day whereas others are to be used in different intervals.

Table 9.4 Nicotine replacement therapy used for tobacco cessation [8, 22–24]

Preparation	Dosage	Administration	Adverse effects	Advantage	Disadvantage
Nicotine gum					
2, 4 mg (Flavored with mint and that one similar to chewing tobacco)	<25 cig = 2 mg every 1–2 h	Chew and Park method (Chew until a tingling/peppery taste is obtained and park in the gap between gum and inner cheek. Continue till the sensation stops i.e., around 30 min)	Usually safe	Effective in controlling withdrawal symptoms	No significant anti-craving property while not using
	>25 cig = 4 mg every 1–2 h (maximum: 24 gums/day)	No drink 30 min before or after the gum	Mouth Irritation, Jaw fatigue, Dyspepsia hiccup	Concomitant use of tobacco does not cause any significant problem	
	Duration: 12 weeks	Gum can be kept more than 1 h in mouth		Can be initiated without complete stoppage of tobacco use	
	Week 1–6: 1 piece every 1–2 h				
	Week 7–9: 1 piece every 2–4 h				
	Week 10–12: 1 piece every 4–8 h				

Nicotine Patch

21, 14, 7 mg				
>10 cigarettes/day: 21 mg/day	Apply in clean, dry and non-hairy part of the body	Local skin reactions (erythema, pruritus, burning), headache, sleep problem (insomnia/dreams)	Easy, as once per day use	Slow release of Nicotine. User cannot alter nicotine level in case of breakthrough craving
<10 cigarettes/day: 14 mg/day	Press the patch over the skin and press down on the margin		Provides steady nicotine level	Can combine gum or any other NRT along with patch
Duration: 10–12 weeks	One patch per day			
Week 1–6: 21 mg/day or 14 mg/day	Do not stop using patch abruptly			
Week 7–9: 14 mg/day or 7 mg/day				
Week 10–12: 7 mg/day				

Nicotine Lozenge

2, 4 mg				
First cigarette <30 min after waking: 4 mg	Dissolve in mouth over 20–30 min	Hiccups or heart burn	Similar to gum	No role in craving
First cigarette >30 min after waking: 2 mg	Do not bite or chew		Can be used with people having dental problems	
Duration: 12 week	No drink 30 min before or after the gum			
Week 1–6: 1 lozenge every 1–2/h				
Week 7–9: 1 lozenge every 2–4 h				
Week 10–12: 1 lozenge every 4–8 h				
Maximum: 20 lozenges per day				

(continued)

Table 9.4 (continued)

Preparation	Dosage	Administration	Adverse effects	Advantage	Disadvantage
Nicotine Inhaler					
10-mg cartridge delivers 4 mg of nicotine per spray	Usual: 6–16 cartridges/day Initially: 1 cartridge every 1–2 h	Inhaled through the mouth	Mouth and throat irritation	Delivers nicotine rapidly	Frequent puffing
	Duration: 12–24 weeks	Patient should inhale into back of throat or puff in short breaths		Mimics the "hand to mouth" ritual of a cigarette user. Controls the nicotine delivery	Device is visible while using
	Taper in last 6–12 weeks	Not inhaled into the lungs (like a cigarette) but puffed as if lighting a pipe			
		Open cartridge retains potency for 24 h			
		No food or beverages 5 min before or during use			
Nicotine Nasal spray	1 spray (1 mg nicotine) in each nostril	Nasal administration	Nasal irritation	Very fast delivery of nicotine	Local irritation to nasal mucosa
	Initial treatment is 1–2 doses/h, as needed			Most rapid delivery of nicotine	
	Typical dosing is 8–40 doses/day				
	Duration: 12–24 weeks				

Table 9.5 Shows comparison of the efficacy of different pharmacological therapies

Pharmacotherapy	Risk ratio (95 % CI) (Placebo or no treatment: 1)	No. of trials
Any NRT	1.60 (1.53–1.68)	150
Nicotine gum	1.43 (1.33–1.53)	53
Nicotine Patch	1.66 (1.53–1.81)	41
Nicotine Spray	2.02 (1.49–3.73)	4
Nicotine Inhaler	1.90 (1.36–2.67)	4
Nicotine Lozenge	2.00 (1.63–2.45)	6
Bupropion Sustained Release	1.69 (1.53–1.85)	36
Varenicline	2.27 (2.02–2.55)	14
Nortriptyline	2.03 (1.48–2.78)	6
Clonidine	1.63 (1.22–2.18)	6

Adapted from [8, 12, 15]

Effectiveness of NRT

The most recent meta-analysis from the Cochrane Collaboration collating data from 150 RCT studies with over 50,000 participants observed that NRT significantly increases the likelihood of tobacco abstinence compared with placebo (risk ratio [RR] 1.60; 95 % CI, 1.53–1.68). The overall risk of long-term smoking abstinence with different forms of NRT varies from 1.49 for gum to 2.02 for nasal spray (details in Table 9.5) [25]. NRT, when used in the proper dose and duration, increases the long-term abstinence by 50–70 % irrespective of treatment setting or type of counseling or type of behavior therapy. The authors further concluded that, "The effectiveness of NRT appears to be largely independent of the intensity of additional support provided to the individual. Provision of more intense levels of support, although beneficial in facilitating the likelihood of quitting, is not essential to the success of NRT" [25].

Initiation of NRT

The initial dose and type of NRT depends on the number of cigarettes and how early a person takes first smoke as soon as he wakes up in the morning. There are two methods of advising to quit. One is "cold turkey" and the other is gradual reduction over a 2 weeks period. NRT is usually initiated 2 weeks prior to target quit date [26].

Smoking Reduction

Initiating nicotine patch during the phase of smoking reduction in preparation for a target quit date, has been shown to be effective and may improve self-efficacy for quitting. A meta-analysis including seven RCTs (2,767 patients) reported that NRT and behavioral counseling is likely to double long-term quit rate compared to placebo [24, 27].

Dose and Duration of NRT

Smokers using more than 25 cigarettes/day or with a Fagerstrom score for nicotine dependence (FTND) [5] (scale to measure the severity of nicotine addiction) of ≥6 are generally defined as highly dependent. This group needs a higher initial dose of NRT. Nicotine gum of 4 mg is significantly effective in this group. However, a higher nicotine dose patch has not been found to be significantly effective compared to lower dose of patch [15].

Once started, NRT should be used for a minimum of 8–12 weeks and then as long as necessary. Once the tobacco cessation is maintained, the NRT can be tapered as mentioned in Table 9.4 [22–24].

NRT can also be used with the goal of reduction of smoking rather than complete quitting as mentioned above (previous section). In this scenario, the immediate goal can be to reduce cigarette consumption by at least 50 %, and the quitting goal should be reviewed after 3 months [28].

Most of the guidelines recommend use of NRT for 12 weeks or less. The recent studies have looked at the long-term continuation of NRT and the effect on cessation. An RCT comparing 6 months versus 8 weeks showed that longer treatment with nicotine patch was superior [29].

Adverse Effects of NRT

NRT use is usually well tolerated. The three most commonly reported adverse effects of NRT in observational studies were headache, nausea and/or vomiting, and other gastrointestinal symptoms. Orally administered NRT was associated with mouth and throat soreness; mouth ulcers; hiccoughs and coughing. Pooled evidence specific to the NRT patch found an increase in skin irritation (OR 2.80, 95 % CO, 2.28–3.24). Coughing has been observed to be more likely with nicotine nasal spray and nicotine inhaler (OR = 2.89; 95 % CI, 1.92–4.43) [30]. There was no statistically significant increase in anxiety or depressive symptoms associated with NRT use, making it a safer option in comorbid psychiatric disorders [30].

Combination of NRTs

The delivery of NRT varies as per the formulation. The standard practice is to prescribe a single NRT. The combination of long acting nicotine patch (slow release, one in 24 h) along with a short acting formulation (gum, spray, or inhaler) has been found to be effective. The short acting NRTs help in controlling urges and are thereby likely to prevent breakthrough tobacco use in the background of nicotine steady state maintained by long acting NRT. A meta-analysis of NRT combinations compared with either NRT monotherapy or no NRT reported an advantage for combination NRT (RR 1.35; 95 % CI, 1.11–1.63) [15, 24]. Combination of nicotine lozenges+patch and bupropion+lozenge was found to be more effective than monotherapy. This beneficial effect is seen both in research and as well as in primary medical settings [31, 32].

Non-nicotine Pharmacotherapy

Antidepressants

Nicotine withdrawal produces a depression-like state and can precipitate a depressive syndrome. Nicotine may have antidepressant effects that maintain smoking, and antidepressants may substitute for this effect. A number of antidepressants including bupropion, doxepin, fluoxetine, imipramine, moclobemide, nortriptyline, paroxetine, sertraline, tryptophan, and venlafaxine have been studied. The best evidence has emerged for two antidepressants: bupropion and nortryptiline [33].

Bupropion

Bupropion is an atypical antidepressant that has been associated with attenuation of the withdrawal symptoms and decreases the rewarding effect associated with smoking. This is achieved through antagonizing the nicotine receptor sites and inhibiting the reuptake of dopamine and norepinephrine [34]. Sustained release bupropion is commonly used for tobacco cessation.

Effectiveness

Systematic reviews and meta-analyses collating data from 49 RCT studies recommend bupropion as being efficacious for smoking. When used as the sole pharmacotherapy in 36 RCTs ($n=11,140$), bupropion significantly increased long-term (≥ 6 months) smoking abstinence (RR=1.69; 95 % CI, 1.53–1.85). But there is insufficient evidence regarding addition of bupropion with standard dose or high-dose NRT with regard to increase in benefit [33, 35].

Bupropion is equally effective for tobacco cessation in patients who are depressed or predisposed to depression as well as those who are not depressed [36]. In an RCT of 199 smokers with either current or past depression, bupropion or placebo was added to nicotine patch and group cognitive behavioral therapy. Abstinence was associated with increased depressive symptoms, regardless of bupropion treatment. Bupropion appeared to have no effect for improving smoking abstinence when added to nicotine patch and behavioral support for smokers with current depressive symptoms or past depression [37].

Dose and Adverse Effects

The recommended dose is 150 mg at initiation, increased to 150 mg twice a day in a week's time. Bupropion is to be initiated a week to 10 days before the planned quit date.

Although an effective medication, its wide acceptance and use have been limited by side effects that include anxiety, headache, insomnia, and irritability and a rare propensity to induce seizures (contraindicated in prior history of seizure), estimated to occur in 1 out of 1,000 patients. RCTs do not report any severe side effects except risk of seizure. Pharmacovigilance reports from post-marketing surveillance of 698,000 people who have received bupropion for smoking cessation reported a total of 475 serious adverse events (SARs), including 21 deaths. Seizures, angioedema, and serum sickness-like reactions were the most frequently reported SARs. The median time to onset of the adverse effects was within 2 weeks of treatment initiation indicating that prescribers should monitor patients exposed to bupropion more carefully during the first 2 weeks of treatment [38].

Earlier studies had reported unexpected increase in blood pressure as an adverse effect of bupropion. A recent RCT of 4 weeks of placebo or bupropion (in doses of 150, 300, or 400 mg/day) suggests that blood pressure elevations are not common [39].

Nortriptyline

Nortriptyline, a tricyclic antidepressant has been used for smoking cessation. The data from four RCTs suggest results similar to that of bupropion (four trials, OR 2.34, 95 % CI 1.61–3.41) i.e., doubling the chance of quitting. Although a tricyclic, nortriptyline was not associated with any significant side effects in these four small trials.

Nortriptyline is economical and its once-a-day dosing makes it a potentially useful drug that is probably underutilized. Its use has been limited by common side effects, including drowsiness, dry mouth, dizziness, constipation, and cardiac dysrrhythmias in susceptible patients. Typically, nortriptyline is begun 10–28 days in advance of the anticipated quit date and titrated from a starting dose of 10–25 mg a day to 75–100 mg daily.

Other Antidepressants

There were six trials of selective serotonin reuptake inhibitors; four of fluoxetine, one of sertraline, one of paroxetine, one of venlafaxine and one trial of the MAOI. None of these detected significant long-term benefits for tobacco cessation.

Nicotine Partial Receptor Agonists

The use of nicotine partial receptor agonists has been a recent addition for the treatment of smoking cessation. Nicotinic receptors, densely present in the ventral tegmental area of the midbrain, play a vital role in the activation of the reward system and dopamine release. This reinforces the process of nicotine addiction. Agonist drugs help people to stop smoking both by maintaining moderate levels of dopamine to counteract withdrawal symptoms (acting as an agonist) and reducing smoking satisfaction (acting as an antagonist). There are three agents in this group: varenicline, cytisine, and dianicline. Varenicline has been in use for the last 6 years but is expensive. Cytisine is cheaper and is being used in countries like Bulgaria and Poland for the last 40 years [40].

Varenicline

Effectiveness

Systematic reviews and meta-analyses collating data from 14 RCT studies involving 6,166 people recommend that varenicline is effective for smoking [41]. Continuous or sustained abstinence at 6 months or longer for varenicline at standard dosage versus placebo showed an RR of 2.27 (95 % CI 2.02–2.55). A low or variable dose of varenicline was twice more effective than placebo.

Compared to bupropion, abstinence rate at the end of 1 year from varenicline was 1.52 (95 % CI 1.22–1.88, three RCT, 1,622 people). Varenicline was found to be slightly superior to NRT in two trials RR of 1.13 (95 % CI 0.94–1.35; two trials, 778 people).

Recent studies also report the robust effectiveness of varenicline in smokers with smoking-related disorders, i.e., chronic obstructive pulmonary disease (COPD) and cardiovascular disease (CVD). The study involving 714 smokers with stable CVD [42], the abstinence rates with varenicline was six times higher at the end of 12 weeks and continuous abstinence rate for end of year was three times more. In a similar multicentric study on COPD patients [43], the abstinence rate was eight times higher for the initial part (9–12 weeks) and four times greater at a later period (9–52 weeks) compared to placebo. The effectiveness of varenicline beyond 12 weeks and role in subsequent relapse prevention is not clear.

Dose and Adverse effects

Varenicline is usually started a week before the quit date. It is started at 0.5 mg daily for 3 days and then increased to twice daily for 4 days. The medication is then increased to its recommended dose of 1 mg, twice daily. The usual duration is for

3 months and can be continued for the subsequent 3 months if required (if there is partial improvement).

The most common adverse effect reported is nausea. This decreases with the slow titration of the medication. There are two important recent warnings, i.e., cardiac events and behavioral change with varenicline. A meta-analysis reported a small but statistically significant increase in serious cardiovascular adverse events, i.e., ischemia, arrhythmia, congestive heart failure, sudden death or cardiovascular-related death in subjects receiving varenicline [44] (varenicline 1.06 % vs. placebo 0.82 %; OR 1.72; 95 % CI, 1.09–2.71) In view of low absolute increase in risk for serious cardiovascular events, compared with the large benefit for smoking cessation, current opinion appears to suggest varenicline may be used in stable CVD [24].

An increased risk of behavioral change, agitation, depressed mood, and suicidal ideation has been reported with Varenicline. However, a recent meta-analysis (11 clinical trials with over 10,000 participants, 7,000 of whom received varenicline), post-marketing surveillance (80,660 smokers attempting to quit, 10,973 with varenicline) and a latest re-analysis of 17 RCTs of more than 8,027 smokers (1,004 with and 7,023 without psychiatric disorders) did not show any increased psychiatric or behavioral change. The mood changes are comparable to that of NRT [41, 45–47].

Still, in view of possible links of varenicline to serious side effects, i.e., depressed mood, agitation, and suicide, patients need to be in regular observation for mood status.

There is a need for a long-term study (>12 weeks) with regard to its efficacy in smoking and independent community-based study for the associated side effects [41].

Cytisine

Cytisine, a partial agonist, is similar to varenicline in its mechanism. This drug has been in use for quite some time in countries like Bulgaria and Poland. There are at least ten studies including three placebo-controlled reporting its effectiveness [48]. A recent 12 weeks RCT compared cytisine to placebo. The rate of sustained 12-month as well as 7-day point prevalence of abstinence at the 12-month follow-up was significantly high in the cytisine group compared to placebo. The primary outcome, abstinence for 12 months after treatment ended, was 8.4 % in cytisine compared to 2.4 % in placebo group. Cytisine was prescribed for 25 days i.e., six 1.5-mg tablets per day (one tablet every 2 h) for the first 3 days, five tablets per day for 9 days (days 4 through 12), four tablets per day for 4 days (days 13 through 16), three tablets per day for 4 days (days 17 through 20), and two tablets per day for the final 5 days (days 21 through 25) [40]. Cytisine, a low-cost drug, may increase the abstinence rate but there is a need for further studies to establish its effectiveness and safety [41].

Clonidine

Clonidine is an alpha 2 adrenergic agonist and primarily used for hypertension. It suppresses the withdrawal symptoms of nicotine and probably has anti-craving property also, although the exact mechanism is not known. Apart from oral use, the transdermal form has also been tried for tobacco cessation. The overall effectiveness from six RCTs was OR: 1.89 (95 % CI 1.30–2.74) [49]. In spite of the beneficial effect close to other agents, its use is restricted because of side effects especially sedation, fatigue, orthostatic hypotension, dizziness, and dry mouth [50].

Table 9.5 shows comparison of the efficacy of different pharmacological therapies.

Conclusion

Tobacco dependence is widespread, and remains one of the most important causes of preventable morbidity and mortality. The guidelines emphasize definite though modest benefits both of non-pharmacological and pharmacological measures. Clinicians should be aware of the necessity of early detection, should be conversant with simple non-pharmacological measures, and should be able to advise NRT and prescribe medications as and when needed. Even modest benefits can accrue in large beneficial effects on a larger scale.

References

1. Murthy P, Mohan B, Hiremath S. Helping people quit tobacco: a manual for doctors and dentists. New Delhi: WHO, Regional Office South East Asia; 2010.
2. U.S. Department of Health and Human Services. Preventing tobacco use among youth and young adults: a report of the Surgeon General. Atlanta: U.S. Department of Health and Human Services, Centers for Disease Control and Prevention, National Center for Chronic Disease Prevention and Health Promotion, Office on Smoking and Health; 2012.
3. U.S. Department of Health and Human Services. How tobacco smoke causes disease: the biology and behavioral basis for smoking-attributable disease: a report of the Surgeon General. Atlanta: U.S. Department of Health and Human Services, Centers for Disease Control and Prevention, National Center for Chronic Disease Prevention and Health Promotion, Office on Smoking and Health; 2010.
4. U.S. Department of Health and Human Services. The health consequences of involuntary exposure to tobacco smoke: a report of the Surgeon General—executive summary. Atlanta: U.S. Department of Health and Human Services, Centers for Disease Control and Prevention, Coordinating Center for Health Promotion, National Center for Chronic Disease Prevention and Health Promotion, Office on Smoking and Health; 2006.
5. Heatherton TF, Kozlowski LT, Frecker RC, Fagerstrom KO. The Fagerstrom Test for Nicotine Dependence: a revision of the Fagerstrom Tolerance Questionnaire. Br J Addict. 1991;86(9): 1119–27.

6. Shrivastava RK. Training manual for doctors: National Tobacco Control Programme. New Delhi: DGHS, Ministry of Health and Family Welfare; 2011.
7. Mackay J, Eriksen M. The tobacco atlas. Geneva: World Health Organization; 2002.
8. Rigotti NA. Strategies to help a smoker who is struggling to quit. JAMA. 2012;308(15): 1573–80.
9. World Health Organization. WHO Framework Convention on Tobacco Control. Geneva: World Health Organization; 2003.
10. Pine-Abata H, McNeill A, Raw M, Bitton A, Rigotti N, Murray R. A survey of tobacco dependence treatment guidelines in 121 countries. Addiction. 2013;108:1470–5.
11. Rajkumar S, Kaur J, Murthy P, Deshpande S, Shah N, Munish VG. Tobacco dependence treatment guidelines. New Delhi: DGHS. Ministry of Health and Family welfare, Government of India; 2011.
12. Fiore M, Jaen C, Baker T, Bailey WC, Benowitz NL, Curry SJ. Treating tobacco use and dependence: 2008 update. Rockville: US Department of Health and Human Services; 2008.
13. Miller WR, Rollnick S. Motivational interviewing: preparing people to change addictive behaviours. 2nd ed. New York: Guildford; 2002.
14. Shiffman S, Kassel J, Gwaltney C, McChargue D. Relapse prevention for smoking. New York: Guilford; 2005.
15. Himelhoch S, Daumit G. To whom do psychiatrists offer smoking-cessation counseling? Am J Psychiatry. 2003;160(12):2228–30.
16. Boyle RG, Enstad C, Asche SE, et al. A randomized controlled trial of Telephone Counseling with smokeless tobacco users: the ChewFree Minnesota study. Nicotine Tob Res. 2008;10(9): 1433–40.
17. Murthy P, Subodh BN. Current developments in behavioral interventions for tobacco cessation. Curr Opin Psychiatry. 2010;23(2):151–6.
18. Tzelepis F, Paul CL, Walsh RA, McElduff P, Knight J. Proactive telephone counseling for smoking cessation: meta-analyses by recruitment channel and methodological quality. J Natl Cancer Inst. 2011;103(12):922–41.
19. Civljak M, Sheikh A, Stead LF, Car J. Internet-based interventions for smoking cessation. Cochrane Database Syst Rev. 2010;(9):CD007078.
20. Varghese C, Kaur J, Desai NG, et al. Initiating tobacco cessation services in India: challenges and opportunities. WHO South-East Asia J Public Health. 2012;1(2):159–68.
21. Molyneux A. Nicotine replacement therapy. BMJ. 2004;328(7437):454–6.
22. Crane R. The most addictive drug, the most deadly substance: smoking cessation tactics for the busy clinician. Prim Care. 2007;34(1):117–35.
23. Grief SN. Nicotine dependence: health consequences, smoking cessation therapies, and pharmacotherapy. Prim Care. 2011;38(1):23–39, v.
24. Hays JT, McFadden DD, Ebbert JO. Pharmacologic agents for tobacco dependence treatment: 2011 update. Curr Atheroscler Rep. 2012;14(1):85–92.
25. Stead LF, Perera R, Bullen C, Mant D, Hartmann-Boyce J, Cahill K, Lancaster T. Nicotine replacement therapy for smoking cessation. Cochrane Database Syst Rev. 2012:(11):CD000146. doi:10.1002/14651858.CD000146.pub4.
26. Bailey AM, Macaulay T. Pharmacologic approaches to smoking cessation. Orthopedics. 2012; 35(6):505–11.
27. Moore D, Aveyard P, Connock M, Wang D, Fry-Smith A, Barton P. Effectiveness and safety of nicotine replacement therapy assisted reduction to stop smoking: systematic review and meta-analysis. BMJ. 2009;338:b1024.
28. Lingford-Hughes AR, Welch S, Peters L, Nutt DJ. BAP updated guidelines: evidence-based guidelines for the pharmacological management of substance abuse, harmful use, addiction and comorbidity: recommendations from BAP. J Psychopharmacol. 2012;26(7):899–952.
29. Schnoll RA, Patterson F, Wileyto EP, et al. Effectiveness of extended-duration transdermal nicotine therapy: a randomized trial. Ann Intern Med. 2010;152(3):144–51.

30. Mills EJ, Wu P, Lockhart I, Wilson K, Ebbert JO. Adverse events associated with nicotine replacement therapy (NRT) for smoking cessation. A systematic review and meta-analysis of one hundred and twenty studies involving 177,390 individuals. Tob Induc Dis. 2010;8:8.
31. Smith SS, McCarthy DE, Japuntich SJ, et al. Comparative effectiveness of 5 smoking cessation pharmacotherapies in primary care clinics. Arch Intern Med. 2009;169(22):2148–55.
32. Piper ME, Smith SS, Schlam TR, et al. A randomized placebo-controlled clinical trial of 5 smoking cessation pharmacotherapies. Arch Gen Psychiatry. 2009;66(11):1253–62.
33. Hughes JR, Stead LF, Lancaster T. Antidepressants for smoking cessation. Cochrane Database Syst Rev. 2007;(1):CD000031.
34. Mooney ME, Sofuoglu M. Bupropion for the treatment of nicotine withdrawal and craving. Expert Rev Neurother. 2006;6(7):965–81.
35. Mills EJ, Wu P, Lockhart I, Thorlund K, Puhan M, Ebbert JO. Comparisons of high-dose and combination nicotine replacement therapy, varenicline, and bupropion for smoking cessation: a systematic review and multiple treatment meta-analysis. Ann Med. 2012;44(6):588–97.
36. Schnoll RA, Martinez E, Tatum KL, et al. A bupropion smoking cessation clinical trial for cancer patients. Cancer Causes Control. 2010;21(6):811–20.
37. Evins AE, Culhane MA, Alpert JE, et al. A controlled trial of bupropion added to nicotine patch and behavioral therapy for smoking cessation in adults with unipolar depressive disorders. J Clin Psychopharmacol. 2008;28(6):660–6.
38. Beyens MN, Guy C, Mounier G, Laporte S, Ollagnier M. Serious adverse reactions of bupropion for smoking cessation: analysis of the French Pharmacovigilance Database from 2001 to 2004. Drug Saf. 2008;31(11):1017–26.
39. Thase ME, Haight BR, Johnson MC, et al. A randomized, double-blind, placebo-controlled study of the effect of sustained-release bupropion on blood pressure in individuals with mild untreated hypertension. J Clin Psychopharmacol. 2008;28(3):302–7.
40. West R, Zatonski W, Cedzynska M, et al. Placebo-controlled trial of cytisine for smoking cessation. N Engl J Med. 2011;365(13):1193–200.
41. Cahill K, Stead LF, Lancaster T. Nicotine receptor partial agonists for smoking cessation. Cochrane Database Syst Rev. 2012;(4):CD006103. doi:10.1002/14651858.CD006103.pub6.
42. Rigotti NA, Pipe AL, Benowitz NL, Arteaga C, Garza D, Tonstad S. Efficacy and safety of varenicline for smoking cessation in patients with cardiovascular disease: a randomized trial. Circulation. 2010;121(2):221–9.
43. Tashkin DP, Rennard S, Hays JT, Ma W, Lawrence D, Lee TC. Effects of varenicline on smoking cessation in patients with mild to moderate COPD: a randomized controlled trial. Chest. 2011;139(3):591–9.
44. Singh S, Loke YK, Spangler JG, Furberg CD. Risk of serious adverse cardiovascular events associated with varenicline: a systematic review and meta-analysis. CMAJ. 2011;183(12):1359–66.
45. Gunnell D, Irvine D, Wise L, Davies C, Martin RM. Varenicline and suicidal behaviour: a cohort study based on data from the General Practice Research Database. BMJ. 2009;339:b3805.
46. Tonstad S, Davies S, Flammer M, Russ C, Hughes J. Psychiatric adverse events in randomized, double-blind, placebo-controlled clinical trials of varenicline: a pooled analysis. Drug Saf. 2010;33(4):289–301.
47. Gibbons RD, Mann JJ. Varenicline, smoking cessation, and neuropsychiatric adverse events. Am J Psychiatry. 2013. doi:10.1176/appi.ajp.2013.12121599.
48. Etter JF. Cytisine for smoking cessation: a literature review and a meta-analysis. Arch Intern Med. 2006;166(15):1553–9.
49. Gourlay SG, Stead LF, Benowitz NL. Clonidine for smoking cessation. Cochrane Database Syst Rev. 2004;(3):CD000058.
50. Herman AI, Sofuoglu M. Comparison of available treatments for tobacco addiction. Curr Psychiatry Rep. 2010;12(5):433–40.

Chapter 10
The Abuse of Agents Used to Induce or Maintain General Anesthesia: Intravenous Hypnotics and the Halogenated Hydrocarbons

Ethan O. Bryson

Key Points

- Intravenous hypnotic agents
- Halogenated hydrocarbons

Introduction

The agents used to induce or maintain general anesthesia have been shown time and time again, in multiple studies involving both humans and animals, to carry considerable abuse liability. These drugs are capable of producing pleasurable sensations and altering consciousness in a manner that some find pleasing. They have a demonstrated ability to reinforce drug-taking behaviors, can produce tolerance, and many are associated with the development of a withdrawal syndrome, yet these drugs are not very well controlled. Many are not scheduled by the DEA and those that are been given the least restrictive schedule IV status. These drugs are almost universally available in unsecured hospital supply rooms or anesthesia carts and few facilities keep specific usage records. As with most drugs of this type, abuse remains most evident in the healthcare professionals with access and knowledge, though there may be a trend towards abuse by laypersons as more people outside the medical professions become aware of these drugs. Because of their narrow therapeutic index, reports of misuse almost always come to light after the death of the individual.

E.O. Bryson, M.D. (✉)
Department of Anesthesiology and Psychiatry, Icahn School of Medicine
at Mount Sinai, New York, NY, USA
e-mail: ethan.bryson@mountsinai.org

© Springer Science+Business Media New York 2015
A.D. Kaye et al. (eds.), *Substance Abuse*, DOI 10.1007/978-1-4939-1951-2_10

Intravenous Hypnotic Agents

Propofol

Propofol (2,6-diisopropylphenol, Figs. 10.1 and 10.2) is an intravenous anesthetic agent first synthesized in 1977 which has been in clinical use in human and veterinary medicine since 1986 [1, 2]. Propofol is widely used for the rapid induction of general anesthesia and for moderate to deep sedation for painful or uncomfortable procedures. Though not considered to have enough abuse liability to be scheduled as a controlled substance by the US Drug Enforcement Agency, recreational use was reported shortly after the drug was brought to market. Initial reports of nonmedical use primarily involved medical professionals with access and an understanding of propofol's effects, but recent reports suggest that recreational use of propofol has expanded outside the healthcare setting [3]. Despite a significant potential for abuse, propofol remains unclassified and the drug is freely available in the hospital setting.

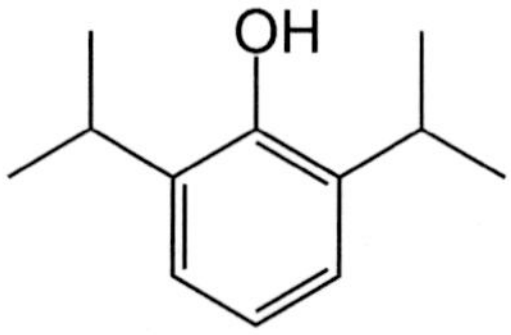

Fig. 10.1 Chemical structure of Propofol (2,6-diisopropylphenol). With permission from *Frost EAM, Bryson EO. Propofol Abuse. In: Bryson EO, Frost EAM Editors, Perioperative Addiction. Springer Science and Business Media, NY: New York, 2011 © Springer 2011* [10]

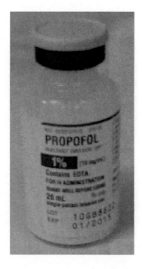

Fig. 10.2 Propofol, an oil at room temperature, is insoluble in water and packaged as a lipid emulsion for injection. Because of its milky white coloring, propofol has been called "milk of amnesia" and the practice of propofol abuse "chasing the white rabbit"

Properties

Propofol is a central nervous system (CNS) depressant that works by activating the chloride current at the gamma-aminobutyric acid (GABA) type A receptor, inhibiting the function of the N-methyl-D-aspartate (NMDA) receptor and modulating calcium influx through slow calcium channel ions [4, 5]. It is an oil at room temperature, insoluble in water, and packaged as a lipid emulsion capable of supporting bacterial growth. Because of this some formulations contain disodium edentate or sodium metabisulphate, which functions as an antifungal or antibiotic. It is a short-acting agent with little or no residual effects, which begins to work rapidly after administration. Patients begin to lose consciousness within one circulation time. The drug causes dose-dependent hypotension and cardiorespiratory depression, as well as some degree of bradycardia. Depending on the dose, consciousness returns after 5–10 min as the drug redistributes from the active site in the CNS into the bodies lipid depots. Patients have reported a broad spectrum of feelings after propofol administration ranging from a general feeling of well-being to elation, euphoria, and sexual disinhibition [6].

Abuse Potential

As with most drugs that have abuse potential, propofol enhances the levels of dopamine in the areas of the brain associated with reward, reinforcing the behaviors associated with obtaining and injecting the drug [7]. Propofol causes dopamine release and inhibits reuptake in presynaptic nerve terminals in the reward circuitry of the mesocorticolimbic system [8]. As well, propofol has been shown to induce a significant expression of the transcription factor Delta FosB [9]. Similar expression of this transcription factor is seen with other drugs of abuse, such as nicotine and alcohol, suggesting that modulation of gene expression of Delta FosB in the nucleus accumbens (NAc) may also be associated with the development of propofol addiction [10]. Propofol-induced upregulation of Delta FosB accumulates in the NAc and this protein may persist for weeks before it degrades.

Propofol, in aerosolized form, is present in detectable amounts in the healthcare environment [11]. Since even nanomolar amounts of propofol can stimulate glutamate transmission to dopamine neurons, chronic environmental exposure in healthcare professionals who administer the drug or care for patients receiving it may increase the risk for abuse and/or addiction [12, 13].

Propofol has been shown to be rewarding even in individuals without a history of drug abuse [14]. When healthy volunteers were administered either propofol or intralipid in a discrete-trials choice procedure subjects either chose propofol because they liked the subjective effects of the drug such as feeling "spaced out" or "high" or chose the intralipid because they disliked the "dizziness" and "confusion" associated with propofol administration.

The biochemical and pharmacokinetic mechanisms of action of propofol contributes to its abuse potential and the physical and psychological effects make it attractive as a recreational drug [15, 16]. Current evidence supports the possibility of tolerance to and also withdrawal from propofol, further enhancing its abuse potential [17, 18].

Abuse Prevalence

The first case of propofol abuse was published in 1992 and involved an anesthesiologist [19]. It makes sense that almost all early cases of propofol abuse involved medical personnel as these people had both access to the drug and an understanding of the drug's effects. An editorial accompanying this case report suggested that propofol, if not scheduled, should be stored in an access-restricted system [20]. Despite this early concern, many hospitals still place no more restriction on access to propofol than to other uncontrolled medications commonly found in the anesthesia carts. Free access is especially prevalent if office based anesthetic practices. Many reports of propofol abuse have surfaced in the 20 years since this first case was published. Most involve medical personnel but increasingly reports of propofol abuse have been discovered in nonmedical personnel. Because of the narrow therapeutic index of the drug and the unfortunate reality that self-administration almost always occurs without the benefit of qualified medical personnel standing by to rescue after an unintended overdose, death by propofol has become more and more common [21–23]. In most cases death is not directly due to propofol itself but rather from respiratory failure after rapid injection.

Historically, access to this drug and familiarity with its properties and administration determined who was more likely to abuse and become addicted to propofol. Ten years after the first report of propofol abuse the first reported case of propofol dependency in a layperson reported [24]. This individual had received propofol as treatment for tension headaches administered by an anesthesiologist, presumably enjoyed the experience, subsequently identified propofol as the drug and was able to obtain more for personal use from various veterinarians. Since it is not a controlled drug, persons motivated to obtain and use propofol can do so quite easily, as one case report of a layperson obtaining the drug via Internet sales and subsequently self-administering it demonstrates [25].

Propofol abuse appears to be on the rise. The decade from 1997 to 2007 experienced a fivefold surge in the incidence of propofol abuse in academic anesthesiology programs [26]. During this period, one or more incidents of propofol abuse or diversion were reported by 20 % of programs in the United States. Currently the incidence of propofol abuse among anesthesia providers is estimated to be 1 in every 1,000 anesthesia providers per decade. Even in this population, individuals who should have a strong working knowledge of the drugs pharmacokinetics and therapeutic index, death resulted in 28 % of reported cases.

The propofol addict is still more likely to be a healthcare professional, especially an anesthesiologist or CRNA, despite the increasing numbers of laypersons presenting to treatment centers after propofol abuse. As well, persons who abuse propofol are more likely to be female, have a history of depression and/or have suffered early life trauma, and have a high frequency of biological relatives with substance abuse or dependence [27].

Management Issues

Propofol is rapidly redistributed when administered as a bolus and the "high" experienced does not last very long at all. The patient who has been abusing propofol must continually readminister the drug to get or to stay high. Each dose carries with it the risk for death or serious injury and rapid self-administration in the absence of respiratory assistance or control of blood pressure may result in cardiac arrest or anoxic brain injury. Trauma related to falls after bolus administration, frequently involving the nose or face are common. Multiple, often infected, puncture wounds may be present in chronic abusers of propofol and the same issues that arise with any form of chronic intravenous drug use are applicable: infection with HIV, hepatitis C, and other blood-borne diseases. Chronic aspiration during repeated periods of apnea and loss of protected airway reflexes may lead to pneumonia or pneumonitis.

High doses of propofol or prolonged infusions have been associated with sudden death (propofol infusion syndrome) characterized by the occurrence of lactic acidosis, rhabdomyolysis, and cardiovascular collapse [28]. Increased serum levels of tumor necrosis factor alpha (TNF) and interleukin-10 (IL-10) resulting from prolonged exposure can cause diffuse areas of myocardial band necrosis [29]. The chronic propofol abuser may be at risk for sudden death related to spontaneous malignant dysrhythmias [30]. The development of ST-segment elevation in leads V1–V3 (Fig. 10.3) may precede the development of hypotension, metabolic acidosis, prolonged QT interval, idioventricular rhythm, ventricular fibrillation, and renal failure [31–34].

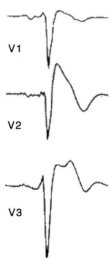

Fig. 10.3 Troublesome electrocardiographic findings suggestive of increased risk for sudden death in the chronic propofol abuser: Note the coved type ST elevation, J-point elevation, gradually descending ST segment and negative T-waves in the anterior precordial leads

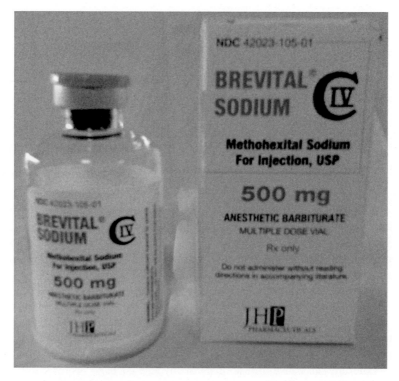

Fig. 10.4 Methohexital is available as a freeze-dried powder that must be reconstituted with sterile water prior to administration

Other Intravenous Hypnotic Agents

Methohexital

Methohexital (Fig. 10.4) is an intravenous hypnotic barbiturate derivative used for the induction of general anesthesia. Because of its rapid onset and short duration (similar to propofol), it is ideal for shorter cases requiring brief periods of general anesthesia. Though it enjoyed widespread use in the past in both surgery and dentistry, methohexital is now primarily used for the induction of general anesthesia prior to electroconvulsive therapy (ECT).

Methohexital is a schedule IV drug in the US Controlled Substances Act, meaning that even when used as indicated it may be habit forming and that it has the potential to produce dependence of the morphine type if it is abused. Methohexital intoxication can mimic some of the characteristics of alcohol, including euphoria, elation, and inhibited behavior. As with all barbiturates, in dependent persons withdrawal can occur 12–20 h after the last dose and may be life threatening.

Despite the fact that methohexital has significant abuse potential, as evidenced by reinforcement and self-administration during discrimination studies in rhesus monkeys [35–37], to date no reports of abuse of this drug by humans have been published.

Thiopental

Sodium thiopental is an intravenous hypnotic barbiturate developed and first used clinically in the 1930s which has been used for a variety of indications including as an induction agent for general anesthesia, to maintain a medically induced coma, as a "truth serum" during interrogations, as well as for euthanasia and execution. At one time sodium thiopental was the primary drug of choice for the induction of general anesthesia and is considered a core medicine in the World Health Organization's "Essential Drugs List" which specifies the minimum medical requirements for a basic healthcare system. Because the use of thiopental in the United States included capital punishment by lethal injection, the UK introduced a ban on the export of thiopental to the United States in December 2010. These restrictions were based on "the European Union Torture Regulation (including licensing of drugs used in execution by lethal injection)" and reflected the EUs disapproval of capital punishment in all circumstances. Because it could not guarantee the Italian government that it would not be used for lethal injections, Hospira stopped production of sodium thiopental from its plant in Italy in January 2011 and it is no longer available for clinical use.

   Thiopental is a schedule III drug in the US Controlled Substances Act, meaning that the drug has a potential for abuse greater than methohexital and other non-scheduled drugs, and that abuse may lead to moderate or low physical dependence or high psychological dependence. Despite its abuse potential, thiopental is rarely used as a recreational drug, and misuse remains uncommon and opportunistic. A single case report from 1998 describes the fatal use of thiopental in combination with multiple other drugs [38].

Etomidate

Etomidate is an intravenous hypnotic carboxylated imidazole derivative used for the induction of general anesthesia. Because of its short duration of action, it is some-times also used for sedation or general anesthesia for short procedures such as reduction of dislocated joints, tracheal intubation, and cardioversion, especially in hemodynamically compromised patients. Developed in 1964, etomidate has been in clinical use in the United States since 1983.

   Etomidate is not a controlled drug. It functions as a modulator at $GABA_A$ receptors [39] in a similar fashion to other injectable anesthetics with abuse potential, yet abuse is almost nonexistent and there has been only published report of recreational use of this drug since its discovery. In this 2012 report, a Washington state paramedic with a substance abuse problem self-injected the drug while on duty and was found to be significantly impaired shortly thereafter [40].

Halogenated Hydrocarbons

The inhaled anesthetics (Fig. 10.5) isoflurane (2-chloro-2-(difluoromethoxy)-1,1,1-trifluoro-ethane), sevoflurane (1,1,1,3,3,3-hexafluoro-2-(fluoromethoxy)propane), desflurane (1,2,2,2-tetrafluoroethyl difluoromethyl ether), enflurane (2-chloro-1,1,2,-trifluoroethyl-difluoromethyl ether), and halothane (2-bromo-2-chloro-1,1,1-trifluoroethane) are halogenated ethers used for the induction and maintenance of general anesthesia. Volatile liquids at room temperature, each is capable of producing surgical levels of anesthesia, even at low inspired partial pressures. They are chemically similar to other volatile substances of abuse [41] (Table 10.1) but as they were developed specifically for use in humans they lack the considerable toxicity associated with abuse of these types of inhalants. Despite this, inhalation of these drugs without the controlled use of a calibrated vaporizer (as is almost always the case when these drugs are used for recreational purposes) leads to a wide range of blood concentrations in the user and dose-related toxicity.

Properties

All of the inhaled anesthetic agents in use today share similar chemical properties. They are all volatile liquids at room temperature, have relatively low boiling points, and low solubility in blood allowing for a rapid induction and recovery from general anesthesia. The majority of the drug (95–98 %) is eliminated unchanged by the lungs, with the remaining drug metabolized by the liver before being excreted by

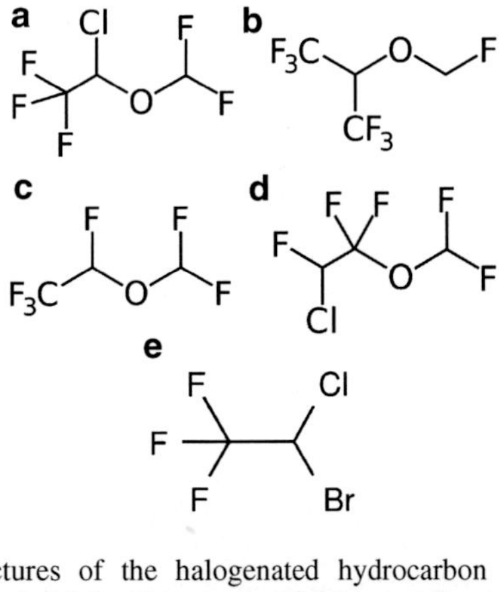

Fig. 10.5 Chemical structures of the halogenated hydrocarbon anesthetics: (**a**) *isoflurane (2-chloro-2-(difluoromethoxy)-1,1,1-trifluoro-ethane)*: (**b**) *sevoflurane (1,1,1,3,3,3-hexafluoro-2-(fluoromethoxy)propane)*: (**c**) *desflurane (1,2,2,2-tetrafluoroethyl difluoromethyl ether)*: (**d**) *enflurane (2-chloro-1,1,2,-trifluoroethyl-difluoromethyl ether)*: (**e**) *halothane (2-bromo-2-chloro-1,1,1-trifluoroethane)*

Table 10.1 Commonly abused household and industrial products

Cigarette lighter fluid	Butane, an aliphatic hydrocarbon
Model glues and rubber cement	Hexane, an aliphatic hydrocarbon
Mothballs	Naphthalene, an aromatic hydrocarbon
Toilet bowl freshener	An aromatic hydrocarbon
Resins and lacquers	Benzene, an aromatic hydrocarbon
Adhesives and paint thinner	Toluene, an aromatic hydrocarbon
Room air freshener	Butyl-isobutyl nitrate, an alkyl nitrate
Nail polish remover	Acetone, a ketone
Paints	Methyl n-butyl ketone
Spray paint	Methyl isobutyl ketone and toluene, an aromatic hydrocarbon
Bottled fuel	Propane, an aliphatic hydrocarbon
Gasoline	Octane, an aliphatic hydrocarbon and benzene, an aromatic hydrocarbon
Dry cleaning agent and spot remover	Trichloroethylene, an alkyl halide
Freon and aerosol propellants	Trichlorofluoromethane, an alkyl halide
Laboratory solvent	Diethyl ether

the kidneys. Though we do not yet fully understand how the potent volatile anesthetics produce anesthesia, muscle relaxation, and analgesia, several investigations have been conducted in attempts to elucidate their mechanisms of action. They have been shown to interact with gamma-aminobutyric acid (GABA) gated chloride channels [42], 5-hydroxytryptamine type 3 (%-HT3) receptors [43], and have been shown to exhibit nonselective actions on a number of ion channels in much the same manner as other nonmedical inhaled agents [44].

Abuse Potential

Though the inhaled anesthetics are primarily used therapeutically, these agents have the potential for recreational use as well and cases of inhaled anesthetic abuse have been reported since the mid-nineteenth century [45]. They produce behavioral effects similar to ethanol in low concentrations [46] (feeling drunk, confused, heavy or sluggish, sedated or having difficulty concentrating) and act as CNS depressants in higher concentrations [47]. Healthy volunteers exposed to different concentrations of sevoflurane in a controlled experimental setting reported subjective effects indicative of abuse liability such as feeling "high, good, and elated" associated with pleasant thoughts and euphoria [48]. Exposure to the volatile anesthetic agents activates mesolimbic dopamine neurons, and may be the mechanism whereby the drug activates reward pathways to encourage abuse. Several studies have shown that the volatile anesthetic agents have reinforcing effects and abuse liability-related subjective effects, as well as the ability to generate tolerance and dependence, suggesting that the potential for abuse of these agents by persons with access (medical staff and other hospital employees) exists [49].

Abuse Prevalence

Abuse of the volatile anesthetic agents is less prevalent than abuse of the injectable drugs but has occurred for as long as these agents have been commercially available. Much of what we know comes from the few case reports that have been published over the last few decades. Persons who abuse volatile agents in general typically do so with the intent to quickly reach an intense level of intoxication. This is achieved by inhaling the concentrated vapors in an enclosed space using a variety of methods. Though less effective than other methods, simply inhaling deeply over an open container of the liquid while "sniffing" the agent does produce some degree of intoxication. Higher blood levels of the drug, and more intense intoxication, can be achieved by placing the volatile agent into a plastic or paper bag and placing the bag over the nose and mouth while hyperventilating, an act called "bagging." Most often, however, the volatile agents are abused through the practice of "huffing" the agent. "Huffing" involves soaking a piece of gauze in the anesthetic agent and holding it up to the mouth so that the vapors are inhaled orally. When done alone, if the agent soaked cloth does not fall away from the mouth once the patient becomes intoxicated, each breath delivers more of the agent to the lungs creating a very real danger for overdose and death. When abused in this manner, blood levels of the volatile agent rapidly rise and create an intense feeling of euphoria, which quickly dissipates as the lipophilic agents are redistributed from the CNS to fat.

Of the potent volatile agents used for inhalational anesthesia today, sevoflurane (Fig. 10.6) is the one most often abused. Unlike the other volatile agents, sevoflurane has a relatively pleasant odor. It is frequently used for mask inductions, primarily in pediatric patients who will not tolerate intravenous placement prior to induction of general anesthesia, and is well tolerated (less breath-holding, low incidence of bronchospasm or laryngospasm) making it a logical choice among persons wanting to abuse the available inhaled anesthetics. Because abuse typically involves "huffing," reports of sevoflurane abuse almost always involve the death of the user. As with most obscure pharmaceuticals, knowledge of and access to the drug are the main determinants of who actually abuses the drug. This person is usually a healthcare professional such as a physician or nurse [50], though in one report a 17-year-old who worked at a veterinary clinic was able to divert and subsequently abuse the drug [51]. Though less frequently abused, isoflurane (Fig. 10.7) has abuse potential and reports of recreational use by hospital employees, in one case an operating room assistant [52] and others [53, 54] have typically resulted in death. Desflurane (Fig. 10.8) is considerable noxious when inhaled and is frequently associated with breath-holding and laryngospasm when used for inhalational inductions. Though it is reasonable to assume that it shares some of the abuse

Fig. 10.6 Sevoflurane is the most often abused of the inhalational agents due to its somewhat sweet and tolerable odor

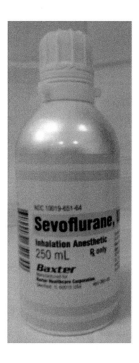

Fig. 10.7 Isoflurane is less frequently abused but reports have associated recreational inhalation with death

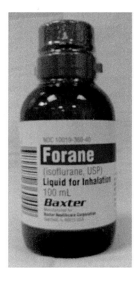

liability of the other inhaled anesthetics, its objectionable qualities make it less likely to be abused when other volatile agents are available, and no reports of desflurane abuse have surfaced as of 2013.

Though rarely used in humans in the developed countries anymore, the older volatile anesthetic halothane (Fig. 10.9) remains commercially available in some markets.

Fig. 10.8 Desflurane is the most noxious of the inhaled agents currently in use. As of 2013 no reports of desflurane abuse have been published

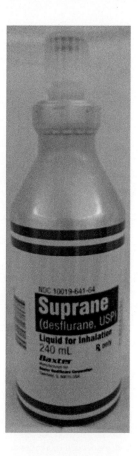

Fig. 10.9 Halothane is rarely used in the developed countries since the advent of more modern (and safer) inhaled anesthetics but some commercial preparations remain available

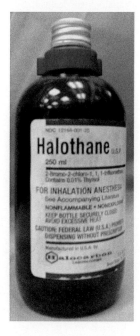

Fig. 10.10 Enflurane was first used clinically in 1966. Though it is no longer in common use, it is still available and reports of abuse have been published as recently as 2002

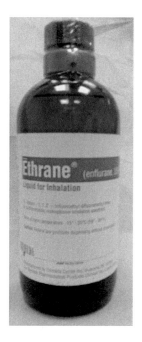

In a recent case of volatile anesthetic abuse, a pharmacist in the UK was discovered after having used a full-face military gas mask to recreationally inhale halothane [55]. It is unclear how this individual was able to obtain a fully functional modern military gas mask, though it is clear he was able to obtain the halothane from his place of employment where it was not very well controlled. Apparently the individual had made a habit of inhaling halothane, as indicated by chronic-specific inflammatory changes in the person's liver, the initial stage of halothane hepatitis, discovered at autopsy [56]. Though early reports suggest halothane can be effectively used for homicide [57] and suicide [58], unintentional death related to recreational use is more common. As with the other inhaled anesthetics, the abuse of halothane almost always involves hospital personnel [59].

First developed in 1963, enflurane (Fig. 10.10) is a structural isomer of isoflurane with similar properties. It was first used clinically in 1966 and though it was used widely during the 1970s and 1980s, it is no longer in common use. As with the other commercially available halogenated ethers, enflurane has been associated with recreational inhalation and unintended death [60–62]. One of the more interesting reports of enflurane abuse involved an episode of driving under the influence of the drug [63]. In this case a 42-year-old physician anesthesiologist was observed huffing enflurane using a handkerchief while parked in his car and subsequently driving into a truck that was stopped at a red light in front of him.

Management Issues

Halogenated hydrocarbon anesthetic agents function as CNS depressants. The effects of the volatile anesthetic agents are similar, regardless of minor differences in chemical structure, and depend primarily on the amount of agent inhaled. During abuse, these agents are typically not administered under controlled circumstances so there is a wide variation in actual blood concentration. In some instances blood concentrations may exceed what would be lethal levels of agent if maintained at that concentration for an extended period of time. At lower doses peripheral vasodilatation, with compensatory tachycardia and the potential for orthostatic hypotension, occurs. As more of the agent is inhaled and drug levels increase, myocardial contractility decreases, further exaggerating hypotension. At higher doses bradycardia, decreased cardiac output, and sudden death may occur. Malignant arrhythmia induced by an acute catecholamine surge in a patient whose myocardium has been sensitized to epinephrine by hydrocarbon inhalation is more commonly associated with halothane use but could potentially occur with unregulated self-administration of the more modern volatile anesthetics.

The volatile anesthetics are lipophilic, easily cross the blood–brain barrier, and have the potential to cause widespread effects throughout the central and peripheral nervous system. Though abuse of these agents is rare enough that it has not been demonstrated, it is theoretically possible that chronic abusers of these anesthetic agents could develop permanent neurologic damage. It is believed that most if not all of the abused inhaled agents have the potential to be neurotoxic if present in the right concentration [64]. Specific concerns in the chronic inhalant abuser include the development of cognitive dysfunction, dementia, encephalopathy, hallucinations, nystagmus, sensorimotor peripheral neuropathy, slurred speech, ataxia, seizures, and coma [65].

Patients who abuse the volatile anesthetic agents chronically may suffer from direct injury to pulmonary tissues. Inflammation of the lungs caused by chronic exposure or chronic aspiration can result in cough, chemical pneumonitis, bronchospasm (even in persons with a history of reactive airway disease) and interference with the ability of the anesthetic gas analyzer to accurately measure end-tidal anesthetic concentrations during surgery [66]. Common effects on the gastrointestinal system include nausea, vomiting, diarrhea, and hepatotoxicity. Chronic abusers have the potential to develop transaminitis, hepatitis, renal tubular acidosis, kidney stones, and glomerulonephritis. Anemia, leukopenia, leukemia, and aplastic anemia, though rare, are recognized sequelae of inhalant abuse [67].

Conclusions

The agents used to induce or maintain general anesthesia have considerable abuse potential as well as a well-documented history of misuse by both medical professionals and laypersons. The intravenous hypnotics and the halogenated hydrocarbons alike are not very well controlled. Anyone with access, some curiosity, and the propensity towards substance abuse could potentially abuse these agents. Sadly, because of the chemical properties of these drugs, such abuse often results in the unintended death of the user. Serious consideration needs to be given to the scheduling status of these drugs, with the goal of reclassification and tighter inventory control.

References

1. Eger EI. Characteristics of anesthetic agents used for induction and maintenance of general anesthesia. Am J Health Syst Pharmacol. 2004;61 Suppl 4:S3–10.
2. Short C, Bufalari A. Propofol anesthesia. Vet Clin North Am Small Anim Pract. 1999;29(3): 747–78.
3. Wilson C, Canning P, Caravati EM. The abuse potential of propofol. Clin Toxicol (Phila). 2010;48(3):165–70.
4. Karowski MD, Koltchine VV, Rick CE, et al. Propofol and other intravenous anesthetics have sites of action on the gamma-aminobutyric acid type A receptor distinct from that for isoflurane. Mol Pharmacol. 1998;53:530–8.
5. Kingston S, Mao L, Yang L, et al. Propofol inhibits phosphorylation of N-methyl-D-aspartate receptor NR1 subunits in neurons. Anesthesiology. 2006;104:763–9.
6. Brazzalotto I. Effects of propofol. Ann Fr Anesth Reanim. 1989;8:388.
7. Pain L, Gobaille S, Schleef C, et al. In vivo dopamine measurements in the nucleus accumbens after nonanesthetic and anesthetic doses of propofol in rats. Anesth Analg. 2002;95:191–6.
8. Keita H, Lecharny JB, Henzel D, et al. Is inhibition of dopamine uptake relevant to the hypnotic action of iv anesthetics? Br J Anaesth. 1996;77:254–6.
9. Xiong M, Zhang C. Molecular basis of propofol addiction. In: IARS annual meeting 2009, San Diego; 2005 (also identified in; Campton MG. Anesthesiology news. Molecular basis of propofol identified. Vol 35: 5; 1).
10. Frost EAM, Bryson EO. Propofol abuse. In: Bryson EO, Frost EAM, editors. Perioperative addiction. New York: Springer; 2011.
11. Merlo LJ, Goldberger BA, Kolodner D, et al. Fentanyl and propofol exposure in the operating room: sensitization hypotheses and further data. J Addict Dis. 2008;27(3):67–76.
12. Li KY, Xiao C, Xiong M, et al. Nanomolar propofol stimulates glutamate transmission to dopamine neurons: a possible mechanism of abuse potential? J Pharmacol Exp Ther. 2008; 325(1):165–74.
13. Mc Auliffe PF, Gold MS, Bajpai L, et al. Second-hand exposure to aerosolized intravenous anesthetics propofol and fentanyl may cause sensitization and subsequent opiate addiction among anesthesiologists and surgeons. Med Hypotheses. 2006;68(5):874–82.
14. Zacny JP, Lichtor JL, Thompson W, et al. Propofol at a subanesthetic dose may have abuse potential in healthy volunteers. Anesth Analg. 1993;77(3):544–52.
15. Roussin A, Monastrue JL, Lapeyre-Mestre M. Pharmacological and clinical evidences on the potential for abuse and dependence of propofol: a review of the literature. Fundam Clin Pharmacol. 2007;21(5):459–66.
16. Monroe T, Hamza H, Stocks G, Scimeca PD, Cowan R. The misuse and abuse of propofol. Subst Use Misuse. 2011;46:1199–205.
17. Soyka M, Schutz CG. Propfol dependency. Addiction. 1997;92(10):1369–70.
18. Bonnet U, Harkener J, Scherbaum N. A case report of propofol dependence in a physician. J Psychoactive Drugs. 2008;40(2):215–7.
19. Follette JW, Farley WJ. Anesthesiologist addicted to propofol. Anesthesiology. 1992;77: 817–8.

20. Ward CF. Substance abuse, now and for some time to come. Anesthesiology. 1992;77: 619–22.
21. Kranioti EF, Mavroforou A, Mylonakis P, Michalodimitrakis M. Lethal self-administration of propofol (Diprivan). A case report and review of the literature. Forensic Sci Int. 2007;167(1): 56–8.
22. Klausz G, Rona K, Kristof I, et al. Evaluation of a fatal propofol intoxication due to self-administration. J Forensic Leg Med. 2009;16(5):287–9.
23. Iwerson-Bergmann S, Rosner P, Kohnau HC, et al. Death after excessive propofol abuse. Int J Legal Med. 2001;114(4–5):248–51.
24. Fritz GA, Niemczyk WE. Propofol dependency in a lay person. Anesthesiology. 2002; 96:505–6.
25. Strehler M, Preuss J, Wollersen H, et al. Lethal moxed intoxication with propofol in a medical layman. Arch Kriminol. 2008;217(5–6):153–60.
26. Wischmeyer PE, Johnson BR, Wilson JE. A survey of propofol abuse in academic anesthesia programs. Anesth Analg. 2007;105(4):1066–71.
27. Earley PH, Finver T. Addiction to propofol: a study of 22 treatment cases. J Addict Med. 2013;7(3):169–76.
28. Stelow EB, Johari VP, Smity SA, Crosson JT, Apple FS. Propofol associated rhabdomyolysis with cardiac involvement in adults: chemical and anatomic findings. Clin Chem. 2000;46: 577–81.
29. Vernooy K, Delhaas T, Cremer OL, et al. Electrocardiographic changes predicting sudden death in propofol-related infusion syndrome. Heart Rhythm. 2006;3:131–7.
30. Riezzo I, Centini F, Neri M, et al. Brugada-like EKG pattern and myocardial effects in a chronic propofol abuser. Clin Toxicol. 2009;47:358–63.
31. Robinson JD, Melman Y, Walsh EP. Cardiac conduction disturbances and ventricular tachycardia after prolonged propofol infusion in an infant. Pacing Clin Electrophysiol. 2008;31(8): 1070–3.
32. Bebarta VS, Summera S. Predictor of mortality in suspected propofol infusion syndrome-Brugata electrocardiographic pattern. Crit Care Med. 2009;37(2):795–6.
33. Jorens PG, Van der Eynden GG. Propofol infusion syndrome with arrhythmia, myocardial fat accumulation and cardiac failure. Am J Cardiol. 2009;104(8):1160–2.
34. Riera AR, Lichida AH, Schapachnik E, et al. Propofol infusion syndrome and Brugada syndrome electrocardiographic phenocopy. Cardiol J. 2010;17(2):130–5.
35. McMahon LR, Coop A, France CP, Winger G, Woolverton WL. Evaluation of the reinforcing and discriminative stimulus effects of 1,4-butanediol and gamma-butyrolactone in rhesus monkeys. Eur J Pharmacol. 2003;466:113–20.
36. Broadbear JH, Winger G, Woods JH. Self-administration of methohexital, midazolam and ethanol: effects on the pituitary-adrenal axis in rhesus monkeys. Psychopharmacology (Berl). 2005;178:83–91.
37. Koffarnus MN, Hall A, Winger G. Individual differences in rhesus monkeys' demand for drugs of abuse. Addict Biol. 2011;17:887–96.
38. Gaillard Y, Pepin G. Evidence of polydrug use using hair analysis: a fatal case involving heroin, cocaine, cannabis, chloroform, thiopental and ketamine. J Forensic Sci. 1998;43(2): 435–8.
39. Vanlersberghe C, Camu F. Etomidate and other non-barbiturates. Handb Exp Pharmacol. 2008;182(182):267–82.
40. Paramedic tampered with drugs. Spokane, WA:EMS Village; 11 October 2012.
41. Balster RL. Neural basis of inhalant abuse. Drug Alcohol Depend. 1998;51:207–14.
42. MacIver BM. Abused inhalants enhance GABA-mediated synaptic inhibition. Neuropsychopharmacology. 2009;34:2296–304.
43. Lopreato GF, Phelan R, Borghese CM, Beckstead MJ, Mihic SJ. Inhaled drugs of abuse enhance serotonin-3 receptor function. Drug Alcohol Depend. 2003;70:11–5.
44. Bieda MC, Su H, MacIver MB. Anesthetics discriminate between tonic and phasic gamma-aminobutyric acid receptors on hippocampal CA1 neurons. Anesth Analg. 2009;108:484–90.

45. Weintraub M, Groce P, Karno M. Chloroformism—a new case of a bad old habit. Calif Med. 1972;117(1):63–5.
46. Bowen SE, Balster RL. Desflurane, enflurane, isoflurane, and ether produce ethanol-like discriminative stimulus effects in mice. Pharmacol Biochem Behav. 1997;57:191–8.
47. Bowen SE, Balster RL. A direct comparison of inhalant effects on locomotor activity and scheduled-controlled behavior in mice. Exp Clin Psychopharmacol. 1998;6:235–47.
48. Walker DJ, Beckman NJ, Zacny JP. Reinforcing and subjective effects of the volatile anesthetic, sevoflurane. Drug Alcohol Depend. 2004;76:191–201.
49. Smith RA, Winter PM, Smith M, Eger EI. Tolerance to and dependence on inhalational anesthetics. Anesthesiology. 1979;50:505–9.
50. Levine B, Cox D, Jufer-Phipps RA, Li L, Jacobs A, Fowler D. A fatality from sevoflurane abuse. J Anal Toxicol. 2007;31:534–6.
51. Caltrell FL. A fatal case of sevoflurane abuse. Clin Toxicol. 2008;46:918–9.
52. Pavlic M, Haidekker A, Grubwieser P, Rabl W. Fatal accident caused by isoflurane abuse. Int J Legal Med. 2002;116:357–60.
53. Dooper MM, Beerens J, Brenninkmeijer VJ, Gerlag PG. Fatal intoxication after ingestion of isoflurane. Neth J Med. 1988;33:74–7.
54. Kuhlman JJ, Magluilo J, Levine B, Smith ML. Two deaths involving isoflurane abuse. J Forensic Sci. 1993;38:968–71.
55. Krajcovic J, Novomesky F, Stuller F, Straka L, Mokry J. An unusual case of anesthetic abuse by a full-face gas mask. Am J Forensic Med Pathol. 2012;33:256–8.
56. Kaplan HG, Bakken J, Quadracci L, et al. Hepatitis caused by halothane sniffing. Ann Intern Med. 1979;90:797–8.
57. Madea B, Musshoff F. Homicidal poisioning with halothane. Int J Legal Med. 1999;113:47–9.
58. Spencer AE, Green NM. Suicide by ingestion of halothane. JAMA. 1968;168:702–3.
59. Spencer JD, Raasch FO, Trefny FA. Halothane abuse in hospital personnel. JAMA. 1976;235(10):1034–5.
60. Lingenfelter RW. Fatal misuse of enflurane. Anesthesiology. 1981;50:603.
61. Jacob B, Heller C, Daldrup T, Burrig KF, Barz J, Bonte W. Fatal accidental enflurane intoxication. J Forensic Sci. 1989;34(6):1408–12.
62. Walker FB, Morano RA. Fatal recreational inhalation of enflurane. J Forensic Sci. 1990;35(1):197–8.
63. Musshoff F, Junker H, Madea B. An unusual case of driving under the influence of enflurane. Forensic Sci Int. 2002;128:187–9.
64. Bryson EO, Frost EAM. Marijuana, nitrous oxide and other inhalants. In: Bryson EO, Frost EAM, editors. Perioperative addiction. New York: Springer; 2011.
65. Kurtzman TL, Otsuka KN, Wahl RA. Inhalant abuse by adolescents. J Adolesc Health. 2001;28:170–80.
66. Sicinski M, Kadam U. Monitoring of the anesthetic volatile agent may be impaired in hydrocarbon abusers. Anesthesia. 2002;57:510–1.
67. Broussard LA. The role of the laboratory in detecting inhalant abuse. Clin Lab Sci. 2000;13:205–9.

Chapter 11
Prescription Drug Abuse

Susan Dabu-Bondoc, Amit A. Shah, and Philip R. Effraim

Key Points

- Definition, classification, and pathophysiology
- Prescription drug abuse: diagnosis and management
- Strategies of prevention and managing the problem of prescription drug abuse or diversion

Introduction

Prescription drug abuse is a rapidly growing problem in the United States, declared an epidemic by the Center for Disease Control (CDC) [1]. The easy access of prescription drugs from friends, family, or via the Internet and, the promises of "legal" highs have attracted potential users to the use of these novel substances. The National Institute of Health (NIH) estimates that approximately 20 % of Americans have engaged in the nonmedical use of prescription drugs, making them second only to marijuana as the most commonly used illicit drugs [1–3]. According to the 2009–2010 National Survey on Drug Use and Health (NSDUH) of the US population 12 years of age and older, prescription drugs were the type of substances used by 30 % of all first-time drug-users [4].

The rapid growth and severity of abuse of prescription drugs has attracted the attention of government organizations such as the US Department of Justice and the

S. Dabu-Bondoc, M.D. (✉)
Department of Anesthesiology, Yale New Haven Hospital, Yale School of Medicine, New Haven, CT, USA
e-mail: susan.dabu-bondoc@yale.edu

A.A. Shah, M.D. • P.R. Effraim, M.D., Ph.D.
Department of Anesthesiology, Yale New Haven Hospital, New Haven, CT, USA
e-mail: amit.shah@yale.edu; philip.effraim@yale.edu

© Springer Science+Business Media New York 2015
A.D. Kaye et al. (eds.), *Substance Abuse*, DOI 10.1007/978-1-4939-1951-2_11

Whitehouse's Office of National Drug Control Policy (ONDCP) [3]. To further elucidate this growing issue, government organizations such as NSDUH conducted surveys and continue to implement strategies to prevent the misuse of prescription drugs. Data suggests that close to 70 % of people who use prescription drugs for nonmedical purposes obtain them from friends or relatives, while approximately 5 % obtain them from the Internet or drug dealers [3, 5]. Physicians still remain a major source as they write the prescriptions, often in sufficient numbers, which are available to be diverted to family and friends. Data also suggests that the nonmedical use of prescription drugs is primarily responsible for the increase in illicit drug use from 5 to 12 % between 2005 and 2008 among active duty service members [1, 6]. Additionally, the adolescent population appears to be the most frequently involved in the misuse of prescription drugs [1, 2, 7], with an estimate of one in seven teenagers abusing prescription drugs.

Chronic use of these commonly misused prescription drugs not only can cause overdose and death, but also can lead to tolerance, dependence, withdrawal, and abuse. A report from CDC in 2008 indicated that 20,044 deaths were attributed to prescription drug overdose, of which 14,800 (73.8 %) were due to opioid prescription pain relievers (OPR), an amount greater than the number of overdose deaths from heroin and cocaine combined [8]. Majority of these deaths were listed as unintentional. Between 1999 and 2008, overdose deaths from OPR have increased fourfold. Correspondingly, sales of OPR have also quadrupled between 1999 and 2010 [9]. Also of note, it has been estimated that about 39% of all opioids were prescribed, administered, or continued to come from the emergency department (ED). Many of the people who die from overdose are not in the patients to whom prescriptions are written, evidence that prescribed medications are diverted and abused, and often not by the patient himself.

This chapter is aimed to educate all levels of healthcare providers on the impacts of prescription drug abuse on patient care. It begins by delineating the differences between misuse, abuse, tolerance, and dependence, and identifying those patient populations who may be active or at highest risk of abuse. It then classifies the varying pharmacologic and pathophysiologic impacts of the chronic use of the most commonly misused drugs. Lastly, it discusses the various established or evolving therapies or strategies, that aid people who may be suffering from prescription drug abuse, as well as the current medicolegal policies directed to curb this rapidly growing problem.

Definition, Classification, and Pathophysiology

Prescription drug abuse can be described as the use of a medication in a way different than the way it was prescribed, or use without a prescription. Such use can lead to a spectrum of disorders including addiction, dependence, and tolerance. Tolerance can be induced with chronic administration of many prescription drugs. It is an adaptation characterized by dose escalation in order to maintain adequate drug efficacy. Physical dependence is an adaptation characterized by manifestation of a withdrawal/abstinence syndrome that occurs when administration of the inciting medication is abruptly stopped, the dose is reduced, or the level of the drug in the blood is reduced. Both physical dependence and tolerance are neurobiological and pharmacological phenomena. These phenomena should be distinguished from addiction, which is a psychological and behavioral syndrome, influenced by many factors including genetic, psychosocial, and environmental. Addiction is characterized by compulsive use of the drug despite potential harm, impaired control, and craving for the drug.

The most commonly abused prescription drugs include pain relievers, stimulants, and tranquilizers/sedatives. Studies estimate that the percentage of the population that has used these kinds of medications outside of prescribed guidelines are 13.5 %, 7.2 %, 8.5 %/2.9 % respectively. Among prescription drugs, opioids are not only the most frequently abused, but also are associated with the most dramatic and serious consequences of prescription drug abuse. The Drug Enforcement Administration (DEA) estimated that seven million Americans abuse pharmaceuticals, leading to a more than 300 % spike in overdose deaths from oxycodone alone from 2005 to 2010. The latest 2008 statistics from the CDC suggest that in recent years, this abuse has contributed to a significant increase in the amount of deaths, totaling 11,528 in 2007, and over 30 % increase in ED visits due to overdose [10–12]. Nevertheless, abuse of sedatives and stimulants is also significant. Abuse of stimulants has become particularly common among students and other young adults. Pain relievers known to have abused include codeine, propoxyphene, meperidine, morphine, fentanyl, hydromorphone, oxycodone, hydrocodone, methadone, and pentazocine.

Opioid abuse is found in 9–41 % of chronic pain patients. Most studies suggest that addiction per se is not common in acute, chronic, and cancer pain treatment. Although the increase in availability of prescription opioids may have led to an increase in their diversion into the illicit market, it has been noted that the increased medical use of opioid analgesics to treat pain does not appear to contribute to increase in the health consequences of opioid analgesic abuse. Additionally, pain itself is not found to be an independent factor for abuse of pain medications, and that majority of legitimate pain patients do not abuse their analgesic medication.

Other medications known to be abused on a significant scale on the streets include Methoxetamine (MXE) and Alprazolam (Xanax) [13]. MXE is an analog of ketamine ("special K"), and both drugs share structural similarity with phencyclidine (PCP). Popular in the United Kingdom, MXE has the potential for wider use via sales in the Internet. Information is limited about its users or patterns of abuse other than that the drug can be injected intravenously.

Of the three major classes of prescription drugs that are abused: opioids, sedatives, and stimulants, opioids are associated with the highest rate of mortality. CDC reports that increases in mortality due to drug overdose is parallel to geographic location and timing, with high rates for prescription of opioids. Aside from overdoses and mortality, the chronic nonmedical use of prescription drugs can pose a challenge to healthcare providers, particularly when unrecognized. Based on the

Table 11.1 Percentage of population reporting more than 100 days of nonmedical use of prescription drugs stratified by population within the last 12 months[a]

Population stratification	Painkillers	Stimulants	Tranquilizers
Total	0.8	0.2	0.2
Male	1	0.3	0.2
Female	0.6	0.2	0.3
Age 12–17	1	0.2	0.2
Age 18–25	1.7	0.4	0.6
Age 26–34	1.3	0.4	0.4
Age 35–49	0.7	0.2	0.2
Age 50+	0.2	0.1	0.1
Married	0.4	0.1	0.1
Widowed	0.2	0.1	0.1
Div/Sep	1	0.4	0.2
Never married	1.4	0.5	0.5
<High school	1.2	0.3	0.3
High school/GED	1	0.3	0.3
1–3 years of college	0.8	0.3	0.2
4+ years of college	0.2	0.1	0.1
Full-time employment	0.7	0.1	0.2
Part-time employment	0.7	0.2	0.3
Unemployed	2	1	0.8
Other/non-labor force	0.7	0.3	0.2
Pregnant	0.8	0.8	0.2
Nonpregnant	0.9	0.3	0.4
White	0.8	0.3	0.3
Black/African–American	0.8	0.1	0.2
Native American/Alaskan Native	3	0.1	0.6
Native Hawaiin/Pacific Islander	0.4	0.6	1.3
Asian	0.1	0	0.1
Mixed race	0.7	0.3	0.3
Hispanic	0.7	0.2	0.1

[a]Data summarized from 2011 NSDUH survey results [7]

most recent NSDUH data from 2011, Table 11.1 presents stratified population data on those who reported over 100 days of the nonmedical use of the prescription drugs described above within the last year. Deaths from opioid painkillers have continued to increase [9], and in 2010 alone, nonmedical use of prescription painkillers was reported by 12 million Americans.

The prescription medications most often abused fall into the class of pain medications. Specifically, they are often opioid analgesics - the opioid agonists. Opioids produce analgesia thru binding to target G-protein coupled receptors that are located primarily in the brain and spinal cord. This, in turn, results in analgesia via inhibition of the release of excitatory transmitters from the primary afferent nerve, and via inhibition of pain transmission nerve in the dorsal horn of the spinal cord. Three major classes of the opioid receptor have been identified: mu, delta, and kappa; however, the majority of currently available opioid analgesics act primarily at the mu receptor (MOR).

At a molecular level, analgesia is achieved by binding of the opioid receptor leading to the activation of the associated G-protein. This G-protein couples the receptor to the other mechanisms to achieve three main effects: (1) closure of presynaptic voltage-gated calcium channels to reduce transmitter release (2) hyperpolarization and therefore inhibition of post-synaptic neurons by opening potassium rectifying channels; and (3) phosphorylation of the receptor by G-protein coupled receptor kinases (GRK), followed by binding of arrestin. This last action leads to desensitization of the receptor and subsequent internalization from the plasma membrane, which in essence terminates the action generated by MOR binding. Disruption of this process is thought to be important in the gradual loss of effectiveness of mu-opioids sometimes observed with repeated administration (tolerance).

After becoming desensitized, the MORs need to be internalized and dephosphorylated in order to be re-sensitized and be capable of returning to the cell membrane to generate another signal. Although there is much debate on the topic, it has been posited that some agonists such as morphine are less efficient at causing internalization which may in turn lead to continued signaling and thus to disproportionate cellular adaptations, such as downregulation of the number of receptors on the membrane and prolonged lowering of cyclic-AMP levels. The net result of these cellular changes is decreased ability to generate inhibition of pain signals, consequently patient experiencing increased pain, requiring higher amount of the drug to achieve same level of efficacy.

Use of opioids often leads to rapid tolerance and eventually to physical and psychosocial dependence. Physical dependence and withdrawal due to opioid use results from upregulation of the cyclic aminophosphorylase (cAMP) pathway at the locus ceruleus. Unlike addiction, which is a pathologic process, physical dependence is a natural expected physiologic response that can occur with use of not only opiates but also with benzodiazepines, antidepressants, corticosteroids, diabetic, cardiac or other medications, and alcohol. Tolerance is also a normal expected physiologic response that can occur with exposure to opiates or certain classes of drugs or substances like alcohol. Administering the drug daily in increasing doses makes addiction to opioids occur more rapidly. Abrupt cessation, rapid dose reduction resulting in decreasing blood level of the drug, and/or administration of an antagonist produce a withdrawal syndrome that is manifested by diaphoresis, nausea, vomiting, abdominal cramps, convulsions, or death. Chronic opioid use leads to cross tolerance to anesthetic and other depressant drugs as a result of chronic receptor stimulation. It is important to note that these prescription medications, though capable of producing physical dependence, may not necessarily be associated with the disease of addiction. A heroin addict for example, is both physically dependent and addicted to the narcotic, while the patient taking opiates is physically dependent, but not necessarily addicted. Both will experience withdrawal if the drug is abruptly stopped, and both can exhibit tolerance to the drug.

Benzodiazepines exert their effects by indirectly decreasing the excitability of neurons via the gamma-aminobutyric acid (GABA) receptors. The GABA receptor has one benzodiazepine-binding site and two GABA-binding sites. The binding of benzodiazepines to the GABA-A receptors leads to an increase in the affinity of the GABA for its receptor, which, in turn, results in increased conduction of chloride ions. The mechanism of how tolerance to benzodiazepines develops is poorly understood. Currently, it is thought that whereas tolerance to the sedative and anticonvulsant properties of these drugs can develop rather quickly, tolerance to the anxiolysis and amnestic effects develop considerably more slowly, if they develop at all.

There are several proposed mechanisms underlying the development of tolerance to benzodiazepines. These mechanisms include that with long-term use, benzodiazepines lose the ability to increase their affinity to the receptor for GABA; perhaps secondary to a change in the subunit composition of the GABA-A receptor, or because of alterations to the receptor such as phosphorylation. Another proposed mechanism is that with chronic exposure, the expression of the GABA-A receptors is downregulated throughout the brain. A third proposed mechanism is that since the GABA system and glutamate system provide inhibitory and excitatory effects on the brain respectively, and are in fine balance, chronic-increased GABAergic activation might lead to compensatory sensitization of the glutaminergic transmission, eventually restoring balance.

Prescription Drug Abuse: Diagnosis and Management

Patients with a history of drug abuse or drug addiction can be classified into three categories: those who are actively involved in drug use, those with a history of prior drug abuse, and those in methadone or suboxone maintenance programs. Evaluation of the drug-abusing patient must be comprehensive in all three key aspects of patient's problem: primary clinical problem (e.g., pain or other clinical entity), addiction, and psychiatric component. Evaluation of addiction should include a determination of which substances were used by the patient and the duration of use; a history of prior substance abuse treatment; an assessment of the severity of the patient's substance abuse problem and the extent of the patient's involvement treatment programs; an assessment of the patient's level of motivation to change; the duration of sobriety if in recovery; and how sobriety is maintained. In this population, it is not uncommon for pain, substance abuse, and psychiatric problems to act synergistically and lead to development of complex, difficult to manage syndromes. Consulting or involving substance abuse specialists such as psychiatry and/or an addiction-medicine professional may often be needed to clarify the diagnosis and complete the evaluation. Current or past history of a personality, anxiety, mood, or psychotic disorder warrants a psychiatric referral and evaluation. Careful chronology may reveal if one component (pain versus psychological disorder versus addictive disorder) is exacerbating or causing another. Table 11.2 enumerates the various criteria used in diagnosing substance abuse and substance dependence as published in *Diagnostic and Statistical Manual of Mental Disorders*, 4th ed. (DSM-IV) [14].

Table 11.2 Diagnostic criteria of substance abuse and dependence in DSM-IV

A. Substance abuse
− Maladaptive pattern of substance use leading to clinically significant impairment or distress, manifested by at least one of the following, occurring within a 12-month period, and symptoms have never met the criteria for substance dependence
1. Recurrent use resulting in failure to fulfill major role obligations at work, school, or home (Examples: Substance-related poor work performance, repeated absences, suspensions, expulsion from school, neglect of children or household)
2. Recurrent use in physically hazardous situations such as driving a vehicle or operating a machine
3. Recurrent substance-related legal problems such as substance-related misconduct leading to arrests
4. Continued use despite substance use related persistent or recurrent social or interpersonal problems (Examples: arguments with spouse about consequences of intoxication, physical fights)
B. Substance dependence
− A maladaptive pattern of substance use, leading to clinically significant impairment or distress, as manifested by three or more of the following, occurring at any time in the same 12-month period:
1. Tolerance—as defined by either of the following:
(a) Need for markedly increased amounts of the substance to achieve intoxication or desired effect
(b) Markedly diminished effect with continued use of the same amount of the substance
2. Withdrawal—as manifested by either of the following:
(a) The characteristic withdrawal syndrome for the substance
(b) The same or closely related substance is taken to relieve or avoid withdrawal symptoms
3. The substance is often taken in larger amounts or over a longer period than was intended
4. There is a persistent desire or unsuccessful efforts to cut down or control substance abuse
5. A great deal of time is spent in activities necessary to obtain the substance (e.g., visiting multiple doctors or driving long distances), use the substance, or recover from its effects
6. Important social, occupational, or recreational activities are given up or reduced because of substance abuse
7. The substance use is continued despite knowledge or having a persistent or recurrent physical or psychological problem that is likely to have been caused or exacerbated by the substance (e.g., current cocaine use despite recognition of cocaine-induced depression)

Diagnostic and Statistical Manual of Mental Disorders, 4th ed. (DSM-IV). Washington, DC: American Psychiatric Association, 1994 [14]

Assessing severity of abuse is, as established in DSM-IV criteria, based on the number of adverse consequences resulting from use. The signs of prescription drug abuse, in contrast to that of illicit abuse, often are subtle, and may need a combination of multiple observations. Not all the criteria in the DSM-IV, however, would be

Table 11.3 The CAGE-AID Questionnaire

1. C—Have you ever felt that you ought to cut down on your drinking or drug use?
2. A—Have people annoyed you by criticizing your drinking or drug use?
3. G—Have you ever felt bad or guilty about your drinking or drug use?
4. E—Have you ever had a drink or use drugs first thing in the morning to steady your nerves or to get rid of a hangover (Eye opener)? [15]

applicable in the chronic pain patient, and in fact some have been a source of confusion in diagnosing addiction. The form of addiction seen in the patient with pain is often not the same as the type seen in the street addict. The requirement in the DSM-IV criteria for substance dependence about giving up or decreasing social, occupational, or recreational activities because of substance abuse often is not found in the pain patient with dependence. Unlike the illicit addict, the pain patient does not usually compromise their lifestyle e.g., drive long distances to seek drugs, or involve himself in criminal activity or drug diversion. Also, the classic sign of compulsive opioid use may not be apparent in the pain patient because opioid is prescribed and is readily available.

Two relatively easy subjective drug screening questionnaires practical for daily use include: (a) validated screening test using a single question: "How many times in the past year have you used an illegal drug or used a prescription medication for nonmedical reasons?" [15], (b) CAGE-AID (Adapted to Include Drugs) is a modification of the four-question tool utilized to detect potential alcohol abuse (Table 11.3) [16].

In Table 11.4, guidelines for prescribing drug with abuse liability in patients with history of addiction are recommended. Setting clear rules and expectations, signing an agreement between physician and patient are ways to prevent abuse or misuse. Current evidence indicates that patients adhering to controlled substance agreements and not displaying obvious dependency behavior do not abuse either illicit or licit drugs. Using feedback from the patient to set the dose is prudent. Patients can be asked to bring in all original medication bottles with or without medication including the date they are filled, the prescribing physician and the dispensing pharmacy, the number of pills dispensed, and the number of remaining pills. Monitoring for lost or stolen prescriptions and obtaining random urine screens may also be helpful. Unnecessary escalation of opiate doses may be avoided by the use of adjunctive medications as necessary. Documentation is key to prevent confusion, and overprescription. Good practice dictates seeing the patient as frequently as needed, working with significant others as well as any close family member. Knowing how to withdraw the patient from the medication is important, as well as, bringing patient in for unscheduled visits. P.R.N. medications need to be limited to prevent drug-seeking behavior.

Detection in the individual's system depends on the drug or combination of drugs involved. Toxicology or Urine drug screening (UDS) is an important tool in collecting objective information about a patient's opioid use, and can be a helpful clinical adjunct to identify aberrant behavior and to monitor opioid use in addiction or diversion. UDS tests, however, have several limitations. Immunoassay screening,

Table 11.4 Guidelines for prescribing drug with abuse liability in pain patients with history of addiction

1. Set clear rules and expectations for you and the patient, have both sign an agreement
2. Set the dose of the medication at the appropriate level to treat the condition, and titrate as necessary
3. Use feedback from patient to set dose
4. Give enough medication plus rescue doses
5. Ask patient to bring in all original medication bottles with or without medication: date filled, pharmacy, prescribing physician, number of pills dispensed, number of remaining pills
6. Monitor for lost or stolen prescriptions
7. Obtain random urine screens
8. Know the drugs for which the laboratory screens
9. Use adjunctive medications as necessary
10. Document, document, document
11. See the patient as frequently as needed
12. Work with significant others or closed family members
13. Know how to withdraw the patient from the medication
14. Know the pharmacology, duration of action, and parenteral to oral conversion ratio of the drugs being prescribed
15. Bring patient in for unscheduled visits
16. Obtain release to contact other healthcare providers
17. Limit p.r.n. medications since this promotes drug-seeking behavior
18. Adequately treat the condition and trust the patient to avoid problems of pseudoaddiction

Adapted from: Schnoll SH, Weaver MF. Addiction and pain. Am J Addict. 2003; 12 Suppl 2: S27-35 [27]

the most common UDS, has frequent false positive results and typically requires confirmation by gas chromatography–mass spectroscopy (GC–MS), which is typically a time consuming process. UDS cannot detect past abuse and also has difficulty detecting fentanyl use. DOA immunoassays do not detect opioids such as propoxyphene, oxycodone, hydrocodone, oxymorphone, hydromorphone, or tramadol. It is also not unusual for Methylphenidate to be not detected by DOA immunoassays. Opioid-specific immunoassays and GC–MS often require special testing and ordering but are commercially available to detect opioids.

Practitioners believe that all patients with chronic nonterminal pain who were treated with opioids should be subjected to random urine screening. This belief has been supported by survey studies demonstrating that about 40 % of the patients with chronic non-cancer pain who were treated with opioids were found problematic, and about half of these problematic cases were identified through toxicology screening. The physician is, nevertheless, the caregiver ultimately responsible for determining the severity of the prescription drug abuse in his practice, and makes the decision on whether toxicology would be utilized on a routine or an occasional basis.

Management of drug effects is directed at the specific substance used. Intoxication with opioids may be treated with naloxone, while intoxication with stimulants (e.g., methylphenidate), may be managed with benzodiazepines. Successful use of benzodiazepines in anxiety tends to improve function over time. When these medications work well with anxious patients, their anxiety improves substantially and often remits, and over time they may need lower rather than higher doses. It is very important that patients be made aware that chasing their anxiety with as-needed use may actually be of harm.

Methadone therapy remains one of the primary treatments of prescription drug abuse. The newer and increasingly popular treatment is the use of buprenorphine. The approval by DEA and FDA of the office-based use of buprenorphine to treat opioid addicts expanded the treatment options for abuse of prescription medications. The Drug Addiction Treatment Act of 2000 inflated the avenues for the treatment of opioid dependence in the United States from specially licensed buprenorphine facilities to physicians' private offices, where Schedule III–V drugs can be prescribed. Opioid substitution has now been monitored by the Substance Abuse and Mental Health Administration and, expansion of treatment to private practice creates opportunities to provide comprehensive care for addicted patients. In France since February 1996, general practitioners have also been allowed to prescribe buprenorphine in high dosage for maintenance treatment of major opioid addiction. As an alternative to methadone in pregnancy, buprenorphine has been validated by several naturalistic studies in France, where outpatient physicians can treat with buprenorphine without specialized training; up to 70,000 patients annually have received the medication on an outpatient basis since the 1996 liberalization of policies.

Buprenorphine (Suboxone) is prescribed by clinicians for the treatment of narcotic addiction or of pain in patients with history (documented or otherwise) of addiction. When patients with narcotic addiction let their narcotic level fall below their threshold, they begin to experience profound withdrawal syndrome that constitutes sweats, cramps, diarrhea, mood swings, and agitation. Buprenorphine both structurally and clinically provides an alternative to treating legitimate chronic pain patients with a predisposition to addiction. Buprenorphine's clinical efficacy results from its unique molecular structure: it is a partial mu-opioid agonist and a weak antagonist. Its high affinity for the mu receptor and its slow dissociation [17] results in a long duration of action and an analgesic potency 25–40 times greater than morphine, as well as, decreased tolerance because of loss of opioid receptors from the cell surface. The main reason the drug is considered in populations with addictive predisposition is its safety profile. In physically dependent individuals, acute cessation of buprenorphine may lead to withdrawal syndromes that appear to be milder than those seen with morphine [18]. Although suboxone can be displaced by higher doses of narcotics, it generally holds patients at a level that curbs withdrawal and craving, while it keeps them from moving up their narcotic level when they take perioperative opioid medications. The other unique feature of suboxone is its having a peak ceiling effect, therefore patients will not step up their narcotic level even if they take more than the recommended daily dose, which is another great advantage of the drug in deterring its abuse potential. Careful titration of perioperative narcotics with appropriate monitoring for side effects remains the mainstay of treatment. Typically, specialists recommend that suboxone be stopped for 2–3 days before elective surgery to make traditional opiates be more effective as its level falls. Patients are prescribed short-acting opiates such as Percocet for 2 days to ward off withdrawal as they stop taking suboxone in anticipation of elective surgery. Intra- and immediately postoperatively, opiates are continuously titrated to effect, and may use or combine with regional anesthesia or field blocks or with nonnarcotic analgesics. Alternatively the provider may continue suboxone into the perioperative period. Patients are transitioned back to their suboxone around the time they are moved off their postoperative narcotics. To avoid withdrawal symptoms, the patient needs to be at their prior narcotic level when they restart suboxone.

Naltrexone is thought to possibly play a role in relapse prevention, and it has been utilized for maintenance after an initial taper with buprenorphine. Naltrexone was used, in one small Australian study, for a detoxification protocol during pregnancy and showed favorable results. Naltrexone implant is currently being studied and initial results seem promising.

Oxymorphone is a semisynthetic opioid analgesic that may be a new treatment option for use in the illicit or licit substance-abusing patient, and for use during opioid rotation. Approximately 6–8 times more potent than morphine, it is a powerful opioid agonist that is marketed in oral form (Opana, Opana ER) in 5, 10, 20, and 40 mg tablets, as a suppository (Numorphan) in 5 mg, or as an injectable hydrochloride salt in 1 mg doses. For patients with addictive disorder, it is an option for the relief of moderate to severe pain, as a preoperative medication to alleviate apprehension, maintain anesthesia, and as an obstetric analgesic. It may be given in 0.5 mg increments up to a total of 2 mg especially in patients who have required at least 4 mg of hydromorphone. The extended release formulation is designed to continuously release drug during the 12-h period and its pharmacokinetic properties are consistent with its use for around the clock therapy. A steady state is typically achieved within 3 days with a relatively stable plasma concentration. Having both the extended and immediate release formulations provide flexibility in dosing that is useful when converting patients from different opioids.

Strategies of Prevention and Managing the Problem of Prescription Drug Abuse or Diversion

The increase in incidence of opiate abuse in the United States has been attributed to a number of reasons. The easy access of prescription drugs from friends, family or via the Internet and, that OPRs are a legally available alternative to illicit substances that provide euphoria have attracted potential users to the use of these substances. Many chronic pain patients are likely to either abuse their pain medications or sell them to others [19]. Identification of patients on chronic pain medications with a high potential for abuse is an arduous responsibility physicians face in managing prescription drug abuse.

Several strategies have been proposed and initiated by CDC to curtail the epidemic of prescription drug abuse. One that may have potential major impact is the use of Prescription Drug Monitoring Programs (PDMPs). They are state-run electronic databases designed to track the prescribing and dispensing of controlled prescription medications to patients. PDMP databases enable physicians to determine if patients have received excessive or unusually high amounts of controlled medications and therefore can adjust their prescribing decisions appropriately. Databases allow information access on whether patients obtain prescriptions from many different physicians or multiple states, and therefore would make control of "doctor shopping" [20] possible. CDC also recommended that PDMPs be linked to electronic health-records systems for the purpose of better integration of the health providers' day-to-day practices. Many hospitals have already adopted many of these recommendations, and professional organizations (e.g., American College of Emergency Physicians) have supported the incorporation of PDMP into their members' clinical practice [21].

A few studies have been conducted to measure the impact of the statewide PDMPs, and have demonstrated that they positively influence physician prescribing practices, however, another investigation found that states with PDMPs already in place had no significant decrease in the number of overdose mortalities from opioids [22]. While PDMPs have the potential to be an effective means of appropriately managing prescribing of controlled pain medications, more data and clinical research is needed to assess the impact of statewide PDMPs.

Another strategy proposed for curbing prescription drug abuse or diversion is formulary restriction (FR). Formulary restriction has been a subject of debate by experts. While FR is direct and simple, and could encourage first-line use of alternative treatments or encourage careful evaluation & clinical review to avoid rash prescribing, the use of FR has several drawbacks. Experts argue that certain patients who legitimately need the prescriptions for therapeutic purposes are likely to be harmed by FR. Additionally, it is generally viewed that formulary restriction are likely be more effective with new cases versus managing chronic cases, with patients abusing multiple substances, or with patients with prior history of one or more abuse relapses. There is also a concern that requiring preauthorization for certain medications such as benzodiazepines may lead to prescribing of less effective anxiolytics as a result of trying to obviate the preauthorization process.

Cognitive behavioral therapy (CBT) can provide an alternative therapy to patients who are on anxiety medications. The basics of CBT entails education about anxiety, the role of avoidance or exposure, the harmful effects of as-needed use of benzodiazepines or other anxiety medications, the core elements of breathing retraining, and cognitive restructuring. In CBT, patients on alprazolam or other anxiety medications are made cognizant that medication blood level fluctuations can in and of itself contribute to anxiety, and that chasing their anxiety with as-needed use may actually be harmful. In a successful behavior therapy, the patient becomes more tempered to the effects of anxiety over time. There is a consensus among experts that CBD may work in getting patients off benzodiazepines or amphetamines but not those on opiates, by providing alternative treatments and skillfully managing any withdrawal syndrome. Stimulants and attention-deficit hyperactivity disorder (ADHD) prescriptions have been shown to be somewhat more effective than alternative agents, unlike the benzodiazepines, which do not have superior efficacy to antidepressants for anxiety. CBT appears to be most appropriate to utilize when it is certain that a specific medication is either less effective and/or safe than alternatives, or more expensive than an equally safe and effective alternative. There is a general consensus that benzodiazepines are overprescribed and that behavioral therapies such as CBT, are underutilized.

Physician education is another important strategy to control the prevalence of OPR abuse. Physicians must avoid prescribing large numbers of leftover opioids. CDC has suggested a nationwide mandatory prescriber education requiring healthcare providers to train in appropriate prescribing of opiates prior to obtaining controlled substance registration from the DEA [19]. Other plans of action listed in the Presidential 2011 report include collaboration with medical boards to institute required educational curricula in health professional schools, use of continuing medical education programs to teach the safe and appropriate use of OPR, and collaborating with the American College of Emergency Physicians to develop evidence-based clinical guidelines that establish best practices for opioid prescribing in the ED [23]. NIDA and multiple National Institutes of Health (NIH) centers (e.g., Centers of Excellence for Pain Education coordinated by the NIH Pain Consortium), developed core curricula for healthcare providers to improve the treatment of pain by focusing on patient assessment, treatment planning, and treatment monitoring. It is believed that education of health professionals will help reduce the over-reliance on opioids, and will facilitate considering other forms of treatment such as CBT, as well as multiple other somatic treatments such as NSAIDs, TENS units, nerve blockade, etc. in their clinical practice. NIDA is helping to develop physician-friendly online screening tools (NIDAMED program), and works with other federal agencies to incorporate substance abuse screening in the Centers for Medicare & Medicaid Services (CMS) electronic health records.

Education of both the patient and the public is important as well. The administration began working on regulations for people and institutions to dispose of unused prescription drugs, this legislation was signed into law by the president in October 2010. Through public and patient education, vigilance among every friend and family member with access to the medicine cabinet must be highlighted as a very important tool to prevent diversion.

Other recommendations to control OPR abuse include implementing regulations against "pill mills" (rogue pain clinics) and practitioners who dispense prescription drugs unscrupulously or unethically. The DEA has worked alongside state and municipal law enforcement agencies to shut down rogue pain clinics and prosecute the physicians that work for them. The agency also has cracked down pharmaceutical abuse by targeting distributors and pharmacies. Several states have instituted regulations against pill mills and penalties against healthcare workers that violate state guidelines for prescribing or dispensing controlled substances.

And lastly, as CDC recommended that states have improved access to substance abuse treatment programs, several federal and statewide efforts to increase access to

substance abuse treatment programs have been initiated. These include: (1) passing
the Affordable Care Act that requires coverage for substance abuse services by
health insurance plans [24] expanding funding for substance abuse treatment, making Naltrexone (Vivitrol) more easily available to clinicians by allowing pharmacies
to bill Medicaid directly for reimbursement [25], (2) legislating more access of substance abuse treatment, e.g., Congress passed (2006) legislation that increased the
limit of patients per physician to receive Buprenorphine (Suboxone), another drug
in detoxification from opiates, from 30 to 100 (Ohio expands), and (3) by increasing
service reimbursement rates to Medicaid providers and expanding benefits of state
substance abuse program by including outpatient substance abuse treatment [26].

Currently our armamentarium for managing and preventing prescription drug
abuse is still limited. Our limited ability to objectively classify chronic pain, anxiety, and attention disorders calls for more research in the mechanisms of such conditions to arrive at new or improved approaches for evaluating and managing these
disorders. As major barriers in time and reimbursements for cognitive services
abound, tendency for clinicians to rely more on medications remain. There is a
strong need to focus on implementation of high-quality care for pain, anxiety, and
attention conditions in order to achieve better patient outcomes such as ones with
less abuse of medication and less diversion.

References

1. Office of National Drug Control Policy. Epidemic: responding to America's prescription drug abuse crisis. http://www.whitehouse.gov/ondcp/prescription-drug-abuse. Accessed 30 March 2013.
2. NIH: National Institute on Drug Abuse. Prescription drug abuse. http://www.nlm.nih.gov/medlineplus/prescriptiondrugabuse.html#cat59. Accessed 30 March 2013.
3. Dabu-Bondoc S, Zhang R, Vadivelu N. Managing pain in the addicted patient. In: Vadivelu N, Urman R, Hines R, editors. Essentials of pain management. New York: Springer; 2011.
4. Substance Abuse and Mental Health Services Administration. State estimates of substance use and mental disorders from the 2009-2010 National Surveys on Drug Use and Health, NSDUH Series H-43, HHS Publication No. (SMA) 12-4703. Rockville: Substance Abuse and Mental Health Services Administration; 2012.
5. Results from the 2009 National Survey on Drug Use and Health (NSDUH): national findings, SAMHSA; 2010.
6. Department of Defense. 2008 Department of Defense survey of health related behaviors among active duty military personnel. 2009. http://www.tricare.mil/2008HealthBehaviors.pdf
7. United States Department of Health and Human Services, Substance Abuse and Mental Health Services Administration, Center for Behavioral Health Statistics and Quality, National Survey on Drug Use and Health. ICPSR34481-v1. Ann Arbor: Inter-university Consortium for Political and Social Research [distributor]; 2011. doi:10.3886/ICPSR34481.v1.
8. Chakravarthy B, Shah S, Lotfipour S. Prescription drug monitoring programs and other inter-ventions to combat prescription opioid abuse. West J Emerg Med. 2012;13(5):422–5.
9. Centers for Disease Control and Prevention (CDC). Vital signs: overdose of prescription opi-oid pain relievers–United States, 1999–2008. MMWR Morb Mortal Wkly Rep. 2011;60(43): 1487–92.

10. U.S. Department of Justice. National Drug Intelligence Center: national drug threat assessment 2011. Product no. 2011-Q0317-001; 2011.
11. Warner M, Chen LH. Increase in fatal poisonings involving opioid analgesics in the United States, 1999–2006. NCHS data brief, No. 22. Hyattsville: CDC; 2009.
12. SAMHSA, Office of Applied Studies, DAWN. The Dawn report: trends in Emergency Department visits involving nonmedical use of narcotic pain relievers; 2010.
13. Goodnough A. Abuse of Xanax leads a clinic to halt supply. New York Times; 14 Sept 2011. http://www.nytimes.com/2011/09/14/us/in-louisville-a-centers-doctors-cut-off-xanax-prescriptions.html. Accessed 15 April 2013.
14. Diagnostic and statistical manual of mental disorders, 4th ed. (DSM-IV). Washington, DC: American Psychiatric Association; 1994.
15. Smith PC, Schmidt SM, Allensworth-Davies D, Saitz R. A single-question screening test for drug use in primary care. Arch Intern Med. 2010;170(13):1155–60.
16. Brown RL, Rounds LA. Conjoint screening questionnaires for alcohol and other drug abuse: criterion validity in a primary care practice. Wis Med J. 1995;94(3):135–40.
17. Jasinski DR, Pevnick JS, Griffith JD. Human pharmacology and abuse potential of the analgesic buprenorphine: potential agent for treating narcotic addiction. Arch Gen Psychiatry. 1978; 35:501–16.
18. Heel RC, Brogden RN, Speight TM, et al. Buprenorphine: a review of its pharmacological properties and therapeutic efficacy. Drugs. 1979;17:81–110.
19. Baehren DF, Marco CA, Droz DE, Sinha S, Callan EM, Akpunonu P. A statewide prescription monitoring program affects emergency department prescribing behaviors. Ann Emerg Med. 2010;56(1):19–23.
20. Centers for Disease Control and Prevention. Prescription painkiller overdoses at epidemic levels. 2011. http://www.cdc.gov/media/releases/2011/p1101_flu_pain_killer_overdose.html?sourc. Accessed 15 April 2013.
21. Center for Disease Control and Prevention (CDC). CDC grand rounds: prescription drug overdoses—a U.S. epidemic. MMWR Morb Mortal Wkly Rep. 2012;61(1):10–3.
22. Paulozzi LJ, Kilbourne EM, Desai HA. Prescription drug monitoring programs and death rates from drug overdose. Pain Med. 2011;12:747–54.
23. The White House. Epidemic: responding to America's prescription drug abuse crisis. http://www.whitehouse.gov/sites/default/files/ondcp/policy-and-research/rx_abuse_plan.pdf. Accessed 4 July 2011.
24. The White House. Substance abuse and the Affordable Care Act. http://www.whitehouse.gov/ondcp/healthcare. Accessed 4 July 2013.
25. Welsh-Huggins A. Ohio expands use of anti-narcotic treatment. http://www.sfgate.com/news/article/Ohio-expands-use-of-anti-narcotic-treatment-3681973.php. Accessed 4 July 2012.
26. Levin A. Congress lets M.D.s treat more buprenorphine patients. Psychiatry News. 2007;42:4.
27. Schnoll SH, Weaver MF. Addiction and pain. Am J Addict. 2003;12 Suppl 2:S27–35.

Chapter 12
Cocaine Abuse

Emily Kahn, Hosni Mikhael, and Nalini Vadivelu

Key Points

- Production and forms of cocaine
- Pharmacokinetics and metabolism
- Testing
- Pharmacodynamics and effect
- Addiction
- Toxicity
- Cocaine and pregnancy
- Withdrawal and treatment

Introduction

Cocaine dependence continues to be a significant public health problem in the United States, with about 1.6 million current cocaine users and over 600,000 new cocaine users in the past year. Of this number, about 1.1 million are said to be dependent on or have abused cocaine in the past year [1]. It is estimated that 25 million people in the United States have used cocaine at least once [2]. Cocaine abuse remains one of the leading causes of drug-related emergency department visits and hospital admissions [3].

E. Kahn, M.D. (✉) • H. Mikhael, M.D.
Department of Anesthesiology, Yale-New Haven Hospital, New Haven, CT, USA
e-mail: emily.kahn@yale.edu; hosni.mikhael@yale.edu

N. Vadivelu, M.D.
Department of Anesthesiology, Yale University, New Haven, CT, USA
e-mail: nalinivg@gmail.com

© Springer Science+Business Media New York 2015
A.D. Kaye et al. (eds.), *Substance Abuse*, DOI 10.1007/978-1-4939-1951-2_12

The leaves of the coca plant were used as early as 3000 BC to increase energy, reduce fatigue and hunger. In the medical world, cocaine was introduced in the late 1800s as a local anesthetic with powerful vasoconstrictive properties useful in limiting surgical blood loss [4]. Medicinal use of cocaine is now limited in practice as it has been replaced by agents that can provide the same local anesthetic and vasoconstrictive effects without the addictive and abuse risks that cocaine carries [5].

Production and Forms of Cocaine

Cocaine is acquired from the plant, *Erythroxylum coca*, which is almost exclusive to the South American region. The two predominant forms of cocaine abused are a cocaine powder, which is a cocaine salt (cocaine hydrochloride, commonly known as "coke"), and a solid form, which is a cocaine free base (commonly known as "crack"). To derive the drug from the plant, the leaves of the plant are soaked in solvents, frequently gasoline, to extract the coca base. Since cocaine is a weak alkaline compound it can combine with various acidic compounds to form a salt. Once the coca paste is obtained from the leaves the liquid solution is pressed out. A powder form of cocaine is then obtained by precipitating the coca paste using an acid, commonly hydrochloric acid, to form cocaine hydrochloric salt, which is the powder form of cocaine commonly used. This powder form is water-soluble and can be readily ingested via inhalation through the nares mucosa or dissolved in water and injected intravenously. It can also be well absorbed through any mucous membrane including oral administration. However, this powder form cannot be smoked as it has a high melting point and will decompose when heated [3]. In order to smoke cocaine, the powder substance is further converted into its base form by dissolving the cocaine salt in an alkaline solvent (a mixture of water and a base, such as baking soda) and allowing it to dry into a hard rock-like state [5]. This form of cocaine is known as "crack" due to the characteristic noise made when it is heated into this form and when it is smoked. It is almost a pure cocaine base and is highly addictive. It is also the cheapest form of cocaine to make and buy and therefore the most commonly abused form of cocaine [3, 4]. Cocaine has many common street names including Snow, Nose Candy, Bernice, Dama Blanca, Baseball, Blow, and Gold Dust [3].

Pharmacokinetics and Metabolism

Ingestion of cocaine through smoking "crack" cocaine versus intranasal use of cocaine is often preferred by addicts due to the more rapid onset and greater intensity of effect by the former route [6]. When inhaled, smoked cocaine has a peak effect within 3 min but a somewhat short duration of about 15 min. The IV route will have an onset within 60 s, peak at 5 min, and will last up to 60 min. Intranasal use has a slower onset with effects starting within 5 min and peaks around 20 min.

The effects from intranasal use will last for 90 min. Cocaine taken orally is the slowest route of administration with an onset by 20 min, peak effect after 60–90 min, and will last for about 3 h [4, 7].

Cocaine is an ester-type local anesthetic. As such, cocaine's ester link is metabolized via plasma and hepatic cholinesterases into metabolites benzoylecgonine and ecgonine methyl esters. This rapid hydrolysis of cocaine by plasma cholinesterases accounts for its short half-life [3]. However, any user with impaired hepatic function or those with genetic polymorphisms in plasma cholinesterase can have prolonged effect following cocaine use due to decreased metabolism. There are decreased levels of plasma cholinesterases in pregnancy which accounts for the potential prolongation of cocaine's effect with pregnancy. Cocaine metabolites are then excreted in urine where they can remain detected for up to 72 h after acute use [4, 8].

Testing

Cocaine can be tested for in any type of biologic specimen (blood, urine, hair, perspiration, mecomium, saliva, and amniotic fluid). Cocaine itself has a very short half-life in plasma of about 1 h (ranges from 0.5 to 1.5 h). Its metabolite, benzoylecgonine is more commonly tested, as it has a longer half-life of about 6 h. A urine sample test is most commonly used. The urine test will usually remain positive for up to 3 days after acute use and can stay positive for up to 2 weeks with chronic cocaine use. The urine test can start detecting benzoylecgonine in about 1–4 h following cocaine use. Testing for the metabolite benzoylecgonine has the added advantage that there are no other known drugs that could lead to a false positive when its presence is assessed. The initial screening test is done by an enzyme immunochemical assay which has a high sensitivity but lower specificity. Consequently gas chromatography/mass spectrometry (GC/MS) is used to confirm its presence following positive immunoassay results [5, 7]. Since the screening tests look for cocaine's metabolite, the positive result cannot be used to differentiate acute intoxication from recent use [3].

Pharmacodynamics and Effect

The effects of cocaine are varied secondary to its various physiologic and pharmacologic properties. Local anesthesia is attained via the inhibition of nerve conduction in peripheral nerves. This is achieved by a competitive inhibition of voltage-gated sodium channels in the neuron membrane thus blocking depolarization and preventing saltatory nerve conduction. Cocaine has strong vasoconstrictive properties primarily secondary to direct stimulation of alpha-adrenergic receptors in arterial wall smooth muscle. Additionally cocaine has been associated with an increase in endothelin-1 (a potent vasoconstrictor) and a decrease in nitric oxide (a vasodilator) blood concentration which may also contribute to cocaine's vasoconstrictive properties [5]. The vasoactive properties of cocaine may persist past the acute intoxication phase in drug use. This is thought to be secondary to two of its metabolites, benzoylecgonine and ecgonine methylester, which may persist for over 24 h after use. This can be significant enough to also cause delayed or recurrent coronary vasoconstriction.

In addition to its alpha-adrenergic effect, cocaine also acts as a sympathomimetic agent. This is primarily a result of its potent inhibition of the dopamine-, norepi-nephrine-, and serotonin-reuptake transporters in the presynaptic terminal [6]. Cocaine has also been found to inhibit the action of monoamine oxidase which is responsible for metabolizing these adrenergic peptides within the synapse. The combination of these actions (decreased reuptake with decreased metabolism) will result in a prolonged effect of action of these substrates following their release. The net result is an extended activation of the sympathetic nervous system peripherally, and since cocaine readily cross the blood–brain barrier, an increase in excitatory neurotransmitters centrally [8]. The impact peripherally includes an increase in heart rate, blood pressure, cardiac contractility, and a characteristic mydriasis. Due to the increase in sympathetic tone, this places the body in a high metabolic state with increased heat production. This combined with increased motor activity, decreased heat dissipation due to vasoconstriction, and affects on the hypothalamic heat regulation center, significant hyperthermia can result [3, 9]. Centrally the increase in serotonin and dopamine results in a feeling of euphoria, well-being, and an increase in self-confidence, arousal, and energy. The euphoria is believed to be primarily the result of greater stimulation of dopamine receptors in the mesolimbic and mesocortical areas of the brain [7]. At higher doses it can produce agitation and delirium [5]. With long-term use cocaine tends to cause irritability, aggressive and stereotyped behavior, and a paranoid-like psychosis [6].

Addiction

The predominance of the dopaminergic system in feelings of euphoria is well proven. In general, psychoactive drugs that cause addiction do so by increasing dopamine within the nucleus accumbens. It is believed that the central euphoric effects of cocaine are primarily due to an increase in extracellular dopamine levels via the inhibition of reuptake and metabolism following its release into the synaptic cleft. In fact, cocaine has been found to bind directly to the dopamine transporter itself [10]. This is also believed to play a central role in its addictive properties as a significant drop in cortical dopamine levels has been demonstrated during withdrawal [6].

Cocaine addiction differs from that seen with opioids and barbituates in that it does not cause the true physical dependence seen with these other illicit substances. However, the euphoric high produced by cocaine is tremendously rewarding and therefore the drug-seeking behavior of the cocaine abuser is similar to that seen with other drugs of abuse [2]. The feeling of euphoria that comes with acute cocaine intoxication changes to dejection and despair as the acute "high" dissipates.

The feeling of ecstasy is once again reinstated with further drug use. The rapid alteration between bliss and misery is what will lead most users into a "binge" pattern of use, where the drug is repeatedly used in successive intervals until either the supply or the user is drained [11]. With chronic repetitive use, cocaine will gradually deplete dopamine stores in the presynaptic terminal due its inhibition of the reuptake transporters. In addition, there will be up-regulation of postsynaptic dopamine receptors in response to the lower levels released. This depletion of dopamine will produce feelings of depression and anergia. It will also cause cravings for further cocaine use. Further compounding this, the addicted user develops a tolerance to the cocaine-induced euphoria. This necessitates the use of larger and larger doses of cocaine to achieve the same effects [7, 11].

Toxicity

There is no set lethal or toxic dose of cocaine that can be measured in the blood. In addition there is no specific plasma concentration of cocaine that can be deemed safe [8]. The greatest incidence of cocaine-related morbidity and mortality occurs within 60–120 min after use. Thus a patient presenting with symptoms related to acute cocaine intoxication should be monitored until the acute phase subsides [11].

Cardiovascular Toxicity

The link between cocaine use and cardiotoxicity has been well studied and proven. Forty percent of emergency department visits resulting from cocaine use are due to cocaine-induced chest pain [3]. Cocaine's strain on the heart is a result of its sympathomimetic properties. Cocaine causes coronary vasoconstriction while simultaneously increasing blood pressure, heart rate, and cardiac contractility. This increase in cardiac oxygen demand while decreasing its supply readily explains the high incidence of chest pain associated with cocaine use. Chronic cocaine use is also linked to the development of progressive coronary atherosclerosis. This can be especially profound in young patients who develop premature atherosclerosis who otherwise demonstrate little to no other cardiac risk factors. This is especially important as frequent cocaine use accounts for 1 of every 4 nonfatal myocardial infarctions in young persons below the age of 45 [12].

Cocaine also triggers platelet aggregation and induces the production of plasminogen activator inhibitor increasing the risk of thrombosis. The net effect of accelerated atherosclerosis combined with increased risk of thrombosis is a predisposition to the development of myocardial infarction with long-term use [2]. Chronic cocaine use has also been found to cause structural changes, most commonly left ventricular hypertrophy, and wall motion abnormalities which result when ischemic changes occur [13]. Additionally, through its interference with nerve conduction via the inhibition of sodium-conducting channels, cocaine can cause cardiac dysrhythmias as well. There is no specific arrhythmia linked with cocaine use although lower doses have been associated with bradycardias while higher doses with tachydysrhythmias. This can range from sinus tachycardia, supraventricular tachycardia, atrial fibrillation/flutter, ventricular fibrillation/flutter, premature ventricular contractions (PVCs), or torsades de pointes [3].

The patient presenting with cocaine-related chest pain must be approached with caution. Chest pain following cocaine use can be the result of myocardial ischemia or infarction, aortic dissection (due to increased shear forces from catecholamine surge), pneumomediastinum or pneumothorax (following crack-cocaine use) [3]. While an underlying serious cardiovascular event must be considered in these patients, the clinical approach remains a challenge. The diagnostic penumbra stems from the fact that chest pain remains one of the most common adverse symptoms reported by users, which as explained above, is often a product of the demand ischemia on the heart that results from cocaine use itself [14]. Though often related to cocaine-induced vasospasm, the risk of accelerated atherosclerosis and thrombosis in this group is significant as well. About 6 % of cocaine-related chest pain presentations are in fact due to myocardial infarction (MI) [15]. Further complicating the workup, an electrocardiogram (ECG) remains unreliable as a diagnostic tool in differentiating between benign cocaine-associated chest pain versus an acute ischemic event. The sensitivity for a positive ECG finding in the diagnosis of an acute MI in this patient population has been reported to be as low as 36 %. An acute myocardial infarction can occur in a significant number of these patients while having normal or nonspecific ECG findings. Additionally there are many patients with cocaine-associated chest pain that will meet diagnostic criteria for an acute ST-elevation infarction without having a true MI [14, 16]. Cardiac biomarkers may also confuse the picture, as cocaine use can also cause rhabdomyolysis resulting in elevated creatine kinase levels. Therefore troponins will be the most sensitive biomarkers for cocaine-associated MI. In general the workup for a patient presenting with cocaine-associated chest pain should comply with same standards used in the evaluation of any patient with a suspected acute coronary syndrome. However, it is essential to keep in mind how cocaine use impacts these testing results and thus subsequent interventions [17].

The current guidelines recommend intravenous benzodiazepines as part of the early first-line interventions for cocaine-associated chest pain. Benzodiazepines provide anxiolysis, which will help mitigate cocaine's neuropsychiatric manifestations, and can temper the intense sympathetic tone improving hemodynamics. Benzodiazepines have been proven to be effective, often as a monotherapy agent, in the relief of cocaine-associated chest pain. Further therapeutic intervention is based on the results of the diagnostic workup and patient symptomatology. If chest pain is relieved with benzodiazepines, in the absence of positive ECG findings or cardiac biomarkers, aggressive treatment to normalize hypertension and tachycardia is not needed as they will improve as the effects from cocaine intoxication subside. In a patient who has persistent chest pain or those with definite ACS, hypertension should be corrected with nitroglycerin or nitroprusside. These agents have the desired anti-hypertensive effects and in addition have been found to reverse cocaine-induced coronary artery vasospasm. If further therapeutic agents are needed for blood pressure management, intravenous phentolamine is recommended. Phentolamine, a pure alpha-antagonist, will cause vasodilation and has also been shown to reverse coronary vasospam following cocaine use. Calcium-channel blockers can also be used in patients whose hemodynamics does not improve following benzodiazepines and nitroglycerin. The important difference in management of cocaine-associated chest pain versus other ACS is the contraindication of beta-blockade in the setting of cocaine-use [16, 18].

The contraindication of beta-blockers stems from the physiologic basis of how cocaine induces its hemodynamic effects including coronary artery vasoconstriction. The vasoconstriction of the coronary vessels from cocaine is primarily mediated by increased stimulation of alpha-adrenergic receptors in the vessel walls. Beta-adrenergic stimulation has a predominantly vasodilatory effect on the coronal vessels. Consequently, the use of beta-blockers will leave the alpha-stimulation unopposed and exacerbate the coronary vasoconstriction and worsen the hypertension [3, 16]. This has been proven in two human studies and multiple experimental and animal studies demonstrating increased coronary vasoconstriction, as well as, an increased risk of seizures and overall mortality when beta-blockade is given in the setting of acute cocaine intoxication. Theoretically, use of a nonselective beta-blocker, such as labetalol, which will block both alpha- and beta-receptors should preclude these undesirable effects as it should avoid the unopposed alpha-stimulation. However the beta-blocker effects of labetalol are greater than its alpha-blocking effects and it has not been found to reverse cocaine-induced vasoconstriction and is still associated with increased risk of seizure and death in animal models [19]. This is an ongoing topic of debate in the literature. Recent retrospective studies looking at outcomes of patients who were treated for acute coronary syndrome and then later (through delayed results of toxicology screens) found to be positive for cocaine found improvement in hemodynamics (heart rate and blood pressure both lowered), with no increase in adverse outcomes [14, 20]. More information is still needed before the safety of beta-blockade in this patient population can be assured, and as explained above, remains contraindicated in the acute setting. Following resolution of the acute event, use of beta-blockers can be considered for patients with evidence of coronary artery disease or left ventricular dysfunction on an individual basis weighing the risks and benefits, especially since recurrent use in this population is high.

Thrombolytic therapy, which is included in first-line therapy for non-cocaine-related ACS also carries a relative contraindication in this patient population. Given the significant hypertension associated with acute cocaine use, these patients are also at greater risk for an acute intracranial hemorrhagic event. Only in patients with a confirmed diagnosis of STEMI who cannot receive a percutaneous coronary intervention should thrombolytic therapy be initiated.

In large doses cocaine can lead to hypotension, arrhythmia, and cardiovascular collapse with sudden death [4]. This is thought to be due to profound shifts in sodium concentrations due to cocaine's effect on these channels. By inhibiting the voltage-gated sodium channels, the rate of depolarization and amplitude of the action potential within the sino-atrial pacemaker can be reduced. This slowing of conduction can lead to cardiac dysrhythmias. In addition, this can interfere with depolarization throughout the heart's conduction system which can lead to ventricular standstill and sudden death in massive doses [7, 8]. This risk of severe cardiotoxicity from cocaine use is greater in those who use cocaine chronically. While these users develop tolerance to the euphoric effects of cocaine with chronic use (prompting the use of larger and larger doses), only partial tolerance to cocaine's sympathomimetic effect develops. Thus the massive dose of cocaine that may be ingested by this population in order to achieve the desired euphoric effects puts them at a much greater risk for a fatal cardiovascular event [7].

Pulmonary

Respiratory complications from cocaine use are primarily seen with smoked cocaine. Thermal injury to the oropharynx and airway, including thermal epiglottitis, has been shown from smoking "crack," or free base cocaine. Crack-cocaine has been found to be a powerful airway irritant (in part due to the contaminants inhaled with it) and can cause significant bronchoconstriction. In patients with preexisting conditions, such as Asthma, this can be fatal [9]. "Crack lung" refers to a myriad of acute pulmonary findings following inhalation of freebase cocaine. This involves acute dyspnea, hypoxia, and pulmonary edema. In addition it can present with hemoptysis, fever, and even respiratory collapse. Lung pathology in these users usually shows alveolar damage with evidence of alveolar hemorrhage and eosinophilic infitrates [4]. Pulmonary edema in these patients often represents underlying alveolar hemorrhage and patients can present with hemoptysis as their primary complaint. This is often self-limited and will remit with cessation of further cocaine. This can occur with any route of cocaine administration and is likely due to ischemic injury from vasoconstriction resulting in interstitial and alveolar hemorrhage. Pneumothorax and pneumomediastinum have also been reported and may be the result of harsh coughing fits that occur with inhalational use or from the deep inspirations taken following inhalation to increase absorption of the drug [5]. There have also been reports of pulmonary hypertension with chronic use [9]. Ischemic injury to the nasopharynx and oropharynx occur with chronic use of cocaine powder due to its local vasoconstrictive properties. This results in epistaxis, nasal septum perforations, and ulcerative lesions of the oropharynx [21].

CNS Toxicity

Cocaine has also been found to be neurotoxic with chronic use. One proposed mechanism for its neurotoxicity is through a cocaine-mediated increase in calcium in dopaminergic neurons. The increased intracellular calcium then activates phospholipases which in turn increase dopamine efflux from the neuron terminal. When activated over prolonged periods of time, the increase in intracellular phospholipase metabolism causes an increase in free radical formation. The end result is neuronal loss over time with chronic cocaine use [2].

Given the increase in excitatory neurotransmitters that results from cocaine use, seizures have been associated with both acute and chronic cocaine use. They are more common in chronic abusers but can occur with acute use, especially with first-time use [8]. It also lowers the seizure threshold so that in patients with a known seizure history, cocaine use increases their risk of seizure by twofold. Most often these seizures are tonic-clonic in nature and are isolated single events that resolve without treatment. They can however, forewarn of a potentially fatal event especially when there are multiple seizures associated with a cardiac dysrhythmia, hyperpyrexia, or acidosis [8, 9].

Cocaine use also increases the risk of both hemorrhagic and ischemic cerebrovascular accidents. Intracranial hemorrhage and infarction is most likely related to the profound hypertension with impaired cerebral autoregulation that can result with cocaine intoxication [8]. While the risk of hemorrhagic stroke is greater in patients with a preexisting vascular abnormality (such as an aneurysm or an arteriovenous malformation), it can also occur in patients with normal cerebral vasculature as well. Cerebral ischemia results from cocaines potent vasoconstriction of cerebral arteries and is more common with chronic use [9, 11].

Movement disorders, such as choreoathetosis and akathisia are not uncommon with chronic abuse. With chronic use there can be a central dopamine depletion and even degeneration of dopamine nerve terminals resulting in Parkinsonian-like motor dysfunction [8]. The cocaine-induced changes in cerebral serotonin levels are believed to be the cause of disorders in sleep and wakefulness in people who use cocaine chronically and during cocaine withdrawal [11].

Gastrointestinal, Renal, and Musculoskeletal Toxicity

Cocaine use has been linked to ischemic injury of the GI tract. This can be severe enough to result in gastric or small bowel ulceration and perforation. Gastrointestinal ischemia is thought to be the result of intense vasoconstriction and possibly thrombosis of the gastric mesenteric vasculature [5]. Since the cells lining the gastric mucosa and small bowel readily become ischemic with reductions in their blood flow, ischemia could rapidly result when blood flow is compromised. In very high doses cocaine can also function as an anticholinergic agent and thus interfere with gastric motility and emptying. This further increases risk of gastric ulceration and perforation due to prolonged exposure to gastric acid [8]. The patients who present with cocaine-induced ischemia or perforation will often be younger patients (versus the 48–65 year old age group who more commonly suffer from peptic ulcer disease) and it is usually within 3 days of last cocaine use [21]. Like other stimulants, cocaine also acts as an appetite suppressant. This can lead to poor nutritional status with chronic use [8].

Cocaine use has also been implicated in causing acute renal failure and infarction. Most commonly acute renal failure from cocaine use is the indirect result of acute tubular necrosis secondary to cocaine-induced rhabdomyolysis. Rhabdomyolysis in the setting of cocaine toxicity can occur by vasoconstriction induced ischemia, muscle injury resulting from hyperthermia or cocaine-induced seizures, or by direct muscle toxicity [8, 9]. Renal injury and even infarction can also result from vasoconstriction or thrombosis of renal arteries. Cocaine is also thought to be directly nephrotoxic by causing alterations in glomerular matrix synthesis and metabolism resulting in increased oxidative stress in the kidney itself [22].

Cocaine and Alcohol: A Deadly Combination

When cocaine and ethanol are consumed together, they produce a metabolite cocaethylene which is deadlier than either cocaine or ethanol alone [2]. Cocaethylene has a more intense inhibition of dopamine reuptake than cocaine does, which produces a greater "high" while minimizing feelings of dysphoria. The euphoria produced by cocaethylene also last longer than that achieved by cocaine alone. The prolonged effect achieved can be explained at a pharmacologic level as cocaethylene has a longer half-life than cocaine itself, $t\frac{1}{2}$ of 150 versus 90 min of cocaine. In addition to the euphoric effects of cocaethylene, it also acts as a sympathomimetic agent and thus causes a more pronounced increase in heart rate, blood pressure, and coronary vasoconstriction, with a further increase in myocardial oxygen demand [2]. What is more, the use of ethanol with cocaine interferes with cocaine metabolism thus further compounding its effect. The end result is a greatly enhanced cardiotoxicity when cocaine and ethanol are used compared to either one alone. In fact, the combination has been shown to increase the risk for cardiac events by 40-times with a 25-times increased risk for sudden death [4]. This effect will occur when even a small amount of cocaine is used in the presence of ethanol [15]. This is especially important to be aware of as 50–90 % of cocaine users will simultaneously ingest ethanol during their cocaine binges [3].

Cocaine and Pregnancy

Cocaine use with pregnancy places the pregnant mother at increased risk. It increases risk of miscarriage, preterm labor, cardiac events (hypertensive crisis, myocardial infarction), and placental abruption. This is thought to be the result of cocaine-induced vasoconstriction which will decrease placental blood flow and cause fetal ischemia [8]. In addition, since those who abuse cocaine during pregnancy tend to be of lower socioeconomic status they are more likely to have little to no prenatal care. Furthermore, since plasma cholinesterase activity is reduced in pregnancy this decreases the pregnant woman's ability to metabolize cocaine which can lead to a prolonged effect when used during pregnancy.

Cocaine readily passes through the placenta and can also be passed through the mammary gland and into a breastfeeding mother's milk. Cocaine is associated with increased risk of intrauterine growth retardation and low birth weight, congenital malformations (especially of the CNS and cardiac system), mental retardation, and delayed development. There can also be strong drug dependence in newborns [2, 7].

Withdrawal and Treatment

Cocaine withdrawal is not life-threatening. It is also not consistent. In several studies of inpatients monitored following cocaine cessation, many did not exhibit any signs or symptoms of withdrawal [11]. The diagnostic criteria for cocaine withdrawal include dysphoric mood with two or more associated symptoms: fatigue, vivid or unpleasant dreams, insomnia or hypersomnia, increased appetite, psychomotor retardation or agitation. For the diagnosis to be made, these symptoms must cause distress or impairment in normal functioning and must not be due to another medical or psychiatric condition [23].

Typically following the termination of cocaine use, in the first several hours the patient will "crash" with feelings of anxiety, depression, drug craving, exhaustion, and hypersomnolence [9]. Following this, the "dopamine washout" that occurs centrally with long-term cocaine use will cause cravings for the drug, as well as a more protracted depressed mood with anhedonia.

There are no current medications specific for the treatment of cocaine addiction or dependence, or from cocaine withdrawal. There is good evidence showing that cocaine abusers are at greater risk for having major psychological and psychosocial impairments [15]. Treatment of these underlying disorders is recommended once identified. Multiple studies have looked at the efficacy of using benzodiazepines, anti-depressants, and even stimulants in cocaine-dependent patients; however none has proven to have consistent clinically significant effect in this population [11, 16].

References

1. Substance Abuse and Mental Health Services Administration. Results from the 2012 National Survey on Drug Use and Health: summary of national findings. NSDUH series H-46 (HHS publication no. (SMA) 13-4795). SAMHSA; 2013.
2. Pincus MR, Abraham NZ. Toxicology and therapeutic drug monitoring. In: McPherson RA, Pincus MR, editors. Henry's clinical diagnosis and management by laboratory methods. 22nd ed. Philadelphia: Saunders; 2011.
3. Goldstein RA, DesLauriers C, Burda AM. Cocaine: history, social implications, and toxicity–a review. Dis Mon. 2009;55(1):6–38.
4. Cain MA, Bornick P, Whiteman V. The maternal, fetal, and neonatal effects of cocaine exposure in pregnancy. Clin Obstet Gynecol. 2013;56(1):124–32.
5. Zimmerman J, Alapat P. Cocaine. In: Vincent JL, editor. Textbook of critical care. 6th ed. Philadelphia: Elsevier/Saunders; 2011. p. 1379–81.

6. Camí J, Farré M. Drug addiction. N Engl J Med. 2003;349(10):975–86.
7. Boghdadi MS, Henning RJ. Cocaine: pathophysiology and clinical toxicology. Heart Lung. 1997;26(6):466–83.
8. White SM, Lambe CJT. The pathophysiology of cocaine abuse. J Clin Forensic Med. 2003;10(1):27–39.
9. Glauser J, Queen JR. An overview of non-cardiac cocaine toxicity. J Emerg Med. 2007;32(2): 181–6.
10. Mariani JJ, Levin FR. Psychostimulant treatment of cocaine dependence. Psychiatr Clin North Am. 2012;35(2):425–6.
11. Mendelson JH, Mello NK. Management of cocaine abuse and dependence. N Engl J Med. 1996;334(15):965–72.
12. Qureshi AI, Suri FK, Guterman LR, Hopkins LN. Cocaine use and the likelihood of nonfatal myocardial infarction and stroke: data from the third National Health and Nutrition Examination Survey. Circulation. 2001;103(4):502–6.
13. Brickner ME, Willard JE, et al. Left ventricular hypertrophy associated with chronic cocaine abuse. Circulation. 1991;84(3):1130–5.
14. Finkel JB, Marhefka GD. Rethinking cocaine-associated chest pain and acute coronary syndromes. Mayo Clin Proc. 2011;86(12):1198–207.
15. Schwartz BG, Rezkalla S, Kloner RA. Cardiovascular effects of cocaine. Circulation. 2010;122(24):2558–69.
16. Afonso L, Mohammad T, Thatai D. Crack whips the heart: a review of the cardiovascular toxicity of cocaine. Am J Cardiol. 2007;100(6):1040–3.
17. Rang HP, Dale MM, Ritter JM, Flower RJ, Henderson G, editors. Rang and Dale's pharmacology. 7th ed. Edinburgh: Elsevier; 2012. p. 584–91.
18. National Guideline Clearinghouse (NGC). Management of cocaine-associated chest pain and myocardial infarction. A scientific statement from the American Heart Association Acute Cardiac Care Committee of the Council on Clinical Cardiology. Agency for Healthcare Research and Quality (AHRQ). http://www.guideline.gov/content.aspx?id=12951. Accessed 4 Sept 2013.
19. McCord J, Jneid H, Hollander JE, et al. Management of cocaine-associated chest pain and myocardial infarction: a scientific statement from the American Heart Association Acute Cardiac Care Committee of the Council on Clinical Cardiology. Circulation. 2008;117(14):1897–907.
20. Ibrahim M, Maselli DJ, Hasan R. Safety of β-blockers in the acute management of cocaine-associated chest pain. Am J Emerg Med. 2013;31(6):989.
21. Shanti CM, Lucas CE. Cocaine and the critical care challenge. Crit Care Med. 2003;31(6): 1851–9.
22. Bemanian S, Motallebi M, Nosrati S. Cocaine-induced renal infarction: report of a case and review of the literature. BMC Nephrol. 2005;6:10.
23. American Psychiatric Association. Cocaine-induced disorder. diagnostic and statistical manual of mental disorders, fourth edition, text revision (DSM-IV-TR). 4th ed. Arlington: American Psychiatric Association; 2000.

Chapter 13
Management of Acute and Chronic Drug Abuse of Amphetamines

Sahra Lantz-Dretnik, Michal Czernicki, and Sreekumar Kunnumpurath

Key Points

- Amphetamines
- Mode of action
- Clinical effects by system (pharmacodynamics)
- Pharmacokinetics
- Acute amphetamine intoxication

Introduction

Amphetamine was first discovered in the 1800s, although its medical use was not recognised until 1929, when biochemist Gordon Alles was searching for an alternative decongestant and bronchodilator to ephedrine. After publishing his works [1–3], amphetamine salts were patented and by 1933, amphetamines were advertised as over-the-counter inhaler in the form of Benzedrine Inhaler, a tube containing 325 mg of oily amphetamine base [4]. By 1937, the American Medical Association (AMA) approved advertising of "Benzedrine Sulfate", racemic amphetamine tablets for narcolepsy, postencephalitic Parkinsonism and minor depression [5].

S. Lantz-Dretnik, M.B.B.S., B.Sc. (Hon.), F.R.C.A. (✉)
St George's Hospital, Blackshaw Road, London, SW17 0QT, UK
e-mail: slantzdretnik@doctors.org.uk

M. Czernicki, F.R.C.A., F.F.P.M.R.C.A., M.D.
Department of Anesthesia and Pain Management, Nottingham University Hospital
in United Kingdom, 3 Melrose Gardens, Nottingham, Nottinghamshire, UK
e-mail: mczernicki@yahoo.com

S. Kunnumpurath, M.B.B.S., M.D., F.F.P.M.R.C.A., F.R.C.A., F.C.A.R.C.S.I.
Department of Anesthetics and Pain Management, Epsom and St. Helier University Hospitals
NHS Trust, Wryth Lane, SM5 1AA Carshalton, UK
e-mail: skunnumpurath@gmail.com

© Springer Science+Business Media New York 2015
A.D. Kaye et al. (eds.), *Substance Abuse*, DOI 10.1007/978-1-4939-1951-2_13

Amphetamines grew in success and in the Second World War, it was used to combat "battle fatigue". It is said to have caused psychosis-like aggression in some soldiers. Given such widespread use, not surprisingly, significant abuse of amphetamines quickly developed. By the 1960s, a study based in Newcastle suggested that enough amphetamines were dispensed to supply more than 1 % of the total population with 60 tablets per month and that between 20 and 25 % of these patients were addicted or dependent to some degree [6, 7].

The World Drug Report 2013, by the United Nations, suggests that the market for amphetamine-type stimulants is expanding. Its use appears globally widespread with 0.7 % of the world's population aged 15–64 having abused amphetamines in the preceding year. Methamphetamine continues to be the mainstay of seized drugs, crystalline methamphetamine in particular with 8.8 ton seized, the highest level during past 5 years suggesting imminent threat [8]. Use appears to vary with gender and race. Recent studies have found correlations between personality traits (risk taking and reward sensitivity) and responses to amphetamine use [9].

Amphetamine has many street names including speed, uppers, crystal meth, ice and white and most types are categorised as a Class B drug in the UK and a Schedule II drug in the US. However, methamphetamine is considered a Class A drug.

Amphetamines

Amphetamine is a psychostimulant drug of the phenethylamine class that increases the activity of dopamine, serotonin and noradrenaline in the brain. Its clinical use includes treatment for narcolepsy and Attention Deficit Hyperactivity Disorder, but it remains a common recreational drug. It elevates users mood, making them euphoric and chatty, heightens libido, makes users resistant to fatigue enabling them to dance and stay awake for hours. It also causes loss of appetite, which is why amphetamine remains a common ingredient in weight loss tablets. However, it may also cause anxiety, aggression and psychosis. Recreational doses are generally far larger than prescribed therapeutic doses, and recreational use therefore carries far greater risk and far more serious side effects [1].

Epidemiology

In the United States, amphetamine is characteristically used by single white men, aged 20–35 years who typically are unemployed [10]. Data from rural populations reveal that Caucasians use amphetamines significantly more than African Americans [11]. However, amphetamine use is becoming more common among women and other ethnic groups.

Reasons for why fewer women than men use amphetamines may be explained by the action of oestrogen within the CNS. Women in their late follicular phase, when oestrogen levels are high and progesterone levels are low, were more likely to report "unpleasant stimulation" when exposed to amphetamine. This effect was not observed in the early follicular phase, when both hormone levels are low [12].

Pharmacology

Amphetamine is a 1-phenylpropan-2-amine or $C_9H_{13}N$ and exists as two enantiomers: the levorotary form levamfetamine and dextrorotary form dexamfetamine, presented as a powder. The dextrorotary form is several times more potent than the levorotary form. The powder can be mixed with water to make tablets or put into capsules for oral administration, the only route used in therapeutic settings. Recreationally, it is also commonly insufflated, injected or administered rectally.

Mode of Action

Amphetamine causes its behavioural effects by neurotransmitter modulation [13] in particular but not exclusively through effects on dopamine, serotonin, noradrenaline, acetylcholine and glutamate [14–18].

Studies have shown that amphetamine increases the amount of dopamine, noradrenaline and serotonin in the synaptic cleft in certain parts of the brain enhancing the post-synaptic neuronal response [14, 18–20]. There are multiple mechanisms of how amphetamine increases neurotransmitter levels, firstly amphetamine is similar in structure to these neurotransmitters and can therefore enter the synapse via various neurotransmitter transporting system and diffusion across the membrane, activating Trace Amine-Associated Receptor 1 (TAAR1). This causes neurotransmitter efflux and reuptake inhibition, increasing neurotransmitter concentrations [14]. Secondly, amphetamine acts as substrate for Vesicular MonoAmine Transporter 2 (VMAT2) and when taken up by VMAT2, causes vesicle release of dopamine, noradrenaline and serotonin [11]. In addition, amphetamines also inhibit monoamine oxidase, the enzyme responsible for intracellular breakdown of these neurotransmitters.

Elevated catecholamine levels lead to a state of increased arousal and decreased fatigue, whilst increased dopamine levels at synapses in the CNS are implicated in movement disorders [21], schizophrenia and euphoria. High levels of serotonin may play a role in the hallucinogenic and anorexic [22] aspects of amphetamines. Other serotonergic and dopaminergic effects may include resetting the thermal regulatory circuits in the hypothalamus and causing hyperthermia. The hyperthermia produced by amphetamines is similar to that of the serotonin syndrome.

Amphetamine also causes elevated levels of acetylcholine, particularly in the hippocampus, caudate nucleus, prefrontal cortex, nucleus accumbens and basal ganglia. This is thought to be due to its effect on dopamine receptor 1 and 2 (D_1, D_2) and may explain at least in part the nootropic (memory enhancing) effects of amphetamine [15]. Extracellular concentrations of glutamate have also been found to be enhanced in the mesocorticolimbic projection, particularly the nucleus accumbens, an area implicated in reward and pleasure following amphetamine use [16, 17].

The effects of amphetamines on the brain appear to be site specific and appear to be linked with the presence of TAAR1 and its associated monoamine transporters [14].

Physiological adaptation occurs through downregulation of receptors. This tolerance and an accompanying psychological tolerance [23] can lead to escalating use of the drug and increased toxicity [24]. Chronic use can lead to a depletion of neurotransmitter stores and a paradoxical reverse effect of the drug, a wash out.

Clinical Effects by System (Pharmacodynamics)

Cardiovascular: Inotropic and chronotropic effects on the heart leading to tachycardia and in large doses may induce arrhythmias [25]. The vasoconstrictive properties lead to increase in systolic and diastolic blood pressures and may result in coronary vasospasm [26]. Patient may complain of palpitations. Long-term use can lead to myonecrosis and dilated cardiomyopathy [26].

Respiratory: Through stimulation of medullary respiratory systems, causes increase respiratory rate and tidal volume by stimulation of medullary respiratory systems. Only clinically important in chronic users where it may lead to pulmonary hypertension [27, 28].

Genito-urinary: Acute urinary retention may occur secondary to increased sphincter tone. The commonly seen dehydration post large recreational doses may cause acute kidney injury (AKI), potentially complicated further if rhabdomyolysis occurs following acute amphetamine toxicity. AKI can cause further fluid and electrolyte imbalances with its own consequences. Erectile dysfunction may also occur.

Metabolic: Acute toxicity may lead to hyperthermia.

Central Nervous System: Pupils appear dilated and user may complain of blurred vision, headache and dizziness. Seizure threshold is reduced, one study from San Francisco suggests that approximately 25 % of all drug-induced seizures were secondary to amphetamine use [29].

Gastrointestinal: May cause diarrhoea, constipation or weight loss.

Skin: Diaphoresis, erythematous painful rashes, flushing.

Psychological: Psychosis which may present itself as paranoia, hallucinations and delusions. A Cochrane review in 2009 suggested as many as 15 % of amphetamine induced psychosis failed to recover completely, whether this results from unmasking underlying disease is unclear. Other common effects include increased libido, alertness, self-confidence, sociability, irritability, aggression, grandiosity and repetitive and obsessive behaviour including restlessness.

Pharmacokinetics

Routes of Administration

When taken orally, amphetamines have low bioavailability. The effects appear within the first 15–60 min following administration, peaking 2–3 h later [30]. Taken orally, many of the common impurities in street amphetamine can be dealt with via first pass metabolism. Whilst it is the safest route of administration, it produces a less intense effect albeit longer lasting.

Insufflation or snorting of amphetamine results in an increased bioavailability of up to 75 %, giving a more intense effect apparent within minutes, however more short lived. It is a popular way of taking amphetamine recreationally.

The practice of injecting amphetamine intravenously or subcutaneously remains common in some parts of the world, popular due to its intense immediate effect [31–33]. Although the effects are short lived, it is the most dangerous route, partly due to unpredictability of effect and in part due to complications associated with lack of aseptic injection techniques.

Rectal administration, referred to as "plugging" on the street, has not been studied in academic studies and therefore any evidence is anecdotal. Through drug forums online, it is suggested that it has better bioavailability compared to the oral route but worse than insufflation.

Methamphetamine may also be smoked.

Distribution, Metabolism and Excretion

About 15–40 % of amphetamine is bound to protein in the plasma and has a half-life of 11–13 h. It undergoes metabolism in the liver by CYP450[2], producing a variety of metabolites, some of which are biologically active such as hippuric acid, noradrenaline, parahydroxyamphetamine and *p*-hydroxynoradrenaline. Amphetamine is renally excreted with a proportion of the drug being excreted unchanged. About 70 % is cleared in 24 h, but this process depends on urinary pH. The p*K*a of amphetamine is 9.8, therefore when the urine is more basic, less is excreted. Apparent half-life and duration of effect increase with repeated use and accumulation of the drug [34, 35].

Amphetamine can be detected in serum and urine up to 48 h after ingestion.

Acute Amphetamine Intoxication

Patients with amphetamine intoxication often are identified by a change of mental status alone with or without associated injury and/or illness. Common presenting complaints in acute amphetamine toxicity are summarised in Table 13.1. Common signs and symptoms of acute intoxication are summarised in Table 13.2.

Table 13.1 Common presenting complaints in acute amphetamine toxicity	
	• Seizures
	• Hypertension
	• Tachyarrhythmias
	• Hyperthermia
	• Psychosis
	• Stroke (through hypertensive crisis or vasospasm)
	• Trauma associated with risk taking behaviour
	• Sepsis
	• Death

Table 13.2 Common signs and symptoms

• Chest pain
• Palpitations
• Shortness of breath
• Urinary retention
• Hyperthermia
• Change of mental status including agitation, aggression, euphoria, disorientation, mydriasis, headache, dyskinesia, formication, seizures, symptoms of stroke, coma, bruxism
• Nausea and vomiting
• Dry mouth
• Diaphoresis

With chronic use, you are likely to encounter a malnourished, anorexic patient with poor skin with possible cellulitis, abscesses, phlebitis or vasculitis with intravenous user and poor dentition ("Meth" teeth)

Table 13.3 Differential diagnosis

1. Acute coronary syndrome
2. Anxiety
3. Other substance toxicity (anticholinergics, antihistamine, caffeine, cocaine, hallucinogens, MDMA, monoamine oxidase inhibitors, mushrooms, sympathomimetics)
4. Chorea
5. Delirium
6. Encephalitis/meningitis
7. Electrolyte imbalances
8. Hypoglycaemia
9. Psychosis
10. Subarachnoid haemorrhage
11. Withdrawal syndromes

Physical examination

Particularly neurological and cardiovascular signs, physical examination findings may demonstrate a variety of symptoms, particularly CNS and cardiovascular symptoms. Small modification of the basic amphetamine molecule produces compounds with variable effects on target organs, i.e. methamphetamine produces prominent central nervous system effects with minimal cardiovascular stimulation (Table 13.3).

Further Inpatient Care

Admission is appropriate for monitoring and treatment of any serious sequelae of amphetamine intoxication. A patient with stable vital signs who exhibits paranoid psychosis and has no evidence of cardiac, cerebral, renal, hepatic or pulmonary complications of amphetamine use may need to be transferred to a psychiatric hospital for observation and treatment.

Outpatient Care

Patients may require follow up for any complications following acute intoxication or chronic amphetamine use. Referrals for outpatient detoxification centres or for management of addictive behaviours may also be necessary if the patient is compliant.

Chronic Abuse Sequelae

An individual who misuses amphetamine long term is likely to develop vitamin deficiencies, appear pale and malnourished and have one of several skin disorders. Dentition is poor and individuals who chronically use amphetamines intravenously are at risk of infection and vascular injury. Amphetamine misusers may have suffered complications as a consequence of acute toxicity including myocardial infarction, stroke or AKI. Cardiovascularly, long-term use can lead to myonecrosis and dilated cardiomyopathy [26], further complicated by pulmonary hypertension [27, 28]. They are at high risk of mental health problems, particularly psychosis.

Special Patient Groups

Use of amphetamines in pregnancy may cause fetal abnormalities, fetal growth retardation, miscarriage, prematurity and stillbirth. This is due to serotonergic action of amphetamines on peripheral vasculature which leads to vasoconstriction, which is especially problematic in placental vessels [36].

Serotonin Syndrome

Serotonin syndrome is a potentially life-threatening drug reaction that may occur following amphetamine use. It is due to excess serotonergic activity in the CNS and peripheral serotonin receptors causing cognitive, autonomic and somatic effects and may cause anything from mild symptoms to causing death [37]. There is no diagnostic test and treatment is supportive.

Summary

Although initially used to treat nasal congestion and battle fatigue, amphetamine is today used in treatment of narcolepsy, ADHD and weight loss. However, it is a common recreational drug with 0.7 % of the world population between 15 and 64 having used it in the past year. Acute amphetamine intoxication is potentially life threatening with several serious medical sequelae. It is imperative that clinicians manage well in the acute setting, but also keeps an open mind as its presentation carries a wide differential diagnosis. Amphetamine is a highly addictive drug with rapidly increasing tolerance. Chronic misuse results in serious medical and psychiatric health problems, which often leads to premature death (Fig. 13.1).

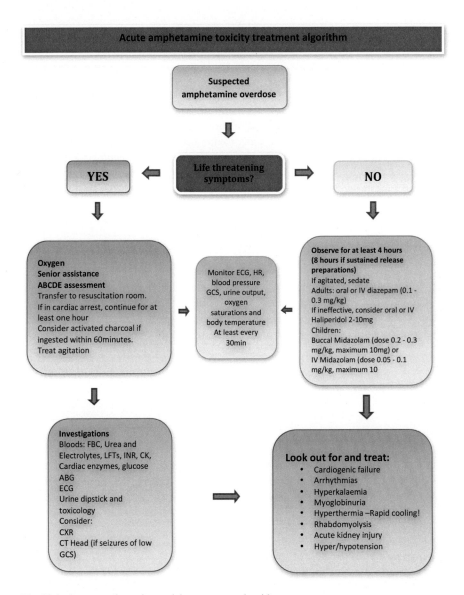

Fig. 13.1 Acute amphetamine toxicity treatment algorithm

References

1. Trevor AJ, Katzung BG, Kruidering-Hall MM, Masters SB. Chapter 32. Drugs of abuse. In: Trevor AJ, Katzung BG, Kruidering-Hall MM, Masters SB, editors. Katzung & Trevor's pharmacology: examination & board review. 10th ed. New York: McGraw-Hill; 2013.
2. Miranda-G E, Sordo M, Salazar AM. Determination of amphetaminoe, methamphetamine, and hydroxyamphetamine derivatives in urine by gas chromatography-mass spectrometry and its relation to CYP2D6 phenotype of drug users. J Anal Toxicol. 2007;31(1):31–6. PMID 17389081.
3. Piness G, Miller H, Alles G. Clinical observations on phenylethanolamine sulfate. J Am Med Assoc. 1930;94:790–1.
4. AMA Council on Pharmacy and Chemistry. Benzedrine. J Am Med Assoc. 1933;101:1315.
5. AMA Council on Pharmacy and Chemistry, Present status of benzedrine sulfate. J Am Med Assoc. 1937;109:2064–9.
6. Kiloh LG, Brandon S. Habituation and addiction to amphetamines. Br Med J. 1962;2(5296): 40–3.
7. Brandon S, Smith D. Amphetamines in general practice. J Coll Gen Pract. 1962;5:603–6.
8. World drug report; 2013.
9. White TL, Lott DC, de Wit H. Personality and the subjective effects of acute amphetamine in healthy volunteers. Neuropsychopharmacology. 2006;31(5):1064–74.
10. Huang B, Dawson DA, Stinson FS, Hasin DS, Ruan WJ, Saha TD, et al. Prevalence, correlates, and comorbidity of nonmedical prescription drug use and drug use disorders in the United States: results of the National Epidemiologic Survey on alcohol and related conditions. J Clin Psychiatry. 2006;67(7):1062–73.
11. Borders TF, Booth BM, Han X, Wright P, Leukefeld C, Falck RS, et al. Longitudinal changes in methamphetamine and cocaine use in untreated rural stimulant users: racial differences and the impact of methamphetamine legislation. Addiction. 2008;103(5):800–8 [Medline].
12. Justice AJ, De Wit H. Acute effects of d-amphetamine during the early and late follicular phases of the menstrual cycle in women. Pharmacol Biochem Behav. 2000;66(3):509–15.
13. Bidwell LC, McClernon FJ, Kollins SH. Cognitive enhancers for the treatment of ADHD. Pharmacol Biochem Behav. 2011;99(2):262–74.
14. Miller GM. The emerging role of trace amine-associated receptor 1 in the functional regulation of monoamine transporters and dopaminergic activity. J Neurochem. 2011;116(2):164–76.
15. Brodie B. Effects of cocaine and amphetamine on acetylcholine release in the hippocampus and caudate nucleus. *Publisher Medical*. Department of Neuroscience, University of Cagliari, Italy. Accessed 5 June 2013.
16. Stuber GD, Hnasko TS, Britt JP, Edwards RH, Bonci A. Dopaminergic terminals in the nucleus accumbens but not the dorsal striatum corelease glutamate. J Neurosci. 2010;30(24):8229–33. doi:10.1523/JNEUROSCI.1754-10.2010. PMC 2918390. PMID 20554874.
17. Gu XL. Deciphering the corelease of glutamate from dopaminergic terminals derived from the ventral tegmental area. J Neurosci. 2010;30(41):13549–51.
18. Eiden LE, Weihe E. VMAT2: a dynamic regulator of brain monoaminergic neuronal function interacting with drugs of abuse. Ann N Y Acad Sci. 2011;1216:86–98.
19. Sulzer D. How addictive drugs disrupt presynaptic dopamine neurotransmission. Neuron. 2011;69(4):628–49. doi:10.1016/j.neuron.2011.02.010. PMC 3065181. PMID 21338876.
20. Kuczenski R, Segal DS. Effects of methylphenidate on extracellular dopamine, serotonin, and norepinephrine: comparison with amphetamine. J Neurochem. 1997;68(5):2032–7.
21. Downes MA, Whyte IM. Amphetamine-induced movement disorder. Emerg Med Australas. 2005;17(3):277–80.
22. Wappler F, Roewer N, Kochling A, Scholz J, Loscher W, Steinfath M. Effects of the serotonin2 receptor agonist DOI on skeletal muscle specimens from malignant hyperthermia-susceptible patients. Anesthesiology. 1996;84(6):1280–7.

23. Murray JB. Psychophysiological aspects of amphetamine-methamphetamine abuse. J Psychol. 1998;132(2):227–37.
24. Karch S. The problem of methamphetamine toxicity. West J Med. 1999;170(4):232.
25. Westfall DP, Westfall TC. 12: adrenergic agonist and antagonists. In: Brunton LL, Chabner BA, Knollmann BC, editors. Goodman & Gilman's pharmacological basis of therapeutics. 12th ed. New York: McGraw-Hill; 2010. p. 277–334.
26. Jacobs W. Fatal amphetamine-associated cardiotoxicity and its medicolegal implications. Am J Forensic Med Pathol. 2006;27(2):156–60.
27. Albertson TE. Amphetamines. In: Olson KR, Anderson IB, Benowitz NL, Blanc PD, Kearney TE, Kim-Katz SY, Wu AHB, editors. Poisoning & drug overdose. 6th ed. New York: McGraw-Hill Medical; 2011. p. 77–9.
28. Chin KM, Channick RN, Rubin LJ. Is methamphetamine use associated with idiopathic pulmonary arterial hypertension? Chest. 2006;130(6):1657–63.
29. Alldredge BK, Lowenstein DH, Simon RP. Seizures associated with recreational drug abuse. Neurology. 1989;39(8):1037–9.
30. Angrist B, Corwin J, Bartlik B, Cooper T. Early pharmacokinetics and clinical effects of oral D-amphetamine in normal subjects. Biol Psychiatry. 1987;22(11):1357–68.
31. Robson P, Bruce M. A comparison of 'visible' and 'invisible' users of amphetamine, cocaine and heroin: two distinct populations? Addiction. 1997;92(12):1729–36.
32. Luna CG. Use and abuse of amphetamine-type stimulants in the United States of America. Rev Panam Salud Publica. 2001;9(2):114–21.
33. Peters A, Davies T, Richardson A. Increasing popularity of injection as the route of administration of amphetamine in Edinburgh. Drug Alcohol Depend. 1997;48(3):227–34.
34. Shargel L, Wu-Pong S, Yu A. Applied biopharmaceutics & pharmacokinetics. 6th ed. New York: McGraw-Hill; 2012.
35. Flomenbaum NE, Goldfrank LR, Hoffman RS, Howland MA, Lewin NA, Nelson LS. Goldfrank's toxicologic emergencies. 8th ed. New York: McGraw-Hill; 2006.
36. Uvnas-Moberg K, Hillegaart V, Alster P, Ahlenius S. Effects of 5-HT agonists, selective for different receptor subtypes, on oxytocin, CCK, gastrin and somatostatin plasma levels in the rat. Neuropharmacology. 1996;35(11):1635–40.
37. Boyer EW, Shannon M. The serotonin syndrome. N Engl J Med. 2005;352(11):1112–20.

Chapter 14
Herbal Supplements and Abuse

Karina Gritsenko, Iyabo Muse, and Amaresh Vydyanathan

Key Points

- Commonly used herbs and supplements
- Other emerging drug of abuse

Introduction

Centuries ago, plants were the predominate agents used for medicinal purpose. In about "1920 standardized pharmaceutical drugs began to replace herbal medicines in the US and were found to have a greater pharmacological benefit and profitability" [1]. Thus, there was a decline in the use of herbal medicine for over 70 years. However, in 1994 after the introduction of the Dietary Supplement Health and Education Act (DSHEA) passed by congress, allowing manufacturers to market their herbal products without evidence of safety or efficacy, a resurgence of herbal supplements and drugs usage was noticed [2]. "In a 2007 National Health Interview Survey (NHIS) Alternative Medicine Supplement showed that 17.7 % of US adults compared to 2.5 % adults in 1990 reported using herbs and other naturally occurring non botanical supplements" [3]. Even till today, some cultures such as Asian, Russian, Native American, and African cultures still rely on herbs as the primary source of healing.

A. Gritsenko, M.D. (✉) • I. Muse, M.D.
Department of Anesthesiology, Montefiore Medical Center—Albert Einstein College of Medicine, 111 East 210th Street, Bronx 10467, NY, USA
e-mail: karina.gritsenko@gmail.com; bunmi.muse@gmail.com

A. Vydyanathan, M.B.B.S., M.S.
Assistant Professor of Anesthesiology Fellowship Co-Director Regional Anesthesia and Acute Pain Medicine Montefiore Medical Center, 3400 Bainbridge Ave, LL 400, Bronx, NY 10467, USA

© Springer Science+Business Media New York 2015
A.D. Kaye et al. (eds.), *Substance Abuse*, DOI 10.1007/978-1-4939-1951-2_14

In the US, there have been few evidence-based studies that have been done to evaluate the efficacy, safety, and drug interactions of herbal supplements with pharmaceutical drugs. In an effort to improve knowledge of these botanical supplements, the National Center for Complementary and Alternative Medicine (NCCAM) was created to establish dedicated botanical research centers. The US Food and Drug Administration (FDA) has also recently been involved in laying down ground rules for Good Manufacturing Practices (GMPs) for dietary supplements. Even with the assistance of these organizations, there have been few to no systematic data about the side effects of herbal drugs on surgical patients and how ingestion can alter medical management. There are only few articles present that show side effects and complications in humans and most are from case reports [4, 5]. Thus, the focus of this chapter is to describe some of the most common herbal drugs and supplements used in the US, their side effects, drug interactions, and how it may change medical, anesthetic, and surgical management in patients. There will also be a discussion of Cannabis abuse and the new generation of related herbal substances which have been produced and exploited by certain people in today's society.

Commonly Used Herbs and Supplements

According to data from NCCAM, there are "over 120 conventionally used pharmaceuticals derived from plant species" [1, 6]. Some drug names with their plant derivatives used by various medical specialists are listed in Table 14.1. In addition, Table 14.2 displays the list of commonly used herbs and supplements according to the US National Library of Medicine (NLM). It is important to understand the common uses as well as potential risks with regards to these commonly used substances. The following will include a detailed description of some common agents [7–10].

Table 14.1 Examples of conventional medications with plant origins

Drug	Herb common name (Latin name)
Atropine	Belladonna (*Atropa belladonna*)
Codeine	Poppy (*Papaver somniferum*)
Colchicine	Autumn crocus (*Colchicum autumnale*)
Digoxin	Foxglove (*Digitalis purpurea*)
Ephedrine	Ephedra (*Ephedra sinica*)
Reserpine	Rauwolfia (*Rauwolfia Serpentina*)
Salicylic acid	Willow bark (*Salix purpurea*)
Scopolamine	Jimson weed (*Datura stramonium*)
Taxol	Pacific view (*Taxus brevifolia*)
Vincristine	Madagascar periwinkle (*Catharanthus roseus*)

Modified from Saper RB. Overview of herbal medicine and dietary supplements. UptoDate http://www.uptodate.com/contents/overview-of-herbal-medicine-and-dietary-supplements?source=search_result&search=Complementary+and+alternative+medicine&selectedTitle=2%7E150#subscribeMessage

Table 14.2 Commonly used herbs in the US: side effects[a]

Herbs	Botanical/Latin name	Percentage	Side effects
Fish oil		37.4	Nausea, "fishy taste" after burping
Echinacea		19.8	Tachyphylaxis, unpleasant taste, hepatotoxicity, affect CYP450
Flax seed oil	Linum usitatissimum	15.9	
Ginseng	Panax ginseng, Panax quinquefolius	14.1	Insomnia, hypoglycemia, vomiting, prolonged bleeding time
Ginkgo biloba		11.3	Platelet dysfunction, possible serotonin syndrome w/MAOIs
Garlic	Allium sativum	11.0	Halitosis, GI upset
Coenzyme Q-10	Ubiquinol, ubiquinone	8.7	Nausea, vomiting, heartburn
Fiber or psyllium		6.6	
Green tea pills	Camellia sinensis	6.3	
Cranberry	Vaccinium macrocarpon, Vaccinium oxycoccos	6.0	Heart burn
Saw palmetto	Serenoa repens	5.1	GI symptoms, headache, bleeding, acute pancreatitis
Soy supplements	Glycine max	5.0	
St. John wort	Hypericum perforatum	Minimal	Photosensitivity, restlessness, dry mouth, dizziness, GI symptoms, serotonin syndrome, fatigue, induces CYP450 system
Ephedra/Ma haung	Ephedra sinica	Banned in US	Hypertension, tachycardia, cardiomyopathy, stroke, arrhythmia
Valerian	Valeriana officinalis	Minimal	Oversedation, hepatotoxicity
Kava Kava	Piper methysticum	Minimal	Hepatotoxicity, dermopathy, oversedation, affects CYP450
Ginger	Zingiber officinale	Minimal	Time

Some data acquired from Kaye AD, et al.: J Clin Anesth 12:468–471, 2000 and National Library of Medicine (NLM)
[a]Cannabis/Marijuana is discussed separately

Ginseng (Panax quinquefolius, Panax ginseng)

Ginseng is one of the species of the perennial plants belonging to the genus *Panax*. It is mostly found in cooler climate like North America and eastern Asia [11]. Ginseng has been used to improve a person's energy, reduce body's reaction to stress, and to improve cancer related fatigue. It has also been used in men with sexual dysfunction due to its stimulatory effect [11]. Like most herbal supplements, the FDA has not evaluated Ginseng for safety, effectiveness, or purity.

Side Effects/Overdose

Some of the documented side effects include insomnia (most common), allergic reaction (skin eruption), nausea, vomiting, headaches, hypoglycemia, hypertension, hypotension, breast pain, irritability, and bleeding. It has been said that the drug is relatively safe in large amounts however with gross overdose symptoms of nausea, vomiting, irritability, restlessness, urinary and bowel incontinence, delirium, convulsion, and seizures can be noted [8, 9].

Drug Interactions

Ginseng may cause mania in depressed patients who mix the drug with their antidepressant. A study has also shown Ginseng to have adverse drug reactions with Phenelzine and Warfarin. It alters coagulation thus causing increase in bleeding. It could also decrease blood alcohol levels [10]. Thus, a complete history should be obtained from the patient to prevent intraoperative and postoperative surgical complication due to bleeding.

Ginkgo biloba

Ginkgo was first used by Chinese physicians to treat problems such as asthma, digestive disorders, vascular problems, dementia, sexual dysfunction, visual loss, and macular degeneration [12, 24]. Ginkgo leave extracts thru animal studies have been shown to inhibit the binding of platelet-activating factor (PAF) to its membrane receptor thus inhibiting platelet aggregation [13, 25]. There are two active components of Ginkgo: terpene lactones and ginkgo flavone glycosides. Both components have been studied in animal studies and they have shown some neuroprotective properties including decreased glucose utilization in brain areas mediating somatosensory processing and vigilance [14, 26].

Side Effects/Overdose

Ginkgo biloba has antiplatelet and antithrombotic effects thus it can possible interact with other anticoagulants such as warfarin, NSAIDs, and aspirin leading to increased risk for spontaneous hemorrhage and bleeding. Other studies show that Ginkgo may reversibly inhibit monoamine oxidase A and B thus caution should be taken in patients taking other antidepressants due to the risk of potentiating a serotonin syndrome (agitation, hyperthermia, diaphoresis, tachycardia, and rigidity) [14, 26].

Drug Interactions

Look at (side effects/overdose).

Coenzyme Q-10 (Ubiquinol, Ubiquinone, Ubidecarenone)

Coenzyme Q-10 is used to treat myopathy caused by statin treatments. There are three small randomized trials that have shown a benefit of CoQ-10 in patient taking statin and who have muscle pain [15, 27]. CoQ-10 has also been shown to be beneficial in infants with encephalomyopathy [16, 28]. The drug has been shown to lower the systolic pressure (by 17 mmHg) and diastolic pressure (by 10 mmHg) in a hypertensive patient [17, 29].

Side Effects/Overdose

There are few side effects to this drug. These are nausea, vomiting, heartburn, skin irritation, hypoglycemia, and hypotension in patients also taking other antihypertensive medication [17, 29].

Drug Interactions

Coenzyme Q10 as mentioned earlier lowers blood pressure. Thus, care should be taken when combining other antihypertensive medications such as beta blocker, ace inhibitors, and calcium channel blockers. In addition, caution should be taken in patients with diabetes and those taking other herbs or supplements that lower blood glucose.

Saw Palmetto (Serenoa repens)

Saw palmetto berry was first used by the Egyptians in the fifteenth century B.C. to treat urinary symptoms in men. "Then in the early 1700s, Native Americans in Florida used saw palmetto to treat prostate gland swelling and inflammation, testicular atrophy, and erectile dysfunction" [18, 30]. Today, saw palmetto is still used to treat BPH. Its active component contains purified lipid soluble extract that contains about 90 % fatty acids, long chain alcohols, and sterols. The mechanism of this herb is unknown, although there have been several proposals such as acting as an antiandrogenic; decreasing the receptors for estrogen, progesterone, and androgen [19, 31]. Another purpose includes inhibition of type 1 and type 2 isoenzymes of 5-alpha-reductase [18, 30].

Side Effects/Overdose

There are mild side effects such as headaches, nausea, and dizziness seen with ingestion of saw palmetto berry. However according to a few case reports, intraoperative bleeding [20, 32] and acute pancreatitis [21, 33] have been observed in patients taking the herb.

Drug Interactions

There are no drug interactions reported in studies or case reports.

Garlic (Allium sativum)

Garlic is an herb used in everyday food and sometimes used as a treatment for certain disorders. The main active ingredient in garlic is allicin. It contains sulfur, and crushing the clove activates the enzyme allinase, which then converts allin to allicin [22, 34]. Garlic has been used as a lipid lowering agent to treat hypercholesterolemia, as antihypertensive, antiplatelet, antioxidant, and has been shown to have some fibrinolytic actions [23, 35]. Because of its inductive property on CYP450 system, garlic may potentiate the effects of anticoagulant agents such as warfarin, heparin, or aspirin thus causing abnormal bleeding in patients. As for its lipid lowering properties, data from a large randomized trial released in 2007 compared three different garlic preparations (raw, powdered, and aged garlic extracts at a daily dose approximately equivalent to one 4 g clove) and placebo in 192 adults with LDL-C concentrations ranging from 130 to 190 mg/dL (3.36–4.91 mmol/L). Patients were treated 6 days per week for 6 months, and the data showed no significant effect on LDL-C or other lipid levels as compared to placebo. Thus, it might not be worth using garlic as a primary agent for treating hyperlipidemia [24, 36].

Side Effects/Overdose

The most common side effects mentioned is halitosis and GI discomfort (i.e., nausea, vomiting, abdominal pain).

Drug Interactions

There is a possibility of increase in bleeding time and more anticoagulation in patients who combine garlic with other anticoagulant drugs such as warfarin, heparin, Plavix, and aspirin. As previously mentioned, garlic induces cytochrome P450 system thus augmenting the effects of these drugs [23, 35]. Thus, there is a higher risk of surgical bleeding perioperatively and postoperatively. Surgeons, regional, and pain prevention anesthesiologist must be mindful of this history when performing surgery, blocks, or placing epidurals/spinal anesthesia.

St. John Wort (Hypericum perforatum)

St. John wort is a five petal yellow flower that dates back to the sixth century where the missionary St. Columba carried a piece of St. John's wort to protect against demonic possession and "evil spirits" [25, 37]. In recent times, St. John wort has been used to treat sleep-related disorders, depression, and anxiety [26, 38]. There are several active compounds in the plant, which includes naphthodianthrones (hypericin, pseudohypericin), flavonoids (quercetin, rutin, and luteolin), hyperforin, several amino acids, and tannins [26, 38]. At first hypericin was thought to be the major active component for St. John's wort in depression; however, it is now believed that hyperforin and related compounds are mostly responsible for St. John's wort's effect on mood. It modulates various neurotransmitter levels including serotonin, norepinephrine, and dopamine [3, 27]. There is several proposed mechanism of actions of this herb. The mechanisms include irreversible inhibition of monoamine oxidase (MAOIs), Y-aminobutyric acid receptor modulation (GABA), calcium channels, and as before mentioned inhibition of serotonin, dopamine, and norepinephrine [28, 39].

Side Effects/Overdose

The most common drug reactions include gastrointestinal symptoms (constipation, nausea), dizziness/confusion, tiredness/sedation, photosensitivity, dry mouth, urinary frequency, anorgasmia, and swelling [29, 30, 40, 41]. Case reports of photosensitivity have been reported in patients taking oral St. John's wort. One case involved a delayed hypersensitivity/photodermatitis following ingestion of herbal tea [29, 40].

Drug Interactions

According to various literature reviews, St. John's wort is contraindicated during pregnancy and lactation since there are inadequate data to demonstrate its safety. Also there have been documented cases of interactions between St John's wort and several medications of different classes which have led to the now diminished use of this herb. Some of the medications include anticoagulants, antiretrovirals, antifungals, immunosuppressive agents, narcotics, and hormonal contraceptives. Because St. John wort is a significant inducer of CYP450 system (3A4, 1A2, 2C9), there is a high risk of serotonin syndrome (hypertonicity, myoclonus, autonomic dysfunction, hyperthermia, hallucinosis) in those patients taking antidepressants (SSRI and MAOIs) and photosensitivity in patients taking tetracycline [30, 41]. For example, there were two case reports of heart transplant rejection in patients who had reduction in cyclosporine levels due to ingestion of St. John wort [31, 42]. Other studies have also shown that the herb reduces the plasma concentration of methadone, oral oxycodone, and thus making it difficult to treat patients with chronic pain and IV drug abusers [32, 43]. Other cases mentioned are of demerol-induced serotonin crisis due to the patient also taking St. John wort at the same time. Due to the multiple drug interactions, the general rule of thumb in the perioperative period is for a discontinuation of St. John's wort for at least 5 days prior to a planned operative procedure [33, 44].

Kava Kava (Piper methysticum)

Kava kava is an herb first used in the South Pacific for centuries to aid in treating anxiety, insomnia (thru sedative properties), menopausal symptoms, epilepsy, and psychosis. Kava is an extract of the *Piper methysticum* plant and its active agents are pyrones, kawain, methysticin, dihydrokavain, and dihydromethysticin [34, 45]. The primary mechanism of the herb on the central nervous system is not well known, however the active agent, pyrones, has been shown to competitively inhibit MAO-B which in turn help treat the symptoms of psychoses [34, 45].

Side Effects/Overdose

The most well-known side effect of Kava is hepatotoxicity. There have been numerous reports of liver failure and hepatotoxicity ranging from after few weeks of ingestion to up to 2 years following ingestion. The reports range from mild elevation of aminotransferases to acute liver failure and death [35, 36, 46, 47]. The patients who develop liver toxicity from Kava are known as "poor metabolizers" which means that they lack the enzyme CYP2D6 which helps break down the active metabolites of the herb [34, 45]. Based upon case reports of serious toxicity, the USFDA issued a consumer advisory in November 2002 regarding kava kava. In addition, in countries like Germany and Australia, kava kava use greater than 3 months is no longer recommended [37, 38, 49, 50]. Other side effects include hallucinations, skin eruptions, antiplatelet effect, and excessive sedation [34, 37, 45, 48].

Drug Interactions

The primary drug interaction that physicians especially anesthesiologist should be aware of is the potentiation of over sedation with the combination of benzodiazepine and barbiturates. The other potential drug interaction is the use of antiplatelet agents (Plavix) and COX inhibitors (ASA, Celebrex) in combination with Kava which may result in a bleeding abnormality. According to theory, kava affects platelets in an antithrombotic manner by inhibiting COX and thus increasing the production of thromboxane [34, 37, 45, 48].

Echinacea

Echinacea also known as coneflowers was first used by Native Americans to treat illness such as cough, sore throat, burns, pain, and snakebites [3, 50]. Today, echinacea is used as prevention and treatment for uncomplicated upper respiratory infections. According to the NHIS, echinacea was the third most common natural product used by adults in the US in 2007 and the most common used in children [39, 51]. There are various active ingredients in echinacea including echinacosides, caffeic acids, alkylamides, polysaccharides, and glycoproteins. It is the alkylamides and polysaccharide substances that produce in vivo immunostimulation properties. This is due to the enhanced phagocytosis and nonspecific T-cell stimulation [40, 52].

Side Effects/Overdose

There are several possible side effects of echinacea. The most common is unpleasant taste. Other side effects include dyspepsia, diarrhea, fever, nausea, vomiting, allergic reaction (anaphylaxis), tachyphylaxis with extended usage (>2 months), and finally hepatotoxicity [30, 41, 42, 53, 54]. Liver toxicity was noted when the herb was taken with other hepatotoxic drugs such as amiodarone, ketoconazole, anabolic steroids, and methotrexate [41, 53].

Drug Interactions

According to one study, there was evidence that echinacea decreases oral clearance of the CYP1A2 system and it also modulates the activity of CYP3A isoenzyme at both the hepatic and intestinal sites. Thus, caution should be taken with drugs such as lovastatin, clarithromycin, cyclosporine, diltiazem, estrogens, and others because the drug levels may become abnormally elevated due to inactivity of both CYP1A2 and CYP3A system [43, 55]. In addition taking benzodiazepine with echinacea may increase sedation in a patient. Echinacea is also contraindicated in patients with autoimmune disorders and pregnant women. However, there has been no study that showed increase in fetal risk or maternal risk in women who took echinacea. The one cohort study that was performed in Toronto did not show an increase in fetal demise or any birth defect [44, 56]. As for autoimmune disorder, there have been a combination of three cases of reported exacerbation of autoimmune disease, two cases were of pemphigus vulgaris, and one case of renal tubular acidosis due to Sjogren's syndrome [45, 57].

Cannabis/Marijuana

Cannabis is the most commonly used illicit drug used in the world [12, 46]. It is derived from the cannabis plant, cannabis sativa. It grows naturally in tropical and temperate climates of the world. However, it can be cultivated indoors by the use of indoor hydroponic technology [13, 47]. The primary active substance in cannabis is delta-9 tetrahydrocannabinol (Δ9-THC) commonly known as THC. There are three main forms of cannabis: marijuana, hashish, and hash oil. The most abused form is marijuana. It is made from dried flowers and leaves of the plant. Although the least potent, marijuana is common in young adults age <29 and it is usually smoked in hand-rolled cigarettes (known as "joints") or in special water pipes called ("bongs") [13, 47]. Some users of this drug have developed an addiction /physical dependence to the herb due to the unpleasant withdrawal symptoms after cessation of the drug. Thus, there are growing concerns about the increasing production and use of a new generation of synthetic cannabinoid (SC) agonist (e.g., JWH-018, CP 47,497) marketed as natural herbal incense mixtures under brand names such as Spice and K2 [14, 48].

As mentioned earlier, cannabis use can lead to abuse or physical dependence. Abuse occurs when a person continues to use a drug that results in poor daily life functioning, interpersonal difficulties, or legal difficulties. On the other hand, physical dependence refers to the continuous use of substance even though the patient is aware that he or she will continue to have physical or psychological problems. In addition, the patient needs larger amount of the substance to get "high," there is an unsuccessful effort to limit substance use and during attempts the patient develops physiological withdrawal [15, 49].

Clinical Presentations with Intoxication

The signs of intoxication include the feeling of getting "high" which is displayed by: euphoria, pleasurable feeling, and a decrease in anxiety, alertness, depression, and tension, increased sociability, the sensation that colors are brighter and music is more vivid. In addition, high doses or potent cannabis products may cause hallucinations, mystical thinking, increased self-consciousness, and depersonalization may occur, as well as transient grandiosity, paranoia, and other signs of psychosis. Cannabis use also decreases reaction time and impairs attention, concentration, and short-term memory [16, 50]. In preoperative and intraoperative management of a patient, one can postulate that a patient maybe intoxicated with Marijuana when there is physiologic sign of tachycardia, hypertension, tachypnea, conjunctiva injection, dry mouth, or increase in appetite postoperatively. With this information, the physician should have a plan to prevent and treat the patient if withdrawal symptoms develop.

Clinical Presentations with Withdrawal

Cannabis withdrawal symptoms are not life threatening however they are very unpleasant and sometimes hard to treat. According to a US epidemiologic survey, in all cannabis users who did not abuse other substances, about 44 % reported two or more withdrawal symptoms upon cessation of cannabis, and 34 % reported three or more symptoms [17, 51]. The most common withdrawal symptoms were fatigue, yawning, hypersomnia, psychomotor retardation, anxiety, and depression. The symptoms begin on the first or second day of abstinences, peaks between day 2 and 6, and often resolves within 7–14 days [18, 52]. The use of delta-9 tetrahydrocannabinol (D9-THC), the active agent in cannabis has been shown to reduce and even prevent cannabis withdrawal symptoms [19, 53]. Dronabinol, a cannabinoid used to treat anorexia and nausea and vomiting was found to be better than placebo in reducing withdrawal symptoms in marijuana abusers [21, 55]. Other than these drugs, the treatment of withdrawal is supportive care.

New Generation of Synthetic Cannabinoid

National debate continues to occur about legalization of cannabis for recreational use. For the first time in history, in a Pew Research Center poll released last month, a majority of Americans (52 %) favored legalization of marijuana. The state of Washington and Colorado are the only two states that have legalized the use of marijuana for recreation. However, there are 18 states that have legalized medical marijuana use, such as for cancer pain control 1. The states include Alaska, Arizona, California, Colorado, Connecticut, Washington DC, Delaware, Hawaii, Maine, Massachusetts, Michigan, Montana, Nevada, New Jersey, New Mexico, Oregon, Rhode Island, and Vermont. Recently, due to the increasing dependence of cannabis and the desire to get "high," a new generation of synthetic cannabinoid (SC) agonist is now been produced and sold to the public as "natural herbal incense or potpourri under various brand names such as 'Spice' or 'K2'" [14, 48]. There is no doubt that the illegalization of marijuana has played a role in the increase demand and sales of the drug in the black market. The compounds generated with the most interest are JWH-018, CP 47,497, cannabicyclohexanol, and JWH-073. The labels on these substances only states that they contain a mixture of psychoactively inert herbs and aromatic extracts sprayed with SC compounds. According to several studies, it has been shown that a cannabis-like effect occurs after smoking this agents (SC products), which includes alteration in mood, perception, tachycardia, hypertension, hyperventilation, diaphoresis, acute onset of cough, nausea, vomiting, and seizures [14, 48]. Thus, it is imperative for the physician to be aware of these agents and to perform a thorough physical and detail medical history.

Other Emerging Drug of Abuse

Kratom, the Thai name for the plant *Mitragyna speciosa Korth* is a new herbal drug sold widely on the internet even though it has been illegal in Thailand since 1946 and in Australia since 2005 [22, 56]. The leaves of *Mitragyna speciosa* have been used in Thailand for its opium-like effect and its ability to prevent fatigue. It also has been used to treat cough, diarrhea, muscle pain, hypertension, and morphine addiction [23, 57]. Currently, there are no studies done that explain the impact of the drug on the human body, thus medical providers should lie on the side of caution and inform their patient of the possible danger of the herbal supplement.

Conclusion

Herbal supplements are a billion dollar business. There have been few to no rules and regulations in this market. Thus, medical providers are the first line of information and knowledge for the public. Therefore, a physician should obtain all data relevant to the proper, safe management of their patients such that they must include the detailed list of synthetic drugs and nonpharmacological drugs such as herbal supplements to avoid devastating injury and possible death.

References

1. Blumenthal M, editor. The ABC clinical guide to herbs. New York: American Botanical Council; 2003.
2. Goldman P. Herbal medicines today and the roots of modern pharmacology. Ann Intern Med. 2001;135:594.
3. Barnes PM, Bloom B, Nahin RL. Complementary and alternative medicine use among adults and children: United States, 2007. Natl Health Stat Report 2008:1.
4. Humberston CL, Akhtar J, Krenzelok EP. Acute hepatitis induced by kava kava. J Toxicol Clin Toxicol. 2003;41(2):109–13.
5. Naik SD, Freudenberger RS. Ephedra-associated cardiomyopathy. Ann Pharmacother. 2004;38(3):400–3.
6. National Center for Complementary and Alternative Medicine. Expanding Horizons of Health Care: Strategic Plan 2005-2009. NIH publication no. 04-5568. National Center for Complementary and Alternative Medicine; NIH, Bethesda; 2005.
7. Saper RB. Overview of herbal medicine and dietary supplements (Table 1). UptoDate. http://www.uptodate.com/contents/overview-of-herbal-medicine-and-dietary-supplements?source=search_result&search=Complementary+and+alternative+medicine&selectedTitle=2%7E150#subscribeMessagehttp://www.umass.edu/cnshp/faq.html
8. Chen JK, Chen TT. Chinese medical herbology and pharmacology. Los Angeles: Art of Medicine Press; 2004.
9. Izzo AA, Ernst E. Interactions between herbal medicines and prescribed drugs: a systematic review. Drugs. 2001;61(15):2163–75.
10. Ginseng. Wikipedia. http://en.wikipedia.org/wiki/Ginseng#cite_ref-CMHP_3-1
11. New York: United Nations Office on Drugs and Crime (UNODC). UNODC, *World Drug Report*—2009. New York: United Nations Office on Drugs and Crime; 2009.
12. Pizzorno JE, Murray MT. A textbook of natural medicine. Seattle: John Bastyr College Publications; 1985.
13. Saper RB. Clinical use of Gingko Biloba. Uptodate.com Topic 1387, April 4, 2013.
14. Rosenson RS, Baker SK. Statin myopathy. Uptodate.com Topic 6833, April 2013.
15. Salviati L, Sacconi S, Murer L, et al. Infantile encephalomyopathy and nephropathy with CoQ10 deficiency: a CoQ10-responsive condition. Neurology. 2005;65(4):606.
16. Rosenfeldt FL, Haas SJ, Krum H, Hadj A, Ng K, Leong JY, Watts GF. Coenzyme Q10 in the treatment of hypertension: a meta-analysis of the clinical trials. J Hum Hypertens. 2007;21(4):297–306.
17. Saper RB. Clincal use of saw palmetto. Uptodate.com Topic 1388.
18. Barrette EP. Use of saw palmetto extract for benign prostatic hyperplasia. Alternative Med Alert. 1998;1:1.
19. Cheema P, El-Mefty O, Jazieh AR. Intraoperative hemorrhage associated with the use of extract of Saw Palmetto herb: a case report and review of literature. J Intern Med. 2001;250(2):167.

20. Wargo KA, Allman E, Ibrahim F. A possible case of saw palmetto-induced pancreatitis. South Med J. 2010;103(7):683.
21. Ness J, Sherman FT, Pan CX. Alternative medicine: what the data say about common herbal therapies. Geriatrics. 1999;54:33–43.
22. Fleischer L. Anesthesia and uncommon diseases: expert consult. In: Kaye AD, editor. Mineral, vitamins, and herbal supplement. New York: Elsevier; 2012. p. 470–88.
23. Gardner CD, Lawson LD, Block E, et al. Effect of raw garlic vs commercial garlic supplements on plasma lipid concentrations in adults with moderate hypercholesterolemia: a randomized clinical trial. Arch Intern Med. 2007;167:346.
24. Hobbs C. St. John's wort—ancient herbal protector. Pharm Hist. 1990;32:166.
25. Jellin JM, Gregory PJ, Batz F, Hitchens K, et al. St. John's Wort. Pharmacist's letter/prescriber's letter natural medicines comprehensive database. 8th ed. Stockton: Therapeutic Research Faculty; 2006. p. 1180–4.
26. Müller WE, Singer A, Wonnemann M, et al. Hyperforin represents the neurotransmitter reuptake inhibiting constituent of hypericum extract. Pharmacopsychiatry. 1998;31 Suppl 1:16.
27. Cott JM, Misra R. Medicinal plants: a potential source of new psychotherapeutic drugs. In: Kanba S, Richelson SE, editors. New drug development from herbal medicines in neuropharmacology, vol. 5. New York: Brunner/Mazel; 1998.
28. Newall CA, Anderson LA, Phillipson JD. Herbal medicines: a guide for health-care professionals. London: The Pharmaceutical Press; 1996.
29. Hughes EF, Jacobs BP, Berman BM. Complementary and alternative medicine. In: Tierney LM, McPhee SJ, Papadakis MA, editors. Current medical diagnosis and treatment. New York: Lange Medical/McGraw-Hill; 2004. p. 1681–703.
30. Ruschitzka F, Meier PJ, Turina M, et al. Acute heart transplant rejection due to Saint John's wort. Lancet. 2000;355:548.
31. Nieminen TH, Hagelverg NM, Saari TI, et al. St John's wort greatly reduces the concentrations of oral oxycodone. Eur J Pain. 2010;14(8):854–9.
32. Ang-Lee MK, Moss J, Yuan CS. Herbal medicines and perioperative care. J Am Med Assoc. 2001;286:208.
33. Jellin JM, Gregory PJ, Batz F, editors. Kava. Natural medicines: comprehensive database. 4th ed. California: Therapeutic Research Faculty Stockton; 2002. p. 759–61.
34. Stickel F, Baumüller HM, Seitz K, et al. Hepatitis induced by Kava (Piper methysticum rhizoma). J Hepatol. 2003;39:62.
35. Pittler MH, Ernst E. Systematic review: hepatotoxic events associated with herbal medicinal products. Aliment Pharmacol Ther. 2003;18:451.
36. Jellin JM, Gregory PJ, Batz F, editors. Kava. Natural medicines: comprehensive database. 5th ed. California: Therapeutic Research Faculty Stockton; 2003. p. 788–91.
37. Forget L, Goldrosen J, Hart JA, editors. Herbal companion to AHFS DI. Bethesda: American Society of Health-System Pharmacists; 2000.
38. Hobbs C. Enchinacea: a literature review. HerbalGram. 1994;30:33.
39. Grimm W, Muller HH. A randomized controlled trial of the effect of fluid extract of Echinacea purpurea on the incidence and severity of colds and respiratory infections. Am J Med. 1999;106:138–43.
40. Miller LG. Herbal medicinals. Arch Intern Med. 1998;158:2200–11.
41. Blumenthal M, Gruenwald J, Hall T, et al., editors. German commission E monographs: therapeutic monographs on medicinal plants for human use. Austin: American Botanical Council; 1998.
42. Gorski JC, Huang SM, Pinto A, et al. The effect of echinacea (*Echinacea purpurea root*) on cytochrome P450 activity in vivo. Clin Pharmacol Ther. 2004;75:89–100.
43. Gallo M, Sarkar M, Au W, et al. Pregnancy outcome following gestational exposure to echinacea: a prospective controlled study. Arch Intern Med. 2000;160:3141.
44. Soon SL, Crawford RI. Recurrent erythema nodosum associated with Echinacea herbal therapy. J Am Acad Dermatol. 2001;44:298.
45. Logan JL, Ahmed J. Critical hypokalemic renal tubular acidosis due to Sjögren's syndrome: association with the purported immune stimulant echinacea. Clin Rheumatol. 2003;22:158.

46. National Cannabis Prevention and Information Center in Australia. http://adai.uw.edu/marijuana/factsheets/whatiscannabis.htm
47. Gunderson EW, Haughey HM, Ait-Daoud N, et al. "Spice" and "K2" herbal highs: a case series and systematic review of the clinical effects and biopsychosocial implications of synthetic cannabinoid use in humans. Am J Addict. 2012;21:320–6.
48. American Psychiatric Association. Diagnostic and statistical manual of mental disorders. 4th ed. Washington, DC: American Psychiatric Association; 2000.
49. Ashton CH. Pharmacology and effects of cannabis: a brief review. Br J Psychiatry. 2001;178:101.
50. Hasin DS, Keyes KM, Alderson D, et al. Cannabis withdrawal in the United States: results from NESARC. J Clin Psychiatry. 2008;69:1354.
51. Budney AJ, Hughes JR, Moore BA, Vandrey R. Review of the validity and significance of cannabis withdrawal syndrome. Am J Psychiatry. 2004;161:1967.
52. Hart CL. Increasing treatment options for cannabis dependence: a review of potential pharmacotherapies. Drug Alcohol Depend. 2005;80:147–59.
53. Haney M, Hart CL, Vosburg SK, et al. Effects of THC and lofexidine in a human laboratory model of marijuana withdrawal and relapse. Psychopharmacology (Berl). 2008;197:157.
54. Levin FR, Kleber HD. Use of dronabinol for cannabis dependence: two case reports and review. Am J Addict. 2008;17:161.
55. Maurer HH. Chemistry, pharmacology, and metabolism of emerging drugs of abuse. Ther Drug Monit. 2010;32:544–9.
56. Suwanlert S. A study of kratom eaters in Thailand. Bull Narc. 1975;27:21–7.
57. Lin JH. Evaluating the alternatives. J Am Med Assoc. 1998;279:706.

Chapter 15
Opioids and Substance Abuse

Matthew Verne Satterly and Magdalena Anitescu

Key Points

- What are opioids?
- Opioid receptors
- Opioid regulation and scheduling
- Illicit versus licit use
- Risks for abuse of opioids
- The widespread use of opioids
- Epidemiology
- Patterns of and predispositions to abuse
- Methods to combat abuse

What Are Opioids?

Opioid refers to a class of medications that include the most potent analgesics or painkillers available. They are used in all aspects of health care from intraoperative therapy for surgical procedures to outpatient use to control acute and chronic pain. An opioid is a synthetic or semisynthetic compound as distinct from an opiate, which is naturally occurring. Opium, harvested from the poppy plant *Papaver somniferum*,

M.V. Satterly, M.D.
Department of Anesthesiology, Center for Advanced Medicine, Western Anesthesia Associates, Pain Management Center, Washington University School of Medicine, 4921 Parkview Place, Suite 14-C, St. Louis, MO 63110, USA
e-mail: mattsatterly@gmail.com

M. Anitescu, M.D., Ph.D. (✉)
Department of Anesthesia and Critical Care, University of Chicago Medical Center, 5513 South Kimbark Avenue, Chicago, IL 60637, USA
e-mail: MAnitescu@dacc.uchicago.edu

© Springer Science+Business Media New York 2015
A.D. Kaye et al. (eds.), *Substance Abuse*, DOI 10.1007/978-1-4939-1951-2_15

contains several opiates including codeine and morphine. Morphine, the prototypical opioid, was the first alkaloid derived from a plant source to be used for medicinal purposes around the turn of the nineteenth century. Since that time, roughly a hundred distinct opioids have been discovered. An endogenous opioid is one of several molecules occurring naturally in the human body and binding to the opioid receptor, a common site of action for all the agents mentioned earlier.

Opiate use dates back thousands and likely even tens of thousands of years. Fossilized poppy seeds dating back as far as 30,000 years ago suggest the use of opium by Neanderthal man. Ancient Sumerian artifacts circa 4000 BC contain images of the opium poppy. Dating back to 1500 BC, the Ebers Papyrus describes the use of opium to stop children from crying. In 1799 Friedrich Serturner discovered the primary active ingredient in opium and named it morphine for the Greek god of dreams, Morpheus. It wasn't until 1973 that a graduate student used radioactive morphine to find receptors in the brain to which opioids bind and exert their effect. The subsequent discovery of enkephalins (Greek for "in the head") and endorphins (endogenous morphine) proved that there were opioid compounds that occur naturally in the body with effects similar to those found with externally administered opioids.

Opioids have numerous effects in the human body, some of which are therapeutic like relief from pain. Opioids are also used for cough suppression. Heroin was first marketed as a nonaddictive cough suppressant until it was discovered that when it was quickly broken down to morphine in the body, it was twice as potent. Other effects can be detrimental such as decreased bowel motility. Opioids are used to treat diarrhea, but the same mechanism of action may lead to constipation during treatment for pain. Other adverse effects of opioids are respiratory depression, itching, and nausea and sedation. A sense of euphoria from recreational use of these medications leads some people to use them solely for that purpose.

Opioid Receptors

There are four known types of opioid receptor. Each was named for the pharmacological agent used to characterize and identify them. Morphine lent its first letter, subsequently changed to its Greek counterpart, mu, to the mu receptors (MOP). MOPs are found throughout the nervous system, with certain locations serving as an explanation for their functions. The ventral tegmenal area is intimately involved in the sense of euphoria and reward produced by opioids and other substances [1]. Opioid receptors in the periaqueductal gray area are thought to contribute to analgesia along with receptors in the substantia gelatinosa in the spinal cord. The MOP produces respiratory depression when the sensitivity of the central and peripheral chemoreceptors to hypercapnia is reduced. In high enough doses, respiratory rate may be reduced to zero, causing death from an opioid overdose. There are ten or more variants of the MOP, and three have been well characterized and studied. To MOP1 is attributed analgesia and physical dependence. To MOP2 is attributed respiratory depression, reduced GI motility, physical dependence, and the sense of euphoria. To MOP3 is attributed vasodilatory properties. In one experiment in which MOP was deleted from the genetic sequence of mice (MOP knockout mice), morphine caused no respiratory depression or analgesia [2]. The effects of MOP are not limited to the central nervous system but are also found in the periphery. In the GI tract they inhibit peristalsis, leading to either constipation or decreased diarrhea.

The kappa opioid receptor (KOP) has analgesic properties as well but does not affect the respiratory drive. This property has led researchers to target the KOP subtype to improve analgesia without the risk of respiratory depression. Unfortunately the kappa receptor mediates dysphoria and has psychotomimetic effects [3].

The delta opioid receptor (DOP) can affect analgesia, although less so than the MOP. DOP contributes to physical dependence and has antidepressant effects. Higher doses cause depression and lower doses may antagonize the depressant effects of opioids that target other receptor subtypes.

The nociceptin opioid receptor (NOP) was given its name from its primary agonist, nociceptin. Nociceptin is thought to be an endogenous antagonist of dopamine transport, which may explain its effect on reward and mood, as dopamine is intricately tied to these functions. The NOP antagonists have been shown to cause analgesia in animals, and tolerance to classical opioids may be attenuated by NOP antagonism. NOP agonists have mixed effects. Given supra-spinally or given spinally at lower doses, they are hyperalgesic, but at higher doses they produce analgesia. It is thought that the NOP may help to regulate the threshold for pain, because NOP knockout mice show a partial loss of tolerance to morphine.

An agonist is a compound that binds to a receptor and exerts a "typical" response from the receptor. Partial agonists bind but with only a partial execution of downstream function and ultimate effect. The term agonist–antagonist was introduced before multiple opioid receptors were identified and was meant to explain the effects seen in vivo. Nalorphine, for example, has agonist and antagonist effects: it reduces respiratory depression and abuse potential but still has analgesic effects. At higher doses it has dysphoric and psychotomimetic effects. It was later identified as an antagonist at the mu receptor and an agonist at the kappa receptor [1]. Researchers seeking agents with analgesic effects and limited respiratory depression and abuse potential developed naloxone and naltrexone competitive antagonists primarily at the mu receptor and less so at delta or kappa receptors. As antagonists, they reverse or block the primary effects of opioids. Partial agonists and agonist–antagonists may displace full agonists from the receptor site if binding affinity at that receptor is stronger. Antagonists bind to a receptor and prevent or reverse the primary effect of the agonists. The use of antagonists or partial agonists must be carefully considered because they may reverse the effects of agonists suddenly and lead to withdrawal. The use of a short-acting antagonist to reverse potentially fatal respiratory depression must be readministered if the agonist it has to counteract has a longer duration of action. Some compounds have affinity for all receptors, like the endogenous opioids endorphins and enkephalins. Others like buprenorphine have agonist properties at several opioid receptors. At low to intermediate doses they provide analgesia through activity at MOP, but at higher doses, the effect is limited by action at NOP [3].

Opioid Regulation and Scheduling

Opioids and other potentially addictive psychoactive substances were unregulated in the United Stated until the early 1900s when the Food and Drug Act of 1906 was passed. After that such medications could be sold, but only when properly labeled with contents and dosages. The Harrison Narcotics Tax Act of 1914 regulated the production, importation, and distribution of opioids for the first time. The next major reform came with the Controlled Substances Act in 1970. This federal policy regulated the manufacture, possession, and use of certain substances. Drugs were categorized based on their potential for abuse into five different classifications. Drugs with a high potential for abuse and with no accepted medical use in the United States are labeled as schedule I: heroin, marijuana, and LSD. Schedule II medications have a high potential for abuse but have a medical use in the US: cocaine, morphine, and most other potent opioid medications. The weaker opioids such as codeine and hydrocodone mixed with acetaminophen are listed in schedule III. They have a lower potential for abuse than schedule I and II medications. Tramadol is a schedule IV medication with less abuse potential than schedule III medications. Codeine is a schedule II drug in a formulation of > than 90 mg per dose but may be a schedule III, IV, or V when formulated with other agents such as acetaminophen or when in low concentration in cough medicines. Codeine may also be in a higher schedule in some states that want to combat abuse of otherwise less tightly controlled, schedule IV or V formulations. There is much debate over how to classify certain medications and often little sound evidence to back up the ultimate decisions.

Illicit Versus Licit Use

Opioid abuse can take a variety of forms. Heroin, also known as diacetyl-morphine is used in the United Kingdom and other countries in the way we use morphine and other opioids in the United States. In the United States, heroin abuse is pursued entirely through illegal importation and distribution as a "street drug." Prescription medications initially prescribed for a medical purpose can also be abused. There are four potential subpopulations of prescription opioid abusers. The first are those who were given a legitimate prescription and use it in a manner other than that for which it was prescribed. Second, there is the heroin user who substitutes with prescription medications when unable to obtain heroin. Third, there is the polydrug abuser who indiscriminately uses whatever is available. Finally, there are those who have no medical reason to use prescription opioids yet seek them out for recreational use [4].

Opioids can be administered in many forms. Oral preparations including tablets, capsules, and liquids comprise immediate release (IR) or delayed release formulations. The formulations may be controlled release (CR), sustained release (SR), extended release (XR), or long acting (LA). Immediate release formulations have a quick onset of action, generally 15–30 min, but a shorter duration of action, typically

3–4 h. The controlled release formulations sustain duration of action over 8–12 h. Immediate release formulations are suitable for acute pain or for "breakthrough" pain that escalates pain over a patient's baseline pain level. The controlled release formulations control a baseline level of chronic pain, but may find new applications in acute pain. Intravenous opioids have a fast onset but a short duration of action, much like medication administered orally. Intravenous forms also may be used subcutaneously, intramuscularly, or even via an epidural or spinal route. Transdermal patches are placed on the skin for slow release of medication over the course of several days to a week. Preparations for buccal administration for those unable to take oral medications have a rapid onset. Intranasal administration via mist has been implemented for outpatient use. The onset and duration of action of the opioids are intimately correlated with their abuse potential. Generally, the quicker the onset and the more potent the opioid the higher its abuse potential. Therefore, long-acting, slow-releasing agents such as morphine are administered as a treatment for abuse, since they produce the immediate sense of euphoria less than do other opioids.

When the long-acting form of oxycodone was introduced to solve the problem of abuse, abusers of opioids quickly found that by crushing or chewing the tablets the timed-release mechanism was defeated and absorption into the body was rapid to produce the sought after high. Solid or powdered forms used in pills or tablets are liquefied to inject intravenously or underneath the skin in a technique called "skin popping." Transdermal patches, too, may be altered for more immediate effect of the medication.

There is much confusion surrounding the terms misuse, abuse, dependence, tolerance, and addiction. Misuse refers to using the medications for a purpose or in a manner other than that for which they were originally prescribed. Using a drug originally prescribed for pain control as a cough suppressant is one example of misuse. The distinction between misuse and abuse can be a little more difficult. The Diagnostic and Statistical Manual of Mental Disorders, Fourth Edition (DSM-IV), defines abuse as a pattern of substance use leading to significant impairment or distress, as manifested by one or more of the following in a 12-month period failing to fulfill major obligations at school or work, using substances in a hazardous manner, such as while driving, encountering legal problems from substance use, and continued use despite recurrent social or interpersonal problems. Abuse infers use despite adverse consequence. All abuse may be described as misuse, but not all misuse is abuse.

Tolerance describes the need for larger doses of medications over time to achieve the same effect. Pharmacokinetic tolerance refers to the changes in the body that lets less drug make it to its site of action, most commonly from increased breakdown of the drug. Pharmacodynamic tolerance refers to the changes the drug has on the body, such as receptor downregulation, that is, fewer receptors available for binding the drug for effect. Tolerance applies to many drug classes. Tolerance to the analgesic effect but not to respiratory depression is possible. The medication may be abused by increasing the amount taken to achieve pain relief, despite the negative consequences of sedation or respiratory depression. Misuse, increasing the amount above what was prescribed, may become abuse when use continues despite adverse consequences. Dependence and withdrawal are intricately intertwined but should not be confused with tolerance. Withdrawal is a state in which abruptly stopping or even decreasing the dose of a medication leads to effects opposite those for which the drug was taken. The sense of euphoria produced by opioids and resultant constipation may cause dysphoria when discontinued or diarrhea during a period of withdrawal. When cessation produces symptoms of withdrawal, physical dependence exists.

Differentiating between addiction and abuse can also be difficult. The DSM-IV uses substance abuse as a category for addiction. Some individuals make a distinction between abuse and addiction, similar to that between misuse and abuse. There is some indication that the DSM-V will not distinguish between abuse and dependence, in favor of the terms mild, moderate, and severe substance use disorder. Addiction implies the inability to stop. Injecting heroin is abuse and not misuse. But injecting it only once and never again could not be considered addiction.

Seeking out opioids for reasons other than that for which they are prescribed may lead to diversion, or the distribution of the medicines obtained legally to persons without a right to use them. Extension of use results if medications obtained for medical use are taken beyond the doses prescribed. Recreational use is taking medications solely for their euphorigenic effects.

Risks for Abuse of Opioids

The fact that opioids lead to physical dependence makes the propensity for abuse higher than for drugs without this property. Euphoria is a powerful effect that some people find irresistible.

The abuse risk of opioids is influenced by many factors including formulation and pharmacology, marketing, availability, and distribution. The stronger the ability of a drug to alleviate pain, the more liable it is to be abused. It is nearly impossible to separate the risk of abuse from therapeutic effect of opioids since work by a similar neuropharmacological mechanism. Many researchers in the field are calling for a systematic study of different opioids, the agents added to formulations, the routes of administration, and the effects when taken as directed or misused. Without these data it is difficult to determine which opioids are the safest and in which situations some opioids are more likely to be misused or abused and to what extent [4].

Undertreated pain may look like addiction or abuse. Abnormal behavior typically attributed to people abusing medication develops as a direct consequence of inadequate pain management. This phenomenon starts with the inadequate prescription of analgesics or interventions to treat the primary pain stimulus. Pain leads to an escalation of analgesic demands and other associated behaviors to convince others of the pain severity. Requesting increases in dose, running out of pills before the end of the month, seeking out illicit substances, or borrowing pain medications are some behaviors of abusers that result from mistrust between patient and health care team when pain is inadequately treated. The ability to distinguish addiction or abuse from pseudoaddiction is often difficult [5].

The Widespread Use of Opioids

In the 1980s pain was routinely undertreated. The scope of the risks of opioids was not understood, especially for chronic nonmalignant or cancer pain. The risks were underreported and underappreciated. The Federation of State Medical Boards considered punishing doctors for undertreating pain and reassured physicians that large doses of narcotics could be prescribed for medical treatment. In one guide, the Joint Commission on Accreditation of Hospitals (JCAHO or simply the Joint Commission) stated that concerns about addiction, tolerance, and other risks of opioids, including death, were exaggerated. There was no evidence of addiction if patients are given opioids for pain control. These beliefs have been superseded with information obtained from additional studies.

The phrase "pain as the 5th vital sign" was first promoted by the American Pain Society to increase awareness of pain treatment. To combat the undertreatment of pain, pain was promoted to the level of a vital sign deserving the same consideration as blood pressure and heart rate [6].

In 2001, the Joint Commission implemented standards for the assessment and treatment of pain in ambulatory care facilities, behavioral health care organizations, critical access hospitals, office-based surgery practices, and long-term care facilities. The Commission recognized that patients have the right to treatment of their pain. Screening of patients for pain during assessment and afterwards with ongoing reevaluation was recommended. Education for patients and their families about pain management was required. The mandate made it difficult to achieve the goals without carefully balancing the risks and benefits of opioid therapy in certain populations of patients.

Epidemiology

With the US government, regulatory bodies and other groups revealing the undertreatment of pain, the sales of prescription opioids have quadrupled between 1999 and 2010 [7]. Hydrocodone with acetaminophen was the #1 prescribed medication in the United States between 2006 and 2011 accounting for 131.2 million prescriptions in 2010, followed by simvastatin with 94.1 million and lisinopril at 87.4 million [8]. Enough opioid pain relievers were sold in 2010 to medicate every adult American with 5 mg of hydrocodone every 4 h for 1 month [7]. The US constitutes 4.6 % of the world's population but consumed 83 % of the world's oxycodone and 99 % of its hydrocodone in 2007. Americans consume 27.4 million grams of hydrocodone annually compared to 3,237 g by British, French, German, and Italian patients. Although opioids for chronic cancer pain have been well studied and shown to be efficacious, there is little to no evidence that opioids have efficacy for patients with chronic noncancer pain [8]. There is a fairly linear correlation between the increase in the number of opioid prescriptions written and the increase in the abuse of prescription opioids. Over the last several years, prescription opioids have been the fastest growing form of drug abuse and the most common cause of unintentional overdose (see Fig. 15.1) [9].

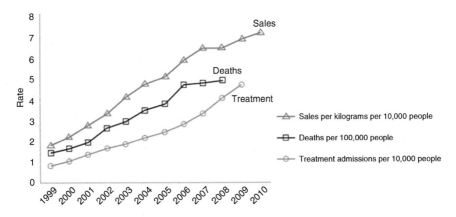

Fig. 15.1 National Vital Statistics System, 1999–2008; Automation of Reports and Consolidated Orders System (ARCOS) of the Drug Enforcement Administration (DEA), 1999–2010; Treatment Episode Data Set, 1999–2009. Accessed from: http://www.cdc.gov/vitalsigns/painkilleroverdoses/ [10]

In 2011, 22.5 million Americans, 8.7 % of the population, had used illicit drugs in the past month. Of the prescription medications abused by 6.1 million people, 4.5 million were opioids, second only to marijuana with 18.1 million users in 1 month. The number abusing prescription opioids was more than the number using cocaine and heroin combined, totaling 1.4 million and 620,000, respectively. Accounting for population growth, the percentage of abusers of opioids was 1.7 % of the population in 2011, down from 2.0 % in 2010 and 2.1 % in 2009 [10, 11]. The misconception is that prescribed medications are safer than illicit drugs or carry less risk. The consumption of prescription pills does not pose the risk of infection from contaminated needles as does heroin, but the effects of powerful opioids are no less dangerous because some are more potent than heroin.

Among young people the use of prescription opioids is growing rapidly. Between 1998 and 2008 substance abuse treatment admissions, because of prescription medications and heroin, increased 51 %. For those between the ages of 12 and 25, the increase was 69 % for heroin and 1,896 % for prescription medications [12, 13].

When data from 2009 were evaluated, nearly 60,000 patients had entered treatment for substance use disorders at 464 facilities in 34 states. Hydrocodone and immediate release oxycodone were the most highly abused medications. After adjusting for prescription volume, hydrocodone and immediate release oxycodone were least often abused on a prescription by prescription basis; methadone and extended release oxycodone were the drugs with the greatest risk for abuse. Morphine and hydromorphone were the most likely to be injected among the prescription opioids.

Given the vast amounts of opioids available for abuse, the question remains, how do those who abuse them obtain them? One survey revealed that among those who used pain relievers nonmedically, 54.2 % got them from a friend or relative and 18.1 % received their prescription from a single physician. Only 3.9 % purchased them from a dealer or stranger. Of those who received opioids from a friend or relative, 81.6 % of the sources had prescriptions from a single doctor. This result dispels the myth that most of opioid prescriptions are diverted to the streets and that abusers are buying them from dealers [11].

In an effort to track providers who are writing prescriptions, the state of California looked at 16,890 workman's compensation claims from 1993 to 2009 in which at least one schedule II medication was prescribed for pain. Just 3 % of the prescribing physicians accounted for 55 % of all the prescriptions of schedule II medications. The top 1 % of prescribers accounted for 33 % of all prescriptions, and the top 10 % accounted for 79 % of them. The top 10 % of injured workers as weighted by total daily morphine equivalents obtained their medications from an average of 3.3 physicians, and the average for all claims was 1.9 % [14, 15]. Primary care physicians were the largest group of opioid prescribers: 42 % of all immediate release and 44 % of long-acting opioids. Specialties identified as pain management, including anesthesiology and physical medicine and rehabilitation, accounted for 6 % of the immediate release and 23 % of long-acting opioids. The remaining drugs were prescribed by surgeons and other specialists [8].

As the toll in dollars and lives exacted has become evident, physicians have become somewhat hesitant to prescribe large doses of opioid medications and refer patients to pain specialists. For the year 2007, and reported in 2009 dollars, it was estimated that prescription opioid abuse cost the US $55.7 billion. Workplace losses totaled $25.6 billion, 46 % of the total amount and included premature death (43.8 %), lost wages due to unemployment (31 %), incarceration (6.9 %), disability and medically related absenteeism (10.2 %), and presenteeism (8 %, the act of attending work while sick or unable to fully perform job duties). The costs added $25 billion (45 % of the total) to the system: excess medical and drug costs (94.9 %), substance abuse treatment (4.5 %), and prevention and research (0.6 %). The costs to the criminal justice system were $5.1 billion (9 %): police protection (29.7 %), legal system (14.1 %), correctional facilities (44.1 %), and property lost because of crime (12.2 %). By comparison, in 2001 total costs were estimated at $11.8 billion. The 2007 figure of $55.7 billion represents an increase of $43.9 billion in just 6 years [16]. An estimate by the CDC in 2011 listed the total cost of opioid abuse to the healthcare system at approximately $72.5 billion annually [17].

Prescription drugs have accounted for most of the increase in death rates since 1999. In 2008 there were 36,450 deaths attributed to drug overdose, just behind the 39,973 deaths from motor vehicle accidents. A drug was specified in 74.5 % of those cases. When a drug was specified, 73.8 % of cases involved prescription opioids [7]. The true numbers of morbidity and mortality from opioid prescriptions are likely underrepresented.

People who see prescription opioids as a "safer" alternative to illicit drugs may be responsible for the surge of misuse and abuse. The number of abusers of prescription opioids far exceeds those who use cocaine or heroin [18]. In 2009, 1.2 million emergency department (ED) visits (an increase of 98.4 % since 2004) were related to misuse or abuse of pharmaceuticals, compared with 1.0 million ED visits from abuse of heroin and cocaine [19]. By 2012 the number of fatalities from drug overdose surpassed fatalities from motor vehicle accidents [20].

A survey by the CDC found that 80 % of patients taking opioid therapy for chronic pain saw a single doctor for treatment and took low dose opioids (<100 mg equivalent daily dosing of oral morphine), 10 % saw a single doctor and took doses ≥ 100 mg morphine equivalent daily, and 10 % saw several doctors and took higher doses. The last group represents a subset of patients who go "doctor shopping" with the intention of misusing, abusing, or diverting opioids. The 80 % of patients treated by a single prescriber for low doses of opioids accounted for only 20 % of overdoses. The other two groups accounted for 40 % each [21]. As the total daily dose of opioid increases, so does the possibility of a negative outcome. A study of 9,940 patients taking long-term opioid therapy for chronic pain found that patients who took ≥ 100 mg had an 8.9-fold increase for overdose [22].

Patterns of and Predispositions to Abuse

The concern of physicians who prescribe opioid therapy is whether the patient will suffer adverse consequences from the therapy. This scenario is all the more important for patients on chronic opioid therapy. It has been estimated that in 2010 more than five million Americans were taking opioid therapy regularly [23]. A Cochrane Review that examined randomized controlled trials of prescription opioids found that only 0.27 % of patients abused opioids [24]. A separate analysis found that 3.3 % of patients had abused their prescriptions, 11.5 % exhibited aberrant drug use behaviors such as losing prescriptions or medications, or running out of pills early, and 14.5 % of the patients in that review had illicit substances in their urine. The discrepancy between the Cochrane review and other studies may be attributed to stringent inclusion criteria for experimental studies. Approximately 20 % of Americans report using prescription opioids for nonmedical use [25].

The characteristics that predispose to abuse could be identified, screening tools could determine those most at risk. When researchers studied 90 prescription opioid abusers receiving treatment, they found that illicit drug use was a major predictor of prescription opioid abuse [26]. Among the patients, 82 % had a parent or sibling who abused drugs or alcohol. Abuse occurs for a variety of reasons. For some it starts after therapy with opioids to treat acute postoperative pain. Others with genetic predisposition to addiction or abuse find the reward from opioid use. In the absence of psychosocial comorbidity or genetic predisposition, prescription opioid abuse is unlikely in a controlled setting and at a stable, effective dose. The risk of abuse is increased with young age at the time of initiation of therapy, severe pain, depression, or other psychiatric illness that is treated concurrently with psychotropic medications [25].

The combination of young age, depression, psychotropic medication, and the degree of impairment from pain increases the risk for abuse by as much as eight times. For a patient with a history of abuse and severe dependence, the risk is increased over 56 times [27]. Prior or concurrent mental illness may lead to an increased rate of abuse [28]. One study of 1,334 patients taking opioid therapy for chronic, noncancer pain found a correlation between depression and opioid misuse.

Patients with moderate to severe depression as defined in the study were 1.8 and 2.4 times more likely to use opioids for nonpain symptoms. Patients with mild, moderate, and severe depression were also 1.9, 2.9, and 3.1 times more likely to self-increase the dose than patients who were not depressed [28].

There is some inconsistency between the effect of population density on abuse and misuse. Some studies show no correlation between the two while others do [29, 30]. One group studied patients treated in New Mexico and used zip codes to map out prescription opioid abuse. In cities where the number of prescriptions written was higher per capita, more patients presented for treatment. In an area close to the Mexican border where the number of prescriptions written was low, abuse numbers still were high. The investigators concluded that geographic information systems can identify clusters of abuse and high availability [31].

The true effect of age on abuse potential is difficult to predict. Some studies show that younger age leads to an increase in abuse, others show no effect of age, and still others that age>75 years puts patients at greater risk. In a study of patients being treated for opioid abuse, 45 % had moderate to severe withdrawal pain, but 75 % of those >45 years of age reported withdrawal symptoms [32]. Risk-taking behaviors in the young and risk aversion in older patients may confound outcomes as well [31, 32].

The diagnosis for which patients receive their prescriptions may influence the rate of abuse. Patients complaining of back pain and headache are likely to become opioid abusers. Those with joint pain and arthritis are less likely. One study found that half of all schedule II opioids were given for minor back injury claims. The efficacy of opioids for this injury has not been well established and is considered questionable by the American College of Occupational and Environmental Medicine. The opioid analgesics for relief of chronic pain may lead to greater disability [15]. The mechanism by which therapy for chronic pain may lead to disability is not well understood [33]. Schedule II medications are associated with a higher rate of abuse than schedule III or IV medications [29]. One study found the abuse rate of tramadol, a schedule IV medication, low, and 97 % of those who abused it had a history of abusing other substances [32].

Methods to Combat Abuse

Given the well-established epidemic of opioid abuse and the toll it takes both financially and physically on those whom it affects, numerous methods for combating the problem have been implemented. These are federally mandated programs, monitoring at the state level, and tools designed to be used by practitioners who prescribe opioids. A set of "universal precautions" for the practice of prescribing opioid medications for pain has been proposed. The ten-step process is as follows: (1) establishing a diagnosis and treating treatable causes including any comorbid psychiatric illness; (2) psychological assessment including risk of addictive disorder; (3) informed consent that includes anticipated benefits and foreseeable risks; (4) a treatment agreement that describes the expectations and obligations of both patient and provider and that establishes limits to enable early identification and intervention around aberrant behavior; (5) pre- and postintervention assessment of pain level and function; (6) a trial of opioid therapy with or without adjunctive medications; (7) reassessment of pain score and function; (8) regular assessment of the "four A's" of pain medicine and effect (analgesia, activities of daily living, adverse events, and aberrant behaviors); (9) a periodic review of the pain diagnosis and comorbid conditions, including addictive disorders; and (10) careful and thorough documentation to reduce medico-legal exposure and risk of regulatory sanction. If a patient's risk is low, medium, or high this information is given to primary care practitioners or to a specialist for assistance with pain management. Side effects from opioids are monitored as is behavior that may indicate misuse or abuse [25, 34].

Opioid contracts require patients to agree to a set of conditions in order to receive treatment with opioids. Patients agree to receive opioids from a single provider and a single pharmacy. Urine drug screens ensure the medications being prescribed are being taken. Some abusers obtain legitimate prescriptions and then sell or trade them to get an illicit drug of choice. Drug screens also detect substances not prescribed to the patient and identify illicit agents or other therapeutic pharmaceuticals that may combine with prescribed drugs. The opioid contract establishes expectations and rules to be followed to continue therapy. Patients are discharged from the care of a provider if the mandates are not maintained.

Insurers may attempt to limit abuse by monitoring or even limiting the number of opioid prescriptions a patient may obtain. Insurers could limit the reimbursement of claims for opioid prescriptions to a designated doctor and a designated pharmacy. Manufacturers of pharmaceuticals can participate in abuse prevention by creating formulations that deter or are resistant to tampering. There are many examples of formulations to deter abuse and misuse [35]. Suboxone, a coformulation of buprenorphine and naloxone (an opioid antagonist), is intended to be taken orally. It is an alternative to methadone for maintenance therapy for those previously addicted to opioids. Studies have shown that alteration of oral suboxone and subsequent intravenous injection produced no euphoria. It is possible that IV administration may still produce euphoria in those not yet physically dependent [28]. Embeda with a naltrexone core surrounded by morphine does not release its core when taken orally. ELI-216, in developmental stages, is extended release oxycodone with naltrexone pellets that do not release when taken orally. Remoxy, a new formulation of oxycodone with a viscous liquid, is intended to resist isolation in alcohol and injecting. There are even formulations of oxycodone that are reformulated with a polymer that resists crushing and turns into a viscous gel when hydrated.

Prescription monitoring programs, at the state level report on prescriptions for controlled substances: what patients are filling, how often, and from which physicians. The primary goal is to identify "doctor shopping." There are several efforts underway to unify reporting among neighboring states and to shorten delays in updating data.

Through the FDA the federal government has authorized the use of risk evaluation and mitigation strategies (REMS) to combat the abuse of prescription opioids. Manufacturers must prove that the benefits of a drug outweigh the risks, and hospitals and providers are required to monitor the dispensing of certain drugs. REMS have been adopted for many different classes of medications including chemotherapeutic agents, immune modulators, antihyperglycemics, antiepileptics and not surprisingly, opioids. Medication guides, communication plans for healthcare professionals, special training or certification for prescribing, and special monitoring are methods employed by REMS. There is a trend for establishing REMS to include all formulations containing fentanyl or oxycodone [36].

Opioid abuse is widespread and not to be taken lightly. There is a real need to balance the obvious beneficial effects of these medications with the sometimes less well-appreciated negative effects. Patients deserve treatment if they suffer from pain. The ideal way to do so is less clear. The euphorigenic effects of opioids are part of alleviating pain and suffering. Physicians who prescribe these medications must be aware of their risks and benefits and take precautions to minimize their misuse and abuse.

References

1. Corbett AD, Henderson HG, McKnight AT, et al. 75 years of opioid research: the exciting but vain quest for the Holy Grail. Br J Pharmacol. 2006;146:S152–62.
2. Mogil JS, Grisel JE. Transgenic studies of pain. Pain. 1998;77:107–28.
3. McDonald J, Lambert DG. Opioid receptors. Contin Educ Anaesth Crit Care Pain. 2005;5(1): 22–5.
4. Zacny J, Bigelow G, Comptom P, et al. College on problems of drug dependence taskforce on prescription opioid non-medical use and abuse: position statement. Drug Alcohol Depend. 2003;69:215–32.
5. Weissman DE, Haddox JD. Opioid pseudoaddiction—an iatrogenic syndrome. Pain. 1989;36(3):363–6.
6. Campbell J. MD Presidential Address, American Pain Society November 11, 1996. http://www.va.gov/;ainmangement/doc/toolkit.pdf. Accessed 26 July 2013.
7. Paulozzi LJ, et al. Vital signs: overdoses of prescription opioid pain relievers—United States, 1999–2008. Morb Mortal Wkly Rep. 2011;60(43):1487–92.
8. Manchikanti L, Abdil S, Alturi S, et al. American Society of Interventional Pain Physicians (ASIPP) guidelines for responsible opioid prescribing in chronic non-cancer pain: part I—evidence assessment. Pain Physician. 2012;15(3 Suppl):S1–65.
9. Grattan A, Sullivan MD, Saunders KW, et al. Depression and prescription opioid misuse among chronic opioid therapy recipients with no history of substance abuse. Ann Fam Med. 2012;10(4):304–11.
10. http://www.cdc.gov/vitalsigns/painkilleroverdoses/. Accessed 26 July 2013.
11. Substance Abuse and Mental Health Services Administration. Results from the 2011 national survey on drug use and health: summary of national findings. NSDUH Series H-44, HHS Publication No. (SMA) 12-4713. Rockville: Substance Abuse and Mental Health Services Administration; 2012.
12. Substance Abuse and Mental Health Services Administration. Office of applied studies: treatment episode data set (TEDS). http://wwwdasis.samhsa.gov/webt/NewMapv1.htm
13. Cleland et al. Substance abuse treatment, prevention, and policy 2011, 6:11. http://www.substanceabusepolicy.com/content/6/1/11. Accessed 26 July 2013.
14. Butler SF, Black RA, Cassidy TA, Dailey TM, Budman SH. Abuse risks and routes of administration of different prescription opioid compounds and formulations. Harm Reduct J. 2011;8.

15. Swedlow A, Ireland J, Johnson G. Prescribing patterns of schedule II opioids in California workers' compensation. California Workers Compensation Institute. www.cwci.org. Accessed 25 June 2013.
16. Birnbaum HG, White AG, Schiller M, et al. Societal costs of prescription opioid abuse, dependence, and misuse in the United States. Pain Med. 2011;12:656–67.
17. Coalition Against Insurance Fraud. Prescription for peril: how insurance fraud finances theft and abuse of addictive prescription drugs. Washington, DC: Coalition Against Insurance Fraud; 2007. http://www.insurancefraud.org/downloads/drugDiversion.pdf. Accessed 26 Sept 2011.
18. Prescription drugs: abuse and addiction. NIH Publication Number 11-4881. July 2001, Revised October 2011. www.drugabuse.gov/sites/default/files/rrprescription.pdf. Accessed 26 July 2013.
19. Substance Abuse and Mental Health Services Administration. Highlights of the 2009 Drug Abuse Warning Network (DAWN) findings on drug-related emergency department visits. The DAWN Report. Rockville: US Department of Health and Human Services, Substance Abuse and Mental Health Services Administration; 2010. http://oas.samhsa.gov/2k10/dawn034/edhighlights. Accessed 3 Oct 2011.
20. Alexander GA, Kruszewski SP, Webster DW. Rethinking opioid prescribing to protect patient safety and public health. J Am Med Assoc. 2012;308(18):1865–6.
21. Centers for Disease Control and Prevention. CDC grand rounds: prescription drug overdoses—a U.S. epidemic. MMWR Morb Mortal Wkly Rep. 2012;61(39):10–3.
22. Dunn KM, Saunders KW, Rutter CM, et al. Opioid prescriptions for chronic pain and overdose: a cohort study. Ann Intern Med. 2010;152:85–92.
23. Boudreau D, Von Korff M, Rutter CM, et al. Trends in long-term opioid therapy for chronic non-cancer pain. Pharmacoepidemiol Drug Saf. 2009;18:1166–75.
24. Noble M, Treadwell JR, Tregear SJ, et al. Long-term opioid management for chronic non-cancer pain. Cochrane Database Syst Rev. 2010;(1):CD006605.
25. Seghal N, Manchikanti L, Smith HS. Prescription opioid abuse in chronic pain: a review of opioid abuse predictors and strategies to curb opioid abuse. Pain Physician. 2012;15:ES67–92.
26. Rigg KK, Murphy JW. Understanding the etiology of prescription opioid abuse: implications for prevention and treatment. Qual Health Res. 2013;23(7):963–75.
27. Boscarino JA, Rukstalis M, Hoffman SN, et al. Risk factors for drug dependence among outpatients on opioid therapy in a large US health-care system. Addiction. 2010;105:1776–82.
28. Edlund MJ, Martin BC, Fan M, et al. Risks for opioid abuse and dependence among recipients of chronic opioid therapy: results from the TROUP study. Drug Alcohol Depend. 2010;112:90–8.
29. Grattan A, Sullivan MD, Saunders KW, et al. Depression and prescription opioid misuse among chronic opioid therapy recipients with no history of substance abuse. Ann Fam Med. 2012;10(4):304–11.
30. Spiller H, Lorenz DL, Bailet EJ, et al. Epidemiological trends in abuse and misuse of prescription opioids. J Addict Dis. 2009;28:130–13.
31. Brownstein JS, Green TC, Cassidy TA, et al. Geographic information systems and pharmacoepidemiology: using spatial cluster detection to monitor local patterns of prescription opioid abuse. Pharmacoepidemiol Drug Saf. 2010;19:627–37.
32. Cicero TJ, Surratt HL, Kurtz S, et al. Patterns of prescription opioid abuse and comorbidity in an aging treatment population. J Subst Abuse Treat. 2013;42:87–94.
33. Katz C, El-Gabalawy E, Keyes KN, et al. Risk factors for incident nonmedical prescription opioid use and abuse and dependence: results from a longitudinal nationally representative sample. Drug Alcohol Depend. 2013;132.
34. Manubay JM, Muchow C, Sullivan MA. Prescription drug abuse: epidemiology, regulatory issues, chronic pain management with narcotic analgesics. Prim Care. 2011;38(1):71.
35. Schneider JP, Matthews M, Jamison R. Abuse-deterrent and tamper-resistant opioid formulations—what is their role in addressing prescription opioid abuse? CNS Drugs. 2010;24(10):805–10.
36. U.S. Food and Drug Administration. Risk evaluation and mitigation strategies for certain opioid drugs; notice of public hearing. April 20, 2009. http://www.fda.gov/OHRMS/DOCKETS/98fr/E9-8992.pdf

Chapter 16
The Multidisciplinary Approach to the Management of Substance Abuse

Andrei D. Sdrulla and Grace Chen

Key Points

- Substance abuse is a chronic, pervasive medical problem commonly associated with comorbid medical and psychiatric disorders.
- Patients with coexisting substance abuse and psychiatric disorders are more difficult to treat and tend to be clinically more severe.
- The role of the physician is to identify those at risk and either to devise a comprehensive treatment plan or to refer the patient to a physician with specialty training in substance abuse.
- The term biopsychosocial refers to treatment programs that incorporate elements of pharmacotherapy, psychological treatments (psychotherapy and behavior therapy), and sociocultural therapy.
- Integrated care programs exist for those with comorbid conditions and research supports improved outcomes over stand-alone programs.
- Numerous pharmacological therapies have been successfully employed to diminish craving and decrease relapse, and there is some evidence to support that combination therapy with other modalities provides added benefit.

Introduction

Substance abuse is a prevalent medical problem. In 2012, 23.9 million Americans were active users, having used illicit substances in the past month, representing approximately 9.2 % of the population aged 12 or older [1]. The treatment of patients abusing substances poses a tremendous problem since addiction is both

A.D. Sdrulla, M.D., Ph.D. (✉) • G. Chen, M.D.
Department of Anesthesiology and Perioperative Medicine, Oregon Health and Sciences
University, 3181 Southwest Sam Jackson Park Road, Portland, OR 97239, USA
e-mail: Sdrulla@ohsu.edu; cheng@ohsu.edu

© Springer Science+Business Media New York 2015
A.D. Kaye et al. (eds.), *Substance Abuse*, DOI 10.1007/978-1-4939-1951-2_16

an acute and chronic problem, and addicted patients quite often have comorbid medical and psychiatric problems. Indeed, substance abuse is associated with various medical conditions, stemming from either direct toxicity (cigarette smoke and lung damage) or from behaviors associated with drug use (injections and risk for acquiring hepatitis and human immunodeficiency virus (HIV)). Cardiovascular disease is strongly associated with tobacco abuse, as are heavy alcohol use and the use of stimulants such as cocaine. Cigarette smoking is the most common cause of lung cancer, the leading cause of cancer death in the United States and globally [2]. Alcohol is a risk factor for developing cancers of the digestive tract, particularly hepatocellular carcinoma that arises in the setting of liver cirrhosis [3]. In addition to liver dysfunction, chronic alcohol abuse is associated with increased risk of developing pancreatitis, which carries a high mortality rate. Cirrhosis can be the sequelae of excessive chronic alcohol intake or can be caused by infection with hepatitis B (40–80 % prevalence among intravenous drug users (IDUs)) or hepatitis C viruses (15–51 % prevalence among IDUs) [4]. Drug abuse has been inextricably linked with HIV/AIDS since the beginning of the HIV epidemic, both due to IDU and to the tendency to trade sex for money or drugs along with unsafe sexual practices [5]. Clinical challenge arises when symptoms of intoxication or withdrawal overlap with those of comorbid medical conditions, and often referral to specialists is required. Myalgia, chills, nausea, vomiting and diarrhea in an opioid abusing patient can represent a manifestation of withdrawal or could be due to an infectious process such as gastroenteritis in a patient with AIDS.

The term "co-occurring disorders" has been used to describe individuals concomitantly having one or more psychiatric diagnoses in addition to one or more substance abuse problems. Approximately 8.9 million adults have co-occurring disorders, and only 7.4 % of these individuals receive treatment for both conditions, with 55.8 % receiving no treatment at all [6]. Certain psychiatric diagnoses are more frequently associated with substance use disorders, for example 40 % of people with unipolar depression have associated with alcohol problem, and 17 % have substance abuse other than alcohol [7]. Bipolar disorder has a lifetime prevalence of substance abuse in more than 40 % of sufferers, whereas patients with bipolar I disorder have a lifetime prevalence of over 60 % [8]. It has been estimated that 65 % of people with one psychiatric disorder have a lifetime history of at least one substance abuse disorder [9]. It is well established that patients with co-occurring disorders are clinically more severe and more difficult to treat than patients with either condition alone [10].

The Role of the Physician in Managing Patients with Substance Abuse

Substance abuse as a disease needs to be regarded similarly as any other chronic condition, such as chronic pain, diabetes, heart disease, and cancer, with periods of exacerbations (intoxication and withdrawal) interspersed with longer periods of remission when sufferers require maintenance therapy. The optimal therapeutic approach depends on where along the continuum of the disease the patients reside, in addition to the abused substance, and medical and psychiatric comorbidities. For example, individuals with severe alcohol dependence require multiple strategies to address the heavy drinking and mitigate the risk of withdrawal, in addition to addressing associated psychosocial and medical complications. In the early phases of addiction treatment, patient with severe disease are best served in inpatient treatment facilities. In these early stages, the goals are to treat the withdrawal and related acute medical conditions. Medical detoxification utilize either an outpatient or inpatient setting, and the inpatient setting is required for conditions such as hepatic insufficiency, acute pancreatitis, bleeding esophageal varices, and decompensated psychiatric conditions. Coexisting psychosocial problems, such as homelessness, warrant admission into inpatient or residential treatment facilities. Once patients have completed the acute detoxification phase and are ready to change their behavior, therapeutic options must be weighed. The vast majority of patients are treated in outpatient facilities, with programs offering a variety of treatment options, including day hospital programs for several hours per day and several days per week.

The role of the physician is to assess the patient and devise a treatment strategy. Some patients are presented to medical care during exacerbations due to health consequences of substance abuse (e.g., withdrawal), while others are legally mandated to seek care. There has been recent interest in screening tools to identify individuals at risk, who are not dependent or addicted, and who could benefit from early intervention [11]. This is different from earlier strategies that focused on universal strategies to prevent use in those who never initiated use, or from referring to treatment those people with the severe abuse or addiction. Evidence suggests that providing screening to those individuals with hazardous levels of substance use, coupled with early intervention, leads to significant improvement in outcomes [12]. Typical elements of intervention are part of a motivational interview, and include personalized feedback regarding the patient's substance abuse, in the case of alcohol compared with norms, risk of injury due to intoxication, physical consequences supported by lab values and negative social consequences supported by screening tests [13]. A review of 361 controlled studies of treatments for alcohol use disorders found that screening and brief intervention was the most effective modality, particularly among those not actively seeking treatment [14]. Early intervention strategies can be applied in the primary care and hospital setting with good success [15]. As of 2011, the federal Centers for Medicare and Medicaid Services began covering the entire cost of screening and brief intervention. Given the high prevalence and the high morbidity of substance abuse, the United States Preventive Services Task Force recommends that clinicians screen all adults aged 18 years or older for alcohol misuse [16] while screening for illicit drug use is not currently recommended [17].

Once patients have been screened and are positive for substance abuse, they should be risk-stratified and an appropriate intervention plan should be formulated. For a patient demonstrating hazardous use, this can be as simple as counseling and ongoing assessment, to brief counseling and a follow-up plan for substance abusing patients and referral to treatment for those who are dependent [18]. Also, substances of abuse should not be regarded as equal, as they have different potentials for harm to the patient and society. Heroin, crack cocaine, and methamphetamine are considered to be the most harmful to the individual, whereas alcohol, heroin, and crack cocaine are considered the most harmful to others [19]. Patients with substance abuse or dependence require specialized in-depth assessment of their problems to better define their problem, provide data for a formal diagnosis, establish the severity, determine appropriate level of care, guide treatment planning, and to define a baseline for future comparisons. This is a very complex and time consuming task, one that involves interviewing the patient, obtaining supporting laboratory tests such as blood and urine drug levels, and obtaining information from family and friends [20]. Primary care physicians have a choice regarding their involvement with the management of the patient's substance abuse problem. This ranges from referring to specialists with experience in substance abuse, to formulating treatment plans and referring to treatment centers, and to providing comprehensive treatment including medical care and pharmacotherapy, depending on expertise and available resources.

Optimally, the treatment plan should be comprehensive and address the medical, psychosocial, and family dimensions; it should include identifying problems, strengths, priorities, goals, and strategies and be formulated in a manner that enables measurement of progress. The patient's condition and goals should shape the structure of the treatment program, such as safe detoxification, development of skills, and an environment to sustain abstinence. The role of the healthcare provider is to perform the initial assessment of the patient and prescribe an appropriate treatment plan that might include additional assessment of patient dimensions outside the scope of practice of that provider. For example, a patient might be referred to a social worker to accurately evaluate the home environment and support structure.

There are allocation guidelines that can be used to match the patient to the appropriate level of care, based on severity of disease, prior treatments, psychiatric impairment, and degree of social stability [21]. The most widely used placement criteria are those of the American Society of Addiction Medicine (ASAM) [22], and are based on a thorough assessment of the patient on six dimensions. The six dimensions (Table 16.1) include: acute intoxication and/or potential for withdrawal, biomedical conditions or complications, emotional, behavioral, or cognitive conditions and complications, readiness to change, potential for relapse and recovery environment. There are five levels of care (Table 16.2), ranging from early intervention (level 0.5) to medically managed intensive inpatient treatment (level IV). The optimal care is the least intensive level that meets the goals of treatment for that patient in a safe and effective fashion (Table 16.3). Patients generally transition from more intensive inpatient based therapy to outpatient modalities, although the opposite can also occur depending on the needs of that particular patient. The length of treatment at a particular level of care depends on the patient achieving the goals

Table 16.1 ASAM placement criteria dimensions

Dimension		Assessment
Dimension 1	Acute intoxication and/or withdrawal potential	Significant risk of severe withdrawal symptoms or seizures
Dimension 2	Biomedical conditions and complications	Any acute or chronic medical illness that might interfere with the current treatment episode
Dimension 3	Emotional, behavioral, or cognitive conditions and complications	Any psychiatric issues, including behavioral or emotional problems that might impede the treatment process
Dimension 4	Readiness to change	Patient's openness to treatment, acceptance of addiction, readiness for change, and motivation for compliance
Dimension 5	Relapse, continued use, or continued problem potential	Patient's ability to cope with cravings, comprehension of relapse triggers, and ability to abstain
Dimension 6	Recovery environment	Current living situation, adequacy of social support network, financial resources, etc.

Table 16.2 ASAM levels of care

Level of care	Treatment
0.5	Early intervention
I	Outpatient
II	Intensive outpatient/partial hospitalization
III	Residential/inpatient
IV	Medically managed intensive inpatient

formulated in the treatment plan. For example, inpatient care would be required for an acutely intoxicated alcoholic patient, completing detoxification until the autonomic (tachycardia, sweating, hypertension) and psychological (anxiety, panic attacks) signs and symptoms have abated and the patient is stable. Alternatively, a patient who is unable to achieve the treatment goals at a prescribed care level, despite adequate participation and due either to lack of capacity or worsening condition, would be moved to a different level or type of service [22]. Studies support the implementation of ASAM criteria for providing appropriate and cost effective treatment [23, 24].

Interestingly, one study did not find a difference in post treatment drinking outcomes for individuals with alcoholism who had been assigned to inpatient, intensive outpatient or outpatient settings, although individuals with high scores on alcohol involvement benefited most from inpatient treatment, whereas those low in alcohol involvement benefited most from outpatient care [25]. Additional prospective studies are needed to examine the effectiveness of matching patients to level of care and to explore mediators of outcomes.

Table 16.3 The ASAM placement criteria

Criteria dimensions	Levels of service									
	Level 0.5 early intervention	OMT opioid maintenance therapy	Level I outpatient services	Level II.1 intensive outpatient	Level II.5 partial hospitalization	Level III.1 clinically managed low intensity residential services	Level III.3 clinically managed medium intensity residential services	Level III.5 clinically managed medium/high intensity residential services	Level III.7 medically monitored intensive inpatient services	Level IV medically monitored intensive inpatient services
Dimension 1: alcohol intoxication and/or withdrawal potential	No withdrawal risk	Withdrawal prevented by OMT	Minimal risk of severe withdrawal	Minimal risk of severe withdrawal	Minimal risk of severe withdrawal	No withdrawal risk	Moderate withdrawal risk (not severe)	Moderate withdrawal risk (not severe)	Moderate risk of severe withdrawal	Severe withdrawal risk
Dimension 2: biomedical conditions and complications	None or stable	None or stable	None or stable	None or stable	None or stable	None or stable	None or stable	Stable; may need medical monitoring	Medical monitoring required	Needs 24 h medical care
Dimension 3: emotional/behavioral conditions and complications	None or stable	None or manageable in outpatient structure	None or stable	Mild severity; needs monitoring	Mild to moderate severity; needs monitoring	None or minimal	Mild to moderate severity	Unable to control impulses	Moderate severity	Severe problems need 24 h psychiatric care
Dimension 4: readiness to change (insight)	Has insight into use affecting goals	Requires structure therapy to progress	Cooperative, but needs motivation and monitoring	Moderate resistance structure required	Significant resistance; more structure needed	Needs structure to maintain therapeutic gains	Little insight; needs motivating strategies	No insight may not believe treatment is necessary	High resistance and poor impulse control	Not applicable for this level of care
Dimension 5: relapse/continued use potential (automaticity)	Need skills to change current use	High relapse risk without OMT	Able to maintain abstinence	Higher automaticity; needs monitoring and support	Significant automaticity; needs more monitoring and support	Understands relapse, but still needs structure	Higher automaticity requiring 24 h monitoring	Inadequate skills to prevent immediate relapse	Unable to control use with dangerous consequence	Not applicable for this level of care
Dimension 6: recovery environment	Good social support	Supportive recovery environment	Supportive recovery environment	Less supportive structure needed to cope	Environment unsupportive; higher structure improves patient coping	Dangerous environment; structure permits success in recovery	Dangerous environment; structure permits success in recovery	Dangerous environment; structure permits success in recovery	Dangerous recovery environment; structure permits success in recovery	Not applicable for this level of care

With permission from Albanese AP. Management of alcohol abuse. Clin Liver Dis 2012 Nov;16[4]:737–762 [26]

Treatment Resources

Once the treatment plan has been created, the physician has to identify local resources that could best implement the treatment. Directories of resources can be found in multiple places, and most information is now available on the Internet. Most communities have directories of substance abuse treatment facilities, generally maintained by public agencies. Databases include information such as the program services offered, eligibility criteria, cost, and staff qualifications such as language proficiency. The local health department, a council on alcoholism and drug abuse, a social services organization, or volunteers who aid in recovery may produce the directory. All states have alcohol and other drug authorities that provide the licensing and review the state's substance abuse treatment programs, and they often publish and post online the directories of licensed facilities. The National Council on Alcohol and Drug Dependence (NCADD) promotes public understanding of alcoholism and drug addiction as treatable and preventable diseases. NCADD provides resources for patients and families including assessment and interventions on their website (see Table 16.4) and they distribute information on treatment facilities. Lastly, the Substance Abuse and Mental Health Services Administration distributes a National Directory of Drug Abuse and Alcoholism Treatment and Prevention Programs that is available on their website with links to state-run programs.

Treatment Models

Most modern treatment programs are multidisciplinary, with integrated medical, psychological, and sociocultural aspects. Medical therapy consists of medications to decrease symptoms and prevent relapse. Psychological treatments address emotional

Table 16.4 Resources for the treatment of substance abuse

Authority	Information included	Website
Local health department, a council on alcoholism and drug abuse, a social services organization, or volunteers in recovery	Program services (e.g., type, location, hours, and accessibility to public transportation), eligibility criteria, cost, and staff complement and qualifications, including language proficiency	Local health department website
State level alcohol and drug authority	Publishes a statewide directory of all alcohol and drug treatment programs licensed in the state	State level websites
National Council on Alcohol and Drug Dependence	Assessment or referral for a sliding scale fee and distributes free information on treatment facilities nationally	http://www.ncadd.org
Substance Abuse and Mental Health Services Administration	National directory of drug abuse and alcoholism treatment and prevention programs	http://findtreatment.samhsa.gov

and motivational components of substance abuse and include psychotherapy and behavior therapy. Sociocultural therapy focuses on providing a social context conducive to abstinence. Given the pervasive nature of substance abuse, most patients can benefit from treatment in all three aspects and most treatment programs include aspects from each modality. The term "biopsychosocial" has been used to refer to programs that include all of these components [26, 27].

Less intensive programs consist of counseling, either individual or group sessions, and family and couples therapy. Most patients enroll in counseling programs after completing more intensive inpatient or outpatient treatments. There are numerous programs that incorporate elements such as educational, support-related, and therapeutic or focused on skill development.

Self-help groups (SHG), support groups consisting of individuals who share a common problem such as specific type of substance abuse, and who meet regularly to exchange information and develop supportive relationships, improve the quality of their lives. SHGs provide a venue for patients to share their feelings in safe and non-judgmental environments, develop interpersonal, self-efficacy and coping skills, increase motivation for abstinence, and identify new activities and goals. Most clinicians do not view SHGs as formal treatment programs, however they provide a valuable support structure that can enhance recovery, thus SHGs should be a component of a patient's therapy at any stage of disease [28].

The largest and most widespread SHG is Alcoholics Anonymous (AA), a group that was established in 1935 and is based on 12 guiding principles that include admission over lack of control, recognizing a higher power that can provide help, examining past errors and making amends with the help of a sponsor, learning to live a new life and helping others suffering from the same addiction and 12 traditions such as emphasis on community welfare, defining the membership to the group and mission of the group, including the anonymity foundation of the group (www.aa.org). AA estimates that in the United States there are 1.3 million members and 59,000 groups, and a worldwide membership of 2.1 million with over 110,000 groups. The success of AA spawned the creation of similar groups for other substances of abuse, such as narcotics anonymous and cocaine anonymous. For persons with dual diagnosis (comorbid psychiatric and substance abuse problems), who often have difficulties relating and bonding to other members, a similar 12 step fellowship program exists, named Double Trouble in Recovery (www.hazelden.org/web/go/dtr). One of the core elements of 12 step programs is acceptance in a Higher Power, and secular SHG's were established for people seeking groups with less spiritual overtones. These include Secular Organizations for Sobriety (www.sossobriety.org), LifeRing (lifering.org), and Moderation Management (www.moderationmanagement.org). Other groups that offer alternatives to the 12 step programs include SMART Recovery, which emphasizes practical four-point programs as well as online message boards and 24/7 chat rooms for support (www.smartrecovery.org). There is evidence to support participation in SHGs, as more frequent participation correlates with maintained abstinence [29]. One study of alcohol-dependent patients enrolled in SHGs after participating in intensive outpatient treatments, found a characteristic dose-response relation, with even modest levels of participation being beneficial [30]. Those who attend SHGs over time are more likely to remain abstinent compared with individuals who stop attending, or those who participated intermittently, even after controlling for the length of formal treatment [31].

Cognitive behavioral therapy (CBT) is a psychotherapeutic intervention that addresses both cognitive processes (dysfunctional emotions) and maladaptive behaviors through systematic, goal-directed procedures. CBT for substance abuse is well defined and has been rigorously studied, with efficacy across the spectrum of substances, including alcohol dependence, cocaine dependence and nicotine dependence [9]. A unique feature of CBT for substance abuse is durability of its effects; patients continue to improve even after completing treatment [32]. In addition to substance use disorders, CBT has proven efficacy for co-occurring disorders including depression and anxiety disorders. When combined with other behavioral and pharmacotherapies, CBT appears to have robust, sustained effects [33].

More recent advances in psychosocial treatment of substance abuse have been motivational interviewing (MI) and motivational enhancement therapy (MET). The premise for these therapies is that most substance abusers lack the motivation to change and that motivation is a crucial component of human intentional behavior change [13]. MI is an integral component of early screening and intervention approaches, as discussed above. MI is seldom given alone, and is often combined with other forms of treatment, including education, self-help manuals, cognitive therapy, skills training, SHG participation, stress management, and specific treatments for the particular setting. Despite some variability in results, MI and MET consistently improved health outcomes, and there is ongoing research to identify the "active ingredients" of motivational interviewing [34].

A large multi-site client treatment matching study did not find differences between cognitive behavioral skills therapy, MET and 12 step facilitation therapy in patients receiving outpatient or aftercare therapy following inpatient or day hospital treatment [35]. The study included 1,726 alcohol-dependent patients who were randomly assigned to one of the three treatment modalities for a period of 12 weeks. All three treatment groups had significant and sustained improvement in drinking outcomes (e.g., alcohol consumption) with minimal difference in outcome by type of treatment. A secondary analysis showed that patients with high anger or hostility scores had better outcomes with MET, as this form of therapy was specifically formulated to reduce resistance to treatment. Patients with low alcohol dependence scores had better results with CBT. A 3-year follow-up revealed sustained benefits with a slight advantage of 12 step facilitation programs [35, 36].

There are other programs that focus on the various aspects of healing, such as having a supportive (therapeutic) community. The therapeutic community approach rebuilds a person's self-esteem and self-image, addressing the needs of the client as a "whole person." This is a shift from engaging only the individual, to instill a greater awareness of the role of the community in the treatment approach. Similarly, network therapy involves and engages people in the patient's social network, committed to the patient's abstinence [37].

A recent randomized trial compared comprehensive substance abuse management with a control strategy. Chronic care management consisted of longitudinal care coordinated with a primary care clinician, MET, relapse prevention counseling, and on-site medical, addiction, and psychiatric treatment, social work assistance, and referrals (including mutual help). The control group received a primary care appointment and a list of treatment resources, including a telephone number to arrange counseling. Over a 12-month period, chronic care management did not increase self-reported abstinence, and the only subgroup analysis that was significant was alcohol dependence, in which chronic care management was associated with fewer alcohol problems [38].

Integrated Care

Given the medical and psychiatric complexities of substance abusing patients, the best health outcomes are achieved when there is an integrated repertoire of indicated specialties, such as substance abuse care, general primary care, subspecialty care and psychiatric care. The concept of integrated programs involving pharmacotherapy and psychosocial therapy has evolved as a means to provide patients with combined services and improve adherence, and to prevent patients from bouncing between different treatment programs. By providing integrated care, patients have easier access and more individualized care than in stand-alone programs. This was studied in a controlled trial where patients with chemical dependency were randomly assigned either to an integrated model in which primary health care was included within the addiction treatment program, or to an independent model in which primary care and substance abuse treatment were provided separately. Although the abstinence rates were similar between the two groups, the patients with substance abuse related medical conditions were more likely to be abstinent in the integrated care model, and this was true for patients with both medical and with psychiatric related conditions [39]. In a recent systematic review that included 13 studies, integrated programs were found to beneficial for pregnant women with substance abuse, with improvement in child development and most growth parameters. The integrated programs in the systematic review included at least one specific substance use treatment and at least one parenting or child treatment service [40]. Thus, recent studies have consistently shown that integrated care programs are more effective than stand-alone treatment programs for patients with co-occurring disorders [41].

Pharmacological Therapies

In addition to therapy-based interventions, pharmacological therapies should be considered to reduce consumption and to prevent relapse. Alcohol abuse can be addressed with disulfiram, a medication that irreversibly inhibits the enzyme acetaldehyde dehydrogenase, leading to buildup of acetaldehyde and producing highly unpleasant symptoms in patients such as nausea, vomiting, throbbing headache, tachycardia, dysphoria, flushing, hypotension, vertigo and dyspnea. This causes a negative association with alcohol and discourages further consumption. A recent systematic review found that supervised treatment with disulfiram, compared to placebo, no treatment or other treatments, has an effect on short-term abstinence and the number of days until relapse, as well as the number of drinking days [42]. There is only modest evidence supporting the use of disulfiram for the treatment of cocaine dependence [43].

Acamprosate is an agonist at the GABA type A receptors, and an antagonist of NMDA receptors that was FDA approved for the treatment of alcohol dependence in 2004. Studies comparing acamprosate with placebo had mixed results, with some studies showing efficacy, while others did not find benefit [44]. A recent meta-analysis including 24 randomized controlled trials found that acamprosate significantly decreased relative risk of any drinking and increased the cumulative abstinence duration, whereas secondary outcomes such as heavy drinking, and enzyme markers of liver injury did not significantly differ compared to placebo [45].

Other pharmacological treatments for alcohol abuse include topiramate, an antiepileptic, presumed to enhance GABA A receptors, leading to increased inhibition, and by inhibiting glutamatergic excitatory neurotransmission. Topiramate scored better than placebo on all drinking measures in multiple trials [44]. Other less well studied medications include baclofen, ondansetron, sertraline, and aripirazole [26]. Finally, complementary and alternative medicine therapies that have been employed in the management of alcohol abuse include biofeedback and acupuncture, although the evidence for benefit is, so far, not compelling [46].

Recently, there has been interest in combined pharmacotherapy and behavioral treatments for alcohol abuse, and in determining whether the efficacy of treatment can be increased by combining modalities. One study randomized alcohol-dependent patients who had been abstinent for 4 days, to either medical management with acamprosate, naltrexone, both or placebo, with and without behavioral interventions that included aspects of CBT, 12 step facilitation, motivational interviewing and building a support system. The outcomes measured were drinking parameters such as percent day abstinent and time to first heavy drinking (primary outcomes), as well as number of drinks per drinking day, drinks per day, and heavy drinking days per month (secondary outcomes). The results showed that behavioral therapy and naltrexone improved outcomes alone and in combination compared with placebo, however the combination of therapy and naltrexone did not improve outcomes any further [47]. In a large VA study, naltrexone and individual counseling was no better than placebo and individual counseling in the percentage of days on which drinking occurred and number of drinks per drinking day [48].

A small study that compared acamprosate with placebo in patients with concurrent depression and alcohol use disorder found improvement in depressive symptoms and a decrease in the number of drinks during the trial, but the study was not powered to detect superiority versus placebo [49]. Another study investigated sertraline, naltrexone, a combination of both or placebo while receiving weekly CBT in patients with co-occurring depression and alcohol dependence. The patients receiving combination sertraline and naltrexone were abstinent from alcohol and had delayed relapse to heavy drinking and tended to not be depressed by the end of treatment [50]. Pharmacological treatments for opioid abuse have proliferated during the twenty first century especially as the rates of abuse (heroin, hydrocodone and oxycodone) have escalated. Methadone maintenance, available in the United States since the 1970s, has been the mainstay of therapy for opioid dependence. Methadone maintenance treatments have to be managed through licensed opioid treatment program (OTPs). To qualify for admission to an OTP, patients must have documentation of current opioid addiction of at least 1 year's duration, and this requirement is waived for patients recently release from incarceration, previously treated in an OTP within the past 2 years, or who are pregnant. Patients under the age of 18 must have had 2 failed attempts at medically supervised withdrawal and have parental or guardian permission [9]. The efficacy of methadone replacement is well established for patients with opioid dependence [51]. However, methadone treatment is limited to highly regulated environments, restricting the number of patients who would or could seek treatment. The passage of the Drug Addiction Treatment of 2000 amended the Controlled Substances Act to allow qualified physicians to prescribe FDA-authorized schedule III, IV, and V medications. Buprenorphine was FDA approved in 2002 for the treatment of opioid dependence, and remains the only medication meeting criteria for office-based opioid treatment. Buprenorphine is a partial agonist of the mu-opioid receptor that is highly lipophilic with excellent sublingual bioavailability, long and variable half-life with once a day dosing, and low potential for abuse, making it an important tool for the management and detoxification of narcotic abusing patients [52].

Naltrexone, a competitive antagonist which binds to the mu-, kappa-, and delta-opioid receptors is FDA approved for the treatment of opioid dependence and for alcohol abuse disorders. The evidence for the use of naltrexone for opioid dependence is equivocal, without proven efficacy [53]. The use of naltrexone for alcohol dependence has been studied, and a recent meta-analysis based on 50 randomized controlled trials with 773 patients found that naltrexone reduced the risk of heavy drinking to 83 % of placebo, and significant effects were demonstrated for secondary outcomes (less heavy drinking days, decreased amount of consumed alcohol and decreased enzymatic markers of liver injury) [54]. Patients with a family history of alcoholism tend to respond better to naltrexone and polymorphisms within the mu-opioid receptor gene (A118G polymorphism) are associated with lower relapse rates, but not with differences in abstinence rates [55].

Summary

Substance abuse is a prevalent medical problem that is chronic, pervasive and is associated with medical and psychosocial comorbidities. Substance abuse needs to be regarded similar to other chronic medical conditions such as diabetes and heart disease, with short periods of exacerbation interspersed with longer periods of remission. Current recommendations suggest that all adults should be screened for alcohol abuse, and only those at risk should be screened for non-alcohol substance abuse. There is evidence that early intervention in those with hazardous use is effective, particularly for those not seeking treatment. Once patients screen positive for substance use, they need to be risk-stratified and those showing evidence of substance dependence must be referred to treatment. Different treatment modalities are available including pharmacotherapy, and behavioral and psychosocial models and resources for treatments are readily accessible, including local and state wide directories. The best outcomes are seen when the modalities are combined, and integrated programs are available for those with coexisting disorders.

References

1. Results from the 2012 National Survey on Drug Use and Health: Summary 2012; NSDUH Series H-46, HHS Publication No. (SMA) 13-4795.
2. Jemal A, Thun MJ, Ries LA, Howe HL, Weir HK, Center MM, et al. Annual report to the nation on the status of cancer, 1975-2005, featuring trends in lung cancer, tobacco use, and tobacco control. J Natl Cancer Inst. 2008;100(23):1672–94.
3. Thun MJ, Peto R, Lopez AD, Monaco JH, Henley SJ, Heath Jr CW, et al. Alcohol consumption and mortality among middle-aged and elderly U.S. adults. N Engl J Med. 1997;337(24):1705–14.
4. Amon JJ, Garfein RS, Ahdieh-Grant L, Armstrong GL, Ouellet LJ, Latka MH, et al. Prevalence of hepatitis C virus infection among injection drug users in the United States, 1994-2004. Clin Infect Dis. 2008;46(12):1852–8.
5. Parikh N, Nonnemacher MR, Pirrone V, Block T, Mehta A, Wigdahl B. Substance abuse, HIV-1 and hepatitis. Curr HIV Res. 2012;10(7):557–71.
6. Substance Abuse and Mental Health Services Administration. Office of Applied Studies, National Survey on Drug Use and Health, 2008 and 2009.
7. Grant BF, Stinson FS, Hasin DS, Dawson DA, Chou SP, Ruan WJ, et al. Prevalence, correlates, and comorbidity of bipolar I disorder and axis I and II disorders: results from the National Epidemiologic Survey on Alcohol and Related Conditions. J Clin Psychiatry. 2005;66(10):1205–15.
8. Pettinati HM, O'Brien CP, Dundon WD. Current status of co-occurring mood and substance use disorders: a new therapeutic target. Am J Psychiatry. 2013;170(1):23–30.
9. Ruiz P, Strain EC, Lowinson JH. Lowinson and Ruiz's substance abuse: a comprehensive textbook. 5th ed. Philadelphia: Wolters Kluwer Health; 2011.
10. Nunes EV, Civic Research Institute. Substance dependence and co-occurring psychiatric disorders: best practices for diagnosis and clinical treatment. Kingston: Civic Research Institute; 2010.
11. Fleming MF, Mundt MP, French MT, Manwell LB, Stauffacher EA, Barry KL. Brief physician advice for problem drinkers: long-term efficacy and benefit-cost analysis. Alcohol Clin Exp Res. 2002;26(1):36–43.
12. Babor TF, Higgins-Biddle JC. http://whqlibdoc.who.int/hq/2001/who_msd_msb_01.6b.pdf. 2013.
13. Miller WR, Rollnick S. Motivational interviewing: preparing people for change. 2nd ed. New York: Guilford Press; 2002.
14. Miller WR, Wilbourne PL. Mesa Grande: a methodological analysis of clinical trials of treatments for alcohol use disorders. Addiction. 2002;97(3):265–77.
15. Gentilello LM, Rivara FP, Donovan DM, Jurkovich GJ, Daranciang E, Dunn CW, et al. Alcohol interventions in a trauma center as a means of reducing the risk of injury recurrence. Ann Surg. 1999;230(4):473–80; discussion 480–3.

16. Screening and behavioral counseling interventions in primary care to reduce alcohol misuse. http://www.uspreventiveservicestaskforce.org/uspstf/uspsdrin.htm. 2013.
17. U.S. Preventive Services Task Force Screening for Illicit Drug Use. http://www.uspreventiveservicestaskforce.org/uspstf/uspsdrug.htm. 2013.
18. Shapiro B, Coffa D, McCance-Katz EF. A primary care approach to substance misuse. Am Fam Physician. 2013;88(2):113–21.
19. Nutt DJ, King LA, Phillips LD, Independent Scientific Committee on Drugs. Drug harms in the UK: a multicriteria decision analysis. Lancet. 2010;376(9752):1558–65.
20. A guide to substance abuse services for primary care clinicians center for substance abuse treatment. A guide to substance abuse services for primary care clinicians. http://www.ncbi.nlm.nih.gov/books/NBK64828/
21. Merkx MJ, Schippers GM, Koeter MW, Vuijk PJ, Poch M, Kronemeijer H, et al. Predictive validity of treatment allocation guidelines on drinking outcome in alcohol-dependent patients. Addict Behav. 2013;38(3):1691–8.
22. Mee-Lee D, American Society of Addiction Medicine, Working Group on PPC-2. ASAM (American Society of Addiction Medicine) patient placement criteria for the treatment of substance-related disorders. 2nd ed. Chevy Chase: American Society of Addiction Medicine; 1996.
23. Sharon E, Krebs C, Turner W, Desai N, Binus G, Penk W, et al. Predictive validity of the ASAM patient placement criteria for hospital utilization. J Addict Dis. 2003;22 Suppl 1:79–93.
24. Magura S, Staines G, Kosanke N, Rosenblum A, Foote J, DeLuca A, et al. Predictive validity of the ASAM Patient Placement Criteria for naturalistically matched vs. mismatched alcoholism patients. Am J Addict. 2003;12((5):386–97.
25. Rychtarik RG, Connors GJ, Whitney RB, McGillicuddy NB, Fitterling JM, Wirtz PW. Treatment settings for persons with alcoholism: evidence for matching clients to inpatient versus outpatient care. J Consult Clin Psychol. 2000;68(2):277–89.
26. Albanese AP. Management of alcohol abuse. Clin Liver Dis. 2012;16(4):737–62.
27. Wallace J. The new disease model of alcoholism. West J Med. 1990;152(5):502–5.
28. Mee-Lee D, Shulman G, Fishman M, Gastfriend D, Griffith J, editors. ASAM patient placement criteria for the treatment of substance—related disorders. 2nd ed. Revisited ed. Chevy Chase: American Society of Addiction Medicine; 2001.
29. Connors GJ, Tonigan JS, Miller WR, MATCH Research Group. A longitudinal model of intake symptomatology, AA participation and outcome: retrospective study of the project MATCH outpatient and aftercare samples. J Stud Alcohol. 2001;62(6):817–25.
30. Kelly JF, Stout R, Zywiak W, Schneider R. A 3-year study of addiction mutual-help group participation following intensive outpatient treatment. Alcohol Clin Exp Res. 2006;30(8):1381–92.
31. Kissin W, McLeod C, McKay J. The longitudinal relationship between self-help group attendance and course of recovery. Eval Program Plann. 2003;26(3):311–23.
32. McLellan AT, Lewis DC, O'Brien CP, Kleber HD. Drug dependence, a chronic medical illness: implications for treatment, insurance, and outcomes evaluation. J Am Med Assoc. 2000;284(13):1689–95.
33. Sofuoglu M, DeVito EE, Waters AJ, Carroll KM. Cognitive enhancement as a treatment for drug addictions. Neuropharmacology. 2013;64:452–63.
34. Hettema J, Steele J, Miller WR. Motivational interviewing. Annu Rev Clin Psychol. 2005;1:91–111.
35. Matching alcoholism treatments to client heterogeneity: project MATCH posttreatment drinking outcomes. J Stud Alcohol 1997;58(1):7–29.
36. Matching alcoholism treatments to client heterogeneity: project MATCH three-year drinking outcomes. Alcohol Clin Exp Res 1998;22(6):1300–11.
37. Glazer SS, Galanter M, Megwinoff O, Dermatis H, Keller DS. The role of therapeutic alliance in network therapy: a family and peer support-based treatment for cocaine abuse. Subst Abus. 2003;24(2):93–100.

38. Saitz R, Cheng DM, Winter M, Kim TW, Meli SM, Allensworth-Davies D, et al. Chronic care management for dependence on alcohol and other drugs: the AHEAD randomized trial. J Am Med Assoc. 2013;310(11):1156–67.
39. Weisner C, Mertens J, Parthasarathy S, Moore C, Lu Y. Integrating primary medical care with addiction treatment: a randomized controlled trial. J Am Med Assoc. 2001;286(14):1715–23.
40. Niccols A, Milligan K, Smith A, Sword W, Thabane L, Henderson J. Integrated programs for mothers with substance abuse issues and their children: a systematic review of studies reporting on child outcomes. Child Abuse Negl. 2012;36(4):308–22.
41. Drake RE, Mueser KT, Brunette MF, McHugo GJ. A review of treatments for people with severe mental illnesses and co-occurring substance use disorders. Psychiatr Rehabil J. 2004;27(4):360–74.
42. Jorgensen CH, Pedersen B, Tonnesen H. The efficacy of disulfiram for the treatment of alcohol use disorder. Alcohol Clin Exp Res. 2011;35(10):1749–58.
43. Pani PP, Trogu E, Vacca R, Amato L, Vecchi S, Davoli M. Disulfiram for the treatment of cocaine dependence. Cochrane Database Syst Rev 2010;(1):CD007024.
44. Miller PM, Book SW, Stewart SH. Medical treatment of alcohol dependence: a systematic review. Int J Psychiatry Med. 2011;42(3):227–66.
45. Rosner S, Hackl-Herrwerth A, Leucht S, Lehert P, Vecchi S, Soyka M. Acamprosate for alcohol dependence. Cochrane Database Syst Rev 2010;(9):CD004332.
46. Cho SH, Whang WW. Acupuncture for alcohol dependence: a systematic review. Alcohol Clin Exp Res. 2009;33(8):1305–13.
47. Anton RF, O'Malley SS, Ciraulo DA, Cisler RA, Couper D, Donovan DM, et al. Combined pharmacotherapies and behavioral interventions for alcohol dependence: the COMBINE study: a randomized controlled trial. J Am Med Assoc. 2006;295(17):2003–17.
48. Krystal JH, Cramer JA, Krol WF, Kirk GF, Rosenheck RA, Veterans Affairs Naltrexone Cooperative Study 425 Group. Naltrexone in the treatment of alcohol dependence. N Engl J Med. 2001;345(24):1734–9.
49. Witte J, Bentley K, Evins AE, Clain AJ, Baer L, Pedrelli P, et al. A randomized, controlled, pilot study of acamprosate added to escitalopram in adults with major depressive disorder and alcohol use disorder. J Clin Psychopharmacol. 2012;32(6):787–96.
50. Pettinati HM, Oslin DW, Kampman KM, Dundon WD, Xie H, Gallis TL, et al. A double-blind, placebo-controlled trial combining sertraline and naltrexone for treating co-occurring depression and alcohol dependence. Am J Psychiatry. 2010;167(6):668–75.
51. Mattick RP, Breen C, Kimber J, Davoli M. Methadone maintenance therapy versus no opioid replacement therapy for opioid dependence. Cochrane Database Syst Rev 2009;(3):CD002209.
52. Colson J, Helm S, Silverman SM. Office-based opioid dependence treatment. Pain Physician. 2012;15(3 Suppl):ES231–6.
53. Minozzi S, Amato L, Vecchi S, Davoli M, Kirchmayer U, Verster A. Oral naltrexone maintenance treatment for opioid dependence. Cochrane Database Syst Rev 2011;(4):CD001333.
54. Rosner S, Hackl-Herrwerth A, Leucht S, Vecchi S, Srisurapanont M, Soyka M. Opioid antagonists for alcohol dependence. Cochrane Database Syst Rev 2010;(12):CD001867.
55. Chamorro AJ, Marcos M, Miron-Canelo JA, Pastor I, Gonzalez-Sarmiento R, Laso FJ. Association of micro-opioid receptor (OPRM1) gene polymorphism with response to naltrexone in alcohol dependence: a systematic review and meta-analysis. Addict Biol. 2012;17(3):505–12.

Chapter 17
Evidence-Based Treatments for Substance Use Disorders

David Pilkey, Howard Steinberg, and Steve Martino

Key Points

- Motivational interviewing
- Cognitive behavioral therapy
- Contingency management
- Twelve-step facilitation
- The four treatments and stages of change

Introduction

Substance-related disorders affect large numbers of people. The 12-month prevalence of all substance use disorders approaches 10 % [1]. Alcohol use disorders are most common with 8.5 % of adults meeting criteria within the past 12 months, followed by cannabis use disorders (1.5 %), opioid use disorders (0.37 %), and cocaine use disorders (0.3 %) [1]. Substance-related disorders lead to many negative consequences including familial relationship problems, employment problems, crime, domestic violence, and child abuse. The financial consequences due to lost productivity, health-care costs, and crime-related costs are staggering. The estimated total overall cost related to alcohol is $235 billion and $181 billion for illicit drugs [2, 3].

With these high prevalence rates, consequences, and costs of substance-related disorders, many efforts have been made to bring evidence-based treatments (EBTs) into community treatment programs. While different definitions for

D. Pilkey, Ph.D. (✉) • H. Steinberg, Ph.D. • S. Martino, Ph.D.
Psychology Service, VA Connecticut Healthcare System, 950 Campbell Avenue (116-B),
West Haven, CT 06516, USA

Yale University School of Medicine, Department of Psychiatry, 300 George Street,
New Haven, CT 06516, USA
e-mail: david.pilkey@va.gov; howard.steinberg@va.gov; steve.martino@yale.edu

© Springer Science+Business Media New York 2015
A.D. Kaye et al. (eds.), *Substance Abuse*, DOI 10.1007/978-1-4939-1951-2_17

EBT have existed [4], in general EBTs are treatments that have been shown to improve patient treatment outcomes in more than one randomized clinical trial [5]. In practice, clinicians then use their clinical expertise to apply these treatments in a manner that addresses their patients' unique characteristics, cultures, and preferences to achieve the best outcomes [6]. EBTs typically are seen as the best treatments clinicians have to offer patients, either alone or in combination with other treatments. This chapter describes four well-recognized EBTs for substance-related disorders: motivational interviewing (MI), cognitive behavioral therapy (CBT), contingency management (CM), and twelve-step facilitation (TSF). This chapter will review each treatment's conceptual framework, evidence that the treatment works, how the treatment presumably works (i.e., mechanisms of action), and future directions for treatment development and research. The chapter concludes by placing the treatments in the context of the transtheoretical stages of change model [7] to describe how they fit together or can be combined to fully support the recovery efforts of patients who have substance-related disorders.

Motivational Interviewing

Conceptual Framework

Miller and Rollnick [8, p. 29], the originators of MI, define MI as "a collaborative, goal-oriented style of communication with particular attention to the language of change. It is designed to strengthen personal motivation for and commitment to a specific goal by eliciting and exploring the person's own reasons for change within an atmosphere of acceptance and compassion." The approach is grounded in humanistic psychology, especially the work of Carl Rogers, in that it employs a very empathic, supportive style of interacting with patients and upholds their welfare, best interests, and inherent potential for change. MI is distinct from nondirective approaches, however, in that clinicians' intentionally attend to and selectively reinforce patients' stated motives that support change. Over the course of the interview, clinicians help patients identify these change-oriented motives, elaborate upon them, and resolve ambivalence about change. If successful, patients become more likely to commit to changing their behaviors and initiating a change plan. The quartet of (1) partnering with patients, (2) nonjudgmentally accepting their stance, (3) showing compassion, and (4) evoking the patients' own arguments for change collectively represent the spirit of MI.

Clinicians use a variety of interviewing techniques and strategies to build the patient's motivation over the course of the interview, and they try to match their interventions to the individual's level of motivation. For example, clinicians sometimes move quickly to planning for change with patients who are already committed to it. Extensive exploration of their motives for change might frustrate patients who want to move forward. In contrast, attempting to develop change plans with patients who are not yet ready to change would likely increase their arguments against it. More time would be needed to determine what might make changing matter more or possible; a change plan might not even be developed in this type of session.

This latter interaction illustrates how motives to change (called "change talk") and motives to stay the same (called "sustain talk") can be thought of as opposite sides of the same coin, meaning that if clinicians give insufficient attention to addressing important issues that impede change, patients are likely to raise these issues again during the interview. Concomitantly, clinicians expect patients who initially argue against change to have some intrinsic motivation for change within them. It is the responsibility of the clinicians to look for opportunities to draw it out.

Notably, MI is behaviorally specific and has direction. This means that clinicians need to be clear about what it is that they are trying to motivate patients for. Motivation for change in one area does not guarantee motivation for change in another (e.g., a patient may commit to cocaine abstinence, but not agree to reduce or stop drinking or smoking marijuana or to enter an addiction treatment program). Each behavior may require a separate motivational enhancement process. MI also requires that clinicians take a stance about the preferred direction for change. For addictive behaviors, this decision is relatively clear in that most people would agree that it is ethically sound to enhance motivation for the reduction or cessation of substances that are potentially harmful or hazardous. However, some behavioral issues do not have a clear change direction. For example, decisions about organ donation or pregnancy termination likely would require a nondirective approach in which clinicians suspend their own values or goals and assume a position of "equipoise" (i.e., indifference or no clear attachment to a position or recommendation). In these situations, a patient-centered counseling approach, devoid of evocation, would allow patients to explore their ambivalence without intentional clinician influence.

MI can be administered with varying intensity. Typically patients participate in 1–4 sessions of 20–50 min in duration over the course of 1–3 months, with booster sessions characterizing applications of MI that extend over longer timeframes (e.g., two initial weekly sessions followed by two monthly boosters) [9]. Moreover, MI can be delivered in individual or group formats [10], though group versions of MI have seldom been systematically studied.

Evidence Base

Several recent reviews of the large body of MI research have come to some conclusions about how well MI works across a wide range of problem areas (e.g., alcohol, tobacco, illicit drugs, gambling, diet/exercise, treatment adherence/engagement) [11–13]. The review by Brad Lundahl and his colleagues [12] included 119 studies that isolated the unique effect of MI on treatment outcomes. They showed that across problem areas MI exerted small yet clinically significant effects, consistent with effects produced by other behavior change interventions but in less time. MI also significantly increased people's treatment engagement. The effects were durable, lasting up to 1 year. The largest area of MI research has been in its application to substance use problems. The evidence suggested that compared to other well-established addiction treatments, MI was as effective for treating problematic drinking, marijuana dependence, and other drugs (e.g., cocaine and heroin) and less effective for promoting tobacco cessation.

Mechanisms of Action

MI works through the clinicians' use of four overlapping processes, represented as stair steps, each building upon one another over the course of the interview [8]. In this model, "each later process builds upon those that were laid down before and continue to run beneath it as a foundation" [8, p. 26]. The processes include *engaging* (connecting with patients and establishing a good working relationship), *focusing* (agreeing on the target of motivational enhancement and directing the conversation toward it), *evoking* (drawing out the patients' own motivations for changing the target behavior), and *planning* (developing commitment to change and formulating a specific plan of action). Clinicians move flexibly between these processes in response to their patients and act like guides rather than experts during the MI transaction [14].

Two main sets of MI practices are simultaneously in motion across the four overlapping processes. First, clinicians use core interviewing skills that build rapport, convey empathy, and clarify the goals toward which the patients and clinicians will move together. These skills include asking open questions to invite conversation about a topic, affirming positive aspects of the patient, reflecting what the patient has communicated, and summarizing periodically, often referred to as the OARS of MI. In addition, mapping out an agenda, often through the exchange of information between patients and clinicians, is another core skill used to set a target for motivational enhancement and provide direction in the interview.

Second, clinicians use specific practices to elicit patients' change talk and consolidate commitment. Change talk includes statements that prepare or build motivation for change, such as desire, ability, reasons, or need to make changes in behaviors (DARN), sometimes referred to as preparatory language in that these statements represent the building of motivation that prepares patients to make a commitment to change. Desire statements indicate a clear wish for change ("I don't want my liver disease to get worse" or "I want to get my life back"). Ability statements indicate patients' beliefs that they can change, given their skills and available resources ("I was able to survive war, so maybe I can get my drug use under control"). Reason statements note the benefits of change and the costs of not changing ("I will have better relationships if I stop using" or "If I don't stop drinking, I doubt I can keep my job"). Need statements underscore how the problem behavior interferes with important areas of an individual's life and how changing the behavior would likely improve matters ("I don't even recognize myself; I can't go on like this anymore").

Change talk also includes statements that suggest people are mobilizing themselves for change. These statements involve commitment, activation, and taking steps to change (CAT). Commitment statements convey the stated intention to change ("My quit date will be this Thursday"). Activation statements indicate how people are getting ready to change ("I am going to call the program and see if I can get in"). Statements about taking steps to change are the strongest demonstration of commitment in that the people have put their words into action and are reporting these early efforts to the clinician ("Instead of going to happy hour after work, I went to a meeting").

During the interview clinicians identify the extent to which patients express motivation in each of these areas and, to the extent needed, encourage them to elaborate further or talk about what has not been discussed, in an attempt to draw out more motivations for change. For example, if a patient clearly articulated desire, reasons, and need for change but had not discussed an ability to change, the clinician would ask the patient about his or her capacity or confidence in making a change. The failure to believe in one's capacity to change may override one's belief that making a change is important. Strategically helping the patient feel more able to change would make the most sense in this juncture of the interview. In short, a patient's statements continuously signal the clinician how to conduct the interview, like a navigation system guiding where the clinician and patient will proceed. Terri Moyers and her colleagues [15] have documented how clinicians' use of MI consistent interventions tailored to the patients' motivations causes change talk to increase, which in turn mediates outcome. These findings underscore the importance of clinicians selectively eliciting and reinforcing change talk when conducting MI.

Future Directions

Many questions remain about MI that could be addressed in future research. Given the widespread application of MI, establishing how well MI works with nonaddictive problem behaviors, populations, and varying age groups remains an open question. In particular, the internationalization of MI suggests more study is needed about the efficacy of MI with diverse ethnic and cultural groups. The efficacy of using MI in modalities other than individual treatment (e.g., group, family, or couples) also has not been established. The relative contributions of the fundamental or person-centered strategies and those used for selectively eliciting and reinforcing change talk to MI's effectiveness remain unclear. In addition, more work is needed to identify effective strategies for training clinicians in MI, sustaining adequate clinician performance over time, and linking these training efforts to improved patient outcomes. Finally, innovations in the delivery of MI might make the approach more feasible and acceptable for use in busy clinical settings where it is increasingly being applied. The degree to which MI can be programmed for computer or Web-based applications needs to be established.

Cognitive Behavioral Therapy

Conceptual Framework

CBT for substance-related disorders is a treatment designed to help patients identify situations, thoughts, and emotions which may lead to substance use while also developing their skills to avoid or effectively manage situations in which substance use is likely to occur. The therapy typically is structured, short term, and problem focused, with greatest attention paid to the current difficulties an individual is having in his or her ability to control and stop using substances [16].

CBT is based upon the premise that an individual's learning history involving substance use serves to maintain substance use or contributes to a patient's ongoing relapse risk. The overarching goal of treatment is to systematically help patients break these long-held associations and establish new ways of thinking, feeling, and acting that support nonproblematic substance use [17, 18]. This is done by thoroughly analyzing substance use experiences to identify the antecedents and consequences related to substance use episodes. Additionally, patients learn how to recognize high-risk situations, avoid them when possible, and cope with both internal and external triggers that historically have been associated with substance use.

Marlatt and Gordon's [18] model of relapse prevention has traditionally served as the prototype for the design of many of the cognitive behavioral treatments for substance use problems. Based upon their model, core treatment components of CBT typically include: (1) identification of high-risk situations (interpersonal and intrapersonal) that may trigger substance use, (2) training in how to cope with craving and thoughts about using, (3) development of skills in how to refuse substances, (4) functional analysis of substance use, and (5) facilitating development of nonuse activities. These components of treatment are described in greater detail below.

CBT is a highly collaborative form of therapy. Clinicians and patients work together to identify and prioritize which substance use problems will be the focus of treatment. For example, if a patient describes recurring problems avoiding drug using acquaintances, the clinician would ask the patient if this issue needs to be addressed in the session. Together, they would look at the relapse risk these encounters pose to the patient and decide upon appropriate coping strategies that could be practiced in the session (e.g., avoidance strategies, drug refusal skills, managing thoughts about using) and then applied as needed. In CBT homework assignments are given to patients to promote coping skill development and generalization outside the session. Homework review and substance use monitoring occurs at the beginning of treatment and is used as the basis for ongoing treatment planning. This collaborative approach begins in the first session and sets the tone for a working alliance and sense of shared responsibility in actively addressing the patient's treatment goals.

CBT is typically provided between 12 and 18 sessions and delivered over the course of 3–4 months. While the length of treatment may vary depending upon the complexity of the presenting problems, there is evidence to suggest that briefer treatment formats (fewer than 20 sessions) may prove more effective than longer courses of CBT [19]. CBT may be delivered in both individual and group settings; there is little empirical support for choosing one modality over the other [19]. The format of treatment most often is dictated by availability, patient preferences, and the potential for increased engagement and retention when discussing highly sensitive issues individually vs. when receiving beneficial peer pressure and support in group formats [20].

Evidence Base

There has been a good deal of empirical support for the use of CBT in the treatment of substance use disorders, including the efficacy of CBT for specific substances of abuse (alcohol, cocaine, opiates, marijuana, methamphetamine, polysubstance) [19, 21, 22]. Positive treatment effects are consistent across treatment formats (individual or group) and when used in conjunction with other psychosocial [19] or pharmacological [21] interventions. Studies also have demonstrated continuing patient improvement after treatment ends, sometimes referred to as the "sleeper" effect of CBT [23], though there is mixed support for this in the literature [19, 21]. Meta-analyses of randomized controlled trials of CBT with adult alcohol and illicit drug users have indicated small [19] to moderate [21] effect sizes of treatment overall. When CBT is compared with no treatment controls, a larger effect size is found. Greater CBT treatment effects have been shown for treating alcohol dependence and those with marijuana use disorders than other substance use disorders. Additionally, some evidence suggests women receive greater benefit from CBT than men [19] and that CBT may be less effective with substance-using patients who have cognitive limitations given the treatment's emphasis on learning and retaining complex coping skills [24, 25].

Mechanisms of Action

CBT is based upon the early learning theories of classical and operant conditioning and social learning theory. Within these learning frameworks, an individual's substance use can be viewed as the development and maintenance of a behavior that is reinforced by the pharmacologic effects of the substance used in addition to the related experiences that accompany the use of the substance [17]. In CBT, the associated contextual learning/reinforcement of triggers to use that occur in substance use environments (physical and social) are proposed to be the greatest determinants of future substance use behavior. Therefore, substantial therapeutic effort is devoted to helping the patient weaken this frequently reinforced connection between substance use and the experiences one has with use, while at the same time working to positively reinforce alternative decision making and participation in healthier activities that are incompatible with substance use behavior [17].

Hence, in the early sessions, the clinician and patient strive to understand situational factors that influence the patient's use of substances. This functional analysis of substance use allows for a detailed account of specific situations in which the patient has used, including identifying the potential triggers for use, thoughts and feelings related to the triggers, the subsequent behaviors, and the consequences (positive and negative) of those behaviors. When working with patients to identify the antecedents to substance use, there are five general domains that should be addressed: emotional, cognitive, social, environmental, and physical [20].

For example, in conducting a functional analysis, a patient may identify that an argument with her boyfriend was the main antecedent to a drug use episode. She may cite that she felt "angry and frustrated' and that she thought "He always tells me what to do. I can do what I want." She might describe how these feelings and thoughts led to additional internal dialogue which included her perceived "need" to use and the positive consequence of being able to "escape from the situation" and "show him he can't control me." It would be important to ask about the negative consequences as well, such as feelings of guilt for using, the financial cost of the use episode, and the risk her continued use poses to her relationship. This type of functional analysis is a common treatment component in CBT, in great part because it provides both patient and clinician an accurate depiction of events occurring outside of the thera- peutic environment. Additionally, the breakdown of each component of the single use episode allows for the targeted skills training that is a hallmark of CBT.

The significance of helping patients to develop or to improve coping skills within the context of CBT has been highlighted by a number of authors [18, 20, 26], includ- ing the importance of including both in-session practice and between-session home- work assignments [27]. Individuals seeking substance abuse treatment may have lost previously learned coping strategies due to long-term use and reliance on sub- stances, never having learned appropriate skills to begin with, or due to the presence of life stressors and conditions that may leave an individual with ineffective or harmful coping strategies such as substance use [20]. CBT acts to develop the patients' ability to use effective interpersonal (e.g., refusal of substances, giving and receiving praise and criticism, assertiveness training) and intrapersonal skills (e.g., managing thoughts about using, anger management, decision making) and to improve the quality with which patients enact these skills over time [28].

Future Directions

Across numerous investigations, CBT has been shown to be an effective treatment for individuals with substance-related disorders. However, most of these studies have involved highly trained and supervised clinicians who implement manualized CBT within established research protocols that provide for sufficient time allotted for sessions. These studies have not tested the effectiveness of CBT in traditional substance abuse treatment settings when used by program clinicians and with a wide range of patients. More studies are needed to test the effectiveness of CBT in the real world. Moreover, more work is needed to develop novel and readily acces- sible ways to deliver CBT with integrity to more patients. A recent randomized controlled trial of computer-based treatment for CBT (CBT4CBT) to treat sub- stance use problems [29] provides one promising direction to achieve this aim. Finally, while some recent progress has been made in identifying mechanisms of action within CBT [28], the necessary ingredients of CBT that lead to sustained behavioral change have not been clearly identified. Additional research into the active and most effective components of treatment would allow for a more efficient and potentially more cost-effective provision of care.

Contingency Management

Conceptual Framework

CM is a widely acknowledged behavioral EBT that utilizes reinforcement to change substance use behavior. CM is based on the principles of operant conditioning and behavior modification. Substance use behavior is influenced by many variables, though the reinforcing aspects of substance use such as pleasure, reward, and reduction of negative feelings are particularly potent for most patients. CM attempts to modify the rewards associated with substance use by modifying contingencies. Specifically, this treatment approach provides incentives for achieving verifiable target behaviors such as abstinence from illicit substances, as well as creating disincentives for use. CM has been used to address many abused substances, including cocaine, opiates, alcohol, marijuana, and nicotine [30–34]. It has also been used to address treatment compliant behavior such as attendance [35], treatment goal attainment [36], and vocational productivity [37].

In developing a CM protocol, the clinician must adhere to several important principles: (1) clearly define, objectively quantify, and consistently measure an unambiguous behavioral target; (2) provide rewards of sufficient magnitude and with sufficient frequency; (3) reward the target behavior immediately when it is detected; (4) escalate the value of the reward for patients' continuous success in achieving the targeted behavior to promote longer periods of success; (5) reset the value of the reward back to its original level when the patients do not reach the targeted goal; and (6) reward successful approximations to difficult to achieve behavioral targets [38, 32, 39] Typically the behavioral target of CM is abstinence from a particular substance, though session attendance or medication adherence also is commonly used. The clinician then develops a method method of detecting the target behavior and establishes the frequency of monitoring it. When drug abstinence is the targeted goal, urine toxicology is used 2–3 times per week. When the target behavior is achieved, the patient receives positive reinforcement, most commonly in the form of voucher, prize, or clinic privileges. In a voucher system patients accumulate vouchers in a "clinic-bank account" and may redeem collected vouchers for retail goods or other items of their choosing. Some patients may choose to use vouchers to add minutes to their cell-phone service or to pay for haircuts. In a prize system, a cabinet is stocked with a range of items such as toiletries, food items, CDs, and music players. An example of a clinic privilege is take-home privileges in a methadone clinic [40]. With successive successes, the reinforcement level rises (e.g., the first negative sample earns $2.50, the second $3.75, the third $5.00, etc.) to support sustained abstinence and to escalate the reinforcement value of abstinence in the face of immediate risk of use [35]. When the target behavior is not achieved, the reinforcement is withheld and the value often is reset back to its original level [35, 41]. In Higgins and colleagues [30] seminal study, a voucher system study, participants could receive up to $1,000 worth of goods and typically received about $600. The "Fishbowl" procedure produces similar results at a much reduced cost, about a third of the Higgins and colleagues study [41].

The "Fishbowl" procedure for delivering reinforcement in a more cost-effective manner was developed by Petry and colleagues [25]. This format provides variable reinforcement. The fishbowl or large container is filled with 500 slips of paper. The patient draws slips from the fishbowl to determine the reinforcement. Half of the slips have "Good job" or "Smiley faces" on them. The remainder consists of 42 % small slips, 7–8 % large slips, and 1 jumbo slip. The patient receives prizes for goods in values matching the slips drawn. The prize cabinet is stocked with restaurant gift certificates, bus tokens at the small level; watches, backpacks, arts, and crafts supplies at the large level; and handheld television and a boom box at the jumbo level [32]. Additionally, the number of opportunities to draw increases with each negative urine toxicology provided. Thus, on the first negative urine toxicology the participant draws once and on the second the patient draws twice. This increase continues until the patient is receiving eight opportunities to draw for a negative urine toxicology. If the urine toxicology is not negative, no reinforcement is provided and the number of draw opportunities is reset to one.

Evidence Base

CM is among the most effective interventions to promote abstinence [42]. There have been a number of randomized controlled trials evaluating the effectiveness of various CM protocols. One of the earliest studies conducted by Higgins and colleagues utilized a voucher system for treating cocaine dependence [30]. In this relatively small study the participants who received CM and community reinforcement participated in more treatment, had longer periods of sustained abstinence from cocaine, and used other substances less frequently than those who received 12-step counseling [30]. Following this seminal study a tremendous number of other trials have been conducted to evaluate the use of CM with a range of substance use disorders including alcohol, tobacco, opioids, cocaine, methamphetamine, and other illicit substances. These studies have also evaluated CM with a range of populations including adults, adolescents, opioid agonist therapy participants, and dually diagnosed individuals. There are four notable multiple meta-analyses evaluating CM and all four provide strong support of CM's effectiveness. Griffith and colleagues focused on studies with methadone maintenance populations [43]. All studies provided contingencies based on urinalysis results. The overall weighted mean effect size was .25, a small-to-medium effect size relative to control groups [43]. Lussier and colleagues conducted a meta-analysis focusing on studies using voucher-based reinforcement in both drug-free clinics and in methadone clinics [44]. A similar small-to-medium effect size of .32 was observed. A meta-analysis of CM in the treatment of illicit drugs, alcohol, and tobacco was conducted by Prendergast and colleagues [44]. The mean effect size was again small-to-medium at .43. Moreover, CM was most effective for opiates and cocaine, medium effect size, than tobacco or multiple drugs, small-to-medium [44]. Dutra and colleagues evaluated a range of psychosocial interventions for substance use disorders by conducting a meta-analysis [45]. CM demonstrated the strongest effect of the psychosocial interventions evaluated which included CBT, relapse prevention, group drug counseling, and dialectical behavior therapy [45].

Mechanisms of Action

CM is believed to work through modifying reinforcement. The aim is to develop competing reinforcers to substance use, first through the rewards provided by the intervention, and eventually through the naturally occurring benefits that accrue through abstinence [38]. Higgins and colleagues [46] cite research on animals and in humans indicating that drugs and alcohol act as an unconditional positive reinforcer in a similar way as food, water, and sex. Second, Substance use may as a negative reinforcer through the removal of withdrawal symptoms. Thus, reinforcement is important in the development and maintenance of a substance use disorder. These same principles of reinforcement may be used in treating a substance use disorder [46].

CM facilitates breaking the reinforcement cycle of substance use. In CM alternative healthy incentives provided through vouchers, prizes, or clinic privileges directly compete against the reinforcing properties of substance use. In addition, patients begin to experience the benefits of reducing or abstaining from substance use. Benefits of sobriety may include having more money, feeling better, thinking more clearly, and better relationships with friends and family. Thus, the benefits of achieving and maintaining sobriety are also reinforcing [47].

Future Directions

CM clearly works well and, in some evaluations, has stronger effect sizes and support than other psychosocial interventions. Given this strong level of support, it is surprising that CM is underutilized in clinical practice. Roll and colleagues have identified a number of implementation barriers including poor communication to the treatment community about what CM is, limited awareness of the effectiveness of CM, need to demonstrate cost-effectiveness of CM, and developing and distributing appropriate CM protocols that fit into community practice [48]. Community program administrators and clinicians have raised several concerns, including questions about behaviors to target for reinforcement (primary drug vs. total abstinence, drug use vs. program attendance or treatment goals), costs (magnitude and frequency of rewards, urine screens, staffing), clinical issues (e.g., worries about increased gambling), and philosophy (e.g., appropriateness of paying patients for "what they should be doing") [49, 50]. Addressing these barriers is an ongoing challenge for the successful dissemination and implementation of CM. For example, improved attendance from CM results in improved clinic reimbursement.

Thus, the costs of CM implementation are offset by improved revenues. Moreover, clinicians implementing CM often observe patients shift from a motivation to "win" prizes to motivation to achieve benefits of abstinence such as improved health and improved relationships [49]. These clinicians are more likely to become advocates of the approach and encourage their professional peers to learn more about CM. Clinicians who have been trained in CM have been shown to carry more favorable attitudes toward it than those who are unfamiliar with the approach [50]. These findings suggest CM likely will become a more heavily utilized substance abuse treatment in the future.

Twelve-Step Facilitation

Conceptual Framework

TSF is a manual-guided, professionally delivered approach based on the 12 steps of Alcoholics Anonymous, Cocaine Anonymous, and Narcotics Anonymous. It is designed for use in early recovery from substance use disorders and assumes that addiction is a progressive disease for which the only effective remedy is abstinence from alcohol or drugs, *one day at a time*, consistent with the tenets of the 12 Steps and 12 Traditions [51]. This approach leverages patients' familiarity with 12-step programs, widespread 12-step meeting availability in the community, and clinicians' typically high regard and encouragement for patients to attend 12-step meetings [52, 53]. Moreover, research on 12-step program participation consistently shows associations with improved rates of abstinence, social functioning, self-efficacy, and healthcare utilization [54–59]. Active involvement, beyond mere participation/attendance, is an even stronger predictor of these outcomes [60, 61]. Hence, having a treatment such as TSF to facilitate involvement in 12-step programs is an important therapeutic tool for patients with substance-related disorders.

The primary goal of TSF is to promote alcohol and drug abstinence by emphasizing the patients' need to (1) accept substance dependence as a chronic, progressive disease over which one has no control, (2) surrender or give oneself over to a higher power, in particular, by involving oneself in the fellowship of other recovering alcoholics and drug addicts and seeking their guidance, and (3) actively participating in 12-step meetings and related activities [62, 63]. TSF clinicians assert these 12-step principles to patients within sessions and try to engender strong patient endorsements of total abstinence, early engagement, and active participation in 12-step programs.

TSF is not meant to supplant 12-step program participation. Rather it specifically promotes patient participation in 12-step programs. Clinicians cover core areas within sessions that educate patients about 12 step programs and principles and actively encourage them to complete recovery tasks between sessions. This means that clinicians of TSF must be familiar with 12-step programs; the related literature; and the locations, times, and types of meetings available to patients.

TSF typically is delivered in an individual format, though a group adaptation of TSF has been developed recently [52]. Sessions typically are 50–60 min in length and patients may receive 12–24 sessions over the course of 3–6 months. In addition, conjoint sessions are available to patients with significant others who would like to support the patients' recovery process.

Evidence Base

TSF has been found to be as efficacious as CBT and MI in the treatment of alcohol dependence posttreatment and at follow-up points on most drinking-related outcomes, though with higher rates of continuous alcohol abstinence when compared to CBT or MI at a 1-year follow-up [9, 64]. In addition, TSF and closely related approaches have been shown to be as effective, or more effective, than other approaches among several samples of primary cocaine users [23, 65–67]. Early engagement and active participation in 12-step programs has been found to mediate patient outcomes in TSF [55, 68–70].

Mechanisms of Action

Clinicians in TSF aim to help patients understand the philosophy, traditions, tenets, and steps of 12-step programs; attend meetings; and actively participate in them. The straightforward idea is that early attrition from 12-step meetings or failure to fully engage in them limits the effectiveness of 12-step meetings. By teaching patients about 12-steps programs (e.g., the first three steps of recovery), coaching patients about how to make use of them (e.g., getting a sponsor), and reinforcing essential principles, patients will be more prepared to take advantage of 12-step programmatic resources and supports and thereby garner better treatment outcomes.

To promote these clinical aims, clinicians address five core content areas: (1) introduction to 12-step programs and assessment of substance use/commitment to abstinence; (2) Step 1—acceptance; (3) people, places, and things (habits and routines); (4) Steps 2 and 3—surrender; and (5) getting active in 12-step programs. An additional termination session completes TSF treatment and several elective topics are available for additional sessions: HIV Risk Reduction, The Genogram, Enabling, Emotions—HALT (Hunger, Angry, Lonely, Tired); Steps 4 and 5—Moral Inventories; and Clean and Sober Living.

In TSF, the concepts of acceptance and surrender are central to recovery from substance use disorders and highlighted in the first three steps of the 12-step program. Acceptance means the patients must recognize that they suffer from a chronic and progressive illness of addiction and that they have lost their ability to control their use of alcohol or drugs. Patients also must accept that there is no cure for addiction and that the only viable approach is to be completely abstinent from all mood-altering substances.

Having accepted their addiction and their inability to manage it alone, patients must surrender or reach out to something beyond themselves that can guide them in recovery—the 12 steps of 12-step programs and a higher power (namely, an individually defined force greater than themselves that represents faith and hope for recovery). Surrender also entails the patients' acknowledgment that the fellowship of 12-step programs has helped countless individuals achieve and sustain their recovery and that their best chance for success is to actively participate in these programs. Clinicians of TSF frequently promote these concepts in sessions.

In addition, clinicians encourage patients to complete recovery tasks between sessions that support 12-step program participation and complement material discussed in the sessions. Common recovery tasks include contacting a sponsor, doing service work at a meeting, identifying meetings that will be attended and going to them, reviewing suggested readings from the 12-step literature, going to a 12-step related social activity, or keeping a journal that documents 12-step group attendance and participation, reactions to the meetings, barriers to attendance, etc. As with any substance abuse treatment, patients may struggle with their addictive behaviors between sessions. In TSF, clinicians share with patients strategies to deal with cravings or slips to substance use consistent with 12-step programs. Common strategies include calling a friend, sponsor, or 12-step hotline or going to a meeting.

Future Directions

TSF is an established EBT for substance use disorders. However, the extent to which clinicians can learn to implement TSF with fidelity remains an open question. Work by Sholomskas and Carroll [70] and Campbell and colleagues [71] suggests that community-based substance abuse treatment clinicians have the potential to learn TSF with adherence and competence in their practice settings. However, which training strategies or combination of them are most effective, what the relationship is to patient treatment outcomes, and which clinician characteristics or types of patients might influence TSF delivery needs more investigation. For example, one could imagine patients varying in the degree to which they endorse important 12-step principles (e.g., emphasis on spirituality or higher power, notions of powerless as a key component of recovery), and these differences might affect a clinician's ability to implement TSF with good fidelity. The extent to which clinicians and patients mutually influence treatment fidelity in TSF needs to be established.

The Four Treatments and Stages of Change

The relationship of MI, CBT, CM, and TSF to each other can be understood within the context of the Stages of Change model by James Prochaska and Carlo DiClemente [7]. The Stages of Change model posits that behavior change occurs sequentially across recurring stages. The earlier stages include precontemplation (people are unaware or do not believe there is a problem or need to change it), contemplation (people are ambivalent about recognizing a problem and shy away from changing it), and preparation (people are ready to work toward behavior change in the near future and develop a plan for change). The later stages include action (people consistently make specific changes) and maintenance (people work to maintain and sustain long-lasting change). Tailoring treatment strategies to achieve stage-related tasks is a hallmark of this model (e.g., conducting a cost–benefit analysis for someone contemplating change).

MI naturally fits into the Stages of Change model in that it can be used to help move people from one stage to another, especially in the early stages when patients may not yet fully recognize their substance-related disorder or commit to change it. CM might help patients with pernicious problems of addiction initiate abstinence in the early action stage. Similarly, CBT might be used when patients decide to take action and learn how to maintain less risky use or abstinence through the development of coping and relapse prevention skills. Finally, as part of an action plan and as a means for maintaining a lifestyle change devoid of substance misuse, TSF could help patients build recovery supports through ongoing meeting participation. Finally, MI strategies may be used to attend to wavering motivation as patients take action or try to maintain changes in stressful situations.

The Stages of Change model further illustrates how the EBTs may integrate well with each other and be combined for patient care. For example, MI might be used to engage people in treatment that then teaches them relapse prevention skills. The combining of MI with more action-oriented treatments, such as CBT, is becoming more prevalent. Two examples of this are the Cannabis Youth (CYT) Study and the Combine Study [72–74]. The CYT study combined Motivational Enhancement Therapy (MET) plus CBT in both a 5-session and a 12-session format. In the Combine Study, MI, CBT, and aspects of TSF were combined to form the Combined Behavioral Intervention. Both studies demonstrated the effectiveness of combined treatments and are a promising area for further development.

Conclusions

EBTs for substance-related disorders represent some of the best practices for caring for patients who struggle with addictive behaviors. MI, CBT, CM, and TSF have strong empirical support and are frequently utilized in clinical settings. All four treatments may be applied across different types of substance-related disorders and used within different patient populations. Moreover, these treatments can be combined to maximize their effectiveness by addressing patients' evolving and interacting clinical needs. If the positive effects of MI, CBT, CM, and TSF are to reach more patients, then the field must work to find ways to better teach clinicians how to use these treatments with integrity and sustain high quality practice over time.

Disclosures Drs. David Pilkey, Howard Steinberg, and Steve Martino are supported by the Veterans Affairs Connecticut Healthcare System. In addition, Dr. Martino receives additional support from the Department of Veterans Affairs New England Mental Illness Research, Education, and Clinical Center (MIRECC), by the US National Institute on Drug Abuse R01 DA023230; R01 DA034243, R01 DA027194, and National Institute of Mental Health R25 DA026636. We have no financial interests to report. The views expressed within this chapter are those of the authors and do not represent the views of the VA, NIDA or NIMH.

References

1. American Psychiatric Association. Diagnostic and statistical manual of mental disorders. 5th ed. Arlington: American Psychiatric Association; 2013. dsm.psychiatryonline.org. Accessed 1 Jun 2013.
2. Rehm J, Mathers C, Popova S, Thavorncharoensap M, Teerawattananon Y, Patra J. Global burden of disease and injury and economic cost attributable to alcohol use and alcohol use disorders. Lancet. 2009;373:2223–33.
3. National Drug Intelligence Center. The economic impact of illicit drug use on American Society. Washington, DC: United States Department of Justice; 2011.
4. Miller WR, Zweben J, Johnson WR. Evidence-based treatment: why, what, where, when, and how? J Subst Abuse Treat. 2005;29:267–76.
5. Chambless DL, Ollendick TH. Empirically supported psychological interventions: controversies and evidence. Annu Rev Psychol. 2001;52:685–716.
6. American Psychological Association Presidential Task Force on Evidence-Based Practice. Evidence-based practice in psychology. Am Psychol. 2006;61:271–85.
7. Prochaska JO, DiClemente CC. The transtheoretical approach: crossing traditional boundaries of treatment. Homewood: Dow Jones-Irwin; 1984.
8. Miller WR, Rollnick S. Motivational interviewing: helping people change. 3rd ed. New York: Guilford Press; 2012.
9. Project MATCH Research Group. Matching alcoholism treatments to client heterogeneity: project MATCH posttreatment drinking outcomes. J Stud Alcohol. 1997;58:7–29.
10. Wagner CC, Ingersoll KS. Motivational interviewing in groups. New York: Guilford Press; 2013.
11. Hettema J, Steele J, Miller WR. Motivational interviewing. Annu Rev Clin Psychol. 2005;1:91–111.
12. Lundahl BW, Kunz C, Brownell C, Tollefson D, Burke B. Meta-analysis of motivational interviewing: twenty five years of empirical studies. Res Soc Work Pract. 2010;20:137–60.
13. Smedslund G, Berg RC, Hammerstrom KT, Steiro A, Leiknes KA, Dahl HM, Karlsen K. Motivational interviewing for substance abuse. Cochrane Database Syst Rev. 2011;Issue 5. Art. No.: CD008603.
14. Rollnick S, Miller WR, Butler CC. Motivational interviewing in health care: helping patients change behavior. New York: Guilford Press; 2008.
15. Moyers TB, Martin T, Houck JM, Christopher PJ, Tonigan JS. From in session behaviors to drinking outcomes: a causal chain for motivational interviewing. J Consult Clin Psychol. 2009;77:1113–24.
16. Higgins ST, Sigmon SC, Heil SH. Drug abuse and dependence. In: Barlow DH, editor. Clinical handbook of psychological disorders: a step-by-step treatment manual. New York: Guilford Press; 2008. p. 547–77.
17. Higgins ST. The influence of alternative reinforcers on cocaine use and abuse: a brief review. Pharmacol Biochem Behav. 1997;57:419–27.
18. Marlatt GA, Gordon JR. Relapse prevention: maintenance strategies in the treatment of addictive behaviors. New York: Guilford Press; 1985.

19. Magill M, Ray LA. Cognitive-behavioral treatment with adult alcohol and illicit drug users: a meta-analysis of randomized controlled trials. J Stud Alcohol Drugs. 2009;70:516–27.
20. Carroll KM. A cognitive-behavioral approach: treating cocaine addiction. Rockville: NIDA; 1996.
21. Irvin JE, Bowers CA, Dunn ME, Wang MC. Efficacy of relapse prevention: a meta-analytic review. J Consult Clin Psychol. 1999;67:563–70.
22. Smout MF, Longo M, Harrison S, Minniti R, Wickes W, White JM. Psychosocial treatment for methamphetamine use disorders: a preliminary randomized controlled trial of cognitive behavior therapy and acceptance and commitment therapy. Subst Abus. 2010;31:98–107.
23. Carroll KM, Nich C, Ball SA, McCance-Katz EF, Frankforter TF, Rounsaville BJ. One year followup of disulfiram and psychotherapy for cocaine-alcohol abusers: sustained effects of treatment. Addiction. 2000;95:1335–49.
24. Cooney NL, Kadden RM, Litt MD, Getter H. Matching alcoholics to coping skills or interactional therapies: two-year follow-up results. J Consult Clin Psychol. 1991;59:598–601.
25. Kadden RM, Cooney NL, Getter H, Litt MD. Matching alcoholics to coping skills or interactional therapies: posttreatment results. J Consult Clin Psychol. 1989;57:698–704.
26. Monti PM, Abrams DB, Kadden RM, Cooney NL. Treating alcohol dependence: a coping skills training guide. New York: Guilford Press; 1989.
27. Caroll KM, Nich C, Ball SA. Practice makes progress? Homework assignments and outcome in the treatment of cocaine dependence. J Consult Clin Psychol. 2005;73:749–55.
28. Kiluk BD, Nich C, Babuscio T, Carroll KM. Quality versus quantity: acquisition of coping skills following computerized cognitive behavioral therapy for substance use disorders. Addiction. 2010;105(12):2120–7.
29. Carroll KM, Ball SA, Martino S, Nich C, Babuscio TA, Nuro KF, Gordon MA, Portnoy GA, Rounsaville BJ. Computer-assisted delivery of cognitive-behavioral therapy for addiction. Am J Psychiatry. 2008;165:881–8.
30. Higgins ST, Delaney DD, Budney AJ, Bickel WK, Hughes JR, Foerg F, Fenwick JW. A behavioral approach to achieving initial cocaine abstinence. Am J Psychiatry. 1991;148:1218–24.
31. Preston KL, Umbricht A, Epstein DH. Methadone dose increase and abstinence reinforcement for treatment of continued heroin use during methadone maintenance. Arch Gen Psychiatry. 2000;57:395–404.
32. Petry NM, Martin B, Cooney JL, Kranzler HR. Give them prizes and they will come: contingency management for treatment of alcohol dependence. J Consult Clin Psychol. 2000;68: 250–7.
33. Stanger C, Budney AJ, Kamon JL, Thostensen J. A randomized trial of contingency management for adolescent marijuana abuse and dependence. Drug Alcohol Depend. 2009;105:240–7.
34. Cavallo DA, Cooney JL, Duhig AM, Smith AE, Liss TB, McFetridge AK, Babuscio T, Nich C, Carroll KM, Rounsaville BJ, Krishnan-Sarin S. Combining cognitive behavioral therapy with contingency management for smoking cessation in adolescent smokers: a preliminary comparison of two different CBT formats. Am J Addict. 2007;16:468–74.
35. Petry NM. A comprehensive guide to the application of contingency management procedures in clinical settings. Drug Alcohol Depend. 2000;58:9–25.
36. Iguchi M, Belding MA, Morral AR, Lamb RJ, Husband SD. Reinforcing operants other than abstinence in drug abuse treatment: an effective alternative for reducing drug use. J Consult Clin Psychol. 1997;65(3):421.
37. Wong CJ, Sheppard JM, Dallery J, Bedient G, Robles E, Svikis D, Silverman K. Effects of reinforcer magnitude on data-entry productivity in chronically unemployed drug abusers participating in a therapeutic workplace. Exp Clin Psychopharmacol. 2003;11(1):46.
38. Higgins ST, Budney AJ, Bickel WK, Foerg FE, Donham R, Badger GJ. Incentives improve outcome in outpatient behavioral treatment of cocaine dependence. Arch Gen Psychiatry. 1994;51:568–76.
39. Petry NM, Petrakis I, Trevisan L, Wiredu L, Boutros N, Martin B, Kosten TR. Contingency management interventions: from research to practice. Am J Psychiatry. 2001;20:33–44.

40. Petry NM, Stitzer ML. Contingency management: using motivational incentives to improve drug abuse treatment. Training series no. 6. New Haven: Yale University Psychotherapy Development Center; 2002.
41. Petry NM, Simcic F. Recent advances in the dissemination of contingency management techniques: clinical and research perspectives. J Subst Abuse Treat. 2002;23:81–6.
42. Prendergast M, Podus D, Finney J, Greenwell L, Roll J. Contingency management for treatment of substance use disorders: a meta-analysis. Addiction. 2006;101:1546–60.
43. Griffith JD, Rowan-Szal GA, Roark RR, Simpson DD. Contingency management in outpatient methadone treatment: a meta-analysis. Drug Alcohol Depend. 2000;58:55–66.
44. Lussier JP, Heil SH, Mongeon JA, Badger GJ, Higgins ST. A meta-analysis of voucher-based reinforcement therapy for substance use disorders. Addiction. 2006;101:192–203.
45. Dutra L, Stathopoulou G, Basden S, Leyro T, Powers M, Otto M. A meta-analytic review of psychosocial interventions for substance use disorders. Am J Psychiatry. 2008;165:179–87.
46. Higgins ST, Heil SH, Lussier JP. Clinical implications of reinforcement as a determinant of substance use disorders. Annu Rev Psychol. 2004;55:431–61.
47. Pan S, Gowing L, Li C, Zhao M. Contingency management for substance use disorders. Cochrane Database Syst Rev. 2012;8:1–13.
48. Roll JM, Madden GJ, Rawson R, Petry NM. Facilitating the adoption of contingency management for the treatment of substance use disorders. Behav Anal Pract. 2009;2(1):4.
49. Stitzer ML, Kellogg S. Large-scale dissemination efforts in drug abuse treatment clinics. In: Higgins ST, Silverman K, Heil SH, editors. Contingency management in substance abuse treatment. New York: Guilford Press; 2008. p. 241–60.
50. Srebnik D, Sugar A, Coblentz P, McDonell MG, Angelo F, Lowe JM, Ries RK, Roll J. Acceptability of contingency management among clinicians and clients within a co-occurring mental health and substance use treatment program. Am J Addict. 2013;20:1–5.
51. Alcoholics Anonymous. Twelve steps and twelve traditions. New York: Alcoholics Anonymous World Services; 1981.
52. Daley DC, Baker S, Donovan DM, Hodgkins CG, Perl H. A combined group and individual 12-step facilitative intervention targeting stimulant abuse in the NIDA Clinical Trials Network: STAGE-12. J Groups Addict Recover. 2011;6:228–44.
53. Donovan DM, Wells EA. 'Tweeking 12-step': the potential role of 12-step self-help group involvement in methadone recovery. Addiction. 2007;102 Suppl 1:121–9.
54. Fiorentine R. After drug treatment: are 12-step programs effective in maintaining abstinence? Am J Drug Alcohol Abuse. 1999;25:93–116.
55. Fiorentine R, Hillhouse MP. Drug treatment and 12-step program participation: the additive effects of integrated recovery activities. J Subst Abuse Treat. 2000;18:65–74.
56. Gossop M, Stewart D, Marsden J. Attendance at narcotics anonymous and alcoholics anonymous meetings, frequency of attendance, and substance use outcomes after residential treatment for drug dependence: a 5-year follow-up study. Addiction. 2008;103:119–25.
57. Humphreys K, Moos RH. Encouraging posttreatment self-help group involvement to reduce demand for continuing care services: two-year clinical and utilization outcomes. Alcohol Clin Exp Res. 2007;31:64–8.
58. Kaskutas LA. Alcoholics anonymous effectiveness: faith meets science. J Addict Dis. 2009;28:145–57.
59. Tonigan JS. Benefits of alcoholics anonymous attendance: replication of findings between clinical research sites in Project MATCH. Alcohol Treat Quart. 2001;19:67–78.
60. Owen PL, Slaymaker V, Tonigan JS, McCrady BS, Epstein EE, Kaskutas LA, et al. Participation in alcoholics anonymous: intended and unintended change mechanisms. Alcohol Clin Exp Res. 2003;27:524–32.
61. Weiss RD, Griffin ML, Gallop RJ, Najavits LM, Frank A, Crits-Christoph P, Thase ME, Blaine J, Gastfriend DR, Daley D, Luborsky L. The effect of 12-step self-help group attendance and participation on drug use outcomes among cocaine-dependent patients. Drug Alcohol Depend. 2005;77:177–84.

62. Norwinski J, Baker S. The twelve-step facilitation handbook: a systematic approach to early recovery from alcoholism and addiction. San Francisco: Jossey-Bass; 1992.
63. Norwinski J, Baker S, Carroll KM. Twelve step facilitation manual: a clinical research guide for therapists treating individuals with alcohol abuse and dependence. NIAAA project match monograph series, vol. 1, DHHS Publication No. (ADM) 92-1893. Rockville: National Institute on Alcohol Abuse and Alcoholism; 1992.
64. Project MATCH Research Group. Matching alcoholism treatments to client heterogeneity: Project MATCH three-year drinking outcomes. Alcohol Clin Exp Res. 1998;22:1300–11.
65. Carroll KM, Nich C, Ball SA, McCance-Katz E, Rounsaville BJ. Treatment of cocaine and alcohol dependence with psychotherapy and disulfiram. Addiction. 1998;93:713–28.
66. Crits-Christoph P, Siqueland L, Blaine J, Frank A, Luborsky L, Onken LS, Muenz LR, Thase ME, Weiss RD, Gastfriend DR, Woody GE, Barber JP, Butler SF, Daley D, Salloum I, Bishop S, Najavits LM, Lis J, Mercer D, Griffin ML, Moras K, Beck AT. Psychosocial treatments for cocaine dependence: National Institute on Drug Abuse Collaborative Cocaine Treatment Study. Arch Gen Psychiatry. 1999;56:493–502.
67. Wells EA, Peterson PL, Gainey RR, Hawkins JD, Catalano RF. Outpatient treatment for cocaine abuse: a controlled comparison of relapse prevention and twelve-step approaches. Am J Drug Alcohol Abuse. 1994;20:1–17.
68. Longabaugh R, Donovan DM, Karno MP, McCrady BS, Morgenstern J, Tonigan JS. Active ingredients: how and why evidence-based alcohol behavioral treatment interventions work. Alcohol Clin Exp Res. 2005;29:235–47.
69. McKellar J, Stewart E, Humphreys K. Alcoholics anonymous involvement and positive alcohol-related outcomes: consequences or just a correlate? A prospective 2-year study of 2,319 alcohol-dependent men. J Consult Clin Psychol. 2003;71:302–8.
70. Sholomskas DE, Carroll KM. One small step for manuals: computer-assisted training in twelve-step facilitation. J Stud Alcohol. 2006;67:939–45.
71. Campbell BK, Manuel JK, Manser ST, Peavy KM, Stelmokas J, McCarty D, Guydish JR. J Subst Abuse Treat. 2013;44:169–76.
72. Dennis M, Godley SH, Diamond G, Tims FM, Babor T, Donaldson J, Liddle H, Titus JC, Kaminar Y, Webb C, Hamilton N, Funk R. The Cannabis Youth Treatment (CYT) study: main findings from two randomized trials. J Subst Abuse Treat. 2004;27(3):197–213.
73. Donovan DM, Anton RF, Miller W, Longabaugh R, Hosking JD, Youngblood M. Combined pharmacotherapies and behavioral interventions for alcohol dependence (the COMBINE study): examination of posttreatment drinking outcomes. J Stud Alcochol Drugs. 2008;69(1): 5–13.
74. Moyers TB, Houck J. Combining motivational interviewing with cognitive-behavioral treatments for substance abuse: lessons from the COMBINE Research Project. Cogn Behav Pract. 2011;18(1):38–45.

Chapter 18
Nursing Perspectives in Managing Patients with Substance Abuse

Larissa Galante, Cynthia French, and Kirsten B. Grace

Key Points

- Definition of the nursing approach
- Barriers to caring for patients with substance abuse disorders
- Screening and assessment
- Social support
- Physical assessment and comorbidities
- Alcohol
- Prescription drugs
- Illicit drugs
- Withdrawal
- Psychiatric issues
- Pain management
- Consent
- Nursing specialties and specific roles

"Every patient with substance abuse has a right to be treated with dignity and respect" [1].

L. Galante, M.S.N., B.S.N., C.R.N.A. (✉)
e-mail: larissagalante@hotmail.com

C. French, M.S., B.S.N., C.R.N.A.
e-mail: cyntfre@aol.com

K.B. Grace, M.S.N., B.S.N., F.N.P-C., A.P.R.N.
e-mail: kristen.b.grace@gmail.com

© Springer Science+Business Media New York 2015
A.D. Kaye et al. (eds.), *Substance Abuse*, DOI 10.1007/978-1-4939-1951-2_18

Substance abuse has become a major health hazard in the United States. Caring for patients with addiction presents unique challenges and requires a comprehensive, multidisciplinary approach in which nurses have a critical role. Alcohol and drug abuse can present in a variety of ways and requires individualized management. The provider must consider the scope of substance use and related disorders, conceptual models of addiction, ethical issues, addiction risk stratifications, and clinical recommendations [1]. Through therapeutic communication, nursing interventions, clinical assessment, and building trusting relationships, nurses have significant impact in managing patients with substance abuse.

Definition of the Nursing Approach

The practice of nursing encompasses autonomous and collaborative care of individuals of all ages, families, groups and communities, sick or well and in all settings. It includes the promotion of health, prevention of illness, the care of patients who are ill, disabled or dying [2]. It also involves the diagnosis and treatment of human responses to actual or potential health problems [3]. Nurses provide care individually to patients and as part of a collaborative team that may include other nurses, physicians, social workers, and the patient's social support system such as family and friends. They may encounter patients with substance abuse in varied practice environments such as primary care, community settings, and in hospital settings. Nurses provide support to the patient throughout the initial screening and assessment and as patients move through the treatment process and recovery from substance abuse. They care for patients being treated for other concerns or procedures who may be unwilling to accept treatment for their addiction. Nurses are involved in screening programs to identify problems and also care for patients who have begun a treatment plan to recover from substance abuse. After treatment, nurses are involved in monitoring the recovering patient's progress and help in developing a life without addiction.

Barriers to Caring for Patients with Substance Abuse Disorders

Nurses face unique challenges when caring for patients with substance abuse disorders. A nurse's personal beliefs, values, judgment, and preconceptions can affect his or her ability to work with a person who suffers from addiction, as do cultural and societal biases. Health care providers often have a preconceived, negative opinion of a patient who is a drug user, alcoholic, or addict [4], and this stigma is the major barrier to provision of effective care, both on the side of the nurse as well as the patient. "Stigma is rooted in shame and guilt and it interferes with development of a therapeutic relationship and trust" [5]. Patients who feel that they are being judged are less likely to trust the provider and share their experiences [5]. For example, a systematic review by van Boekel et al found that health professionals have a generally negative attitude towards patients with substance abuse disorders. These attitudes inhibit patients' feeling of empowerment and leads to poor communication between the provider and the patient which diminishes the therapeutic alliance. It can also result in diagnostic overshadowing which leads to misattribution of symptoms of physical illness to substance abuse. The perception that substance abusing patients are potentially violent, manipulative, or poorly motivated may cause feelings of frustration, resentment, and powerlessness among professionals [4]. Nurses may be less motivated to care for patients with history of illicit drugs because they are unwilling or unable to empathize with their patients [6].

The nurse's role in reducing and eliminating stigma is to develop a rapport with the patient and his or her family, to educate them regarding the disease model of addiction, and to provide reasonable alternatives to treatment when appropriate. The ethical nursing principles of autonomy, dignity, beneficence, nonmaleficence, justice, fidelity, and veracity apply to nursing care of patients with addiction [1]. The choice of language used with the patient, as well as in reference to the patient, may also influence willingness to be open with the caregiver. Terms such as "dirty, clean, junkie" may promote feelings of shame and lack of empathy, resulting in the patient feeling judged by the provider and close down communication. Preferred terms include "people with substance use disorders, active addiction" [7].

Healthcare professionals often feel that they are not appropriately trained or prepared and that they lack education and support structures especially when personal exposure to this patient group has been limited. This results in less involvement and a more task-oriented approach in the delivery of care, leading to diminished personal engagement and empathy. Organizational support such as supervision and the option to consult resources increases self-esteem of the nurse, perceived knowledge, feelings of empowerment, willingness, and satisfaction in working with these patients. Nurses should have role support from their facilities and organizations as well as training related to caring for patients with addiction [4].

Screening and Assessment

A critical role of the nurse is to identify and screen patients who may be at risk for or show signs of substance abuse. Most patients with substance abuse disorders seek treatment for other issues, and healthcare professionals are essential in identifying problems in order to make treatment accessible [8]. Approaching this sensitive topic requires tact and clinical skill. Some patients may be cooperative and respond to direct questioning, but other patients may be evasive and minimize their history.

Known risk factors for substance abuse include: physical and sexual abuse, parental substance abuse, parental incarceration, dysfunctional family relationships, peer involvement with drugs or alcohol or serious crime, and smoking tobacco.

Table 18.1 CAGE (cut down, annoyed, guilty, eye opener) questionnaire

1. Have you ever felt you should **cut down** on your drinking?
2. Have people **annoyed** you by criticizing your drinking?
3. Have you ever felt bad or **guilty** about your drinking?
4. Have you ever had a drink first thing in the morning to steady your nerves or to get rid of a hangover (**eye opener**)?

Scoring: Item responses on the CAGE are scored 0 for "no" and 1 for "yes" answers, with a higher score an indication of alcohol problems. A total score of 2 or greater is considered clinically significant Though a score of 2 or greater is clinically significant, a score of 1 or greater may require further evaluations [7]

Signs include sudden changes in physical health, deteriorating performance in school or employment, changes in personality or friends, dress, or involvement in serious delinquency or crime [7]. Any patient taking any analgesic for chronic pain in a primary cares clinic may be at risk for developing prescription drug use disorder (PDUD). Risk factors for PDUD include previous time in jail, pain related limitations, current smoking, family history of substance abuse, white race, male gender, and posttraumatic stress disorder [9].

Screening should be conducted as part of a comprehensive health assessment, and it is recommended that all primary care providers, physicians as well as nurse practitioners, routinely screen all of their patients for substance use disorders. Primary care offers a unique opportunity to identify addiction early in the disease process because patients are seen frequently and develop a relationship with the provider [7]. Routinely screening all patients in a systematic way for substance abuse along with social history, diet, and exercise removes stigma and may also mitigate any personal biases of the nurse. Although many screening tools have not been tested in primary care, the four-question CAGE questionnaire [10] and the Alcohol Use Disorders Identification Test (AUDIT) [11] have been identified as effective. To screen for alcohol problems using a self-administered written questionnaire, a brief instrument like the AUDIT can be used expected reading level and comprehension of written English are not likely to be problematic. The AUDIT screening tool can be self-administered by English speaking and literate patients or can be administered by the clinician. It consists of 10 questions and assesses the rate and frequency of alcohol intake by the patient. If screening will be administered by a clinician, the CAGE, supplemented by the first three quantity/frequency questions from the AUDIT, is recommended. This combination will increase sensitivity for detection of both problem drinking and alcohol dependence because it includes questions about both alcohol consumption and its consequences (Table 18.1) [12].

Nurses working in primary care should periodically screen all patients for alcohol abuse using AUDIT supplemented by CAGE to screen for alcohol abuse. The modified AUDIT-AID may be used to screen for substance abuse. The only screening test for drug use that has been studied in primary care is the CAGE-AID [13].

Although the available screening tests have inherent cultural biases, there is currently insufficient evidence to recommend specific alternative screening instruments for different cultural groups. However, a few special populations should be screened

Table 18.2 CRAFFT (car, relax, alone, forget, friends, trouble) questionnaire

C: Have you ever ridden in a **car** driven by someone (including yourself) who was "high" or had been using alcohol or drugs?
R: Do you ever use alcohol or drugs to **relax**, feel better about yourself or fit in?
A: Do you ever use alcohol or drugs while you are by yourself, **alone**?
F: Do you ever **forget** things you did while using alcohol or drugs?
F: Do your family or **friends** ever tell you that you should cut down on your drinking or dug use?
T: Have you ever gotten into **trouble** while you were using alcohol or drugs?

A "yes" to 2 of the questions would indicate a need for further evaluation and a "yes" to 4 or more should raise suspicion of substance dependence [14]

with additional tests. Substance abuse in adolescents can have serious consequences for the patient both during use and later in life. Adolescents should be screened for substance abuse at least annually. However, since not all adolescents seek care for an annual physical exams, substance abuse should be addressed at all visits, including encounters for acute problems [7]. Adolescents can be screened with the CRAFFT questionnaire which screens for alcohol and substance use (Table 18.2) [14]. CRAFFT differs from CAGE because it is developmentally appropriate for adolescents and screens for both alcohol & drugs. It can be self-administered or administered by a healthcare provider.

Pregnant women and women of child bearing age require more vigilant screening because there is no safe limit of alcohol or drug use allowed during pregnancy [15], and women must be educated about alcohol consumption and pregnancy. Drinking during pregnancy can lead to an array of physical, cognitive, and behavioral defects in the developing brain, most serious of which is fetal alcohol syndrome [16]. Children with FAS have distinct facial features and infants are much smaller than average. Their brains are smaller and have fewer neurons, leading to long-term problems in learning and behavior. CRAFFT, AUDIT-C, and TWEAK are valid screening for substance abuse during pregnancy (Table 18.3) [15]. TWEAK can be used to screen for alcohol use, though it only screens for heavy use [7, 15].

To screen for drug use in women, a nurse can ask "Do you use street drugs?" or may use CRAFFT or the 4P's plus, although there is a cost to use the 4P's plus [15].

The geriatric population also requires special screening. Patients who are older than 60 years should be screened annually and at each major life event (such as the loss of a spouse or after moving to an assisted living or skilled nursing facility) [7]. It is particularly important to screen for alcohol abuse since the signs and symptoms of alcohol abuse (sleep problems, falls, and confusion) can be similar to other conditions that are more common in the geriatric population [7]. The CAGE questions can be used to screen for alcohol abuse in the geriatric population. The Michigan Alcoholism Screening Test - Geriatric Version (MAST-G) was developed specifically for the geriatric population, but it may take considerable time to answer all of the 24 items on the test [17]. Though the AUDIT screening tool has not been validated specifically for geriatric patients, it can be used across cultures and is a reasonable alternative for patients who present with cultural barriers [7].

Table 18.3 TWEAK (tolerance, worried, eye opener amnesia, cut down) questionnaire

T: **Tolerance,** How many drinks can you hold?
W: Have close friends or relatives **worried** or complained about your drinking in the past year?
E: **Eye opener**: Do you sometimes take a drink in the morning when you first get up?
A: **Amnesia:** Has a friend or family member ever told you about things you said or did while you were drinking that you could not remember?
K (C): Do you sometimes feel the need to **cut down** on your drinking?

Scoring: A 7-point scale is used to score the test. The "tolerance" question scores 2 points if a woman reports she can hold more than five drinks without falling asleep or passing out. A positive response to the "worry" question scores 2 points, and a positive response to the last three questions scores 1 point each. A total score of 2 or more indicates the woman is at risk for alcohol abuse

Older adults with chronic health conditions may have prescriptions for a large number of medications. To screen for prescription drug abuse the nurse may such questions as:

"Do you see more than one health care provider regularly? If so, why?
"Have you switched doctors recently? If so, why?"
"What prescription drugs are you taking? Are you having any problems with them?"
"Where do you get your prescriptions filled? Do you go to more than one pharmacy?"
"Do you use any other nonprescription medications? If so, what, why, how much, how often, and how long have you been taking them?" [7].

Answers to questions may change depending upon how the questions are asked. Inquisitions should be open-ended such as, "Please tell me about your drinking". Some clinicians report that assumptive questions may yield a more accurate response, "When was the last time you were high?" may be a better question than "Do you drink?" It may also be helpful to ask "At what age did you first use?" and "How many times did you use last month". It's important to maintain privacy during the screening process so that the patient will understand that his or her responses will be confidential [7]. This assessment may also reveal that a family member has a problem with drug abuse. The relationship between the primary care provider and the patient provides for a unique perspective to support the non-using family member who may be upset, confused on how to proceed, or exhausted of dealing with their loved one's substance abuse without help [7].

The above tools can be used for outpatient as well as inpatient settings. However, in hospital environments such as the emergency room and intensive care units, it may be more difficult to identify substance dependence because of competing clinical goals, urgent admission or surgery, or the patient's inability to communicate. In these situations, obtaining a history from family or friends, the primary care physician, or consulting with specialist services in anticipation of illicit drug use is reasonable [18]. Patients who are communicative should be assessed for substance use. If a patient experiences mental status changes after 2 or 3 days of admission, it may be difficult to differentiate between an acute neurologic change or substance withdrawal. In settings where the patient cannot communicate, laboratory tests such as blood and urine toxicology, CT scans, and other screenings may be warranted. If the clinician suspects intoxication, regardless of the patient's ability to communicate, a blood or urine toxicology examination is appropriate.

Social Support

The North American Nursing Diagnosis Association creates [19] nursing diagnoses, which are actual or potential health problems, that can be identified by the nurse and are amenable to nursing interventions [3]. Some nursing diagnoses relevant to patients with substance abuse include:

- alteration in coping with stress
- self-concept dysfunction
- altered family function

Substance use represents an *alteration in coping with stress*. If a person does not have effective coping mechanisms to deal with stress, he or she may use substances to manage stress rather than using social supports or healthy behaviors. The results of excessive alcohol and drug use are addiction, dependency, psychological problems, physiologic consequences and likely more stress and even less effective coping. Substance abuse may be a manifestation of *self-concept dysfunction* [19]. Persons with low self-esteem and negative self-image find it difficult to change self-destructive behaviors because they are unable to view themselves in a worthy, positive way. Such people may turn to substances for immediate gratification to avoid their negative feelings and thoughts [3].

A normally functioning family meets its developmental tasks and guides members to accomplish individual goals appropriate for age and progress. Substance abuse may lead to *altered family function* as the members of the family develop coping mechanisms to manage the individual who is involved with substance abuse [19]. If a person has alcohol addiction, family members may deny that alcohol is problem in an effort to continue functioning. A spouse or child may become the enabler, a person who can keep the family functioning even at an altered level [3]. The enabler provides care for the person with alcoholism, assumes responsibility for tasks, which that person cannot accomplish, and makes excuses, which allows the individual to continue drinking [20]. Additionally, is it possible for family members to have substance abuse problems of their own.

Drugs are generally more expensive than alcohol, so economic hardship may play a greater role in the family of a drug abuser than in that of someone with alcoholism. Drug use is also less socially acceptable, and the individual may be isolated from the community. Drug testing may prevent the user from holding a job, which affects the family's financial security, and the prevalence of homelessness is higher in this population. If the drug user is incarcerated, this completely disrupts the family unit [3]. A nurse can educate family members the consequences of role alcohol and substance abuse, encourage the user to seek help, or provide community supports to prevent further disruption of the family and to assist with healthy coping mechanisms. This may include support groups or individual psychotherapy.

Domestic violence is prevalent in homes where alcohol or drugs are abused. Women are at increased risk for domestic violence if their male partner has alcoholism. Children are at increased risk of violent behavior by their parents. If a patient is known to have alcohol addiction, it may be appropriate to also educate and assess the partner regarding risk. Child abuse and neglect are more frequent among families where substance abuse is an issue. Become familiar with the laws in the state where the nurse practices is important to report suspected child abuse correctly. Each state has a child abuse hotline to report suspected child abuse and neglect [23].

Physical Assessment and Comorbidities

In addition to a detailed history, a thorough physical assessment for signs and symptoms of complications related to substance abuse should be conducted. Abusing alcohol, prescription medications, and illicit drugs all have acute as well as chronic physical implications which require examination.

Alcohol

Alcohol is the leading cause of preventable death and disease in the United States. Nurses and doctors should assess and council all patients with excessive alcohol consumption in attempts to prevent its significant long-term consequences. When patients who consume alcohol regularly are admitted to the hospital and no longer have access to it, they may display symptoms of withdrawal or develop delirium tremens, a life-threatening complication. Anticipation and identification of withdrawal is critical to effective management.

In surgical patients, alcoholics are at higher risk for postoperative infections, bleeding, heart failure, respiratory issues, and delayed wound healing. It should be anticipated that the patient will begin to show signs of withdrawal in 2–3 days since last consuming alcohol, and if the patient is still admitted, prophylactic benzodiazepines should be given in order to prevent delirium tremens. Patients who are chronic alcoholics may have a decrease in white blood cells which places them at risk for community-acquired pneumonia. It is recommended that patients with alcoholism receive an annual pneumococcal vaccination. Alcoholics are also at risk for osteoporosis, skin sores, and muscular atrophy [24].

There are several cardiac comorbidities associated with alcoholism. In their meta-analysis, Kodama and colleagues found that regular drinking is associated with atrial fibrillation in a dose–response fashion at alcohol levels below current definitions of risky use [9, 25]. Binge drinkers have a significantly higher risk for myocardial infarction [9]. CAD is a leading cause of death of alcoholics. They are at increased risk for hypertension, congestive heart failure, cerebrovascular accidents, and increased levels of low-density lipoproteins [24]. Chronic alcoholics are at risk for cardiomyopathy and weakening of the heart [21]. Patients should be assessed for shortness of breath, peripheral edema, and fatigue.

Gastrointestinal complications are frequent in patients with a history of heavy alcohol consumption. Repetitive vomiting may cause tears in the gastroesophageal junction, and portal hypertension may lead to esophageal varices which can cause life-threatening bleeding. Patients are at increased risk for ulcers especially if taking non-steroidal anti-inflammatory agents or aspirin. The risk of developing pancreatitis increases over time, but only 5 % of people with alcohol dependence will develop pancreatitis [21]. Abstinence from alcohol can slow the progression of pancreatitis and the effects of alcohol on the pancreas can be managed but not reversed. Another increased risk is pancreatic cancer, although this usually occurs in people who have a history of smoking [24].

Liver disease is common in patients with alcoholism. Alcohol is processed in the liver and toxic byproducts of metabolism are responsible for the production of cytokines, inflammatory chemicals of the immune system. With chronic inflammation and tissue injury, cirrhosis ensues, and liver function continues to decline resulting in coagulopathy, ascites, encephalopathy, cirrhosis, portal hypertension esophageal varices, and gastrointestinal bleeding. Additional danger to the liver involves the high-risk lifestyles of heavy drinkers which place them at greater chances of contracting HIV Hepatitis B and C [24].

Women are more vulnerable than men to many of the medical consequences of alcohol consumption. Most notably, they develop cirrhosis, cardiomyopathy, and peripheral neuropathy after fewer years of heavy drinking [26–28]. The national cancer institute has identified alcohol as a risk factor for breast, esophagus, larynx, liver, mouth, and pharynx. Epidemiology reports show that 7 out of 10 people with mouth cancer are heavy drinkers. Research has found that people who drink are also more likely to smoke and the combined effects increase the risk of cancer significantly [21].

Individuals who drink alcohol regularly frequently have nutrient deficiencies and should take vitamin supplements. Folate deficiency due to alcohol's interference with its metabolism can lead to severe anemia and during pregnancy leads to birth defects. Vitamin B tends to be the most deficient, and Vitamin B12 deficiency can lead to peripheral neuropathy and nerve damage. With severe thiamine deficiency, Wernicke-Korsakoff syndrome ensues and patients may experience loss of balance and confusion, and it can also result in permanent brain damage, memory loss, and death. Once this syndrome occurs, patients can no longer take oral thiamine and aggressive intravenous treatment must be initiated [24].

Prescription Drugs

Worldwide use of prescription opioids more than tripled from 1989 to 2009. In 2009, the United States, which accounted for 5.1 % of the global population, was responsible for 56 % of global morphine and 81 % of global oxycodone use [29]. In 2010, 12 million American reported nonmedical use of prescription painkillers in the past year [30]. Between 2004 and 2009, emergency department visits for adverse events due to prescription opioids increased by almost 90 %, with the highest increases for oxycodone and hydrocodone. In 2009, the number of Americans that reported nonmedical use of prescription drugs exceeded those using cocaine, heroin, hallucinogens, and inhalants combined [31].

As use of illegal and prescription opioids increase, more patients will exhibit opioid tolerance. Obtaining information about patient drug use and potential ongoing treatment is critical in constructing an appropriate plan. Inaccurate knowledge of the patient's history with opioids may compromise patient care and satisfaction [32]. This may have financial implications and in a time where patient, now referred to as a customer, satisfaction is critical and starting to become a criteria for hospital reimbursement.

Physiologic implications of prescription drug abuse are variable with different substances. Opioids can result in hypotension, hypoventilation, higher risk of aspiration, and respiratory arrest. Anxiolytics such as benzodiazepines can cause hypotension, hypoventilation, memory loss and other cognitive issues, and abruptly stopping medications can lead to life-threatening withdrawal due to central nervous system hyperactivity and seizures. Stimulants result in increased heart rate, hypertension, seizures, tremors, violence or aggressive behavior, paranoia, and hyperthermia [33]. Milder forms of any or all of the symptoms present with use of each drug may be present and warrants assessment by the healthcare provider.

Illicit Drugs

Patients who abuse illicit drugs are at risk for a myriad of comorbidities. Initial presentations may be severe including organ damage, infectious diseases such as HIV, tuberculosis, hepatitis, associated psychological disorders, and drug specific adaptations such as tolerance, physical dependence, and withdrawal [22]. Medical problems associated with intravenous drug use include malnutrition and cachexia, chronic anemia, cellulitis, AIDs, hepatomegaly, sclerosing glomerulonephritis or kidney failure, aspiration pneumonitis, atelectasis, heroin induced asthma, and pulmonary edema. Cardiac comorbidities include endocarditis of the tricuspic valve, pulmonary and septic emboli and infarctions, increased risk of ectopic activity, atrial fibrillation, and ventricular tachycardia [34].

Inpatient and perioperative management of opioid-dependent patients requires planning for pain management and drug withdrawal. Postoperatively, it is best if no withdrawal attempts are made until the patient has been discharged from the hospital. Patients may be ingesting other compounds used for "cuts" that reduce purity and may cause toxic cardiovascular or neurologic reactions. Methadone has been used since the 1960s to aid in recovery from heroin, but it may be two or more weeks until a treatment reaches an optimal dose. Induction doses should be monitored by a doctor or trained nurse. The aim is to achieve a dose that patients experience minimal intoxication and withdrawal symptoms. The risk of methadone overdose in the induction phase is high whereas the risk is low with buprenorphine.

Table 18.4 Time from symptom to development since last alcohol intake

Symptom	Time (h)
Hand tremor	6–36
Insomnia	6–36
Nausea or vomiting	6–36
Hallucinations or illusions	6–48
Anxiety	6–36
Grand mal seizures	48–96
Autonomic hyperactivity	48–96

Withdrawal

Once a patient ceases intake of the routinely abused substance, whether intentionally for rehabilitation or unintentionally for emergency surgery, the risk of withdrawal ensues. It is important to understand both the physical and psychological factors of drug withdrawal. Symptoms are often so severe that patients return to using drugs to ease the discomfort. Nurses can help patients manage their symptoms and cope during the withdrawal process as they experience anxiety, depression, and suicidal ideations. In patients whose addiction is unknown, nurses are vital in identifying signs of withdrawal. Evaluation and testing should be directed to the systems affected by the patient's substance abuse. Appropriate tests include basic metabolic panel to assess electrolytes, complete blood count to assess anemia, liver function tests, coagulation panel for clotting abnormalities, chest X-ray, electrocardiogram, and blood and urine toxicology screens.

Alcohol Withdrawal

Alcohol withdrawal syndrome (AWS) occurs when a person who regularly drinks large amounts of alcohol considerably reduces the amount consumed or ceases drinking. Current estimates state that 20–25 % of patients admitted to the hospital have alcohol addiction or dependence [35, 36]. Withdrawal from alcohol can be fatal. Mortality was as high as 35 % before the advent of intensive care and advanced pharmacotherapy. Today death rates range from 5 to 15 % [37]. Risk factors for AWS include the number of previous detoxifications, history of prior seizures, history of DT's and a current desire to drink. Signs and symptoms must be clinically significant, not caused by other medical conditions and must include:

1. Cessation or reduction of heavy and prolonged alcohol use
2. The above plus two or more of the following, developing within several hours to a few days after cessation (Table 18.4) [38].

Delirium Tremens is the most severe form of alcohol withdrawal. Characteristics include autonomic hyperactivity and altered mental status. Treatment for this condition

Table 18.5 Pharmacologic management of symptoms

Agent	Treated symptom
NSAIDs	Myalgias, headache and fever
Dimenhydrinate	Nausea and vomiting
loperamide (Imodium)	Diarrhea and abdominal cramps
Benzodiazepines	Acute anxiety
Trazodone	For sleep disturbances
Fluids	Maintain hydration

consists of relieving symptoms and preventing complications. Monitoring vital signs, blood chemistry, and electrolytes vigilantly is critical. Clinicians should also assess liver enzymes for abnormalities as it can interfere with metabolism and excretion of medications. Anticonvulsants and depressants such as valium or lorazepam, along with sedatives, should be administered on a fixed schedule. The effects of these medications on the central nervous system are similar to that of alcohol, and antipsychotics such as haldol may be necessary if the patient presents symptoms of psychosis. Intravenous thiamine to prevent Wernicke-Korsakoff syndrome and encephalopathy, as well as assessing the patient for signs of jaundice and altered liver function, are also part of treatment. This regimen should be followed for a minimum of 1 week and for the duration of the withdrawal. Other important interventions include ensuring a patent airway and intravenous access, encouraging the patient to rest, providing adequate nutrition, and offering emotional support to the patient and the family to reduce anxiety. Upon cessation of withdrawal and completion of other medical treatment, the next step is referral to a short or long-term facility that specializes in addiction. Counseling may assist with psychiatric problems associated with alcoholism. Alcoholic Anonymous, a 12-step program is also very effective in improving patient outcomes [39].

Opiate Withdrawal

Withdrawal from heroin or prescription narcotics is predictable, identifiable, and although it is quite uncomfortable for the patient, it is not life-threatening. Signs and symptoms of opiate withdrawal include drug seeking behavior, mydriasis, piloerection, diaphoresis, rhinorrhea, lacrimation, diarrhea, insomnia, elevated blood pressure and pulse, intense desire for drugs, muscle cramps, joint pain, anxiety, nausea, vomiting, and malaise. Management of withdrawal can be accomplished with clonidine for intranasal users or methadone for intravenous users (Table 18.5).

Opioid withdrawal can occur safely in both inpatient and outpatient settings, and the choice of location is dependent upon the patient's family support, polysubstance abuse, comorbidities, and psychiatric issues. Buprenorphine (Subutex) is the most effective medication for treating opiate withdrawal. It can shorten the length of detoxification but is also used for long-term maintenance similarly to methadone. Patients are more likely to complete withdrawal and experience fewer side effects with buprenorphine when compared to clonidine [40]. Buprenorphine is equally effective as methadone for withdrawal completion, but symptoms resolve more quickly with buprenorphine [41]. Methadone maintenance programs were developed to reduce risk factors associated with a drug abusing lifestyle such as criminal behaviors, reduce needle sharing, and promiscuous behaviors leading to transmission of HIV and other diseases [42].

It is important to note that detoxification does not prevent relapse. Most opiate-related deaths and overdoses occur when the user relapses with taking the same quantity of drugs as prior to detoxification. Intense behavioral therapy and 12-step programs are critical to successful rehabilitation.

Benzodiazepine Withdrawal Syndrome

Benzodiazepine withdrawal is comparable to alcohol and barbiturate withdrawal and can be life-threatening. It is often characterized by severe sleep disturbances, irritability, tension and anxiety, panic attacks, hand tremors, diaphoresis, difficulty with concentration, confusion and cognitive difficulty, dry retching, nausea, weight loss, palpations, headache, muscular pain and stiffness. Symptoms which frequently have a prolonged duration include anxiety, cognitive impairment, depression, various sensory and motor phenomena and gastrointestinal disturbances. Patients using high doses are prone to more serious developments such as seizures and psychotic reactions [43]; administering long-acting benzodiazepines is more effective in treating symptoms. A taper over 8–12 weeks or longer may be indicated in patients who have been using benzodiazepines for several years. The rate of taper is adjusted depending on patient tolerance. Ashton published a comprehensive guide and literature review in withdrawal of Benzodiazepine: The Ashton Manuel *Benzodiazepines: How they work and how to withdraw*, summarizing 12 years of clinical experience, is a comprehensive guide and literature review to help people safely withdraw from benzodiazepines.

Psychiatric Issues

In 2008, an estimated 23.5 million Americans aged 12 and older required treatment for substance abuse. The Substance Abuse and Mental Health Services Administration (SAMSHA) reports that by 2020 mental and substance use disorders will surpass all physical diseases as a major cause of disability worldwide [44]. Drugs are commonly abused among psychiatric patients and may have significant implications for treatment and prognosis. In the acute psychiatric setting, many patients have recently taken substances that may affect their behavior or mental state. Symptoms of substance abuse may resemble psychiatric conditions and it can be difficult for the nurse to discern if the patient is under the influence of drugs or alcohol or suffering from acute psychosis [45]. Patients admitted to a psychiatric unit or emergency department with acute mental or medical illness and an altered mental status must also be assessed for substance intoxication.

Because many patients who abuse substances also have an underlying psychological condition, called dual diagnosis, the needs of these patients are complex. People with dual diagnoses have a higher risk of suicide, victimization, violent behavior, less compliance with medication and treatment, more severe mental health problems, family history of childhood abuse, and involvement in the criminal justice system. An excellent resource titled is *The Dual Diagnosis Good Practice Handbook: Helping practitioners to plan, organize, and deliver services for people with coexisting mental health and substance abuse needs*. The handbook emphasizes including the patient and families in the treatment plan as well as the importance of an interdisciplinary approach and communication to maximize chances of success [46].

Pain Management

It is essential to assess every patient for pain in all practice settings. Pain management is a complex and rapidly expanding field in medicine. When combined with substance abuse or dependence, managing pain can become quite a challenge. "The American society for pain management nursing (ASPNM) and the International Nurses Society on Addiction (IntNSA) hold the position that patients with substance use disorders and pain have the right to be treated with dignity, respect, and the same quality of pain assessment and management as all other patients" [1]. Pain management is a complex and rapidly developing specialty.

Many factors should be considered in a pain management program for patients with a history of substance abuse. Physical dependence, tolerance, addiction, and psychological factors such as anxiety and depression can all influence a patient's experience of pain [22]. Patients are aware of the social stigma surrounding opioid and substance dependence and may be hesitant to share information with providers. Using the methods described in the "Assessment" and "Barriers to Care", through a nonjudgmental approach and establishing a trusting relationship, nurses are able to facilitate acquisition of information. It is also important to explain that knowledge of all substances used, both prescribed and illicit, is necessary in order to provide adequate pain control [47]. These patients, as all others, have a right to privacy and confidentiality.

In surgical patients with a history of substance abuse, pain management should begin in the preoperative period, ideally prior to admission, as identification of opioid tolerance is important in order to anticipate difficult postoperative pain control. Documentation of all routinely used drugs and doses should be known in order to plan for adequate analgesia. Postoperatively, pain scores may be higher and decrease more slowly than in a patient who is not opioid dependent. As with any patient, if reports of pain continues to escalate or does not decline even with intervention and medication, other reasons such as surgical complications should be suspected [47]. The primary principles of pain management in a patient who is tolerant to opioids are optimizing adequate perioperative analgesia, preventing withdrawal, and addressing related social, psychiatric, or behavioral issues. Working with other clinicians though a collaborative, interdisciplinary approach both in the hospital and in the community to promote continuity of care is crucial, as is elaborate discharge planning [48]. Stress from poorly treated pain may trigger relapse or exacerbate an existing addiction. Failure to identify and treat the concurrent condition of pain and substance abuse disorders compromises the ability to treat either condition effectively [1].

Nurses have ethical obligations to evaluate and treat issues associated with unrelieved pain, being cognizant of actual or potential risk of a substance use disorder or addiction, to practice without stigmatization, to correct misconceptions in practice, and to advocate for holistic treatment of patients with pain [1]. Nurses must advocate for the individual patients and consider their unique needs related to pain in the context of substance use disorders. All interdisciplinary healthcare team members are encouraged to engage in therapeutic discussions with each other to explore personal beliefs and attitudes regarding these conditions which may be barriers to providing effective care [5]. A common concern of healthcare professionals is that of drug seeking behaviors. Assessment of realistic causes of pain and using clinical judgment, challenging one's own preconceptions and stereotypes, and communication with other providers are all ways to promote adequate treatment of pain in the opioid-dependent patient [49].

Consent

Patients who are under the influence of drugs or alcohol present legal considerations with obtaining consent. For example, a patient who is intoxicated is not able to give an informed consent because he/she may not be able to understand the risks, benefits, and treatment alternatives. In some states, specific legislation states that no legal recourse will come upon a physician for examining and treating a patient without his or her consent if the patient is intoxicated or under the influence of drugs, or otherwise incapable of providing informed consent. Ability to consent to medical treatment excludes those of unsound mind, related to "natural state, age, shock, anxiety, illness, injury, drugs or sedation, intoxication, or other causes of whatever nature." In states without such statutes, case law supports the underlying philosophy that intoxicated patients are incapable of giving consent. Documentation of the patient's care, along with a therapeutic relationship, will facilitate communication with the patient and other providers, allow evaluation of clinical outcomes and further treatment planning, and reduce medical-legal liability [1].

Nursing Specialties and Specific Roles

Substance abuse nursing is a specialty that deals extensively with addiction and requires specific training. Prior to becoming addiction specialists, nurses often work in psychiatric facilities or substance abuse treatment centers. Upon completion of 2,000 h of addiction-related nursing, they are eligible for certification through an examination administered by the International Nurses Society on Addictions to become a Certified Addictions Registered Nurse (CARN). In this specialty, nurses care for patients in inpatient and outpatient settings including drug treatment centers, psychiatric facilities, methadone clinics, hospitals, and primary care physicians' offices. They are also in demand in rural areas where options for drug treatment and rehabilitation may be limited. The patent population includes all ages and settings such as teenagers undergoing inpatient rehab at residential treatment centers to adults seeking outpatient services [50].

Nurse Practitioners (NPs) are advanced practice nurses that treat patients with substance abuse in a variety of environments. NPs are responsible for routinely screening patients for substance abuse. Nurse practitioners can specialize in gerontology, women's health, pediatrics, neonatology, acute care, family health, and psychiatry. They work in outpatient and inpatient and settings which likely have contact with patients or family members with addictions. Some roles, such as in a primary care setting, allow for developing long-standing relationships with patients and families. They are a crucial part in preventing abuse, recognizing risk factors, and part-taking in treatment plans for managing patients. They may be responsible for performing and ordering tests and exams to assess physiological effects substance abuse as well as referring patients to treatment clinics and specialists in addiction. Nurse practitioners are in a key position to offer treatment options and counseling patients and family members having difficulty coping with their loved ones' addiction.

Psychiatric-Mental Health Nurse Practitioners (PMHNs) are perhaps the most skilled and specialized nurses to provide care for patients with substance abuse. Professional preparation includes mental health promotion, mental illness diagnosis and treatment across the lifespan, although some choose to focus in certain phases of life. PMHNs can also specialize in substance abuse with an addiction focus. They can also be eligible for recognition as a Certified Addictions Registered Nurse. The settings and patient populations are similar to that of the substance abuse nurse described above, but their roles also include in diagnosing, treating, prescribing, and forming and ensuring administration of the treatment plan [51].

Nurse case managers are important members of the addiction recovery team and are involved in the care of the addicted patient from the time of admission to treatment and integration into society as a sober person. They obtain a history, lead coping skills groups and individual patient sessions, facilitate the change process and transition to life without addiction, and assist in facilitating community resources to maximize chances of success. They must have a thorough understanding of the disease of addiction as well as the process of relapse and offer support and skills strategies. The evolution of the addiction nurse case manager's role in an inpatient and outpatient treatment program shows improvements in patient satisfaction and outcome when the nurse was an integral part of the team [52].

The interaction of a Certified Registered Nurse Anesthetist (CRNA) and a patient with substance abuse is generally short-term when the patient requires anesthesia for a procedure or surgery. The focus tends to be on the physiologic implications of acute intoxication and long-term substance abuse as well as the potential pharmacological interactions of the ingested substances with medications. Nearly all abused substances require special anesthetic consideration such as central nervous system excitation or depression. For example, the pharmacological consequences of administering ephedrine or labetalol (agents commonly used to treat intraoperative low and high blood pressure, respectively), or meperidine (a pain medication) can be fatal if the patient has a history of recent or acute cocaine use. It is therefore imperative that the anesthetist is aware of any history of substance abuse as it will certainly affect decisions made during perioperative care.

Certified Nurse Midwives (CNMs) are in the unique position of providing care to not one, but rather two patients who may be affected by the substance abuse of one individual. The nurse midwife may be the first healthcare professional a woman sees when seeking maternal care, and if substance abuse is identified, referral to other specialists and community resources as early as possible is essential due to the potentially devastating implications for the fetus. Traditionally, the parturient with addiction is considered to be a high-risk pregnancy. Much like in the general population of substance abuse, a multidisciplinary approach is especially important, and expectant mothers fear stigma and feel that prenatal care may not be accessible to them due to their addictions [53].

Summary

In a variety of care settings and roles, nurses are an integral part of providing effective care to patients with addiction. Nurses are involved in all aspects of patient care, from screening and assessment to physical examination, administering care, evaluating efficacy of interventions, and serving as advocates. They facilitate the treatment of patients with substance abuse and should be included as part of a cohesive care team to ensure the highest likelihood of patient success. The nurse's role is to form a relationship with the patient and the family, free of stigma, and educate them about the disease and facilitate in therapy [7]. Nurses engage in patient education, assist in transitioning to life without substance use, aid in repairing relationships, and offer psychosocial and emotional support to patients with addiction. With a combination of compassion and knowledge, nurses are prepared to care for individuals and their families in each of these situations based on accepted guidelines and evidence-based practice.

References

1. Oliver J, Coggins C, Compton P, Hagan S, Matteliano D, Stanton M, et al. American Society for Pain Management nursing position statement: pain management in patients with substance use disorders. Pain Manag Nurs. 2012;13(3):169–83.
2. International Council of Nurses. Definition of nursing; April 12, 2010. http://www.icn.ch/about-icn/icn-definition-of-nursing/. Accessed 20 Jun 2013.
3. Craven RF, Hirnle CJ. Fundamentals of nursing: human health and function. Philadelphia: Lippincott Williams & Wilkins; 2003.
4. van Boekel LC, Brouwers EP, van Weeghel J, Garretsen HF. Stigma among health professionals towards patients with substance use disorders and its consequences for healthcare delivery: systematic review. Drug Alcohol Depend. 2013;131(1–2):23–35.
5. McCaffery M, Grimm MA, Pasero C, Ferrell B, Uman GC. On the meaning of "drug seeking". Pain Manage Nurs. 2005;6(4):122–36.
6. Ford R, Bammer G, Becker N. Improving nurses' therapeutic attitude to patients who use illicit drugs: workplace drug and alcohol education is not enough. Int J Nurs Pract. 2009;15(2):112–8.
7. Center for Substance Abuse Treatment. A guide to substance abuse services for primary care clinicians. Treatment improvement protocols (TIP) series 24, SMA 97-3139; 1997.
8. Muhrer JC. Detecting and dealing with substance abuse disorders in primary care. J Nurse Pract. 2010;6(8):597–605.
9. Rastegar DA, Kunins HV, Tetrault JM, Walley AY, Gordon AJ, US Society of General Internal Medicine's Substance Abuse Interest Group. 2012 Update in addiction medicine for the generalist. Addict Sci Clin Pract. 2013;8:6.
10. Ewing JA. Detecting alcoholism: the CAGE questionnaire. JAMA. 1984;252(14):1905–7.
11. Babor TF, Higgins-Biddle JC, Saunders JB, Monteiro MG. AUDIT: the alcohol use disorders identification test: guidelines for use in primary care. Geneva: World Health Organization; 2001. http://whqlibdoc.who.int/hq/2001/who_msd_msb_01.68.pdf. Accessed 10 Aug 2013.
12. Hays RD, Merz JF, Nicholas R. Response burden, reliability, and validity of the CAGE, Short MAST, and AUDIT alcohol screening measures. Behav Res Methods. 1995;27(2):277–80.
13. Brown RL, Rounds LA. Conjoint screening questionnaires for alcohol and other drug abuse: criterion validity in a primary care practice. Wis Med J. 1995;94(3):135–40.
14. Knight JR, Sherritt L, Shrier LA, Harris SK, Chang G. Validity of the CRAFFT Substance Abuse Screening Test among adolescent clinic patients. Arch Pediatr Adolesc Med. 2002;156(6):607–14.
15. Goodman DJ, Wolff KB. Screening for substance abuse in women's health: a public health imperative. J Midwifery Womens Health. 2013;58(3):278–87.
16. US Dept of Health and Human Services. Alcohol Alert. 2004;63.
17. Blow FC, Brower KJ, Schulenberg JE, Demo-Dananberg LM, Young JP, Beresford TP. The Michigan Alcoholism Screening Test—Geriatric Version (MAST-G): a new elderly specific screening instrument. Alcohol Clin Exp Res. 1992;16(2):372.
18. Broyles LM, Colbert AM, Tate JA, Swigart VA, Happ MB. Clinicians' evaluation and management of mental health, substance abuse, and chronic pain conditions in the intensive care unit. Crit Care Med. 2008;36(1):87–93.
19. http://www.nanda.org/
20. McArdle P, Wiegersma A, Gilvarry E, Kolte B, McCarthy S, Fitzgerald M, et al. European adolescent substance use: the roles of family structure, function and gender. Addiction. 2002;97(3):329–36.
21. Montoya ID. The pathology of alcohol use and abuse. Clin Lab Sci. 2013;26(1):15–22.
22. Mitra S, Sinatra RS. Perioperative management of acute pain in the opioid-dependent patient. Anesthesiology. 2004;101(1):212–27.
23. Lazoritz S, Rossiter K, Whiteaker D. What every nurse needs to know about clinical aspects of child abuse. Am Nurse Today. 2010;5(7). August 3, 2013.

24. *New York Times*. Health guide: alcoholism and alcohol abuse, an in-depth report. 2013. http://health.nytimes.com/health/guides/disease/alcoholism/in-depth-report.html. Accessed 20 Jul 2013.
25. Kodama S, Saito K, Tanaka S, Horikawa C, Saito A, Heianza Y, et al. Alcohol consumption and risk of atrial fibrillation: a meta-analysis. J Am Coll Cardiol. 2011;57(4):427–36.
26. Nace EP. Alcohol. In: Frances RJ, Miller SI, Mack AH, editors. Clinical textbook of addictive disorders. 3rd ed. New York: Guilford Press; 2005. p. 75–104.
27. Gordon AJ, Gordon JM, Carl K, Hilton MT, Striebel J, Maher M. In: Gordan AJ, editor. Physical illness and drugs of abuse: a review of the evidence. New York: Cambridge University Press; 2010.
28. Salitz R. Medical and surgical complications of addiction. In: Ries RK, Fiellin DA, Miller SC, Saitz R, editors. Principles of addiction medicine. 4th ed. Philadelphia: Lippincott Williams & Wilkins; 2009. p. 945–67.
29. International Narcotics Control Board. Narcotic Drugs: estimated world requirements for 2013—statistics for 2011. Vienna: United Nations; 2013.
30. Centers for Disease Control and Prevention. Vital signs: overdoses of prescription opioid pain relievers and other drugs among women—United States, 1999–2010. MMWR Morb Mortal Wkly Rep. 2013;62(26):537–42.
31. Substance Abuse and Mental Health Services Administration, Center for Behavioral Health Statistics and Quality. The DAWN report: highlights of the 2009 drug abuse warning network (DAWN) findings on drug-related emergency department visits. 2010.
32. Vaghari B, Baratta MD, Ghandi K. Perioperative approach to patients with opioid abuse and tolerance. Anesthesiol News. 2013;38(6):1–4.
33. Mayo Clinic. 2012. http://www.mayoclinic.com/health/prescription-drug-abuse/. Accessed 12 Jul 2013.
34. Kain Z, Barash PG. Anesthetic implications of drug abuse. ASA Refresher Courses Anesthesiol. 2001;29(1):159–73.
35. Parsons HA, Delgado-Guay M, El Osta B, Chacko R, Poulter V, Palmer JL, et al. Alcoholism screening in patients with advanced cancer: impact on symptom burden and opioid use. J Palliat Med. 2008;11(7):964–8.
36. Repper-DeLisi J, Stern TA, Mitchell M, Lussier-Cushing M, Lakatos B, Fricchione GL, et al. Successful implementation of an alcohol-withdrawal pathway in a general hospital. Psychosomatics. 2008;49(4):292–9.
37. Burns MJ, Lekawa ME, Price JB. Delirium tremens (DTs). April 9, 2013. http://emedicine.medscape.com/article/166032-overview#showall. Accessed 16 Jul 2012.
38. American Psychiatric Association. Diagnostic and statistical manual of mental disorders. 4th ed. Arlington: American Psychiatric Association; 2000.
39. Elliott DY, Geyer C, Lionetti T, Doty L. Managing alcohol withdrawal in hospitalized patients. Nursing. 2012;42(4):22–30; quiz 30-1.
40. Gowing L, Farrell M, Ali R, White JM. Alpha2-adrenergic agonists for the management of opioid withdrawal. Cochrane Database Syst Rev. 2009;(2):CD002024.
41. Kunoe N, Lobmaier P, Vederhus JK, Hjerkinn B, Hegstad S, Gossop M, et al. Naltrexone implants after in-patient treatment for opioid dependence: randomised controlled trial. Br J Psychiatry. 2009;194(6):541–6.
42. Doyon S. In: Tintinalli JE, Kelen GD, Stapczynski JS, Ma OJ, Cline DM, editors. Emergency medicine: a comprehensive study guide. 6th ed. New York: McGraw-Hill; 2004. p. 1071–4.
43. Petursson H. The Benzodiazepine withdrawal syndrome. Addiction. 1994;89(11):1455–9.
44. Substance Abuse and Mental Health Services Administration. Results from the 2010 National Survey on Drug Use and Health (NSDUH): summary of national findings. NSDUH Series H-41, HHS 2011; SMA11-4658.
45. Vaaler AE, Morken G, Fløvig J, Iversen VC, Linaker OM. Substance abuse and recovery in a psychiatric intensive care unit. Gen Hosp Psychiatry. 2006;28(1):65–70.
46. National Mental Health Development Unit. Developing a capable dual diagnosis strategy: a good practice guide. London: Department of Health and National Mental Health Development Unit; 2009.

47. Huxtable CA, Roberts LJ, Somogyi AA, MacIntyre PE. Acute pain management in opioid-tolerant patients: a growing challenge. Anaesth Intensive Care. 2011;39(5):804–23.
48. Roberts L. The opioid-tolerant patient, including those with a substance abuse disorder. In: Macintyre PE, Walker SM, Rowbotham DJ, editors. Clinical pain management: acute pain. 2nd ed. London: Hodder Arnold; 2008. p. 539–56.
49. Sim MG, Hulse GK, Khong E. Clinical practice. Acute pain and opioid seeking behaviour… ninth and final article in a series of case files. Aust Fam Physician. 2004;33(12):1009–12.
50. Williams E. Demand Media. The role of a nurse in drug rehabilitation. 2013. http://work. chron.com/role-nurse-drug-rehabilitation-15460.html. Accessed 12 Aug 2013.
51. American Psychiatric Nurses Association. http://www.apna.org/i4a/pages/index.cfm?pageid= 4792. Accessed 16 Jun 2013.
52. White BK, Bouton LL, Garris SK, Humphreys PT, Miltier JR. The role of the nurse case manager in substance abuse treatment. J Addict Nurs. 1998;10(3):136–41.
53. Economidoy E, Klimi A, Vivilaki VG. Caring for substance abuse pregnant women: the role of the midwife. Health Sci J. 2012;6(1):161–9.

Chapter 19
The Role of the Social Worker

Janet Lucas, Anne Riffenburgh, and Bill Mejia

Key Points

- Teamwork
- Why social work
- Navigating the Minefield
- Assessment
- Care planning and monitoring: an ongoing process

"Bill, we need you. Now!" There was no mistaking the urgency in the unit manager's voice. Bill, the palliative care social worker, excused himself from a department meeting. The unit manager quickly filled him in. The discharge of a patient was spiraling out of control. The nurses had orders to remove the patient's PICC line. He refused. The unit manager explained, "We have to remove the port before he leaves. The patient's a total addict, and he'll just use the PICC line for drugs. Do something. We have to get him out." When Bill arrived on the unit, he found a frail elderly man cowering near the elevator, surrounded by two security guards and a nurse. Bill approached and knelt before the patient, creating a neutral space. Bill said, "Sir, can you tell me what's happening?" The patient replied, "It hurts too much to take out. They're just going to put another one in before my next chemo appointment on Wednesday." Bill asked, "Are you worried that it's going to hurt to remove, just to have another one put in next week?" The patient nodded. Bill extended his hand and said, "I understand. Can I help you back to your room, and then I'll check on this?" The patient agreed.

J. Lucas, L.C.S.W. (✉)
Family Medicine Residency Program, Glendale Adventist Medical Center,
801 South Chevy Chase Drive, Suite 201, Glendale, CA 91205, USA
e-mail: jclucas11@aol.com

A. Riffenburgh, L.C.S.W.
The Huntington Cancer Center, Palliative Care, Huntington Memorial Hospital,
100 West California Boulevard, Pasadena, CA 91105, USA

B. Mejia, L.C.S.W.
Department of Palliative Care, Social Work, and Spiritual Care,
Huntington Memorial Hospital, 100 West California Boulevard, Pasadena, CA 91105, USA

© Springer Science+Business Media New York 2015
A.D. Kaye et al. (eds.), *Substance Abuse*, DOI 10.1007/978-1-4939-1951-2_19

After getting the patient back to bed, Bill conferred with the unit manager and nurse, who then paged the doctor. The doctor confirmed the patient's Wednesday chemotherapy appointment and, while acknowledging the patient's substance abuse history, agreed that removing the portacath was unnecessary. A new order was written, and the patient was discharged before the end of shift.

Introduction

Providing palliative care for patients with a history of substance abuse poses highly charged and unique challenges. The trifecta of death, pain, and addiction can activate deep fears and prejudices in the health care setting. Health care providers are called upon to manage their own emotional reactions and judgments, while striving to provide sound and compassionate medical care. Patients and family members affected by substance abuse carry a legacy of complex psychosocial wounds. Common feelings of anger, loss, betrayal, regret, resentment, and fear often lie close to the surface, readily awakened by the nearness of death. These dynamics create an additional layer of complexity, the suffering within the suffering.

Although there is a marked lack of consensus within the medical community regarding the definition of substance abuse, this chapter will adhere to the following:

Substance abuse (also known as addiction) may be defined as a chronic, relapsing, treatable disease of the brain characterized by compulsive use of a substance, resulting in physical, psychological, or social harm to the user, who continues to use despite that harm [1, 2].

The National Center on Addiction and Substance Abuse reports that "1 in 4 Americans will have an alcohol or drug problem at some point in their lives" [3]. This daunting statistic affects health care providers, who must give weighty consideration to the risks and benefits of utilizing potentially abusable medications, while addressing the complex psychosocial dynamics that accompany a substance abuse history.

Teamwork

The interdisciplinary team provides a well-recognized and recommended approach to caring for palliative care patients [4, 5]. The complicating presence of substance abuse makes the interdisciplinary team indispensable in addressing a tangle of medical, psychosocial, and logistical issues [6–9]. An optimal palliative care team configuration may consist of a physician, nurse, social worker, chaplain, and a mental health professional with expertise in substance abuse [6, 10]. Members of the team bring their unique knowledge and perspective to assessment, care planning, and medical management, helping to ensure that each patient receives individualized, comprehensive, and compassionate care. Mutual support and collaboration enable team members to maintain a sense of efficacy and professional gratification, mitigating the potential for compassion fatigue and burnout.

Why Social Work?

Social work, with its professional focus on person-in-environment, social justice, and the importance of human relationships, is ideally suited to address the issues of substance abuse in palliative care [11]. The social worker obtains a nuanced and comprehensive psychosocial history, advocates for marginalized and vulnerable individuals, and recognizes the power of compassion and empathy as a catalyst for healing. The ability to integrate these core values helps create an atmosphere of dignity, respect, clear boundaries, realistic expectations, and a dedication to patient, family, and staff well-being.

Navigating the Minefield

For members of the palliative care team, the admonition "Know thyself" becomes a tool for survival. As health care professionals, each of us carries a personal history of illness, grief, loss, suffering, and regret. Working in palliative care immerses us in a daily minefield of emotionally activating experiences. When issues of substance abuse compound the clinical picture, the minefield becomes exponentially more explosive. Team members should consider their own personal or family history. Significant unresolved issues may call for intervention. There is much to be said for healing the wounded healer.

The presence of substance abuse highlights human flaws and frailties. Patients and families display a variety challenging behaviors and emotional defenses, which may include:

- Self-harm
- Manipulation
- Noncompliance/pushing limits and boundaries
- Codependence
- Belligerence/hostility
- Victimization
- Impaired insight/judgment
- Unwillingness to explore emotional wounds or accept personal responsibility.

Difficult behaviors can evoke feelings of impatience, frustration, anger, and exhaustion. Our natural tendency is to focus outward on "the other," blaming and labeling, rather than acknowledging and managing our own emotional reactions. Social workers must look within to discover the feelings and core beliefs that challenging behaviors activate.

One palliative care social worker recalls her experience managing strong negative emotions:

> *Our team was working with Mr. H, a lung cancer patient with a long history of heroin abuse. Formulating a care plan proved challenging. We considered Mr. H high-risk for seeking illicit drugs outside the hospital. To ensure his safety, we had Mr. H verbally agree that he would not leave the ward. Two days later, when we approached the bedside, Mr. H appeared somnolent and incoherent. The nurses immediately reported that Mr. H had been absent from his room for over an hour. Our team strongly suspected that Mr. H had obtained street drugs. Experiencing intense feelings of anger and frustration, I did not take my usual place at the head of Mr. H's bed. Instead, I hung back and withheld my usual chipper greeting. Despite his altered mental status, Mr. H immediately commented, "You're mad at me." Taken aback that my feelings were so transparent, I replied, "No. No, I'm not mad." But deep down I knew that Mr. H saw in me what I was reluctant to see in myself.*
>
> *During lunch I processed the interaction with the nurse on our team. I realized that I felt personally betrayed. How could Mr. H do this to us when we were working so hard to help him? Furthermore, my investment in being the always kind and helpful member of the team had been jeopardized.*

Initial emotional reactions often mask unconscious beliefs of inadequacy and incompetency. This social worker first had to acknowledge her feelings of anger and identify the deeper, underlying core issues driving her response. Upon reflection, she realized that she was emotionally invested in the success of the care plan, expecting Mr. H to "follow the rules" and appreciate the care and effort the team had shown him. Rather than acknowledge her frustration and disappointment, the social worker labeled Mr. H as untrustworthy. In truth, the core issue was a need to feel capable and look competent in the eyes of others. Processing her response allowed the social worker to depersonalize Mr. H's behavior, which had little to do with the team or the care plan, and everything to do with his heroin abuse.

Debriefing with a trusted team member provided the social worker with an opportunity to share her experience, acknowledge her feelings, and examine her own core beliefs. Taking time to share and reflect allows social workers and other team members to provide optimal care to patients and themselves.

While all members of the interdisciplinary team encounter emotional triggers, the social worker is often called upon to engage, manage, and resolve the challenges that these issues generate in the health care setting.

Assessment

The social worker's initial task is to conduct an in-depth psychosocial assessment. The presence of substance abuse may already be noted in the patient's medical work-up. For example, a diagnosis of cirrhosis of the liver or smoking-related lung cancer provides overt evidence of a patient's substance abuse history. Often, however, substance abuse remains hidden, requiring skillful identification. The psychosocial assessment identifies common comorbidities associated with substance abuse, including depression, anxiety, mood disorders, and any history of trauma and abuse [12, 13]. These comorbidities serve as "red flags," indicating that further assessment is indicated. However, pursuing a substance abuse assessment can prove daunting.

Health care professionals may shy away from exploring a patient's substance abuse history, fearing an angry and defensive reaction. Combining an engaging, empathic interview style with a nonthreatening, graduated approach can reduce the potential for a hostile response. Asking focused questions, beginning with less-stigmatized substances, such as caffeine and nicotine, and progressing to questions regarding alcohol and prescription/illicit drugs, helps minimize denial and promotes candor [14, 15]. The social worker may start with less personal questions before moving to questions about the patient's own history. Accurate patient disclosure may be encouraged by explaining that people often underreport alcohol and drug use for a variety of reasons, including embarrassment, mistrust, and fear of judgment. The social worker can reassure patients that an accurate history helps prevent undertreatment of symptoms and promotes optimal pain management [14, 16, 17]. In addition, patients may gain a much-needed opportunity to openly share their abuse and recovery narrative.

Despite best efforts to obtain an accurate history, the social worker must remember that denial is a hallmark of substance abuse. Eliciting additional information from friends and family may be useful. Be sure to observe privacy guidelines per HIPAA [18].

Useful measures for identifying patients at risk for abuse of opioids include the Screener and Opioid Assessment for Patients with Pain (SOAPP) [19] or the shorter Opioid Risk Assessment Tool [20]. Patients with a substance abuse history combined with a major medical diagnosis, such as cancer, are subject to higher rates of drug abuse and relapse. In addition, ready access to centrally acting drugs, such as opioids or benzodiazepines, compounds the risk [6, 10]. The presence of a life-threatening or endstage illness can prove overwhelming for even the most functional and emotionally resilient individuals. For patients whose coping skills are fragile or compromised, such situations may reactivate the desire to rely on old patterns of destructive behavior.

To complete an accurate history, the following information may be illuminating:

- Dates and duration of treatment and sobriety
- Desired effects of drugs/alcohol
- Factors that undermined recovery or promoted relapse (include people/events/ triggers)
- Factors that facilitated recovery (include people/events/personal strengths)
- Benefits/gifts of sobriety
- Current level of motivation to maintain sobriety/seek recovery [14, 21].

For some patients, the expectation of sobriety and total adherence to a care plan may be unrealistic. The social worker helps shift the focus from compliance to minimizing the harmful effects of substance abuse [6, 22]. The focus on harm reduction can:

- Decrease consumption
- Decrease the hazards of consumption
- Increase social functioning
- Increase the potential for abstinence [22].

Culture and Special Populations

When assessing for substance abuse the social worker should consider cultural traditions or special groups with which a patient may identify. Attention must also be given to personal demographics such as race, age, sexual orientation/gender identity, and socioeconomic status. Such factors may influence:

- Attitudes about privacy
- Willingness to disclose personal information
- Perceptions of what constitutes a harmful behavior
- Perceptions of when treatment is needed
- Attitudes about pain and pain management
- Acceptance of help
- Capacity to trust health care providers/institutions [21, 23]

While language, race, and ethnicity are commonly noted in a psychosocial assessment, information about less conventional subgroups may receive limited attention. Special populations may include subcultures (e.g., street gangs, LGBT communities), recovery/treatment groups (e.g., 12-step, alternative healing), and nontraditional spiritual communities. Members of subgroups may hold values and beliefs unfamiliar to health care providers, triggering unconscious biases that negatively impact patient care. Clinical observation suggests that health care providers more readily label a questionable behavior as drug related in patients whose social and cultural norms differ from their own [16]. Conversely, patients who uphold or represent conventional traditions or belong to a demographic less commonly associated with substance abuse may receive inadequate assessment and monitoring. Research in health care settings indicates that substance abuse is often underidentified or misdiagnosed in older adults, women, and those with higher incomes, higher education, or private medical insurance [7, 24].

Maintaining self-awareness and respectfully addressing issues of culture and personal identity enables the social worker to develop an enhanced rapport while obtaining valuable insights that can enhance patient care.

A comprehensive substance abuse assessment yields multiple and interrelated psychosocial factors, allowing team members to develop an individualized medical and psychosocial care plan [21, 22]. The most effective care plan acknowledges and integrates a patient's unique perspectives, vulnerabilities, and sources of strength to promote resilience and provide opportunities for healing.

Care Planning and Monitoring: An Ongoing Process

A cornerstone of effective care planning lies in establishing appropriate boundaries to help manage common behaviors associated with substance abuse. Health care providers encounter these substance abuse behaviors (also referred to as aberrant drug-related behaviors) in both the in-patient and out-patient settings. Examples include:

- Aggressively complaining of the need for higher doses, despite ongoing assessment
- Concurrently abusing illicit drugs
- Increasing dosage without physician approval, i.e., "I had to take more and then I ran out."
- Requesting early refills (see above)
- Seeking "emergency" refills after established office hours via on-call or emergency room physicians
- Using multiple medical providers to obtain similar medications
- Treating psychic symptoms with medications intended to treat pain, i.e., "The Norco really calms me down."
- Claiming recurrent prescription losses, i.e., "The movers lost the box that had my medicine in it."
- "Borrowing" or stealing prescription medications, i.e., "I tried my friend's Roxanol, and that worked. I want to change my medicine to that!"
- Demanding specific medications (see above)
- Refusing to use adjuvant medications
- Obtaining prescription drugs from nonmedical sources
- Selling prescription drugs
- Forging prescriptions
- Drug hoarding during periods of reduced symptoms
- Acting entitled, belligerent, or victimized
- Continuously pushing established care plan boundaries [7, 20, 25, 26]

Tip: When documenting a patient's substance abuse behaviors, avoid using pejorative terms such as "drug-seeking" or "manipulative." Such terms may reflect a health care provider's bias and frustration, without yielding useful information to guide patient care. Be specific and use discernment. Cite only those behaviors that directly affect patient care.

The team implements various strategies to manage substance abuse behaviors, which include:

- Clearly stating the goals of care
- Educating patients about their medications—purpose, dosage, risks, and side effects
- Citing expectations of how patients will use their medications
- Clearly explaining how medications and doses may be reevaluated if pain is undertreated
- Establishing and applying consequences if patients misuse or abuse their medications
- Continually reevaluating the care plan

In an outpatient setting, pain agreements are frequently employed to address the specifics of care and consequences outlined above. In an inpatient setting, pain agreements are typically less formal; the agreement is often a verbal one, contracted between the patient and members of the palliative care team and then charted in the medical record. Team members must take extra care to communicate with each other to minimize manipulation and the potential for patients to play one team member off another, a tactic known as "splitting."

Tip: To minimize the potential for splitting, avoid seeing a patient alone. Including another team member communicates to the patient that the team is united and committed to the care plan and established consequences.

Developing the Medical Care Plan

A patient's substance abuse history alerts the team to the risk for potential abuse and helps shape the medical care plan. One of the first issues the team considers is duration of sobriety. For example, a person who has been sober for 20 years with involved family, a religious community or 12-step contacts may be more likely to use prescribed medications appropriately, requiring less monitoring for misuse, than someone who is 6 months out of treatment and socially isolated.

Regardless of the risk of abuse, the team should adhere to the primary goals of palliative care, which are to adequately manage pain and related symptoms and promote quality of life. Consulting an addiction specialist may yield useful strategies and support [2, 6, 10, 14]. Aggressively treating pain and acknowledging that "pain is what the patient says it is" must trump team members' fears of being duped or manipulated. Patients benefit from the assurance that they will receive sufficient medication to relieve their pain [6, 18]. While abuse of medication can lead to substance abuse behaviors, so can the undertreatment of pain, a phenomenon known as pseudoaddiction [2, 6, 27].

Care is taken to tailor pain management strategies to suit specific patient needs. A patient's self-reporting of the sought-after effects of drugs or alcohol helps the team prescribe appropriate medications. The team may be hesitant to prescribe strong, short-acting opioids to someone who has revealed that "the rush of a fix" has served as the driving force for abusing drugs. Extended release formulations may be a better option. For patients who report that they self-medicate "to calm down," the doctor may consider adding an anxiolytic medication to treat anxiety [28]. The social worker participates by introducing psychosocial interventions, critical adjuvants in minimizing the stress response.

To the extent possible, involve patients and families in identifying the goals of the medical care plan [10]. Underscore that they are an integral part of the palliative care team. Creating an atmosphere of mutuality increases cooperation and mitigates the potential for difficult and challenging behaviors. When conflicts erupt, containment is more easily attained when patients and families are invested in the care plan.

The medical care plan is a work in progress, requiring ongoing reevaluation and monitoring. When patients and families push boundaries or display substance abuse behaviors, the team should respond with a balance of structure, flexibility, and compassion [29]. New information and changing impressions must be addressed and reintegrated as the care plan evolves [10]. An effective medical care plan creates a predictable, safe, and nurturing environment that helps counter the chaos, dysfunction, and trauma that often accompanies substance abuse.

Developing the Social Work Care Plan

While intensifying emotional vulnerability and the risk of relapse, a medical crisis may also serve as a catalyst for change and recovery, providing an opportunity for what some clinicians call "accelerated healing." In an atmosphere of heightened distress, those with an extended history of denial or resistance may be willing to acknowledge, address and potentially heal deep psychosocial wounds and damaged relationships.

Intense emotional distress and lingering psychosocial wounds can exacerbate a patient's perception of physical pain [18, 30]. Patients who have used substances as a way of self-medicating emotional pain are especially vulnerable during hospitalization, as they find themselves with limited or no access to alcohol, drugs, and/or nicotine. Even patients with an established history of recovery have an increased risk of relapse when faced with an endstage diagnosis [6, 10]. In addition, identification of depression, anxiety, mood disorders, and any history of trauma/abuse highlights key areas requiring intervention.

Patients benefit from social work interventions designed to:

- Calm overwhelming emotional distress
- Address emotional vulnerabilities and wounds
- Identify emotionally activating experiences and relationships
- Identify areas of resilience and integrate emotional strengths
- Provide an opportunity to learn and reinforce healthy methods of coping
- Offer alternatives to destructive patterns of belief and behavior
- Repair damaged relationships

The social worker upholds and reinforces the social work care plan by:

Practicing self-awareness. Social workers may find unconscious biases reflected in their own body language, facial expressions and speech, unintentionally alienating those they seek to help. Patients and families who feel judged may retreat, physically and emotionally, impeding communication and their willingness to seek or accept support. Social workers must possess self-awareness and an on-going ability to monitor their own assumptions and emotional triggers.

Listening without judgment. Substance abuse includes behaviors that can evoke shame, regret, and self-loathing. When the social worker creates a safe and supportive atmosphere, patients and families may be willing to tell their stories, letting go of distortions and integrating the truth of their personal experiences. Experiencing the compassion and acceptance of another is vital to the healing process.

Maintaining boundaries. The role of the social worker is to support the goals, expectations, and consequences outlined in the medical care plan. Clear boundaries, maintained with compassion and discernment, allow patients and families to feel safe, accept responsibility, and maintain dignity. Patients and families with a substance abuse history can test limits and push boundaries, which may evoke the following inappropriate responses from health care providers:

- Enabling behavior and misplaced compassion, i.e., a health care providers relax or ignore an established boundary, such as no early refills, because they feel that the consequence is "too cruel" or harsh. Rather than supporting the patient, such behavior undermines the care plan and may unwittingly promote further substance abuse behaviors [6].
- Rigidity and inflexibility, i.e., a health care provider fails to recognize that relapse and substance abuse behaviors will likely occur, thus responding with punitive measures, such as withholding pain medication and exhibiting an attitude of disdain and judgment.

The social worker may act as liaison with other health care providers to explain the goals of care and underlying rationale for boundaries and consequences. When all those involved in the patient's care are "on the same page," the care plan is strengthened by consistency and unity of purpose. For health care providers, working together to develop and maintain a mutually agreed-upon care plan promotes interdisciplinary communication, cohesion, and support.

Providing Psychosocial Interventions

The social worker offers a variety of psychosocial interventions, which may include referrals to other qualified practitioners. Availability of services, cost, and individual motivation/receptivity are factors that should be considered. Interventions may include:

- Active listening
- Supportive counseling
- Cognitive-behavioral reframing
- Guided imagery/meditation/breathing/relaxation
- Journaling and bibliotherapy
- Healing touch
- Music, humor, art, and pet therapy
- Prayer
- Yoga
- Acupuncture
- Aromatherapy [18, 31]

Educating. The social worker continually gauges patient and family understanding of the medical situation and care plan. General topics that may require education include:

- Goals, expectations, and consequences outlined in the medical care plan
- Basic information regarding safe and effective pain management strategies
- Distinctions between tolerance, dependence, and addiction
- Instructions for monitoring pain
- Guidelines for communicating with and contacting health care providers
- Tips for navigating the health care system [31]

Patients, who have established sobriety, are in recovery or who have a family history of substance abuse may be reluctant to use centrally acting medications. Resistance may be driven by fear of relapse, judgment from others in their sobriety/recovery support networks, or activation of what they may consider "the family curse" of addiction. Reassurance and clarification may address:

- Dosing: Patients with a substance abuse history may require a higher initial dose or rapid dose escalation due to tolerance [10, 32]
- Therapeutic effect: Opioids taken for pain have a different effect on the central nervous system than when taken for the purpose of "getting high" [6]
- Uncontrolled pain: Suboptimal pain relief heightens the risk of substance abuse behaviors and relapse [6, 10, 14]

Advocating. Advocating for substance abuse patients at the end of life may take a variety of forms. The social worker may:

- Address common, ingrained biases held by health care providers that may interfere with or undermine the care plan
- Intervene with family members who may struggle with the patient's need for medications that carry the potential for abuse
- Provide outreach to sponsors and members of the 12-step community who may adhere to an abstinence-only philosophy
- Negotiate with residential recovery programs, since many are highly reluctant to accept residents with medications that may be abused
- Participate in social action within the larger community to address the needs of those who require substance abuse recovery at the end of life

Providing discharge planning. Start discharge planning early in the hospitalization to establish a safe and effective plan of care for home. Important tasks may include:

- Establishing medications for outpatient use
- Identifying the person who will dispense medications
- Identifying caregivers who can support care plan goals and boundaries
- Identifying family members or others who may undermine care plan goals and boundaries
- Linking patients to appropriate referrals, such as treatment/recovery support programs, sober living, and hospice
- Providing counseling to help patients, family members and caregivers anticipate and cope with emotional triggers and challenging relationships
- Establishing a plan for medical follow-up and support

Reminder: The presence of opioids in the patient's home may provide additional risks and challenges, especially if family members, caregivers, or "friends" also struggle with substance abuse.

Managing conflicts. The extreme stress of endstage illness, compounded by a past history of substance abuse, can lead to behavioral challenges and explosive conflicts at the bedside. Dysfunction and chaos in the patient's life and family system are common. Anger, blame, and mistrust may be directed at the patient, family members, and health care providers. Helpful strategies include:

- Involving patients and families in establishing care plan goals
- Reinforcing that all involved (patient, family, health care providers) share the same goals of relieving pain/symptoms and promoting quality of life
- Maintaining care plan goals and boundaries
- Highlighting that boundaries and consequences are established to promote the patient's safety and well-being
- Redirecting focus from past grievances to the present situation

Patients may respond to care plan consequences with anger resulting from a belief that they are being punished or victimized. Tip: Avoid a defensive, angry response. Avoid bargaining. Instead, employ empathy and underscore the team's commitment to sound patient care: "I know this is very difficult, but this is not a punishment. We are dedicated to your care and well-being. We are upholding these consequences to ensure your safety, which is our first priority."

Combining these strategies with compassion, confidence and clarity of purpose enables the social worker to effectively minimize, defuse, and contain conflict.

> *Mr. V was a 45-year-old Latino male with endstage liver disease. He was unresponsive and on a ventilator. His wife of 15 years, along with his three older sisters, met with the palliative care team. The physician began by asking the family what they knew of Mr. V's diagnosis. Almost immediately, the eldest sister stood up, pointed her finger at Mr. V's wife, and yelled, "This is all your fault. You never took good care of him." The wife rose to face the sister and retorted, "It was all you who let him drink, whenever he wanted to, when he was growing up. You still let him drink whenever he goes over to your house. This is YOUR fault, not mine!" Before the next accusation could be hurled, the social worker intervened. "We are here to discuss the medical situation of your husband and your brother. This is not the time or place for accusations or blame. He needs you all to focus on what's best for him now. I know this is a really difficult time and emotions are running high, but this is our opportunity to come together to make some important decisions about his care. Are you able to do that? Once the social worker felt that the situation was sufficiently defused, he established rules: "No blaming, no raised voices, remain seated, and let's make Mr. V's well-being our top priority." When the social worker finished speaking, he nodded to the physician, who continued the discussion. Later the physician confided, "I didn't know what to do when they started yelling. I wanted to crawl under the table. Thanks for taking the lead."*

The family meeting may serve as a crucible for conflict. Family members often enter the meeting with emotions charged, ready to ignite. Anger and blame defend against deeper issues of guilt and sadness. The social worker used his calm, authoritative presence to contain a potentially explosive situation, which enabled the meeting to move forward.

The following vignette provides a further example of how compassionate authority and ground rules provide structure and boundaries, creating a safe space for grief and healing.

Miss H was a 36-year-old Latina woman with a long history of alcohol abuse, who was admitted to the ICU for management of sepsis and liver failure, and placed on a ventilator. Miss H came from a large supportive family, consisting of her parents, four siblings, aunts, uncles and cousins. In addition, Miss H had a six-year-old son, who was being raised by her brother, the child's court-appointed guardian. For 10 days the family watched Miss H's slow and steady decline. On day 11, with support from the palliative care team, the family made the decision to remove Miss H from the ventilator and allow her to die. As the social worker headed to the ICU waiting room to meet with the family and the rest of the palliative care team, she heard shouting. She was taken aback, as previous interactions with family members had gone smoothly. The man doing much of the shouting turned out to be Miss H's ex-boyfriend and the father of her son. Mr. R hurled several ugly epithets at the women in the family, prompting the chaplain to call security. Two officers arrived immediately. The palliative care physician responded by requesting that "everyone to sit down, take a breath and stop the name calling." He did this twice. Finally, he drew his chair close, faced Mr. R and said, "I need you to understand that this is your final opportunity to say goodbye to the woman that you once loved and who is the mother of your child. If you're able to remain calm and refrain from name calling, the social worker will take you to the bedside, where you can spend some time with her. Can you do this? If not, these two officers will escort you out of the hospital now. Mr. R composed himself and replied, "I want to see her." The social worker and Mr. R headed to the ICU. Once separated from the others, the social worker extended her hand, introduced herself and asked his name. Referring to him by name, she prepared Mr. R for what he would see when he entered the room. The social worker remained just inside the doorway while Mr. R approached the bedside and spoke quietly to Miss H. When he finished, the security officers escorted him from the hospital. An hour later, Miss H died. To her family's relief, the extubation was unnecessary. After her death, the chaplain provided spiritual support to family members, offering oil, which they used to anoint her body, in a peaceful, meaningful ritual.

As this vignette illustrates, the team's ability to effectively manage conflict was a pivotal factor in creating and maintaining an environment that supported dignity and emotional healing, ensuring that the needs of each family member, including Mr. R, were met.

Summary

The "suffering within the suffering" of those touched by substance abuse poses special challenges to health care providers. The legacy of psychosocial wounding and the nearness of death can evoke intense memories and feelings in patients and families, triggering emotional reactivity and destructive patterns of coping. The social worker is uniquely positioned to address these challenges, working with the interdisciplinary team and other health care providers to foster self-awareness, collaboration, compassion, communication, discernment, and flexibility—characteristics easy to espouse but difficult to implement. When these characteristics are combined with the individual gifts and skills of team members, the results can be powerful: pain and symptom management is optimized, the risk for substance abuse and relapse is reduced, and the opportunity for psychosocial healing is enhanced. The highest values of palliative care are honored: comfort, dignity, and healing at the end of life.

References

1. Oliver J, Coggins C, Compton P, Hagan S, Matteliano D, Stanton M, St. Marie B, Strobbe S, Turner H. American society for pain management nursing position statement: pain management in patients with substance use disorders. Pain Manage Nurs. 2012;13(3):169–83.
2. Rinaldi R, Steindler E, Wilford B, Goodwin D. Clarification and standardization of substance abuse terminology. JAMA. 1988;259:555.
3. The National Center on Addiction and Substance Abuse at Columbia University. Califano calls for fundamental shift in attitudes and policies about substances abuse and addiction. Press Releases 2007. http//www.casacolumbia.org/templates/PressReleases.aspx?articleid=487&zoneid=65. Accessed 7 May 2007.
4. Bascom PB. A hospital-based comfort care team: consultation for seriously ill and dying patients. Am J Hosp Palliat Care. 1997;14(2):57–60.
5. Ryan A, Carter J, Lucas J, Berger J. You need not make the journey alone: overcoming impediments to providing palliative care in a public urban teaching hospital. Am J Hosp Palliat Care. 2002;19(3):171–80.
6. Passik SD, Portenoy RK, Ricketts PL. Substance abuse issues in cancer patients. Part 2. Oncology. 1998;12(5):729–34; discussion 736, 741–2.
7. Crowther J, Fainsinger R. Incorrect diagnosis and subsequent management of a patient labeled with cholangiocarcinoma. J Palliat Care. 1995;11(4):48–50.
8. Lawlor P, Walker P, Bruera E, Mitchell S. Severe opioid toxity and somatization of psychosocial distress in a cancer patient with a background of chemical dependence. J Pain Symptom Manage. 1997;13(6):356–61.
9. McCorquodale S, De Faye B, Bruera E. Pain control in an alcoholic cancer patient. J Pain Symptom Manage. 1993;8(3):177–80.
10. Kemp C. Managing chronic pain in patients with advanced disease and substance-related disorders. Home Healthc Nurse. 1996;14(4):255–63.
11. National Association of Social Workers. Code of ethics, Washington, DC: National Association of Social Workers; 2008. http://www.socialworkers.org/pubs/code/code.asp. Accessed 20 Apr 2013.
12. Grant B, Stinson F, Dawson D, Chou P, Dufour M, Compton W, Pickering R, Kaplan K. Prevalence and co-occurrence of substance use disorders and independent mood and anxiety disorders. Arch Gen Psychiat. 2004;61:807–16.
13. Khantzian E, Treece C. DSM-III psychiatric diagnosis of narcotic addicts. Arch Gen Psychiat. 1985;42:1067–71.
14. Kirsh K, Passik S. Palliative care of the terminally ill drug addict. Cancer Invest. 2006;24:425–31.
15. Passik S, Olden M, Kirsh K, Portenoy R. Substance abuse issues in palliative care. In: Berger A, Shuster J, Von Roenn J, editors. Principles and practice of palliative care and supportive oncology. 3rd ed. Philadelphia: Lippincott Williams & Wilkins; 2007.
16. National Cancer Institute. PDQ substance abuse issues in cancer. Bethesda: National Cancer Institute; 2011.
17. Savage S. Addiction in the treatment of pain: significance, recognition, and management. J Pain Symptom Manage. 1993;8(5):265–78.
18. Kinzbrunner B, Policzer J. End-of-life care: a practical guide. 2nd ed. New York: McGraw Hill; 2011. p. 174–81.

19. Butler S, Budman S, Fernandez K, Jamison R. Validation of a screener and opioid assessment measure for patients in pain. Pain. 2004;112:65–75.
20. Webster L, Webster R. Predicting aberrant behaviors in opioid-treated patients: preliminary validation of the opioid risk tool. Pain Med. 2005;6(6):432–42.
21. Center for Substance Abuse Treatment. Screening, assessment, and treatment planning for persons with co-occurring disorders. COCE overview paper 2. DHHS Publication No. SMA 06-4164. Rockville: Substance Abuse and Mental Health Services Administration and Center for Mental Health Service; 2006.
22. Lushin V, Anastas J. Harm reduction in substance abuse treatment: pragmatism as an epistemology for social work practice. J Soc Work Pract Addict. 2011;11:96–100.
23. Center for Substance Abuse Treatment. Substance abuse treatment: Addressing the specific needs of women. Treatment improvement protocol series (TIP) No. 51. Rockville, MD: Substance Abuse and Mental Health Services Administration and Center for Mental Health Services; 2009.
24. Center for Substance Abuse Treatment. Substance abuse among older adults. Treatment improvement protocol series (TIP) No. 26. Rockville: Substance Abuse and Mental Health Service Administration and Center for Mental Health Services; 1998.
25. Passik SD, Portnoy RK, Ricketts PL. Substance abuse issues in cancer patients. Part 1: prevalence and diagnosis. Oncology. 1998;12(4):517–21.
26. Lucas J, Gurvich T. Chronic pain protocol. Glendale Adventist Family Practice Residency Program; 2011. Unpublished.
27. Weissman D, Hadddox J. Opioid pseudoaddiction—an iatrogenic syndrome. Pain. 1989;36: 363–6.
28. Podymow T, Trumbull J, Coyle D. Shelter based palliative care for the homeless terminally ill. Palliat Med. 2006;20(2):81–6.
29. Reisfeld GM, Paulien G, Wilson GR. Substance abuse disorders in the palliative care patient. 2nd ed. Fast facts and concepts. April 2009; 127. http://www.eperc.mcw.edu./EPERC/FastFactsIndex/ff_127.htm.
30. Zara C, Baine N. Cancer pain ad psychosocial factors: a critical review of the literature. J Pain Symptom Manage. 2002;24(5):526–42.
31. Keefe FJ, Abernethy AP, Porter LJ, Campbell LC. Nonpharmacologic management of pain. In: Berger A, Shuster J, Von Roenn J, editors. Principles and practice of palliative care and supportive oncology. 3rd ed. Philadelphia: Lippincott Williams & Wilkins; 2007.
32. Kaplan R, Slywka J, Slagle S, Ries K. A titrated morphine analgesic regimen comparing substance users and nonusers with AIDS-related pain. J Pain Symptom Manage. 2000;19(4): 265–73.

Chapter 20
Physical Medicine and Rehabilitation in the Opioid Addicted Patient

Michael N. Brown

Key Points

- The use of exercise and movement therapy and opioid addiction recovery
- Treating the opioid addicted patient in pain
- Behavioral modification approaches during physical rehabilitation
- Multidisciplinary consensus concerning "taking the heat off the clinician"
- Exercise and activity prescription
- Exercise therapy in the back pain patient
- Physical therapy modalities
- Manual and manipulative therapies

Introduction

The utilization of physical medicine services which include physical therapy (PT), occupational therapy (OT) as well as the use of physical medicine and rehabilitation principals can be an important adjunct in providing a multidisciplinary rehabilitation of the opioid addicted patient. Common principals of treatment and recovery of opioid addiction include a three-pronged therapeutic regimen: Physical, mental, and spiritual. Physical medicine, which includes PT and OT services as well as other complementary services, can be used as part of the opioid recovery process by taking advantage of the physiologic and psychological effects of exercise and movement therapies. For the purpose of this discussion the opioid addicted patient will be divided into three categories. The first is the opioid addicted with no pain. The second are those with some pain or intermittent pain and finally those with chronic

M.N. Brown, M.D., D.C. (✉)
12601 116th Ave. NE., #110 Bellevue, WA 98004, USA

10 Harris Court, Building A, Suite #1, Monterey, CA 93940, USA
e-mail: drbr1@aol.com

© Springer Science+Business Media New York 2015
A.D. Kaye et al. (eds.), *Substance Abuse*, DOI 10.1007/978-1-4939-1951-2_20

severe pain. It will be assumed that this population has comorbidities, which may include issues with stress, anxiety, and depression. Services of physical medicine rehabilitation professionals potentially could be employed to assist in the treatment of all three of these patient categories. The treatment of comorbid pain states in the opioid addicted population can be problematic. This article will review a number of basic principles in rehabilitative movement and exercise. We will also review physical medicine, manual medicine, and physical therapy modalities as well as some recent advances in these modalities that could potentially be employed in the treatment of various pain states that can be complicated to manage in this patient population. In the "no pain population," physical medicine services tend to focus on exercise, movement therapy, and mind-body integration methodologies as a means to change behavior and physiology. In the pain states the focus is on specific diagnosis, specific therapy taking into consideration, the patient may be in a hyperalgesic state. In addition, certain behavioral characteristics of this population need to be addressed during the course of care.

The Use of Exercise and Movement Therapy and Opioid Addiction Recovery

Regardless of whether or not the patient participating in an addiction recovery program has comorbidities of pain or not, basic principles of exercise and movement prescription can be helpful to enhance recovery. The use of poly-modal treatment methods and techniques that incorporate methods to deal with stress, anxiety, depression, deteriorating health and the neural biologic changes initiated by opioid use can be addressed by utilizing exercise as an intervention. It is, in fact becoming commonplace to use exercise and movement therapies in opioid recovery programs. The reason for this increasing popularity is that although methadone maintenance treatment may be a "gold standard" of opioid dependence treatment, its use and success is limited [1]. If one is only going to employ the use of opioid replacement as a means of therapy in this population it leads to longer duration of participation in recovery programs and a lesser chance of retention and overall success [2]. A promising adjunct for opioid agonist programs is to address some of these limitations by the utilization of exercise [3]. Adjunctive interventions such as exercise can improve and augment opioid agonist treatment outcomes, including drug abstinence, quality of life, and physical health. Exercise can improve mood, overall quality of life, while reducing other substance use. Poor adherence and dropout of programs frequently prevent individuals from taking advantage of the many physical and mental health benefits of exercise [3].

The benefits of exercise is well-established in terms of both mental health and physical health which includes cardiovascular, health related quality of life and risk of chronic disease [4]. Exercise can simultaneously deal with the common comorbidities of anxiety and depression by lowering anxiety and the risk of depression relapse [5, 6]. Exercise can provide additional benefits to addiction rehabilitation programs such as decreasing the urge to drink alcohol, lessens nicotine withdrawal and cannabis and cigarette craving [7–9]. Exercise provides a more effective means of coping with depression than other substance free activities [10].

Meta-analysis data suggests that exercise should be taught as a means of coping with an individual's stress [11]. Exercise has been known to increase serotonin levels [12]. Exercise programs can improve regulation of stress by improving the body's response to stress and improve mood by providing a feeling of vigor and reduced tension, fatigue, and confusion [3, 13]. Exercise can also introduce socialization in substance abuse programs [14]. Regardless of the immediate successive substitute drugs this process does provide positive reinforcement for utilizing a drug to feel better. Exercise may help to "reset" the stress reactivity for substance abusers, treatment, and the reduce risk of relapse [3]. For these reasons, more exercise should be considered as part of a substance abuse program.

The intensity of exercise requested of participants will need to be carefully considered to avoid risk of injury, overexertion, or development of musculoskeletal complaints. We have addressed this issue in a later section in this chapter but would recommend adherence to the American College of Sports Medicine (ACSM) guidelines as a means of setting the frequency, and intensity of exercise. The guidelines also provide recommendations as to whether or not medical consultation is required before participating in an exercise program. Both the American College of sports medicine and the American Heart Association recommends adults 18–65 years of age to participate in the following: [15]

1. Exercise five times per week at 30 min per session at a moderate intensity (noticeably increased breathing and heart rate) or greater intensity 20 min, 3 days per week.
2. Strength/resistant program 2–3 days per week. One-3 sets of 8–15 repetitions to major muscle groups.
3. Flexibility and stretching 2–3 days per week.

Exercise programs will need to be monitored frequently with reinforcement of importance and benefits of participation.

Treating the Opioid Addicted Patient in Pain

The vast majority of individuals suffering from chronic pain do not go on to develop opioid addiction. However, in the opioid addicted patient, there is a higher prevalence of chronic pain compared to the general population [16, 17]. We know that current or former use of illicit drugs is strongly associated with prescription drug abuse [16, 18]. This adds complexity to the management of chronic pain in these populations. Clinicians have no real guidelines available for management pain in this population. In physical medicine and rehabilitation successful management of chronic pain in patients with opioid addiction requires balancing opioid dependence and addiction with pain relief and restoration of function.

The other obstacle for clinicians to overcome is the ambiguity that most providers face in dealing with the subjective nature of pain and a definitive diagnosis. Berg and her colleagues in 2009 recommended a heuristic (guiding principle contend that identified problems poorly understood domains) method to deal with this problem. She recommended adherence to her decision-making framework to help providers cope with the ambiguous diagnostic and therapeutic decisions across patients in this population [19]. They recommended adopting 1 of 2 decision-making frameworks to determine clinical behavior. The first is prioritizing addiction treatment by emphasizing the destructive consequences of abusing illicit drugs and prescription medications. The other is prioritizing pain management by focusing on the consequences of untreated pain. Identifying the decision-making was shown to shape the providers experience, including their treatment goals, perceptions of the treatment risk, pain management strategies, and tolerance of the ambiguity of dealing with the issues of nonspecific diagnosis and unproven treatment methods [19].

Because of ambiguity many physicians delay in initiating treatment until the completion of diagnostics and more objective evidence becomes available in regard to the source of pain prior to treating or initiating treatment. The truth of the matter is that implementation of physical medicine treatment can be instituted immediately in patients with most pain states without a specific diagnosis initially. For example, utilizing specific therapeutic modalities, movements and exercises for back pain patient within a couple of sessions can be helpful until a definitive diagnosis is made in specific therapeutic intervention implemented. The therapeutic response to some treatment interventions such as the prescription of certain movements can also provide diagnostic criteria to make a definitive diagnosis. One should try to minimize the amount of time that is implemented nonspecific therapies utilized without a specific diagnosis in order to define therapeutic goals and definitive therapeutic intervention. An expert in pain and musculoskeletal diagnosis can be a helpful member of the team, which can prevent wasting valuable resources in the treatment of pain in this population. When choosing physical therapy modalities and patients who are opioid dependent or opioid addicted one also needs to consider that these patients are probably in a "hyperalgesic" state since the long-term use of opioid medications commonly leads to hypersensitivity to painful stimuli [20]. We know that in both animal and clinical studies individuals on long-term opioids correlates with lower pain tolerance [21–23]. Therefore, in making decisions to implement specific physical therapy modalities one needs to be cognizant of the specific diagnosis, consider pathophysiology, and have focused goals and therapeutic directives to a specific treatment direction. The choice of modalities may be influenced because these patients are in a hyperalgesic or hypersensitive pain state. Therefore, we will discuss a number of physical modalities, which may offer better pain management modalities to patients that are hyperalgesic.

Behavioral Modification Approaches During Physical Rehabilitation

Motivational interviewing is not new to those involved in the treatment of opioid addiction [24–27]. Members of the multidisciplinary rehabilitation team participating in physical therapy, occupational therapy, and other allied healthcare practitioners involved in the physical medicine and rehabilitation treatment of pain in the opioid addicted patient should have an understanding of motivational interviewing skills. Motivational interviewing is a method of augmenting the individuals motivation to change problematic behaviors [28]. It is a patient centered counseling style that seeks to help individuals resolve ambivalence about behavioral change. Motivational interviewing has successfully been used in the field of addictions and has recently increased interest as a means of promoting treatment adherence and physical healthcare settings. And more recently adaptations of this approach have been used to improve the wide range of problem behaviors [29–31]. Utilizing combined motivational interviewing with exercise and rehabilitation programs has demonstrated that the patients participating in programs exercise more vigorously and had better long-term outcome than those that did not have combined motivational interviewing as part of their program [32–34]. In the chronic low back pain population combining motivational interviewing with physical therapy approaches has demonstrated enhance motivation and exercise compliance and showed better improvement in physical function and improve disability scores in patients with chronic LBP compared with PT alone [35, 36]. Clinicians providing physical medicine and rehabilitation services may also do well to have brief training in progress of goal attainment program skills. Progress of goal attainment programs (PGAP) was popularized by Sullivan et al. and offer an evidence based and modified motivational interviewing program targeted to reducing disability associated with pain, depression, and chronic health conditions [37–41]. This structured and specific program can be learned quickly by clinicians and modified to the current pain population in current question. Sullivan and his colleagues also provide an approach to identifying catastrophizing behaviors also common with opioid addicted patients and a means of dealing these behaviors, which is commonplace in this patient population [42–44].

Another critical component of providing physical therapy, occupational therapy, and other allied rehabilitation services to this population is curtailing inappropriate communication from the well-intended clinician. An example of this would be a manual therapy practitioner who describes interpretation of physical findings during the course of treatment and make statements such as your vertebra is out of alignment, your back is "out" or "that is the tightest muscle I have ever felt." These statements are commonplace in manual therapy practices and can serve to create misconceptions and false beliefs in this patient population about their physical condition, function, and perceived disability. All members of the rehabilitation team must have a consensus about language and communication before implementing care. It is for this reason that I recommend members of the team to be at least familiar with motivational interviewing skills.

Multidisciplinary Consensus Concerning "Taking the Heat off the Clinician"

Physicians participating in pain management of the opioid addicted patient commonly find themselves negotiating medication dosing schedules, treatment programs, etc. This can often be a daunting task. Having participated in multidisciplinary pain medicine teleconferencing (Tele-pain University of Washington) and making decisions in difficult pain populations I have seen countless occasions the benefits of allowing a multidisciplinary consensus team to make important decisions such as medication dosing schedules, etc. Consensus team conferencing can be done utilizing current modern teleconferencing technology making this process convenient to assemble multiple subspecialty disciplines in a single meeting without them having to leave their offices. By having a consensus this provides a means of "taking the heat off" the clinician who is faced with patients who catastrophize, manipulate, and demonstrate behaviors that are often difficult to deal with in the clinical setting. This also provides a means for the rehabilitative specialist to also participate in providing recommendations for movement, exercise, physical and occupational therapy. The multidisciplinary consensus conferencing process provides strict guidelines for the clinician in this regard, which can often be stress reducing for the caregiver.

Exercise and Activity Prescription

The process of prescribing movement and exercise for the purpose of this chapter will need to be limited to some basic principles and clinical pearls. The specific application of exercise and rehabilitation techniques to the opioid addicted patient in pain patient is a complex topic. However there are a few basic principles that one can follow. The prescription of exercise needs to be proceeded by a healthcare assessment to identify high-risk individuals and to set exertion levels. This provides a means to evaluate baseline values, body weight, body fat which can be used for motivation during the program. A medical clearance may need to be considered for men over 40 and women over 50 or for any individual that may be perceived to be high risk. A brief assessment of risk cardiac risk factors such as HTN, hypercholesterolemia, diabetes, etc. should be considered. A simple risk stratification can be utilized as follows:

- *Apparently healthy*: Asymptomatic, apparently healthy with ≤1 major coronary risk factor
- *Increased risk*: Signs or symptoms suggestive of possible cardiopulmonary or metabolic disease and/or ≥2 major cardiac risk factors
- *Known disease*: No known cardiac, pulmonary or metabolic disease

Typically an exercise program incorporates cardiovascular/aerobic training, resistance training, and flexibility exercises. The exercise prescription should also include the type of exercise, frequency, duration, and intensity. Intensity is based on the goals and objectives of the exercise. Many utilized the percentage of the maximum heart rate (HR_{max}). A common method for setting maximum exercise intensity is the use of maximum heart rate.

$$Max\ HR = 220 - Age.$$

A common practice is to use 70 % of HR_{max} to set the maximum intensity of exercise exertion. This could be modified as response, tolerance, and goals are reevaluated. Utilization of VO_2 max or utilizing METS are other options of setting exercise intensity. Many adopt the ACSM guidelines in providing exercise prescription [45].

Exercise Therapy in the Back Pain Patient

Since it is quite commonplace for low back pain in this population we will address briefly some clinical suggestions for exercise and movement prescription in the back pain patient based on my 30 years of clinical experience. There have been some reported difficulties in determining the specific type of exercise program to prescribe a low back pain patient [46]. A comprehensive discussion of prescribing movement and exercise for various musculoskeletal pain states is clearly not possible within this chapter.

Therefore, I offer the reader some basic approaches that can be incorporated into an algorithm for dealing with the back pain patient in this population. It is not uncommon for clinicians who encounter back pain patients to be told, "I tried physical therapy and their exercises made me worse."

There are many well-intended clinicians in multiple allied professions that prescribe movement and exercise to patients in an attempt to provide rehabilitation services to the back pain patients yet the patient's back pain is aggravated with the prescribed and recommended exercise and movement. This leads to further fear avoidance behavior and perpetuates disability behavior. When this occurs it is usually because they have encountered a well-intended clinician who does not process sufficient skill in the basic foundational principles of prescribing movement to the low back pain patient. It is important to point out that the goal is to be able to prescribe movement and exercise as part of the opioid addiction rehabilitation process and to avoid an individual participating in such a program placing barriers to why they cannot participate in exercise by stating that the exercise "makes them worse." Most clinicians retreat with regard to the recommending movement and exercise once they are told; it makes the patient worse and they cannot participate. This discussion is not about efficacy of a specific therapeutic approach and its ability to "resolve" a back pain problem. This discussion is focus on a specific methods that the clinician can utilize to provide a method to be able to get the back pain patient to participate in exercise without aggravating their back pain condition or pain. My recommendations in using the strategies described below are a means to teach patients that they in fact can participate in exercise and movement. A critical and foundational principal in dealing with the opioid addictive patient is to promote "the internal locus of control." These patients need to be less dependent on external sources of pain relief such as an opioid medication and more self-reliant on movement and self-care that they can provide for themselves. For that reason I would like to introduce the reader to two basic approaches to the back pain patient that will help clinicians in dealing with this patient population with back pain.

The McKenzie Approach

I would like to begin this discussion with a typical case scenario of how and when this unique approach to the back pain patient could be utilized in a specific clinical setting:

Case: A 42-year-old Caucasian male is participating in an opioid rehabilitation program for heroin addiction. He has a previous history of episodic lower back pain. More recently he has developed low back pain with pain radiation into his right buttock and proximal leg. The pain typically remains above the knee but occasionally can radiate into the calf. He has entered a opioid rehabilitation program and now is requesting pain medications for his back and leg complaints. His back complaints are constant and overshadowing the focus of his rehabilitation process. The staff trying to maintain focus on behavioral modification and opioid rehabilitation feels they have little options for management of the pain. The patient reports that PT has made him worse in the past. He states he cannot tolerate any of the pain adjuvant medications that he has tried for this problem in the past. A pain medicine specialist consultation was called but his recommendations provided little real assistance in management. Dr. Thatsbetter is requested to see him. He places him in a prone position and requests that he places hands under his chest, relax his back and buttock and press his chest up off the floor extending his back. The patient protests stating that the movement will worsen his pain. The doctor reassures him and explains the purpose of the movement. The patient reluctantly performs the extension movement and reports movement to be painful. The physician reinforces the importance of the movement and the patient repeats the end range motion in extension. On the fourth repetition the patient states the pain was not as bad as it was with the first repetition. With each repetition he is able to extend his back somewhat further and with less pain. The patient is then requested to stand up and he then begins to walk about the room reporting complete resolution of his leg pain and reduction in his back pain. He is instructed to repeat these movements every 2 h for a period of a day and given specific posture and preventative exercise instruction. Each time the patient repeats these maneuvers he begins to experience further improvement. The patient is encouraged to continue the exercise and the purpose of these exercises is reinforced with further education. No further intervention is then required for his ongoing back pain during the course of his rehabilitation program.

The following case presentation is a consultation I participated in with an inpatient in the hospital admitted for drug rehabilitation. This scenario represents a situation where the patient is experiencing a specific episode of discogenic back pain. McKenzie, a physical therapist from New Zealand provided a means of categorizing back pain syndromes based on the symptomatic response to end range loading [47, 48]. He also provided a means of teaching the patient how to prevent future back pain episodes [49]. Although I have not found the majority of his categorization system all that helpful, the patient presenting with "derangement syndromes" as depicted above is one of the most helpful and simplistic interventions for back pain that I have encountered in my 30-year career. This particular syndrome is commonplace in the back pain population. When this syndrome is recognized specific corrective movement can be prescribed that both provide relief immediately for the patient as well as provides preventative strategies for future difficulties. The movement prescribed and the methods utilized can be mastered by the nonspine specialist clinician evaluating the low back pain patient in an opioid rehabilitation program. The example above where the patient has reduced leg pain and/or reduction of back pain with end range movement represents a phenomenon described as "centralization."

Generally this occurs with lumbar spine extension movement and therefore rather than going into all of the details of the areas of movement testing I recommend the reader to request only spinal extension as the clinical testing tool and prescribe movement as noted below.

The lumbar disc is a common source of low back pain. Disruptions in the annulus can allow movement and entrapment of a portion or fragment of the nucleus pulposus into annular disruptions causing persistent back pain that often fails conservative treatment and typically does not respond to opioid management. A fragment of the nucleus can become entrapped in the laminar rings of the annulus causing the patient to have episodes of incapacitating back pain. The pain worsens with sitting. The patient will experience difficulties making the transitional movement from sitting to standing as the spine moves from a flexed position to a lordotic position. As the patient rises, the posterior aspect of the disc space narrowing was normally with standing. This entraps the nuclear fragment causing increased pain until eventually after a few moments the nucleus begins to migrate into a more central position and the symptoms get better and the patient can then walk.

There is an established process of categorizing the patient into 3 basic categories based on the response in range loading introduced by Robin Mackenzie, PT [47, 49, 50]. After years of using this systematic approach personally I share with the reader only the category that is useful for the purpose of this discussion, the category of the derangement syndrome described below. Therefore, the details of the categorization system, as well as interpretation of these categories are too complex for this discussion. What I want the reader to know is the category "the derangement syndrome." The only critical fact that you must know with these patients is whether they "centralize" or not. Prior to performing the movement testing it is important to begin to rate the patient's pain on a 0–10 pain scale and to determine the location of the pain. To begin the examination, ask the patient to go into a prone position and request that they relax the muscles of the back, buttock, and abdomen. Have the patient place their hands under the chest in the "pushup position" as noted in Fig. 20.1. Have the patient pressed with the hands passively extending their back as shown in Fig. 20.1. The patient is requested to do 10 end range spinal extension repetitions. It is helpful to have them hold the extended position for a few seconds before returning back to neutral. This process often requires the patient to get over the fear of performing an extension movement. The patient will more than likely experience some discomfort in the lower back initially when performing the first few repetitions. If the patient experiences increased pain radiation into the lower extremity when performing this

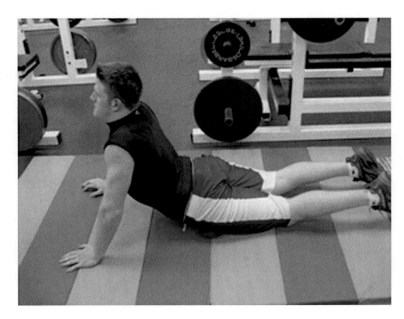

Fig. 20.1 The patient placing their hands under the chest in the "pushup position." The patient presses with the hands passively extending the back. The patient is requested to do 10 end range spinal extension repetitions

movement then it is not therapeutic and the movement should be discontinued. If the patient has no leg pain but does describe increased back pain it is important to reassure the patient and have them continue. Within a few repetitions this movement typically becomes easier for the patient and they begin to lose the fear of the movement. Once the patient has completed 10 repetitions, ask them to stand and move about and rate their subjective complaints again on a 0–10 pain scale. Once the patient has completed the movement and is now standing, determine the symptomatic response to this movement. Determine if the patient has no change in symptoms, increase symptoms, or relief of symptoms. If there has been improvement, identify whether the improvement has been in leg pain, back pain, or both. Patients will often describe that the muscles of the back feeling more relaxed if the movement is therapeutic.

If they have relief of leg pain but no improvement in back pain this is still a centralization phenomenon and the movement is considered therapeutic. If they have relief of low back pain the maneuver is also considered a centralization phenomenon [51–53]. If they have no change in the pain or have worsening pain then my advice to the reader is to discontinue the movement. The interpretation of that response is too complex for the purpose of this chapter. I remind the reader that the patient may experience worsening symptoms in the back upon the initial several repetitions and as long as the pain does not radiate peripherally or into the leg then the testing should continue.

If the patient does in fact experience improvement of symptoms then the patient is asked to repeat these 10 movements several hours through the day. They are requested to remain out of sustained flexion positions or sitting with poor posture without a back support. As the patient improves the frequency of the exercises can be decreased. This process is not only a physical medicine intervention but is psychosocial intervention as well. The patient has gone from a position of fear avoidance and seeking opioid medications and outside sources for pain relief to a position where they now have the "internal locus of control." They are now able to begin to control their own symptoms without using pharmaceutical agents. Frequently in patients who are on opioid medications, I ask the patient what is the degree of symptomatic relief they obtain with opioids. The answer is typically 20–30 %. If the patient has a "derangement syndrome," I then ask the patient what was the degree or percent of relief when performing the movement, they will commonly state 50–70 %. I then take the opportunity for a teaching moment. Not all patients have discogenic back pain. The patient may have more pain arising from the facet joints for example, which will not respond favorably to this movement. There are however a significant number of patients with back pain who does respond to this movement and it is critical for anyone examining the back pain patient to initially know whether they centralize or not before beginning the process of making recommendations for care. The utilization and implementation of this simple strategy can be taught to physician extenders, allied healthcare clinicians, and primary care physicians within several hours and can be utilized in both the inpatient and outpatient opioid rehabilitation programs to provide control of low back pain.

Another example of utilizing the McKenzie approach would be the hospitalized patient. A common scenario would be an opioid dependent patient hospitalized for a procedure or illness and lies in a hospital bed and begins to complain of worsening severe back pain unresponsive to any medications provided. They remain in a hospital bed with the head of the bed elevated. This places the lumbar spine in a flexed position and neither the patient nor the caregivers have any idea that the hospital bed physician is the source of the problem. I have been called in on countless occasions for consultations as a pain physician for inpatients with this exact scenario. Because many of these patients have undergone surgical procedures in the abdomen or have IV lines and other barriers to having the patient do the examination process I simply write an order to have the patient remain out of bed as much as possible. I explain to them if they are in bed they should avoid elevating the head of the bed and placing their lumbar spine in a sustained flexed position. I submit an order to have a sling back wheelchair brought into the patient's room for them to sit and watch TV, eat and do the ADLs. The simple process of prescribing a sling back wheelchair causes the patient to have to sit in an upright lordotic position. I often remove the lounge chairs which place the patient in a flexed position and also worsen the problem. The sling back wheelchair has unique features that place the buttock in a more posterior position during seating and provides a support to the lumbar lordosis. I explain the reasons for this and the following day and definitely the patient's mysterious back pain is usually improved or resolved. Utilizing this simple physical medicine approach rather than a pharmaceutical approach frequently allowed me to provide more relief for a patient that I could ever achieve using pain medications.

In closing, the phenomenon of centralization has both diagnostic and therapeutic value and can determine prognosis and provide a means for the patient to rapidly reverse their own back pain repeatedly when needed [53–56]. Well-trained clinicians with advanced skills using the system can subcategorize patient's using this movement and can actually predict findings on discography [56].

The "Neutral Spine Stabilization" Approach

Another concept and prescribing exercise and movement to the back pain patient is the concept of "neutral spine stabilization" [57, 58]. If the patient complains that they have had their pain worsened when participating in an exercise program you can for the most part count on the fact that they have not been educated and directed through a progressive neutral spine stabilization exercise program. If this patient does not demonstrate a centralization phenomenon as described previously my advice to the reader is to direct these patients into a "neutral spine stabilization program" as another means of exercise. In this program the patient will be taught to hold their spine and pelvis in the most pain-free and balanced position and to hold that position with cocontraction of transverse abdominis muscles, paraspinal muscles, and intrinsic muscles of the spine. Simultaneously while holding this position simple and controlled movements are then introduced. A trained practitioner then monitors the patient to see if they have the ability to maintain the "neutral spine position" during the simple movements. If the patient does not have sufficient muscular control to maintain neutral position the complexity of the movement is reduced and the patient practices this control under the hands of the training clinician until they master the method of maintaining the neutral spine position in each of the prescribed exercises. As the patient demonstrates mastery and control over maintaining a balanced and neutral spine position the movements and exercises are increased in complexity progressively through the program. The neutral spine position is taught to the patient in various positions including sitting, standing, recumbent prone and supine positions as well as later more challenging positions such as the "plank position." Because the patient is progressed through the program based on their ability to maintain a neutral and balanced position there is virtual complete control over the patient's symptomatic management and response to exercise. If they are performing a movement that flares her pain they have been simply progressed to rapidly or have been asked to perform a movement that they were unable to control and the program can be modified appropriately. If a patient proclaimed they have had exacerbation of pain performing exercises all clinician needs to do is inquire as to their knowledge of neutral spine positioning and the details of the specific movements that have been requested for them to do during the course of their exercise program to determine why these patients have had treatment failure with exercise. Inevitably the pain exacerbation with exercise has been caused by the fact that the patient has not yet mastered the techniques and needs more reinforcement and training or the patient has not been taught these basic principles and the therapist or clinician involved does not have adequate training to handle this patient.

The point of this discussion is to provide a means where the opioid addicted patient in pain can participate in exercise programs since movement and exercise should be part of the rehabilitation process. There are still question as to whether or not this specific approach is the most efficacious approach to "resolve" a back pain problem. This often requires a multimodal approach as well. The point of this discussion is not how to resolve the back pain problem but how to get the patient to exercise and remove the barriers that patients in pain place on clinicians and excuses as to why they cannot participate. The neutral spine stabilization exercise program resolves this barrier. The focus of this process is improved function and to improve functional abilities through core strength, stability, and endurance. The focus is not to resolve the pain; however improved pain often accompanies the functional improvements derived in participating. A neutral spine stabilization program is another psychosocial intervention because it teaches the patient how to exercise and improve the overall conditioning and reinforces the internal locus of control. It provides a means for the patient to exercise, which reduces opioid dependence as previously described without exacerbating their premorbid back pain condition. This process should be integrated with behavioral modification, careful communication, and motivational interviewing which are important adjuncts to stabilization program. Having had an opportunity to work in spine rehabilitation for over 30 years and having had an opportunity to see numerous modified stabilization programs that are available in the industry I believe the most appropriate, and simplistic approach that clinicians can learn this type of exercise stabilization training is the approach described by Stewart Magill, PhD [58–60]. I find his systematic approach the best documented, and most practical approach to prescribing stabilization training exercises to back pain patients.

Participating in pool exercise or hydrotherapy programs can also be helpful in prescribing exercises and movements for the chronic pain patient. One still has to be cautious about the movement and exercise prescription in water. For example, a patient with back pain, facet arthrosis, and stenosis may not do well utilizing free-style swimming in a prone position because patients often attempt to hold the head up out of the water with the spine extended. This patient may do much better unweighted with the buoyancy belt upright in the water simulating walking and running movements or lying in a supine position doing backstroke and kicking with the spine maintained in a more flexed position. Other precautions need to be taken such as the use of buoyant exercise devices such as filled water bottles. These may produce undue stress on the rotator cuff and shoulder in certain patients with shoulder pathology. Water and hydrotherapy programs also need to be well thought out and the physical demands requested of the patients participating in a program need to be consistent with known diagnosis and pathology. In addition, I typically always teach the patient neutral spine positioning and neutral spine techniques before entering the water and how to maintain neutral spine positions with exercising in pools.

In summary, we have provided two basic approaches to prescribing exercise in the back pain patient. We discussed the importance of determining initially whether or not the patient demonstrates centralization phenomenon. If the patient's back pain centralizes and demonstrates a directional preference utilizing the "McKenzie approach" may be a simplistic means of prescribing exercise to control the patient's symptoms.

The second approach is to consider a "neutral spine stabilization" approach where patients participating in a rehabilitation program as well as clinicians; overseeing such a program will be much better assured that the patients will maintain compliance because movements are progressed based on the patient's ability to maintain a neutral spine and stable position during all movements. This process should prevent exacerbations of back pain when participating in such programs.

Physical Therapy Modalities

As we have discussed, the use of physical medicine principles and methods can be an adjunct to providing a multidisciplinary rehabilitation approach to the opioid addicted patient. The patient with no pain can utilize the exercise approaches described above. When comorbidity of pain occurs with opioid addiction there is always an interest in searching for nonpharmaceutical alternatives. I offer the reader a few examples of physical therapy modalities as well as a few advances that have been made using physical modalities for treating pain and providing analgesia. Of all of the modalities used in physical medicine today I have chosen to review electrotherapy specifically since these modalities target hyperalgesic states and utilize neurophysiologic principles that address the hyperalgesic state more than other modalities used in physical medicine today.

Before we begin this discussion of physical therapy modalities it is important to remind the reader that the application of physical agents and or modalities is only a small component in the comprehensive rehabilitative approach to a pain complaint. It is critical for an accurate diagnosis as well as a well thought out program of management for the specific diagnosis in order to be cost-effective. All clinicians within the current healthcare delivery system have seen the significant socioeconomic impact of improperly directed medications, inappropriate interventions, and ineffective physical medicine treatment for the wrong diagnosis. The cost of treating pain just in the USA alone has exceeded $560–$635 billion annually [61].

The initial encounter for the purpose of considering physical therapy modalities and agents requires the same careful history, physical, and accurate assessment to determine strategies that will be used in management modalities as it does with any treatment intervention. When choosing physical modalities in patients who are opioid dependent or opioid addicted one may need to consider that the patient is probably "opioid hyperalgesic" wherein the long-term use of opioid medications has led to a hypersensitivity to painful stimuli [2]. We know that in both animal and clinical studies individuals on long-term opioids correlate with lower pain tolerance [21–23]. Therefore, in making decisions to implement specific physical therapy modalities one needs to be cognizant of the specific diagnosis, consider pathophysiology, and have focused goals and therapeutic directives to apply a specific modality. The choice of modalities may be influenced because these patients are in a hyperalgesic or hypersensitive pain state.

Electrotherapies

History of electrotherapy dates back to rudimentary applications involving electric rays for migraine headaches by Egyptians [62]. Modern electrotherapy is closely related to the discovery use of modern physics including patterns of magnetic field studied by Faraday [62]. Galvanic current was quickly utilized as a method to treat pain. This led to many forms of electrotherapy and many questions about the mechanisms by which electric current relieves pain. Melzack and Wall in 1965 provided us the "gait control" theory which provided us early understanding of mechanisms of pain relief generated by periods electrotherapy devices [63].

Today, we understand there may be many mechanisms by which electrotherapy provides symptomatic relief from pain as well as affecting microcirculation, contractile tissues, edema, and enhanced wound healing [62, 64]. This discussion of electrotherapy is not meant to be a comprehensive discussion of physics, biochemistry, and complex physiology involved in electrotherapy but will be limited to a practical discussion of various electrotherapy devices utilized in the treatment of pain and rehabilitation by modern physical medicine practitioners. We will forego discussions of electrotherapy techniques such as low voltage galvanic stimulation and its use with iontophoresis, high voltage galvanic stimulation, and numerous other electrotherapy modalities that have fallen out of favor in the treatment of pain. We will make some attempt to interject clinical evidence in the use of these modalities but I will take an authors privilege and also provide some empirical experience with the use of these modalities that I feel may be helpful.

Types of Electrotherapy Devices

Transcutaneous electrical nerve stimulation (TENS): It is currently one of the most commonly used forms of electroanalgesia. Since this is such a commercially popular modality we will discuss this modality in more detail. There are hundreds of clinical reports describing TENS utilized in many conditions such as low back pain, myofascial pain, sympathetically mediated pain, osteoarthritis, bladder incontinence, neurogenic pain, postsurgical pain, and visceral pain. TENS has been the subject of multiple systematic reviews and meta-analysis discussions with an ongoing debate as to whether TENS is more effective than placebo [65–68]. My empirical experience mimics clinical studies, in that although I have had some successes, my empirical results utilizing this modality have been inconsistent and often disappointing. Despite this there are important electro-therapeutic principals that are helpful for clinicians utilizing this modality to understand. The first is consideration of the basic science in regard to potential mechanism of action of TENS on pain.

1. Gate theory of Melzack and Wall [63]. The classic theory and the one most commonly tested on board exams is the gait control theory of Melzack and Wall where they theorized that the CNS can only interpret and transmit one form of sensory stimulus at a time. Therefore, stimulation of larger diameter and

Fig. 20.2 Gate theory of
Melzack and Wall [63]

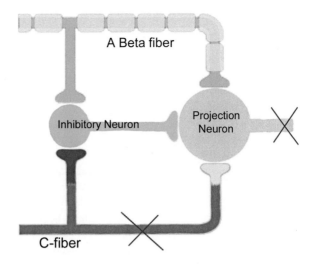

myelinated A-beta fibers carrying touch sensation when stimulated may create
an inhibition of the slower conducting C- and A-delta fibers thereby "closing the
gait to pain perception to the brain" (Fig. 20.2).
2. Opiate-mediated control theory via endogenous endorphins, enkephalins, dynorphins [69].
   Studies have demonstrated increased beta endorphin and met-enkephalin with
   low-frequency TENS which is reversed by naloxone [70]. These are thought to
   be mediated through micro-opioid receptors. High-frequency TENS analgesia is
   not reversed by naloxone, implicating a naloxone-resistant, dynorphine-binding
   receptor.
3. Local vasodilation of blood vessels to ischemic tissues [71].
4. Stimulation of acupuncture points causing a sensory analgesic effect [72].
5. Direct inhibition of an abnormally excited nerve.

Contemporary TENS units typically have symmetric biphasic wave with no
polar affect; therefore there is no positive or negative leads or polarity to the leads.
Because of this it typically does not matter which lead is placed in a specific location as it does with typical DC/galvanic current stimulators. There are several
parameters to choose from one applying TENS.

1. Waveforms: Some units have the choice of waveforms typically square or spiked.
   Typically the square waveform has been noted to be less irritating to the skin
   since it approaches a sine waveform. It is also thought to be more helpful for
   neural pathology, neuropathic pain and is probably better for hypersensitive and
   chronic pain patients [73]. Despite these basic principles of TENS there is no
   clear evidence of a physiologic benefit of any specific waveform.
2. Frequency or rate: Typically higher frequency rates 80–120 cps are considered
   more effective in stimulating large myelinated fibers and therefore probably
   more effective in treatment of acute pain or more rapid pain relief.

Table 20.1 TENS (Transcutaneous electrical nerve stimulation) guide

Pulse width (µs)	Indications
50	Large myelinated fibers responding more effectively (sensory-touch)
100–150	Normal neuromuscular system
200	Small myelinated fibers responding more effectively

Lower frequencies <100 cps typically 1–20 cps more effectively stimulate small unmyelinated fibers. This works by increasing endorphins production, and thus the analgesia typically will follow the stimulation. Therefore this may be more effective in neuropathic pain states. So when high frequency is not noted to produce desired effect one should try changing to a lower frequency.

3. Pulse width or duration: This is the length of time the current is actually acting on the patient in each individual pulse. This is measured typically in microseconds (µS). There may be a number of choices on a TENS unit. A basic guide is noted in Table 20.1 [73, 74].

4. Amplitude or intensity

   TENS units of intensity range from 1 to 100 mA.

   The "ideal intensity" is always to patient tolerance and comfort. Unlike microcurrent TENS is only effective with the patient actually feels stimulus; thus the intensity may need to be increased when the body accommodates to electrical current conduction. One may start with one intensity and because of accommodation the intensity and the sensation may go away. The patient may need to increase intensity so that he once again feels the stimulation.

ESTIM and interferential current therapy: Interferential current and modern electrical muscle stimulation are actually old technologies that have been around for many years but are still available and have some utility (Fig. 20.3). Many years ago we utilized electrical muscle stimulation at relatively low frequencies using a technique called sinusoidal current stimulation. The specific physics behind this technique is not important but conceptually this involved low-frequency current, which provided significant skin resistance. Because of the skin resistance it was necessary to increase the current sufficient to cause a muscle contraction. This also causes some discomfort at the stimulation site. It was later discovered that medium frequency currents around 4,000 Hz rather than 50 Hz broke skin resistance with much greater ease and created a smoother stimulation. With no skin resistance companies began to blend sinusoidal current to stimulate muscle contraction with medium frequency current to break skin resistance and provide a smooth and comfortable method to cause muscle contraction. This provided a combination of electroanalgesia and a means of contracting muscles to either fatigue muscles to relax muscle spasm or to tone muscle based on duration of stimulation intensity, frequency, etc. Another technology that emerged at that time was a technique where we placed four electrodes on the body. Two of the electrodes A1 to A2 and two additional electrodes B1 to B2. They were placed in the configuration noted to the right where there was a difference

Fig. 20.3 Interferential current therapy

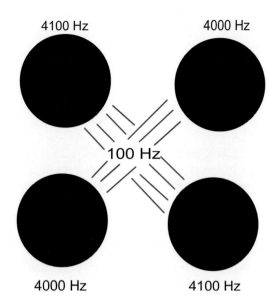

in frequencies between A1/A2 and B1/B2. When two different frequencies were used and the transmission of the current was crossed at the intersection it resulted in a central "beat current" that resonated at the difference between the two frequencies. Because of the crisscross sitting or interference pattern set up, this technique received its neck name "interferential current." An over simplified explanation of this would be two currents interfering with each other as they crisscross currents resulting in a central "beat current" that occurs at the intersection. The theory is if the difference in current is 80–100 Hz the patient will experience more electroanalgesia. If the difference results in lower frequency such as 5–30 Hz then on provides more control over edema, promote circulation, etc. Interferential current machines have become available in smaller and more inexpensive units that can now be prescribed for the patient to perform at home. Electrical muscle stimulation units are also commonplace to be used at home by the patient with some basic training.

H-wave: It eventually became available and also became popular among physical therapist, chiropractors, and physicians. All of these companies manufacturing electrotherapy devices claim to provide proprietary wave links, frequencies, and methods of stimulation that provide unique therapeutic benefit. H-wave therapy uses a "blend" of current frequencies and stimulation that provides a combination of smooth muscle stimulation, a method to promote circulation, and electroanalgesia. This technology is simple to use and is also a unit that is commercially available as a prescription for patient to take home and use as a means of stimulating electroanalgesia as well as other therapeutic benefits. There are some small studies suggesting H-wave provides a means of treating neuropathic pain, improving function and reducing need for pain medication [75–77].

Camamare: As a pain physician and someone who is constantly searching for nonpharmaceutical alternatives for pain management this technology may hold great promise in the treatment of neuropathic pain specifically. I have had an opportunity to utilize this modality in treatment of various neuropathic pain states in the cancer pain population. My empirical experience continues to stimulate my interest in this modality. Although this has been utilized in Italy for some time it has been just over the last few years that this has gained interest in the USA by pain physicians. They also report proprietary electrotherapy stimulation as a means in which this produces its effect. The unique nature of this method of treatment stems from placing surface electrodes outside a region of allodynia, CRPS, or neuropathic pain. Electrodes placed away from the region of neuropathic pain generate what the company states is a "no pain signal" on the surface of the skin and described the clinical fact as a pain "scrambler therapy" [78]. The stimulation is able to interfere with pain signal transmission by mixing a "no pain" signal into a transmission channel for the purpose of masking the existing pain information [78, 79]. It has been my empirical experience that patients with allodynia and neuropathic pain can experience improved allodynia and neuropathic pain during the initial treatment session. The most important component of this treatment is its ability to maintain sustained relief for longer and longer periods of time with repeated treatment exposure. In a pilot study Marneo et al. described scrambler therapy provided relief of chronic neuropathic pain better than guidelines based drug management [80]. It has also been used in the treatment of neuropathic pain states secondary to chemotherapy-induced peripheral neuropathy in cancer pain patients. The report sustained relief in both acute and chronic pain states as well as improvement in quality of life indicators in these patients [81]. Most importantly observations of cessation of pain medications in as much as 72 % of patients treated and 28 % of patients with reduced pain medication dosing after treatment have also been reported [82].

The technology describes generating via surface electrodes artificial neuron "packets" or strings of information that is recognized as a "non-pain signal" as previously described. This is developed through a series of algorithms within the instrument, which creates an adaptation of the perception, which can be decoded as a dominant stimulus by a means of over modulation of the endogenous bio potentials. The latter condition gives rise to a favorable adaptation of algogenic sensitivity. The hypothesized learning mechanism of the pain sensory system now becomes "remodeled" to the non-pain scrambler information resulting in a gradual rise in the subjective pain threshold [83]. One of the disadvantages to the specific electrotherapy technology happens to be the high cost of the equipment and the lack of recognition and reimbursement by healthcare insurance companies. Therefore the patient has to have the economic resources typically the pain out of pocket for this modality of treatment. Despite this, I believe, as further research emerges describing the efficacy of this method of treatment, this modality offers significant potential for the treatment of neuropathic pain states.

Micro-electrical neural stimulation (MENS): Microcurrent also represents a rather unique electrotherapy modality that can have some value as a nonpharmaceutical method for pain management. Unlike traditional TENS which only works by stimulation of A-beta fibers in the skin works to inhibit pain by the gait control mechanism. MENS therapy is quite different. TENS uses milliamperes current whereas

MENS uses micro-amperage current. Once again MENS also delivers unique electrotherapy current, wavelength, frequency, etc. A typical microcurrent pulse is about 0.5 s, which is 2,500 times longer than a typical pulse width of a TENS unit. MENS uses micro-amperage, which is 1,000 times less than TENS. MENS also utilizes direct-current rather than alternating current and typically is administered through two electrodes or probes where current passes between them. My initial introduction to this modality was in 1982 where the dogma at that time was that microcurrent therapy increased ATP production by 500 % in cells [84].

MENS was also thought to duplicate what was thought to be a natural endogenous current flow used by the body to repair tissues and promote healing. MENS has been used effectively to treat pain [85–87]. It has been used with modest effects and non-specific back pain in a randomized clinical control trial [88]. MENS has also been shown to enhance wound healing [64, 89]. MENS stimulation ranging from 200 to 800 µA has shown 200–350 % faster healing rates, with stronger tensile strength of scar tissue and antibacterial effects [90]. Some clinicians experienced with this modality are reporting clinical results with frequency specific MENS in treating fibromyalgia and neuropathic pain states [91, 92]. MENS machines have become commercially available as small portable units that can be used at home and certainly are units that could also be used in the inpatient opioid rehabilitation setting.

ELECTROSLEEP—Cranial-Electro Stimulation (CES): It is yet another unique electrotherapy application that may have utility in dealing in an opioid rehabilitation program. CES was initially studied for insomnia and called electrosleep therapy; it is also known as Cranial-Electro Stimulation and Transcranial Electrotherapy [93, 94]. It has been proposed that CES focuses on the hypothalamic region and may result in elevating the brains levels of serotonin, norepinephrine, and dopamine and decrease its level of cortisol [95, 96]. It also has been reported to increase alpha and decrease delta brain waves on EEG. CES basically utilizes MENS electrodes that are placed on the cranium during sleep typically clipped to the ear or placed on the mastoid region. Since the complaints of insomnia, anxiety, and depression are commonplace in opioid addicted patients especially when participating in both inpatient or outpatient rehabilitation programs, CES may offer a unique nonpharmacological approach to assisting with sleep and anxiety [97–99]. CES has also been used for the treatment of chronic pain [100, 101]. CES is still an FDA Class III device and more studies are needed to prove efficacy of this treatment and quality studies are needed to be able to evaluate this modality utilizing meta-analysis techniques [102].

Manual and Manipulative Therapies

Manual medicine techniques, which include manipulation, mobilization, and numerous soft tissue mobilization and massage techniques represent a basic foundational treatment modality in physical medicine. Like many other healthcare disciplines there is a highly varied level of expertise and clinical outcomes in disciplines utilizing manual medicine principles. Despite this, manipulation and soft tissue mobilization techniques do represent nonpharmaceutical methods of treatment of both chronic and acute pain states and could potentially be utilized as a replacement alternative to opioid pain in the opioid addicted population. A review of the literature on this topic would require an entire chapter devoted for this purpose. Speaking as a clinician dual licensed in both medicine and chiropractic I have a unique perspective on this subject. There are as many manipulative therapy techniques as there are clinicians practicing. Because of the varied methods and levels of skill of individual practitioners it makes the study of the efficacy of manual therapy difficult at best. Rather than an exhaustive review of the literature I am going to take an authors prerogative to discuss empirical experience and practical application that I think will be helpful for the reader.

In the non-pain opioid addicted patient manual therapy plays no significant low in opioid rehabilitation. However, in the opioid addicted patient with pain manual therapy can be of some assistance in certain circumstances. There are many musculoskeletal peripheral joint and spine complaints that are quite amenable to manual therapy. Manual therapy techniques including the prescription of therapeutic movements as I have already addressed in the exercise portion of this chapter can be a way of integrating multidisciplinary care to some musculoskeletal and pain states in the opioid addicted patient in pain. Manual therapy and manipulative therapy techniques are commonly used by chiropractors, osteopathic physicians, and certain physical therapist with advanced training. A practitioner of manual therapy armed with appropriate communication skills, behavior modification understanding, motivational interviewing skills can play an important role in specific circumstances on the multidisciplinary team that can assist in reinforcing nonpharmaceutical methods of pain management. When the rehabilitation team is dealing with a difficult opioid addicted patient in pain, manual therapy could be one of the approach which is considered as a nonpharmaceutical approach to helping a patient get through a difficult time. The manual therapy approach probably provides better short-term resolution to problems and long-term changes at this still can be used as an important adjunct in the treatment process.

In summary, the implementation of physical medicine and rehabilitation methods of treatment and principles is an important adjunct to the multimodal/multidisciplinary management of the opioid addicted patient. It offers countless nonpharmaceutical approaches to improve outcomes in patients who were not in pain by using exercise or as a means to assist in the multidisciplinary treatment of pain in this patient population. Many barriers have to be over, in the rehabilitation process, which will include in the future access to rehabilitation professionals in the era of utilization restriction in healthcare.

References

1. Fischer B, Rehm JGK, Kirst M. Eyes wide shut? A conceptual and empirical critique of methadone maintenance treatment. Eur Addict Res. 2005;11:1–14.
2. Hunt G, R M. "Hustling" within the clinic: consumer perspectives on methadone maintenance treatment. 6th ed. London: Sage; 1998.

3. Weinstock J, Wadeon H, VanHees J. Exercise as an adjunct treatment for opioid agonist treatment: review of current research and implementation strategies. Subst Abus. 2012;33:350–60.
4. Penedo F, Dahn J. Exercise and well-being: a review of mental and physical health benefits associated with physical activity. Curr Opin Psychiatry. 2005;18:189–93.
5. DiLorenzo T, Bargman E, Stuckey-Ropp R, et al. Long-term effects of aerobic exercise on psychological outcomes. Prev Med. 1999;28:75–85.
6. Rethorst C, Wipfli B, Landers D. The antidepressant effects of exercise: a meta-analysis of randomized trials. Sports Med. 2009;39:491–511.
7. Ussher M, Sampuran A, Doshi R, et al. Acute effect of a brief bout of exercise on alcohol urges. Addiction. 2004;99:1542–7.
8. Bock B, Marcus B, King T, et al. Exercise effects on withdrawal and mood among women attempting smoking cessation. Addict Behav. 1999;24:399–410.
9. Buchowski M, Meade N, Charbonequ E, et al. Aerobic exercise training reduces cannabis cravings and use in nontreatment seeking cannabis dependent adults. PLoS One. 2011;6:e 17465.
10. Salmon P. Effects of physical exercise on anxiety, depression, and sensitivity distress: a unifying theory. Clin Psychol Rev. 2001;21:33–61.
11. Forcier K, Stroud L, Papaadonatos G, et al. Links between physical fitness and cardiovascular reactivity and recovery to psychosocial stressors: a meta-analysis. Health Psychol. 2006;25:733–9.
12. Wipfli B, Landers D, Nagoshi C, Ringenbach S. An examination of serotonin and psychological variables in the relationship between exercise and mental health. Scand J Med Sci Sports. 2011;21(3):474–81.
13. Puetz T, O'Connor P, Dishman R. Effects of chronic exercise on feelings of energy and fatigue: a quantitative synthesis. Psychol Bull. 2006;132:866–79.
14. Palmer J, Palmer L, Michiels K, Thigpen B. Effects of type of exercise on depression in recovering substance abusers. Percept Motor Skills. 1995;80:523–30.
15. Nelson M, Rejeski W, Blair S, et al. Physical activity and public health in older adults: recommendation from the American College of Sports Medicine and the American Heart Association. Med Sci Sports Exerc. 2007;39(8):1435–45.
16. Ilves T, Chelminski P, Hammett-Stabler C, et al. Predictors of opioid misuse in patients with chronic pain: a prospective cohort study. BMC Health Serv Res. 2006;6(6):46.
17. Jamison R, Kauffman J, Katz N. Characteristics of methadone maintenance patients with chronic pain. J Pain Symptom Manage. 2000;19(1):53–62.
18. Michna E, Ross E, Hynes W, et al. Predicting aberrant drug behavior in patients treated for chronic pain: importance of abuse history. J Pain Symptom Manage. 2004;28(3):250–8.
19. Berg K, Amsten J, Sacaijiu G, Karasz L. Providers' experiences treating chronic pain among opioid-dependent drug users. J Gen Intern Med. 2009;24(4):482–8.
20. Compton P, Athanasos P, Elashoff D. Withdrawal hyperalgesia after acute opioid physical dependence in nonaddicted humans: a preliminary study. J Pain. 2003;4:511–9.
21. Compton P, Charuvastra V, Kintaudi K, Ling W. Pain responses in methadone-maintained opioid abusers. J Pain Symptom Manage. 2000;20:237–45.
22. Compton P, Charuvastra V, Ling W. Pain intolerance in opioid-maintained former opiate addicts: effect of long-acting maintenance agent. Drug Alcohol Depend. 2001;63:139–46.
23. Pud D, Cohen D, Lawental E, Eisenberg E. Opioids and abnormal pain perception: new evidence from a study of chronic opioid addicts and healthy subjects. Drug Alcohol Depend. 2006;82:218–3.
24. Cole B, Clark DC, Seale JP, et al. Reinventing the reel: an innovative approach to resident skill-building in motivational interviewing for brief intervention. Subst Abus. 2012;33(3):278–81.
25. Cowell AJ, Brown JM, Mills MJ, Bender RH, Wedehase BJ. Costeffectiveness analysis of motivational interviewing with feedback to reduce drinking among a sample of college students. J Stud Alcohol Drugs. 2012;73:226–37.
26. Lundgren L, Chassler D, Amodeo M, D'Ippolito M, Sullivan L. Barriers to implementation of evidence-based addiction treatment: a national study. J Subst Abuse Treat. 2012;43:231–8.

27. Pomm HA. Nonpharmacologic strategies for treating the addicted patient in an office-based setting: motivational interviewing. Northeast Fl Med. 2012;36(1):32–6.
28. Miller W, Rollnick S. Motivational interviewing: preparing people for change. 2nd ed. New York: Guilford Press; 2002.
29. Dunn C, DeRoo L, Rivara P. The use of brief interventions adapted from motivational interviewing across behavioral domains: a systematic review. Addiction. 2001;96:1725–42.
30. Burke B, Arkowitz H, Dunn C. The effectiveness of motivational interviewing and its adaptations: what we know so far. In: Miller WR, Rollnick S, editors. Motivational interviewing: preparing people to change addictive behavior. 2nd ed. New York: Guilford Press; 2002. p. 217–50.
31. DeRoo L, Rivara F. Use of brief interventions adapted from motivational interviewing across behavioral domains: a systematic review. Addiction. 2001;96:1725–42.
32. Scales R. Motivational interviewing and skills-based counseling in cardiac rehabilitation: the Cardiovascular Health Initiative and Lifestyle Intervention (CHILE) Study [dissertation]. University of New Mexico. Dissertation Abstracts International 59-03A, 0741; 1998.
33. Scales R, Atterbom HA, Lueker R. Impact of motivational interviewing and skills-based counseling on physical activity and exercise. Med Sci Sports Exerc. 1998;30:92.
34. Scales R, Atterbom H, Lueker R, Gibson AE. Enhancing physical activity in cardiac rehabilitation with stage-matched counseling. Med Sci Sports Exerc. 1999;31:38.
35. Vong S, Cheing G, Chan F, So E, Chan C. Motivational enhancement therapy in addition to physical therapy improves motivational factors and treatment outcomes in people with low back pain: a randomized controlled trial. Arch Phys Med Rehabil. 2011;92(2):176–83.
36. Friedrich M, Gittler G, Arendasy M, Friedrich K. Long-term effect of a combined exercise and motivational program on the level of disability of patients with chronic low back pain. Spine (Phila Pa 1976). 2005;30(9):995–1000.
37. Sullivan MJL, Adams H, Ellis T. A psychosocial risk-targeted intervention to reduce work disability: development, evolution and implementation challenges. Psychol Injury Law. 2013;6:250–7.
38. Sullivan M, Adams H, Rhodenizer T, Stanish W. A psychological risk factor targeted intervention for the prevention of chronic pain and disability following whiplash injury. Phys Ther. 2006;86:8–18.
39. Sullivan M, Adams H. Psychological treatment techniques to augment the impact of physiotherapy interventions for low back pain. Physiother Can. 2010;62:180–9.
40. Sullivan M, Feuerstein M, Gatchel R, Linton S, Pransky G. Integrating psychological and behavioral interventions to achieve optimal rehabilitation outcomes. J Occup Rehabil. 2005;15:485–9.
41. Sullivan M, Stanish W. Psychologically based occupational rehabilitation: the pain-disability prevention program. Clin J Pain. 2003;19(2):97–104.
42. Slepian P, Bernier E, Scott W, Niederstrasser N, Wideman T, Sullivan M. Changes in pain catastrophizing following physical therapy for musculoskeletal injury: the influence of depressive and post-traumatic stress symptoms. J Occup Rehabil. 2013;24:22–31.
43. Sullivan M, Bishop S, Pivik J. The pain catastrophizing scale: development and validation. Psychol Assess. 1995;7:524–32.
44. Sullivan MJL. The Communal Coping Model of pain catastrophizing: clinical and research implications. Can Psychol. 2013;53:32–41.
45. Garber C, Blisser B, Deschenes M, et al. Quantity and quality of exercise for developing and maintaining cardiorespiratory, musculoskeletal, and neuromotor fitness in apparently healthy adults: guidance for prescribing exercise. Med Sci Sports Exerc. 2011;43(7):1334–59.
46. Faas A. Exercises: which ones are worth trying, for which patients, and when? Spine (Phila Pa 1976). 1996;21(24):2874–8; discussion 2878-9.
47. McKenzie R. Understanding centralisation. J Orthop Sports Phys Ther. 1999;29(8):487–9.
48. McKenzie NS. Low back pain. N Z Med J. 1986;99(805):515.
49. McKenzie RA. Prophylaxis in recurrent low back pain. N Z Med J. 1979;89(627):22–3.
50. McKenzie R. Low back pain. N Z Med J. 1987;100(827):428–9.

51. Bybee RF, Olsen DL, Cantu-Boncser G, Allen HC, Byars A. Centralization of symptoms and lumbar range of motion in patients with low back pain. Physiother Theory Pract. 2009;25(4):257–67.
52. Delaney PM, Hubka MJ. The diagnostic utility of McKenzie clinical assessment for lower back pain. J Manipulative Physiol Ther. 1999;22(9):628–30.
53. Donelson R. Is your client's back pain "rapidly reversible"? Improving low back care at its foundation. Prof Case Manag. 2008;13(2):87–96.
54. Donelson R. The McKenzie approach to evaluating and treating low back pain. Orthop Rev. 1990;19(8):681–6.
55. Donelson R, Aprill C, Medcalf R, Grant W. A prospective study of centralization of lumbar and referred pain. A predictor of symptomatic discs and annular competence. Spine (Phila Pa 1976). 1997;22(10):1115–22.
56. Donelson R, Silva G, Murphy K. Centralization phenomenon. Its usefulness in evaluating and treating referred pain. Spine (Phila Pa 1976). 1990;15(3):211–3.
57. Saal JA, Saal JS. Nonoperative treatment of herniated lumbar intervertebral disc with radiculopathy: an outcome study. J Biomech. 1989;14:431–7.
58. McGill SM. Low back disorders. Evidence-based prevention and rehabilitation. Champaign: Human Kinetics; 2007.
59. McGill SM. The biomechanics of low back injury: implications on current practice in industry and the clinic. J Biomech. 1997;30:465–75.
60. McGill SM, Cholewicki J. Biomechanical basis for stability: an explanation to enhance clinical stability. J Orthop Sports Phys Ther. 2001;31(2):96–100.
61. Ponte DJ, Jensen GJ, Kent BE. A preliminary report on the use of the McKenzie protocol versus Williams protocol in the treatment of low back pain. J Orthop Sports Phys Ther. 1984;6(2):130–9.
62. Delisa J, Gans B, editors. Physical medicine and rehabilitation: principle & practice. 4th ed. Philadelphia: Lippincott Williams & Wilkins; 2005. p. 435–6. Chapter 18: Electrotherapy in rehabilitation.
63. Melzack R, Wall P. Pain mechanisms: a new theory. Science. 1965;150(699):971–9.
64. Gardner S, Frantz RA, Schmidt F. Effect of electrical stimulation on chronic wound healing: a meta-analysis. Wound Repair Regen. 1999;7(6):495–503.
65. Nnoaham K, Kumbang J. Transcutaneous electrical nerve stimulation (TENS) for chronic pain. Cochrane Database Syst Rev. 2008;3:CD003222.
66. Fernandez-Del-Olmo M, Alvarez-Sauco M, Koch G, et al. How repeatable are the physiological effects of TENS? Clin Neurophysiol. 2008;119(8):1834–9.
67. Peters K, Carrico D, Burks F. Validation of a sham for percutaneous tibial nerve stimulation (PTNS). Neurourol Urodyn. 2008;28:58–61.
68. Robb K, Bennett M, Johnson M, et al. Transcutaneous electric nerve stimulation (TENS) for cancer pain in adults. Cochrane Database Syst Rev. 2008;3:CD006276.
69. Basbaum A, Fields H. Endogenous pain control mechanisms: review and hypothesis. Ann Neurol. 1978;4(5):451–62.
70. Clement-Jones V, McLoughlin L, Tomlin S, et al. Increased beta-endorphin but not met-enkephalin levels in human cerebrospinal fluid after acupuncture for recurrent pain. Lancet. 1980;2(8201):946–9.
71. Leandri M, Brunetti O, Parodi C. Telethermographic findings after transcutaneous electrical nerve stimulation. Phys Ther. 1986;66(2):210–3.
72. Melzack R, Wall P. The challenge of pain. 2nd ed. London: Penguin; 1988.
73. Kahn J. Principles and practice of electrotherapy. 2nd ed. New York: Churchill Livingstone; 1987.
74. Hecox B, Mehreteab T, Weisberg J. Physical agents: a comprehensive test for physical therapists. Appleton & Lange: Norwalk; 1994.
75. B K, C TJ, Martinez-Pons M. The H-Wave small muscle fiber stimulator, a nonpharmacologic alternative for the treatment of chronic soft-tissue injury and neuropathic pain: an extended population observational study. Adv Ther. 2006;23(5):739–49.
76. Blum K, Chen A, Chen T, et al. The H-Wave device is an effective and safe non-pharmacological analgesic for chronic pain: a meta-analysis. Adv Ther. 2008;25(7):644–57.

77. Blum K, Ho C, Chen A, et al. The H-wave device induces no dependent augmented microcirculation and angiogenesis, providing both analgesia and tissue healing in sports injuries. Phys Sportsmed. 2008;6(1):103–14.
78. Serafini G, Marineo G, Sabato A. "Scrambler Therapy": a new option in neuropathic pain treatment? Pain Clin. 2000;12:271–340.
79. Marineo G, Spaziani S, Sabato A, Marotta F. Artificial neurons in oncological pain: the potential of Scrambler Therapy to modify a biological information. Int Congr Ser. 2003;1255:381–8.
80. Marineo G, Iorno V, Gandini C, Moschini V, Smith T. Scrambler therapy may relieve chronic neuropathic pain more effectively than guideline-based drug management: results of a pilot, randomized, controlled trial. J Pain Symptom Manage. 2012;43(1):877–95.
81. Wan W, Dodson P, Swainey C, Smith T. A trial of scrambler therapy in the treatment of cancer pain syndromes and chronic chemotherapy-induced peripheral neuropathy. J Pain Palliat Care Pharmacother. 2013;27(4):359–64.
82. Marineoa G, Spazianib S. A.F. Sabatoc A, Marottaa F. Artificial neurons in oncological pain: the potential of Scrambler Therapy to modify a biological information. Int Congr Ser. 2003;1255:381–8.
83. Pachman D, Linquist B, Barton D, et al. Pilot study of scrambler therapy for the treatment of chemotherapy-induced peripheral neuropathy. J Clin Oncol. 2012;30:1–2.
84. Cheng N, Van Hoff H, Bockx E, et al. The effect of electric currents on ATP generation protein synthesis, and membrane transport in rat skin. Clin Orthop. 1982;171:264–72.
85. Bauer W. Electrical treatment of severe head and neck cancer pain. Arch Otolaryngol. 1983;109:382–3.
86. Kirsch D, Lerner F. Innovations in pain management: a practical guide for clinicians. In: Weiner R, editor. Electro medicine, vol. 23. Hamburg: Deutsche Press; 1990. p. 1–29.
87. Kulkarni A, Smith R. The use of microcurrent electrical therapy and cranial electrotherapy stimulation in pain control. Clin Pract Alternat Med. 2001;2(2):99–102.
88. Koopman JSVD, van Wijck AJ. Efficacy of microcurrent therapy in the treatment of chronic nonspecific back pain: a pilot study. Clin J Pain. 2009;25(6):495–9.
89. Frick A. Microcurrent electrical therapy heals a recalcitrant wound in a horse. J Equine Vet Sci. 2005;25(11):418–22.
90. Wolcott L, Wheeler P, Hardwicke H, Rowley B. Accelerated healing of skin ulcer by electrotherapy: preliminary clinical results. South Med J. 1969;62(7):795–801.
91. McMakin C, Gregory W, Phillips T. Cytokine changes with microcurrent treatment of fibromyalgia associate with cervical spine trauma. J Bodyw Mov Ther. 2009;9:169–76.
92. McMakin C. Nonpharmacologic treatment of neuropathic pain using frequency specific microcurrent. Pain Practitioner. 2010;20:68–73.
93. Appel CP. Effect of electrosleep: review of research. Goteborg Psychol Rep. 1972;2:1–24.
94. Iwanovsky A, Dodge CH. Electrosleep and electroanesthesia—theory and clinical experience. Foreign Sci Bull. 1968;4(2):1–64.
95. Gilula MF, Kirsch DL. Cranial electrotherapy stimulation review: a safer alternative to psychopharmaceuticals in the treatment of depression. J Neurother. 2005;9(2):7–27.
96. Kennerly R. QEEG analysis of cranial electrotherapy: a pilot study. J Neurother. 2004;8(2):112–3.
97. Klawansky S. Meta-analysis of randomized controlled trials of cranial electrostimulation: efficacy in treating selected psychological and physiological conditions. J Nerv Ment Dis. 1995;183(7):478–84.
98. Winick R. Cranial electrotherapy stimulation (CES): a safe and effective low cost means of anxiety control in a dental practice. Gen Dent. 1999;47(1):50–5.
99. Weiss M. The treatment of insomnia through use of electrosleep: an EEG study. J Nerv Ment Dis. 1973;157(2):108–20.
100. Kirsch D, Smith RB. The use of cranial electrotherapy stimulation in the management of chronic pain: A review. NeuroRehabilitation. 2000;14:85–94.
101. Cevei M, Jivet I. Experiments in electrotherapy for pain relief using a novel modality concept. IFMBE Proc. 2011;36(Part 2):164–7.
102. Barrett S. Dubious claims made for NutriPax and cranial electrotherapy stimulation. QuackWatch (January 28, 2008).

Chapter 21
Appropriate Dispensing of Prescription Medications and Recognition of Substance Abuse: The Pharmacist's Perspective

Adam Marc Kaye and Alan David Kaye

Key Points

- The Role of the Pharmacist
- Risk Evaluation & Mitigation Strategies (REMS)

Introduction

The term "abuse" is often defined in pharmacy circles as either using a medication wrongly or improperly. Medications with abuse potential can be prescribed with the best of intentions, only to be used improperly at the whim of a reckless patient.

We must be aware that some in our profession lack the knowledge of medical standards, current research, ethics, and clinical practice guidelines. The lack of knowledge about risks of addiction, expected levels of dependency, and history of misuse or abuse prevents accurate evaluation of appropriate treatment with controlled substances. Red flags should alert Physicians and Pharmacists to exercise extreme vigilance and to utilize additional diligence before prescribing or dispensing these powerful medications.

A.M. Kaye, PharmD, F.A.S.C.P., F.C.Ph.A. (✉)
Department of Pharmacy Practice, Thomas J. Long School of Pharmacy and Health Sciences, University of the Pacific, Stockton, CA, USA
e-mail: akaye@pacific.edu

A.D. Kaye, M.D., Ph.D., D.A.B.A., D.A.B.P.M., D.A.B.I.P.P.
Departments of Anesthesiology and Pharmacology, Louisiana State University Health Sciences Center, Louisiana State University Interim Hospital, and Ochsner Kenner Hospital, New Orleans, LA, USA
e-mail: alankaye44@hotmail.com

© Springer Science+Business Media New York 2015
A.D. Kaye et al. (eds.), *Substance Abuse*, DOI 10.1007/978-1-4939-1951-2_21

From the perspective of a Pharmacist, any recognition that a patient is not following prescribed directions dictates the required immediate action toward increased monitoring of the patient. The "corresponding responsibility doctrine" requires the Pharmacist to properly assess and to recognize before dispensing, i.e., that a controlled substance is being prescribed for a legitimate medical purpose. The difficulties in making this determination are compounded by possible dishonesty by patients or Physicians knowingly issuing a prescription for illegitimate purposes.

Challenging situations involve the deliberate misrepresentation of pain by patients, which can progress to Physicians unable to or unwilling to properly assess the falsity of their needs for analgesia or their claims of severe or chronic pain. Misuse and other reckless behaviors often include doctor shopping, illicit purchasing from drug dealers, and theft. These inappropriate and illegal behaviors are too often the final passageway to the abyss known as substance abuse.

The Role of the Pharmacist

As Pharmacists, we are considered the last line of defense, ensuring that patients are not prescribed an unsafe medication regimen. As the health systems' last point of contact with the ultimate user of potentially dangerous pharmaceuticals, it is our responsibility to intervene on behalf of the patient if any medication error or excessive drug dosing is detected. These interventions by Pharmacists provide a much needed safety check for patients. Many have been issued a prescription by a Physician in which the prescriber is unaware of the totality of the patient's historical medication regimen.

With the knowledge that patients with and without documented mental health issues often utilize controlled substances for nonmedical uses, the Pharmacist must remain a constant vigilance against dishonest prescribing and utilization of controlled substances. The Drug Enforcement Agency (DEA) along with other federal and state regulators are constantly adjusting rules and regulations in an effort to create guidelines that will allow legitimate pain patients to continue to have access to these pharmaceuticals. As gatekeepers, we are constantly working to develop a way to insure that these medications are issued by prescribers in the usual course of medical treatment, while having safeguards in place to prevent the prescribing and dispensing of these substances. Recognition is clearly the first step to entertain if we are going to discover a way to prevent the illicit use of pharmaceuticals in those attempting to cleverly deceive our healthcare system while hiding their drug-seeking behavior. Almost every state currently has a pharmacy database known as Prescription Drug Monitoring Programs (PDMP), which allow for identification of patients who are also being prescribed substances of abuse by other Physicians within the same state. However, this would not preclude a patient from obtaining a prescription from more than one Physician in another state and until a national database is created, our current system is not optimal in its capacity to recognize all patients who are inappropriately being dispensed these potent agents.

It is important to keep in mind that medications are often prescribed for legitimate indications only to be misused by patients in an attempt of producing well-intentioned larger therapeutic responses. Patients may not be aware or even concerned about the possible dangerous outcomes, which can occur due to this misuse or abuse. Medications being used for sleep, pain relief, or stimulants being used for attention deficit hyperactivity disorder (ADHD) can all have life-threatening consequences when consumed at higher than the recommended levels. To this end, over the counter agents, such as antihistamines can enhance sedation and analgesia but provide additive or synergistic effects resulting in respiratory depression and sedation with resultant morbidity or mortality. Intentionally abusing prescription medications can lead to side effects and risky outcomes including death related to the common patient belief that these agents are able to produce a "safe high" because they are acquired from a Pharmacist instead of on the streets.

While an abundance of theories exist as to how unlawful prescriptions might get filled or over- utilized, safeguards will always be lacking unless strict monitoring of suspicious "orders" and risky "patients" becomes a priority, making the Pharmacist a critical and important player in this process. Increased vigilance along with due diligence is necessary to confirm compliance and cooperation by both Physicians and Pharmacists in detecting and reporting of questionable activities in an effort to prevent patient substance abuse, misuse, and diversion.

It is important for Physicians and Pharmacists to be reminded that many therapeutic agents can produce "euphoric feelings" by taking certain medications and by consuming higher doses or combinations. The ability to "get high" is often a goal of patients with mental health issues. Oversight is needed by all in the healthcare system to prevent patients with risk factors for abuse from acquiring these products. Clearly, the benefits do not outweigh the risks for many due to the risk of consuming higher than prescribed doses of these powerful substances with catastrophic results.

We must keep in mind that all medications can produce adverse events. Without appropriate oversight by the medical community, a patient can die from respiratory depression from abusing prescription opioids, sedatives, and even stimulants and in a typical year, these agents are responsible for approximately 20,000 deaths in the United States. Risks are further evident in those that combine these pharmaceuticals with alcohol or readily available illicit agents.

It is important to remember that many of the patients that ultimately develop controlled substance abuse problems already have a history of mental health issues and commonly have a history of multi-substance abuse which may consist of tobacco, marijuana, and/or alcohol.

Tranquilizers such as barbiturates, benzodiazepines, and non-benzodiazepine-hypnotics are frequently prescribed for anxiety and insomnia. These medications are often utilized by abusers who are looking for a way to "come down" after using cocaine, amphetamines, or other stimulant drugs or in an attempt to better manage their anxiety state.

Example of the prescription class "Benzodiazepines" also known as "Benzos" and "Downers" include the commonly prescribed medications Xanax (alprazolam), Ativan (lorazepam), Klonopin (clonazepam), Valium (diazepam), and Restoril (temazepam).

Other less prescribed agents include those prescribed as sedative-hypnotics Halcion (triazolam), Dalmane (flurazepam), Prosom (estazolam), Doral (quazepam), and those used primarily for anxiety Libium (chlordiazepoxide), Tranxene (clorazepate), and Serax (oxazepam).

Popularity of this class is due to its ability to reduce irritability and agitation associated with recent cocaine or other stimulant. Unpleasant withdrawal from opioids or alcohol is often attenuated by individuals utilizing one or more of these central nervous system (CNS) depressants.

Adverse effects seen with this class include: lack of motor coordination, decreased brain activity, anterograde amnesia, depression, slurred speech, and fatal reactions due to additive respiratory depression when combined with alcohol or opioids without proper monitoring. Tolerance and dependency can also develop secondary to appropriate prescription use or illicit use.

Stimulants have long provided "relief" from fatigue for hundreds of years. Abuse and addiction to this class of medications is well known to health professionals. In recent years reports of designer drugs with either mixed amphetamine or amphetamine-like medications have become popular fodder for the media. Methamphetamine or cocaine-induced crime waves are often described on our television news or on the front pages of our newspapers or magazines. In recent years, new legal requirements were designed and enacted to further restrict the purchases by criminal elements of precursor's pseudoephedrine and ephedrine in an effort aimed at curbing methamphetamine production.

Prescription stimulants indicated for ADHD medications like Adderall (mixed amphetamine salts), Ritalin (methylphenidate), Concerta (methylphenidate extended release) have recently seen a jump in popularity by high school and college students. These medications have in the mind of the abuser, the ability to be able to provide the ability to stay alert long hours for the user to work or to study, combined with a perceived safety not associated with methamphetamines.

The ability of this class of medications to mask fatigue but not prevent exhaustion, may contribute to the dangerous consequences of their use [1]. Reported risks and side effects associated with these products include dangerous increases in blood pressure and/or pulse. Sudden death and serious cardiovascular events are not uncommon in patients using these agents without proper indication. High potential for abuse and dependence may be due to possible changes in the brain which may cause the user to begin to compulsively use or to seek out the medication before spiraling toward a dangerous path to addiction.

Provigil (modafinil) and the single-isomer formulation Nuvigil (armodafinil) are medications classified as anti-narcoleptics or wakefulness promoters. This class of agents is sometimes described as eugeroics due to their ability to produce long-lasting "good arousal." Often prescribed to narcolepsy and shift work sleep disorder (SWSD) patients, its unauthorized usage has recently been seen among individuals interested in enhancing their alertness or in mitigating fatigue. Its popularity may be due to the belief that it may possess less adverse effects than those found in traditional psychostimulants than amphetamine, methylphenidate, or cocaine [2]. Though there are scarce reports of serious modafinil-induced side effects or other adverse reactions, this agent must be evaluated with regard to possible detrimental health outcomes related to prolonged sleeplessness of its users rather than actual toxicity of these agents.

Opioid abuse has been reported for literally thousands of years. One does not have to look far to find reports related to the rampant use of opioids. Prescription opioid abuse is a widespread problem often complicated by over prescribing and diversion by pharmacy employees.

To further complicate things, unethical and opportunistic prescribers have allowed the black market to become flooded with prescription opioids by writing prescriptions without so much as an exam in so called "pill mills." Physicians in hope of financial gain have ignored any consideration for societal consequences of their actions including increases in overdose and addiction; have added to the abuser's relative ease of acquiring and possessing these agents. This proliferation of opioid prescribing has added to the supply available for illegal distribution and increased both ease and profitability of selling these painkillers on the street and via the internet by drug dealers. Pharmacy employees including technicians are also commonly being coerced by gang members, who demand the diversion of opioids from pharmacy supplies.

Opioid analgesics are frequently associated with reports of drug diversion and risks of addiction. Questions about long-term efficacy are also abundant. What is known is that while death from opioid withdrawal is relatively rare, unpleasant complications are extremely common. Anxiety related to CNS hyperactivity, associated with opioid withdrawal, often is the motivation for patients to pursue illicit avenues for acquisition of these analgesics. Popular drugs of abuse include heroin, which has an extremely short duration of action and therefore requires constant fixes or withdrawal will follow, and pharmaceutical medications such as hydrocodone and oxycodone.

When one thinks about teenagers hiding even a single can or bottle of an alcoholic beverage from their parents, it is abundantly clear that dozens if not even hundreds of pills would be even more difficult to detect when hidden. With large quantities of prescribed medications diverted in society, it is easy to understand why illegally sold prescription medications and/or illicit drugs are so easily stolen, transported, and exchanged cheaply in clandestine meetings. In this regard, a dose of Oxycontin often is purchased for $1.00/mg ($10.00–$80.00) while a "fix" of Heroin (diacetylmorphine) can be obtained for as low as 10–15 dollars in almost any city in the United States.

With regard to opioid analgesics, MS Contin, Avinza, Kadian (morphine), Vicodin, Norco, Lortab (hydrocodone), Dilaudid (hydromorphone), Dolophine (methadone), Oxycontin (oxycodone), codeine, Duragesic (fentanyl), Demerol (meperidine), and the non-opioid Ultram (tramadol) and Nucynta (tapentadol) are all readily available on the streets and most can be crushed or snorted to increase a greater euphoric high by essentially increasing bioavailability.

In very recent years, the Food and Drug Administration (FDA), in what is called Risk Evaluation & Mitigation Strategies (REMS) notified drug manufacturers that class-wide REMS would be required for ER and LA opioids [3]. This July 9, 2012, FDA News Alert informed Physicians and Pharmacists of a program involving education programs that would provide "safeguards" to reduce the known dangers

Table 21.1 Abuse deterrent formulations—US market

• *Reformulations*: (*crush/extraction resistant*)
– OxyContin® ER (reformulation launched in 2010)
– Opana® ER (reformulation launched in 2012)
• Exalgo® (Hydromorphone ER-crush/extraction resistant)
• Suboxone® (Buprenorphine/naloxone)
• Embeda® (Morphine/naltrexone-recalled 2011)
• Acurox® (Oxycodone/niacin–irritant/unpleasant systemic)

associated with these powerful medications. These guidelines, if followed, can hopefully help in reducing unintentional overdose resulting from inappropriate prescribing, misuse, and abuse [4]. These programs rely on manufacturers to provide and/or fund physician education and continued Pharmacist's participation involving patient counseling on the risks of opioids. Although voluntary, a movement to require physician education to obtain or renew Drug Enforcement Administration licensing is occurring. Pharmacists are not included in the class-wide REMS per se. Pharmacists play an important role in overall risk reduction and are critical to the success of the class-wide REMS. Some of these are listed in Table 21.1.

To reduce misuse due to destroying the controlled-release dosage form, Purdue Pharmaceuticals reformulated their agent. The new formulation is less likely to be snorted or injected; such that any crushing would result in the drug being inactivated. OxyContin (oxycodone HCl controlled-release), due to the addition of an abuse deterrent encapsulated, highly viscous reformulation is designed to resist common physical manipulation, and chemical challenges to reduce the risk of product abuse, misuse, and their consequences [5, 6].

It is likely that in the coming years, the FDA will make this type of formulation a prerequisite for new opioid agents and a standard for existing opioid analgesics. In fact, at the most recent FDA Anesthesia and Analgesic Advisory Board meeting, a novel extended release hydrocodone preparation was rejected by the committee, not because of lack of efficacy but by strong concerns regarding lack of deterrent formulation. A panel of experts assembled by the US Food and Drug Administration (FDA) voted against recommending approval of the painkiller Zohydro ER (reported December 10, 2010). Concerns over the potential for addiction resulted in the 11-2 vote against approval. The panel said that while the drug's maker, Zogenix, had met narrow targets for safety and efficacy, the painkiller could be used by people addicted to other opioids, including oxycodone. Zohydro contains the opioid hydrocodone. Unlike some hydrocodone products such as Vicodin, Zohydro does not contain acetaminophen [7]. Acura Pharmaceuticals and King Pharmaceuticals were handed a rejection FDA expert panel in April 23, 2010 for their pain drug Acurox. In a 19 to 1 vote, the committee determined that the drug's anti-abuse properties weren't strong enough to warrant approval. In addition to properties that prevent the drug from being abused, Acura and King added niacin to Acurox, which causes uncomfortable flushing if too many pills are taken. Due to concerns that niacin's effects could have been dulled by taking the pills with food, panelists questioned whether it truly is an effective abuse deterrent [8].

Opioids are often prescribed by physicians to treat pain; however, they also can suppress cough and reduce diarrhea. Unfortunately, a problem of substance abuse may exist in some of these patients in which they are really utilizing these powerful medications to maintain an addiction, for off-label reduction of tension or anxiety, or in order to produce sedation and to help with insomnia. As controlled substances, these agents should be recognized as potential life destroyers if prescribing and dispensing is done without careful thought and respect for addiction and abuse.

In addition, we should not downplay the potential of many other classes of pharmacologically diverse agents which can also be abused by some patients. Tramadol, which possesses weak opioid analgesic effects as well as serotonin reuptake inhibitor actions, is often abused with reported unpleasant withdrawal symptoms. Muscle relaxants, including Soma (Carisoprodol) a controlled substance, and Flexeril (Cyclobenzaprine), a noncontrolled substance, are commonly abused as well.

The Medical and Pharmacy communities must work together if "appropriate" prescribing and dispensing is to occur. A well-intentioned Physician may prescribe a controlled substance with the best intentions for what appears to be sound and logical reasons. If a patient had covert motivation for fraud and was interested in selling or diversion, detection may be difficult even with mandatory drug testing. The roles of both the Pharmacist and the Physician are paramount to best understand if illicit activity is occurring. If a Physician suspects that a patient is exaggerating an injury or pain level, insisting that a patient sign an agreement (previously known as a "drug contract", which would include a requirement to use "only" one pharmacy).

It is well known that many opioid prescriptions are related to work-related injuries. It is also common for certain patients to fake injury in hopes of receiving medications to fuel substance abuse. Another difficult determination is to ascertain whether a treated patient is unable to work because of severe pain or because of habituation related to a given medication regimen. It would be helpful and appropriate for a Physician to be alerted by the Pharmacist when a patient is being prescribed opioids as part of an injury, if the patient already had been on pain medications from their primary physician for many years? Physicians may trust claimants exaggerated claims of injuries with little investigational efforts and patients may withhold critical data of other injuries, conditions, or other Physician providers when substance abuse is in play. Subjective complaints of pain with little objective documented medical evidence available to explain the stated levels of pain are common, problematic, and challenging.

Before prescribing opioids long-term, it is appropriate to drug test patients in an effort to verify medication history and the potential for substance abuse, and many Physicians, in particular Pain Physicians are currently doing this. Continual drug testing can confirm that a patient is actually consuming the medications as prescribed, not taking other illicit substances, or selling the drug(s).

Motivation for ongoing request of pain medications can include other factors, many of which revolve around substance abuse. The significance of not having any sick time at work may prompt the employee to falsely manufacture an injury or workers compensation claim so the patient will be paid to stay away from work or have extra time off to stay at home or go to physical rehabilitation.

Physicians often fail to review previous medical records or are not provided with accurate patient history. Some of the reasons include: chemical dependency, addiction, drug-related convictions, rehabilitation stays and treatments, suicide attempts, and previous or current psychiatric issues. Only with accurate patient histories can a Physician be expected to create an effective treatment plan that may allow the patient to become functional to the extent that they were before their injury. The goal should always be the lowest dose of a medication possible to maintain functionality and minimize risk, which includes toxicity and substance abuse.

In addition, patients with exaggerated distress about their pain including either inappropriate anxiety or other irrational thoughts about the true nature of their injury may be at high risk of opioid misuse. Subsequent hyperalgesic risk is also common related to patient's lower threshold for pain as a result of psychological distress and perceived increased pain sensitivity [9].

C-II pain medications are commonly prescribed for back injuries and necessitate patients remaining on these medications until they return to work. Unfortunately, many become dependent as a result of utilizing these medications long-term and become permanently disabled related to feeling unable to function without opioids.

With this knowledge, the Pharmacist should provide an extra observation of a patient's level of discomfort. Feedback can be provided each month in the form of early timing and requests of medication refills and if available database review from the PDMP, which provides comprehensive reporting of patient's prescription history for controlled substances (only within any given state not nationwide). The PDMP is a powerful tool that should be utilized at least a few times a year in patients with low risk for abuse and more frequently in those with warning signs of potential abusive behaviors.

Specific PDMP information that can be provided and sent to the provider including:

1. Patient filling prescriptions from multiple providers for the same or other controlled substances.
2. Patient filling prescriptions at different pharmacies.
3. Patient requesting or filling prescriptions early or claiming that they had to visit urgent care or emergency room due to lost or stolen medications.
4. Being prescribed medication that could be considered contradictory in mechanism: uppers and downers, amphetamines and benzodiazepines for example.
5. Therapeutic duplications including multiple long-acting or short-acting Opioids, sedatives, or hypnotics.
6. Opioid containing cough syrups being prescribed on a regular basis (weekly or monthly over months to years).
7. Frequently filling prescriptions from Dentists-even with regular monthly quantities of prescriptions from pain management physicians.

Recognizing addictive behaviors is incredibly difficult. Spouses, co-workers, Physicians, and Pharmacists are commonly among the shocked and confused onlookers after addiction and abuse are finally recognized. Clinical situations involving individuals with active addictions can be better recognized and treated or at least minimized with education, including comprehensive reviews and books, such as this one.

Recently, our literature has begun to describe techniques utilized by addicts to minimize the effects of drug withdrawal symptomology. For many, this becomes almost as critical and anxiety filled as obtaining the high itself. Patients seek alternative ways to "calm down" after abusing large doses of amphetamines, opioids, and/ or tranquilizers, even after they have run out of their drugs of choice. To prepare for self-treatment of these expected withdrawal symptoms, frequent requests for early refills or reported theft of these agents may be seen from patients. Physicians are rarely aware that many of these peculiar often duplicated requests have illegal and inappropriate intentions.

Patients who consume their supplies of drugs of abuse during a short binge often will attempt to "bridge" their recovery time between fixes. Less-suspicious sedating medications such as Neurontin (gabapentin) and Seroquel (quetiapine) are taken in high doses to provide a restful or less anxiety-filled withdrawal. Gabapentin and other gabapentanoid agents such as pregabalin (Lyrica), Gralise, and more recently developed gabapentin enacarbil extended release (Horizant), do not produce any euphoria and are calcium channel blockers and are not recognized as drugs of abuse. There are used for many neuropathic pain states or restless leg syndrome and have nonscheduled drug status.

Pharmacists are well aware of reports of gabapentanoid agent abuse. As an example, a patient in their twenties was recently prescribed Neurontin in a small two day supply with instructions from a psychiatrist to dispense "only every 48 h due to patient's potential abuse". The patient came back the same day with a prescription for the highest strength "800 mg", #180, with 12 refills. Shockingly, the patient was able to purchase three early refills (1–2 days apart) from the pharmacy before abuse was detected. The patient bypassed the insurance rejections and gladly paid hundreds of dollars for each refill before the Pharmacists, Physician, and ultimately the patient were instructed to cease dispensing and prescribing.

In conclusion, Pharmacists are often the last providers to counsel patients on medications before ultimate consumption. Pharmacists protect the public and society, playing a critical role with regard to drug dispensing in society. Extra care and diligence is required for those with pain states as well as emotional or psychiatric comorbidities. Those who catastrophize their pain symptomatology or who appear to have a reduced sense of life control, mood, anxiety, or mental health issues all need to be aggressively monitored for potential abusive behaviors or at some point, morbidity or mortality will result. Drug monitoring, effective Pharmacist–Physician communication, and pharmaceutical deterrents such as appropriate and effective REMS are all paramount in dealing with substance abuse in society.

References

1. Wagner JC. Abuse of drugs used to enhance athletic performance. Am J Hosp Pharm. 1989;46(10):2059–67.
2. Kim D. Practical use and risk of modafinil, a novel waking drug. Environ Health Toxicol. 2012;27:e2012007. doi:10.5620/eht.2012.27.e2012007. Epub 2012 Feb 22.

3. FDA News Alert: Approved Risk Evaluation and Mitigation Strategy (REMS) for extended-release (ER) and long-acting (LA) opioid medications. http://www.fda.gov/drugs/drugsafety/informationbydrugclass/ucm163647.htm. Accessed 9 July 2012.
4. Matthews ML. Class-wide REMS for extended-release and long-acting opioids: potential impact on pharmacies. J Am Pharm Assoc. 2003;53(1):e1–7. doi:10.1331/JAPhA.2013.12025. 2013 Jan–Feb.
5. Sellers EM, Perrino PJ, Colucci SV, Harris SC. Attractiveness of reformulated OxyContin(R) tablets: assessing comparative preferences and tampering potential. J Psychopharmacol. 2013;27(9):808–16. doi:10.1177/0269881113493364. Epub 2013 Jun 19.
6. Friedmann N, Klutzaritz V, Webster L. Efficacy and safety of an extended-release oxycodone (Remoxy) formulation in patients with moderate to severe osteoarthritic pain. J Opioid Manag. 2011;7(3):193–202. 2011 May–Jun.
7. U.S. Food and Drug Administration (FDA) voted against recommending approval of the pain-killer Zohydro ER on 12-10-2010. http://www.drugfree.org/join-together/addiction/fda-panel-votes-against-recommending-zohydro-for-approval
8. FDA Rejects Acurox by a 19 to 1 vote, questions about whether it truly is an effective abuse deterrent. http://www.fiercebiotech.com/story/19-1-vote-fda-panel-rejects-acurox/2010-04-23. Accessed 23 April 2010.
9. Edwards RR, Wasan AD, Michna E, Greenbaum S, Ross E, Jamison RN. Elevated pain sensitivity in chronic pain patients at risk for opioid misuse. J Pain. 2011;12(9):953–63.

Chapter 22
Methadone: Uses, Abuses, and Metabolism

Andrea Trescot, Natalia Murinova, and Daniel Krashin

Key Points

- History
- Clinical use
- Abuse
- Metabolism
- Drug interactions
- Genetics
- Precautions
- Recommendations

History

Methadone (Dolophine®) is a synthetic opioid which was developed by the Germans during World War II, but not put into widespread use until after the war due to difficulty understanding the proper dosing, difficulties that continue to bedevil prescribers of methadone [1]. Methadone's unique properties make this drug particularly

A. Trescot, M.D. (✉)
Pain and Headache Center, Wasilla, AK, USA
e-mail: drtrescot@gmail.com

N. Murinova, M.D., M.H.A.
Department of Neurology, University of Washington, Seattle, WA, USA
e-mail: nataliam@uw.edu

D. Krashin, M.D.
Department of Psychiatry and Pain and Anesthesia, Harborview Medical Center,
University of Washington, Seattle, WA, USA
e-mail: krashind@uw.edu

© Springer Science+Business Media New York 2015
A.D. Kaye et al. (eds.), *Substance Abuse*, DOI 10.1007/978-1-4939-1951-2_22

well suited to certain uses in medicine, particularly in the areas of chronic pain treatment and in the treatment of opioid dependence. However, it has a large inter-individual variability in response and a narrow therapeutic index, making it potentially very dangerous, and therefore the clinician using methadone must have great skill and knowledge to use it safely.

Clinical Use

Opioid addiction: The federal government has estimated that over 268,000 people are enrolled in methadone maintenance programs for the treatment of opioid dependence [2], while over 720,000 patients use methadone to treat chronic pain [3]. The reasons for this wide use are multiple. The half-life of methadone is long, allowing it to be used as a long-acting medication once a day to prevent withdrawal or 2–3 times a day to treat pain. Methadone for chronic pain is fairly inexpensive, with an estimated cost of $27 for a month supply of ninety 10 mg tablets [4]. However, the oral liquid and IV formulations are significantly more expensive. Methadone also has high bioavailability and lacks neurotoxic metabolites. The N-methyl-D-aspartate (NMDA) receptor antagonism of methadone may also make it less prone to cause hyperalgesia and more effective in treating neuropathic pain.

Chronic pain: Patients with past histories of opioid abuse frequently have significant opioid tolerance and may require higher opioid doses for the management of pain [5, 6]. It should be noted that it is illegal to treat opioid dependence with opioid agonists either for detoxification or opioid maintenance unless they are being prescribed as part of a methadone maintenance program or by a registered Suboxone® (bupernorphone) prescriber. However, pain treatment with opioids is allowable, and prescriptions should be clearly documented as such.

Pregnancy: Methadone is the most commonly used opioid during pregnancy, primarily in opioid-dependent patients such as heroin addicts. Traditionally, these methadone maintenance programs involve once-a-day dosing. According to Jarvis et al. [7], their study of pharmacodynamics showed a higher elimination rate and greater renal clearance of methadone in pregnant compared to non-pregnant opioid-dependent women.

Abuse

Methadone can be abused and diverted just as any other opioid medication, and with the growing use of methadone for pain, growing numbers of overdoses have been observed with methadone [8]. For any chronic opioid therapy patient, but particularly one with red flags such as psychiatric illness or substance abuse history, it is essential to follow best practices in pain management. These include the use of opioid agreements, patient education and informed consent, and the use of prescription monitoring programs. More direct assessments of compliance such as pill counts and urine drug screens should also be used. Patients should use only one provider and one pharmacy to obtain their opioids and need to understand that doctor-shopping and seeking early refills is a violation of the treatment agreement. Long-acting opioids are also recommended to decrease the "pop a pill, feel better" effects of short-acting opioids.

Accidental overdose is a common cause of death with methadone treatment. The long and variable half-life, which results in patients receiving the full effect of a new methadone prescription more than a day after having started a new prescription, potentially results in patients developing sedation and respiratory depression at unexpected times, often at night. The other pitfall in methadone dosing is the non-linear dose–response curve. The ratio of morphine equivalency increases dramatically with dosing, so that methadone potency ranges from three to four times that of morphine at the lowest doses to twelve times morphine at doses of 120 mg/day. Thus, increasing the dose seemingly small increments can greatly increase the opioid potency, and patients on a stable dosing regimen who take an extra methadone tablet in response to increased pain can easily put themselves in the toxic range. Dose titration for methadone should therefore be slow and cautious taking the long time to steady state into account [9]. If the patient on methadone needs additional medication for acute pain, such as after a surgical procedure or trauma, it may be safer to use short-acting opioids along with the standard methadone dose.

Metabolism

Methadone is a unique synthetic opioid, unrelated to standard opioids (leading to its usefulness in patients with "true" morphine allergies). It is a basic and lipophilic drug with an excellent (though highly variable) oral bioavailability (from 40 to 100 %). It can be crushed or dissolved to deliver down an NG tube and is also available in a liquid. The analgesic effects occur within 30–60 min and peak after about 2–4 h, with a half-life of about 22 h, with a range of 4–190 h [10]. Methadone is highly protein bound, primarily to alpha1 acid glycoprotein (AAG), which is an acute-phase reaction protein that can fluctuate widely [11]. Methadone is metabolized in the liver and intestines and excreted almost exclusively in feces, an advantage in patients with renal insufficiency or failure. It may also cause less constipation than morphine [12].

In addition to its mu-opioid receptor activity, methadone is also an antagonist of the N-methyl-D-aspartate (NMDA) receptor. Methadone is a 50/50 racemic mixture of two enantiomers; the R form is more potent, with a tenfold higher affinity for opioid receptors (which accounts for virtually all of its analgesic effect), while S-methadone is the NMDA antagonist. The inherent NMDA antagonistic effects make it potentially useful in severe neuropathic and "opioid-resistant" pain states. The S isomer also inhibits reuptake of serotonin and norepinephrine, which should

Table 22.1 Common *substrates* of CYP enzymes

1A2	2B6	2C19	2D6	3A4
Amitriptyline	Bupropion	Barbiturates	Codeine	Alprazolam
Nabumetone	Methadone	Topiramate	Tramadol	Midazolam
Desipramine	Ketamine	Diazepam	Meperidine	Cyclosporine
Tizanidine	Testosterone	Amitriptyline	Oxycodone	Sildenafil
Imipramine		Imipramine	Hydrocodone	Indinavir
Acetaminophen	**2C9**	Clomipramine	Dextromethorphan	Verapamil
Cyclobenzaprine	Valproic acid	Sertraline	Amitriptyline	Atorvastatin
Clozapine	Piroxicam	Citalopram	Nortriptyline	Lovastatin
Fluvoxamine	Celecoxib	Phenytoin	Doxepin	Digoxin
Theophylline	Ibuprofen	Carisoprodol	Tamoxifen	Amiodarone
Melatonin	Warfarin	Clopidogrel	Amphetamines	Methadone
Duloxetine			Duloxetine	Erythromycin
Caffeine			Metoclopramide	Trazodone
Lidocaine			Propranolol	Fentanyl
Warfarin			Venlafaxine	Buprenorphine
Methadone				

Modified from Indiana University website [16] and Genelex website [17], among others

be recognized when using SSRIs and TCAs. Both forms bind to AAG, but a greater percentage of S-methadone is bound. Although it has traditionally been used to treat heroin addicts, its flexibility in dosing, use in neuropathic pain, and cheap price has lead to a recent increase in its use in chronic pain. Unfortunately, a lack of awareness of its metabolism and potential drug interactions, as well as its long half-life, has lead to a dramatic increase in the deaths associated with this medication.

The metabolism of methadone is always variable. Methadone is metabolized by CYP3A4 primarily and CYP2D6 secondarily; CYP2D6 preferentially metabolizes the R-methadone, while CYP3A4 and CYP1A2 metabolize both enantiomers. CYP1B2 is possibly involved and a newly proposed enzyme CYP2B6 is emerging as an important metabolic pathway [13]. CYP3A4 expression can vary up to 30-fold, and there can be genetic polymorphism of CYP2D6, ranging from poor to rapid metabolism. Methadone is metabolized by CYP3A4 and CYP2B6 to an inactive *N*-demethylated metabolite, 2-ethylidene-1,5-dimethyl-3,3-diphenylpyrrolidine (known as EDDP) [14]. When looking at urine drug toxicology, EDDP levels are, on average, about twice the methadone concentrations, but there is a wide variability in the ratio of methadone to EDDP urine levels that is not concentration dependent [15].

The initiation of methadone therapy can induce the CYP3A4 enzyme for 5–7 days, leading to low blood levels initially, but unexpectedly high levels about a week later if the medication has been rapidly titrated upward; an intestinal CYP3A4 transport enzyme may also be involved. A wide variety of substances can also induce or inhibit these enzymes, or are substrates of these enzymes (Tables 22.1, 22.2 and 22.3) [16–18]. The potential differences in enzymatic metabolic conversion of methadone may explain the inconsistency of observed half-life. Methadone has no active metabolites, and therefore may result in less hyperalgia, myoclonus, and neurotoxicity than

Table 22.2 Common *inducers* of CYP enzymes

1A2	2C9	2C19	2D6	3A4
Carbamazepine	Rifampin	Carbamazepine	Carbamazepine	Carbamazepine
Griseofulvin	Ritonavir	Rifampin	Phenobarbital	Phenytoin
Lansprazole	Barbiturates	Ginko	Phenytoin	Nevirapine
Omeprazole	St. John's Wort		Rifampin	Modafinil
Ritonavir			Dexamethasone	Topiramate
Tobacco				Butabutal
St. John's Wort				St. John's Wort

Modified from Indiana University website [16] and Genelex website [17], among others

Table 22.3 Common inhibitors of CYP enzymes

1A2	2C9	2C19	2D6	3A4
Fluvoxamine	Fluvoxamine	Fluoxetine	Duloxine	Ketoconazole
Ciprofloxin	Paroxetine	Fluvoxamine	Cimetidine	Erythromycin
Mexiletine	Amiodarone	Paroxetine	Sertraline	Mifepristone
Verapamil	Modafinil	Topiramate	Fluoxetine	Nefazodone
Caffeine	Tamoxifen	Modafinil	Haloperidol	Grapefruit
Grapefruit juice		Birth control pill	Methadone	Indinavir
			Paroxetine	Ritonavir
			Quinidine	Verapamil
			Celecoxib	Diltiazem
			Bupropion	
			Ritonavir	
			Amiodarone	
			Metoclopramide	
			Chlorpromazine	

Modified from Indiana University web site [16] and Genelex web site [17], among others

morphine. It may be unique in its lack of profound euphoria, but its analgesic action (4–8 h) is significantly shorter than its elimination half-life (up to 190 h), and patient self-directed re-dosing and a long half-life may lead to the potential of respiratory depression and death.

Drug Interactions

Because of the multiple enzymes involved in methadone metabolism, multiple medicines can cause changes in methadone blood levels. Inducers of CYP3A4 will drop methadone blood levels, and can cause withdrawal symptoms in patients who continue to take their medications. Kell and Musselman [19] described a 50 % decrease in blood levels and a return of headaches in a patient on methadone who took butabutal (a CYP3A4 inducer). More concerning are the CYP3A4 inhibitors, which can cause potentially life-threatening overdoses. For instance, Herrlin et al. [20] described a patient, stable on methadone for 6 years, who noted profound sedation, confusion, and respiratory depression after being treated with ciprofloxacin (an inhibitor of CYP1A2 and 3A4). The inhibition of methadone metabolism can be used therapeutically to deliberately raise blood levels without increasing the dose. DeMaria and Serota [21] reported using fluvoxamine to raise methadone blood levels to avoid opioid withdrawal symptoms in a patient on methadone 200 mg per day but ineffective blood levels. Additional interactions may be seen with venlafaxine (a known CYP3A4 inhibitor) [18]. Cimetidine (but not ranididine), famotidine, omeprazole, esomeprazole, and pantoprazole all inhibit CYP3A4 [22].

Many of the HIV medications have the potential for drug–drug interactions with methadone. Ritonavir inhibits both CYP3A4 and CYP2B6. Efavirenz and nevirapine have been shown to induce both CYP3A4 and CYP 2B6. Twelve methadone-using HIV patients on ritonavir/saquinavir were studied for 24 h; there was a 40 % decrease in S-methadone and a 32 % decrease in R-methadone (though there were no signs of withdrawal in this short study) [23]. Indinavir, a protease inhibitor used to treat HIV infections that is both a CYP3A4 substrate and an inhibitor, did not have a discernable effect on methadone levels when studied in a double-blinded fashion for 8 days.

To make it even more complicated, methadone can induce its own metabolism, at least for the first week [24], and can inhibit CYP2D6, a secondary metabolism pathway [25]. Methadone can be lethal even after a single dose if patient has genetic predisposition to long QTc interval, which can cause a Torsades de Pointe cardiac arrhythmia syndrome. In a case familiar to the author, a patient with undiagnosed congenital prolonged QT interval suffered cardiac arrest after receiving a single methadone dose, surviving only because this occurred in a large medical center and she was immediately able to receive cardiac care. This adverse effect, not shared by other opioids, occurs because methadone binds to the KCNH2 cardiac channel and prolongs the action potential in a dose-dependent fashion [26]. High-dose methadone increases the corrected QT interval [3, 27]. Congenital QT prolongation, high methadone levels (usually over 60 mg per day), and conditions that increase QT prolongation (such as hypokalemia and hypomagnesemia) may increase that risk [28]. In patients with a normal screening EKG, another should be checked once the patient is stable on their dose of methadone to reassess QT interval while on this medication [29, 30].

There is an incomplete cross-tolerance between methadone and other opioids. Even when prescribed in low doses, and used appropriately by individuals experienced with opioids, the long half-life of methadone may be underestimated while dosing is titrated to analgesic effect. In general, better relief is observed with methadone doses that are 10 % of the calculated equianalgesic doses of conventional opioids.

Genetics

Genetic polymorphisms in genes that code for methadone-metabolizing CYP enzymes, the methadone transporter proteins (p-glycoprotein; P-gp), and mu-opioid receptors may explain part of the observed interindividual variation in the pharmacokinetics and pharmacodynamics of methadone.

As describe above, CYP 3A4 and CYP2B6 have been identified as the main hepatic enzymes involved in methadone metabolism. Both of these enzymes are polymorphically expressed. The transport protein P-glycoprotein (p-gp) is genetically coded by the ABCB1 gene, and is an outward transporter at the blood–brain barrier. Methadone is a P-gp substrate, and ABCB1 genetic polymorphisms may also contribute to the interindividual variability of dose requirements. OPRM1 is the gene that codes for the mu-opioid receptor, and genetic variability in the activity of this receptor can affect the analgesia seen with methadone. Therefore, potentially multiple genetic polymorphisms contribute to the high interindividual variability of methadone blood concentrations for a given dose. As an example, Li et al. [31] estimated that, in order to obtain a methadone plasma concentration of 250 ng/mL in a 70-kg patient, doses of racemic methadone as low as 55 mg/day or as high as 921 mg/day might be needed. The clinician must be aware of the pharmacokinetic properties and pharmacological interactions of methadone in order to personalize methadone administration. In the future, pharmacogenetics, at a limited level, can also be expected to facilitate individualized methadone therapy.

Precautions

Although patients typically do not feel a "buzz" while on methadone, it is still a centrally acting agent with the potential for cognitive dysfunction. In 2011, Bramness et al. [32] reviewed personal injury motor vehicle accidents (MVAs) in Norway for a 2.5 year period, linking this information to the Norwegian Prescription Database, and comparing the incidence of MVAs in patient on methadone compared to those not exposed. During the 4,626 person-years observed in patients on methadone, there were 26 MVS, almost all on which were among males. Even when patients on concurrent benzodiazepines were excluded from the analysis, there was still a Standardized Incidence Ratio (SIR) of 2.4, with a 95 % confidence interval of 1.5–3.6, suggesting that males on methadone have an increased risk of MVA.

Recommendations

In 2009, Krantz et al. [3] proposed five recommendations regarding cardiac precautions for providers prescribing methadone. They suggested that:

1. Clinicians should inform patients of arrhythmia risk when they prescribe methadone.
2. Clinicians should ask patients about any history of structural heart disease, arrhythmia, and syncope.
3. Clinicians should obtain a pretreatment electrocardiogram for all patients prior to starting methadone to measure the QTc interval, with a follow-up electrocardiogram within 30 days and then annually. Additional electrocardiography is recommended if the methadone dosage exceeds 100 mg/d or if patients have unexplained syncope or seizures.

4. If the QTc interval is greater than 450 ms but less than 500 ms, clinicians should discuss the potential risks and benefits with patients and monitor them more frequently. If the QTc interval exceeds 500 ms, consider discontinuing or reducing the methadone dose; eliminating contributing factors, such as drugs that promote hypokalemia; or using an alternative therapy.
5. Clinicians should be aware of interactions between methadone and other drugs that possess QT interval-prolonging properties or slow the elimination of methadone.

In this author's practice, methadone has been part of the medication armamentarium for nearly 15 years. Patients who have been deemed good candidates for methadone undergo a detailed counseling session, discussing the risks (drug–drug interactions, lethal arrhythmias, and a slow titration schedule). We obtain a detailed current drug list (including OTC and herbals), and then start the patient on 5–10 mg at night for a week, increased by 5–10 mg per week. The patient is maintained on their short-acting medication for the first month, which is then weaned as the methadone dosing increases. Patients are counseled not to start or stop ANY medications, OTC or prescription, without discussing with us first. They get a baseline EKG, and then another if they are prescribed greater than 60 mg/day of methadone.

Conclusion

For a group of patients, methadone provides superior analgesia with minimal CNS effects and little tolerance. This author has personally had patients on the same dose of methadone for 15 years, and has returned doctors, nurses, policemen, and pharmacists back to full function on methadone. However, there are significant risks with the medication, and clinicians must be careful and cognizant of the potential life-threatening risks.

References

1. Chen KK. Pharmacology of methadone and related compounds. Ann N Y Acad Sci. 1948;51(1):83–97.
2. Substance Abuse and Mental Health Services Administration. Results from the 2010 National Survey on Drug Use and Health: Summary of National Findings. In: US Department of Health and Human Services, editor. Rockville: Substance Abuse and Mental Health Services Administration; 2011.
3. Krantz MJ, Martin J, Stimmel B, Mehta D, Haigney MC. QTc interval screening in methadone treatment. Ann Intern Med. 2009;150(6):387–95.
4. GoodRx. GoodRx Methadone Page. 2013 [updated 2013; cited]. http://www.goodrx.com/methadone
5. Hughes JR, Bickel WK, Higgins ST. Buprenorphine for pain relief in a patient with drug abuse. Am J Drug Alcohol Abuse. 1991;17(4):451–5.
6. Umbricht A, Hoover DR, Tucker MJ, Leslie JM, Chaisson RE, Preston KL. Opioid detoxification with buprenorphine, clonidine, or methadone in hospitalized heroin-dependent patients with HIV infection. Drug Alcohol Depend. 2003;69(3):263–72.

7. Jarvis MA, Wu-Pong S, Kniseley JS, Schnoll SH. Alterations in methadone metabolism during late pregnancy. J Addict Dis. 1999;18(4):51–61.
8. Maxwell JC, McCance-Katz EF. Indicators of buprenorphine and methadone use and abuse: what do we know? Am J Addict. 2010;19(1):73–88.
9. Davoli M, Bargagli AM, Perucci CA, Schifano P, Belleudi V, Hickman M, et al. Risk of fatal overdose during and after specialist drug treatment: the VEdeTTE study, a national multi-site prospective cohort study. Addiction. 2007;102(12):1954–9 [Multicenter Study Research Support, Non-U.S. Govt].
10. Eap CB, Buclin T, Baumann P. Interindividual variability of the clinical pharmacokinetics of methadone: implications for the treatment of opioid dependence. Clin Pharmacokinet. 2002;41(14):1153–93.
11. Garrido MJ, Aguirre C, Troconiz IF, Marot M, Valle M, Zamacona MK, et al. Alpha 1-acid glycoprotein (AAG) and serum protein binding of methadone in heroin addicts with abstinence syndrome. Int J Clin Pharmacol Ther. 2000;38(1):35–40.
12. Moolchan ET, Umbricht A, Epstein D. Therapeutic drug monitoring in methadone maintenance: choosing a matrix. J Addict Dis. 2001;20(2):55–73.
13. Lynch ME. A review of the use of methadone for the treatment of chronic noncancer pain. Pain Res Manage. 2005;10:133–44.
14. Iribarne C, Berthou F, Baird S, Dreano Y, Picart D, Bail JP, et al. Involvement of cytochrome P450 3A4 enzyme in the N-demethylation of methadone in human liver microsomes. Chem Res Toxicol. 1996;9(2):365–73.
15. Leimanis E, Best BM, Atayee RS, Pesce AJ. Evaluating the relationship of methadone concentrations and EDDP formation in chronic pain patients. J Anal Toxicol. 2012;36(4): 239–49.
16. Drug Interaction Table: Abbreviated "Clinically Relevant" Table. [cited 9/21/13]. http://medicine.iupui.edu/clinpharm/DDIs/ClinicalTable.aspx
17. Oesterheld J. Cytochrome P-450 (CYP) Metabolism Reference Table. Seattle: Genelex; 2012 [updated 2012; cited 9/2/13]. http://youscript.com/healthcare-professionals/why-youscript/cytochrome-p450-drug-table/
18. Leavitt SB, Bruce RD, Eap CB, Kharasch E, Kral L, McCance-Katz E, et al. Addiction Treatment Forum: Methadone-Drug Interactions. 2009 [updated 2009; cited]. www.atforum.com/SiteRoot/pages/rxmethadone/methadone.shtml
19. Kell M, Musselman D. Methadone prophylaxis of intractable headaches: pain control and serum opioid level. Am J Prev Med. 1993;3:7–14.
20. Herrlin K, Segerdahl M, Gustafsson LL, Kalso E. Methadone, ciprofloxacin, and adverse drug reactions. Lancet. 2000;356(9247):2069–70.
21. DeMaria Jr PA, Serota RD. A therapeutic use of the methadone fluvoxamine drug interaction. J Addict Dis. 1999;18(4):5–12.
22. Moody DE, Liu F, Fang WB. In vitro inhibition of Methadone and Oxycodone Cytochrome P450-dependent metabolism: reversible inhibition by H2-receptor agonists and proton-pump inhibitors. J Anal Toxicol. 2013;37(8):476–85.
23. Gerber JG, Rosenkranz S, Segal Y, Aberg J, D'Amico R, Mildvan D, et al. Effect of ritonavir/saquinavir on stereoselective pharmacokinetics of methadone: results of AIDS Clinical Trials Group (ACTG) 401. J Acquir Immune Defic Syndr. 2001;27(2):153–60.
24. Peng PW, Tumber PS, Gourlay D. Review article: perioperative pain management of patients on methadone therapy. Canad J Anaesth. 2005;52(5):513–23.
25. Bruera E, Sweeney C. Methadone use in cancer patients with pain: a review. J Palliat Med. 2002;5(1):127–38.
26. Kornick CA, Kilborn MJ, Santiago-Palma J, Schulman G, Thaler HT, Keefe DL, et al. QTc interval prolongation associated with intravenous methadone. Pain. 2003;105(3):499–506.
27. Gil M, Sala M, Anguera I, Chapinal O, Cervantes M, Guma JR, et al. QT prolongation and Torsades de Pointes in patients infected with human immunodeficiency virus and treated with methadone. Am J Cardiol. 2003;92(8):995–7.
28. Krantz MJ, Lewkowiez L, Hays H, Woodroffe MA, Robertson AD, Mehler PS. Torsade de pointes associated with very high dose methadone. Ann Intern Med. 2002;137:501–4.

29. Cruciani RA. Methadone: to ECG or not to ECG…That is still the question. J Pain Symptom Manage. 2008;36(5):545–52 [Meta-Analysis Review].
30. Chugh SS, Socoteanu C, Reinier K, Waltz J, Jui J, Gunson K. A community-based evaluation of sudden death associated with therapeutic levels of methadone. Am J Med. 2008;121(1):66–71 [Comparative Study Research Support, N.I.H., Extramural].
31. Li Y, Kantelip JP, Gerritsen-van Schieveen P, Davani S. Interindividual variability of methadone response: impact of genetic polymorphism. Mol Diagn Ther. 2008;12(2):109–24.
32. Bramness JG, Skurtveit S, Morland J, Engeland A. An increased risk of motor vehicle accidents after prescription of methadone. Addiction. 2012;107:967–72.

Chapter 23
Buprenorphine for Pain and Opioid Dependence

Sanford M. Silverman

Key Points

- Partial agonists and antagonists
- Pharmacology and metabolism
- Buprenorphine preparations
- Safety
- Buprenorphine and precipitated withdrawal
- Buprenorphine and pain

Naturally occurring opiates are derived from the poppy. They include morphine, codeine, and thebaine. Buprenorphine is a synthetic thebaine derivative (Fig. 23.1). It is highly potent whose primary action is partial antagonism at the mu receptor and full antagonism at the kappa receptor. Buprenorphine has an extremely high affinity for the mu receptor; much higher than other opioids to include antagonists such as naloxone. Based on this high affinity, buprenorphine slowly dissociates from the receptor with somewhat milder withdrawal symptoms upon discontinuation in patients who are physically dependent on full agonists such as morphine, heroin, oxycodone, etc.

Partial Agonists and Antagonists

Agonist agents bind to a receptor and stimulate a physiologic process, usually mediated through an intracellular chemical cascade. They have full efficacy at the receptor. Antagonists bind to the receptor and block such activity, exhibiting no efficacy.

S.M. Silverman, M.D. (✉)
Comprehensive Pain Medicine, Florida Society of Interventional Pain Physicians (FSIPP),
100 East Sample Rd., Ste 200, Pompano Beach, FL 33064, USA
e-mail: sanfordsilverman@cpmedicine.com

© Springer Science+Business Media New York 2015   311
A.D. Kaye et al. (eds.), *Substance Abuse*, DOI 10.1007/978-1-4939-1951-2_23

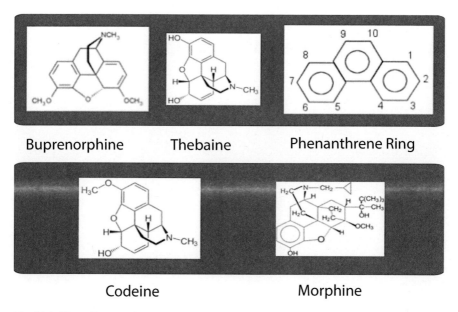

Fig. 23.1 Naturally occurring opiates; thebaine, codeine, morphine. The phenanthrene ring is the central common structure for all opiates and most synthetic opioids

Table 23.1 Properties of partial agonists and antagonists

	Buprenorphine	Pentazocine	Nalbuphine	Butorphanol
Mu receptor activity	Partial agonist	Partial agonist	Antagonist	Partial agonist
Kappa receptor activity	Antagonist	Agonist	Agonist	Strong agonist
Schedule	III	IV	Unscheduled (*Schedule IV in KY*)	IV

Modified from Johnson RE, Fudala PJ, Payne R. Buprenorphine: Considerations for Pain Management. J Pain Symptom Manage 2005;29(3):297-326. [20]

Partial mu receptor agonists are a unique class in that they bind tightly to the mu receptor but only partially activate it, thus having reduced or intermediate efficacy. Partial agonist–antagonists such as nalbuphine, bind tightly to the mu receptor but have no mu efficacy. They also have kappa receptor agonist activity which is thought to be associated with spinal analgesia, sedation, miosis, and psychotomimetic (i.e., dysphoric) effects. These agents are used as analgesics, but have a partial or a ceiling to their analgesic effect, such that escalating the dosage beyond a certain level will only yield greater opioid side effects. The binding properties of partial agonists/mixed antagonists are summarized in Table 23.1.

Pharmacology and Metabolism

Buprenorphine has a rapid onset of action secondary to its high lipophilicity after both sublingual and intravenous administration; approximately 30–60 min and 5–15 min respectively. Buprenorphine penetrates the blood–brain barrier more easily

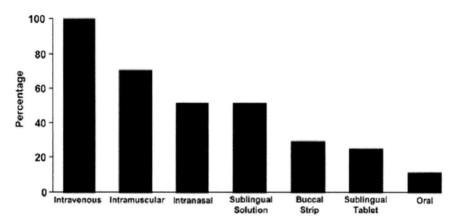

Fig. 23.2 Bioavailability of buprenorphine. *Modified from Johnson RE, Fudala PJ, Payne R. Buprenorphine: Considerations for Pain Management. J Pain Symptom Manage 2005;29(3): 297-326.* [20]

than morphine. The peak effect for sublingual administration occurs around 100 min and the duration is relatively dose related. Its slow dissociation from the receptor is responsible for its relatively long elimination half-life of approximately 37 h.

Buprenorphine is highly bound to plasma proteins and has a relatively high volume of distribution [1]. It is metabolized through the cytochrome P450 system into the active metabolite norbuprenorphine (25 % the potency of buprenorphine). Both buprenorphine and norbuprenorphine are conjugated with glucuronide acid and excreted through the bile. Approximately 15 % of buprenorphine is excreted unchanged in the urine. There is relatively little effect on buprenorphine metabolism in renal failure.

Buprenorphine has poor oral bioavailability secondary to extensive first pass effect by the liver (approximately 10 % oral bioavailability). However, it has superb sublingual bioavailability better than other opioids. It also has very good transdermal bioavailability which has led to various commercial preparations; parenteral, sublingual, and transdermal (Fig. 23.2).

Buprenorphine Preparations

Buprenorphine preparations for the treatment of pain include parenteral (Buprenex® [Reckitt Benckiser Group]) and transdermal (Butrans® [Purdue Pharma L.P.]). For the treatment of opioid dependence, the sublingual formulations include Subutex® (Reckitt Benckiser Group) and generic formulations. Buprenorphine can be formulated with naloxone (Suboxone® [Reckitt Benckiser Group] and Zubsolv® tablets (Orexo AB), which is designed to deter abuse. The reason for this is while buprenorphine is highly bioavailable parenterally or via sublingual administration, *both* buprenorphine and naloxone are poorly absorbed orally. Naloxone is poorly absorbed sublingually but readily absorbed parenterally. Hence, the combined formulation affords efficacy via sublingual administration, but during illicit parenteral use, the naloxone counteracts the effects of the buprenorphine. The single component formulations have been illicitly used in Europe, and in particular Great Britain, which prompted the combined formulation, which is widely utilized in the United States. The single component drug is available for use in patients with documented allergy to naloxone or for opioid dependence during pregnancy, since the combination product with naloxone is considered a class C teratogen.

Physicians who wish to prescribe buprenorphine for the treatment of opioid dependence must meet certain requirements established by SAMHSA/CSAT (Substance Abuse and Mental Health Services Administration/Center for Substance Abuse Treatment).

Qualified physicians must submit notification to SAMHSA/CSAT, and a unique identification is then issued from the Drug Enforcement Administration (DEA) in the form of an "X number," thus providing these physicians 2 distinct DEA numbers.

Initially, a provider is limited to treating not more than 30 patients, but can be increased to 100 with secondary notification to SAMHSA/CSAT.

Sublingual buprenorphine (2 mg, 8 mg) is available in tablet or film and the combination product, Suboxone® is available in 2/0.5 mg, 4/1 mg, 8/2 mg, 12/3 mg (tablet or film). Zubsolv® tablets (Orexo AB) sublingual combination formulation tablets (available in September 2013) in 1.4 mg/0.36 mg and 5.7 mg/1.4 mg strengths as a menthol flavor.

Safety

Buprenorphine demonstrates a ceiling effect on mu receptor activity, such as respiratory depression and analgesia. It has a high therapeutic index relative to morphine (Table 23.2).

Buprenorphine safety has been studied in the treatment of opioid dependence. Heroin addicts were treated with sublingual buprenorphine daily (8 mg) for up to 36 days with no significant morbidity [2]. Buprenorphine was studied in a maintenance therapy program during an observational study [3]. The mortality rate was 4 % (3 of 77). The successful retention rate with respect to treatment was felt to be secondary to the use of buprenorphine. However, comorbidities of cocaine and

Table 23.2 Therapeutic indices for morphine and buprenorphine

Opioid	LD_{50}, Acute (mg/kg)	ED_{50}, Tail Pressure (mg/kg)	Therapeutic index, LD_{50}/ED_{50}
Morphine	306 [237, 395]	0.66 [0.26, 1.6]	464
Buprenorphine	197 [145, 277]	0.016 [0.011, 0.024]	12,313

Modified from: Johnson RE, Fudala PJ, Payne R. Buprenorphine: Considerations for Pain Management. J Pain Symptom Manage 2005;29(3):297-326. [20]

other opiate dependence may have contributed to morbidity and mortality. Buprenorphine was found to have less morbidity and better retention in a study of heroin addicts when it was continued for up to 350 days as opposed to rapidly withdrawn [4]. A randomized controlled study found that buprenorphine had similar efficacy to methadone in a maintenance program for opioid dependence [5].

Buprenorphine and Precipitated Withdrawal

Buprenorphine has a very high affinity for the mu receptor. It competes and subsequently displaces full opioid agonists from the mu receptor. Buprenorphine also has a lower intrinsic activity than a full agonist (partial agonist). When administered to a patient with opioid dependence already utilizing full agonists, this reduced mu receptor activity is experienced by the patient as withdrawal. Therefore, if a patient is currently using a full opioid mu agonist and is *not* in withdrawal, the administration of buprenorphine will *precipitate* withdrawal. Hence, patients must be in some degree of opioid withdrawal in order to be treated with buprenorphine (Fig. 23.3).

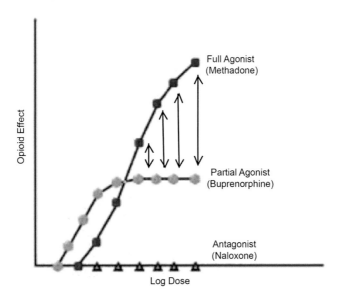

Fig. 23.3 Precipitated withdrawal. If buprenorphine is given to an opioid-dependent patient who is not in withdrawal, the *difference* in activity at the mu receptor between a full agonist and a partial agonist is clinically expressed as opioid withdrawal

Buprenorphine and Pain

Buprenorphine is an effective opioid analgesic with approximately 30 times greater potency than morphine, when administered for acute pain. There is a ceiling effect on both analgesia and respiratory depression. Although buprenorphine has a relatively long half-life, clinical experience shows that the analgesic half-life is shorter and therefore requires multiple doses (twice to three times daily) similar to methadone. In the United States only Buprenex® and Butrans® are approved by the Food and Drug Administration (FDA) for the treatment of pain.

Buprenorphine has been successfully utilized via epidural administration providing good analgesia without significant respiratory depression [6, 7]. It has been shown to provide more prolonged pain relief in postoperative cesarean section patients compared with controls who did not utilize buprenorphine [8]. Buprenorphine can be given subcutaneously to provide postoperative pain control at approximately 30 mcg per hour [9]. It has also been shown to significantly reduce analgesic requirements after knee arthroscopy when intra-articular injection is provided during surgery [10]. The addition of buprenorphine to the local anesthetic in axillary brachial plexus blockade provided significant postoperative analgesia [11].

Transdermal buprenorphine for the treatment of chronic pain was studied in a moderate quality, open-label, parallel-group randomized trial which compared it to extended release tramadol for the management of osteoarthritis of the hip and knee, yielding indeterminate results [12].

Transdermal buprenorphine is indicated for the treatment of chronic pain. In the United States it is available in 5, 10, 20 mcg per hour patches (Butrans®) which provide seven days of therapy. As mentioned, there is a ceiling effect on analgesia and therefore is not recommended for patients who have daily requirements of 80 mg or greater morphine equivalents. It should not be used for the treatment of opioid dependence because even at the maximum dose, 20 mcg per hour corresponds to 0.48 mg daily of buprenorphine. Sublingual buprenorphine provides anywhere from 2 to 12 mg per day (or more, depending on the amount given). The use of buprenorphine to treat opioid dependence corresponds to a relative overdose compared to that for chronic pain. Very low doses of buprenorphine are required for analgesia.

Sublingual buprenorphine is FDA approved for the treatment of opioid dependence requiring a waiver from the DEA and SAMHSA/CSAT. However, it is a schedule III medication and can be used to treat pain, which does *not* require a waiver [13, 14].

The management of acute pain for patients utilizing sublingual buprenorphine for opioid dependence can be challenging. The addition of a full mu agonist to a regimen of buprenorphine will not precipitate withdrawal, however, the converse will. The buprenorphine and full agonist will compete for binding at the mu receptor. This may reduce the efficacy of the full agonist.

This situation is often seen during surgery. If the postoperative analgesic requirements are not significant (i.e. dental extraction, outpatient surgery, expected rapid recovery) then maintenance therapy with sublingual buprenorphine should be continued. However, maintenance therapy will not treat the acute surgical pain.

Non-opioid analgesics should be tried first. Additional sublingual buprenorphine can be added on an as-needed basis to treat the acute pain [15]. If necessary, a full mu agonist can be added and then tapered in the usual fashion while the patient continues his maintenance dose of sublingual buprenorphine.

There are several other strategies for preoperative management that have been recommended for patients who are utilizing maintenance buprenorphine for opioid dependence. These include conversion to a full agonist preoperatively [16]. Also studied was the continued maintenance of buprenorphine throughout the perioperative period with a full agonist used for postoperative pain control, and discontinuation of buprenorphine 72 h prior to surgery with preoperative conversion to a full agonist to eliminate any partial blockade [17]. Sublingual buprenorphine can be used for postoperative pain control [18]. In addition, pain can be controlled with parenteral buprenorphine.

If major surgery is anticipated and postoperative analgesic requirements are significant, then buprenorphine should be discontinued 24–48 h (72 h if higher doses used) prior to surgery. Postoperative pain should be treated with full mu receptor agonists (usually parenterally via patient-controlled analgesia) and the patient discharged on full agonist pain medication. They will then require reconversion (induction) with buprenorphine for the continued treatment of opioid dependence.

Buprenorphine may also have a niche role in the treatment of Opioid Induced Hyperalgesia (OIH). OIH is a state of increased pain caused by chronic long-term use of opioids, usually moderate to high doses. There are several mechanisms that are involved but it is believed that the excitatory neurotransmitter (glutamate) is involved with stimulation of NMDA receptors. It is also felt that spinal dynorphin levels are increased during OIH. Spinal dynorphin is a kappa receptor agonist. Buprenorphine is a kappa receptor antagonist and may have a significant role in breaking the hyperalgesic cycle [19].

In summary, buprenorphine is a unique opioid partial agonist/antagonist which can be used for the treatment of both opioid dependence and pain. There are certain legal ramifications for its use in opioid dependence requiring a waiver from the DEA and SAMHSA/CSAT. The parenteral and transdermal formulations are approved for the treatment of pain, transdermal for chronic pain. The sublingual form is approved for the treatment of opioid dependence and can be used to treat chronic pain as well. It may play a niche role in the treatment of complex chronic pain patients who exhibit repeated tolerance to full agonists or OIH. It is also useful for the treatment of patients who suffer from *both* chronic pain and opioid dependence.

References

1. Elkader A, Sproule B. Buprenorphine: clinical pharmacokinetics in the treatment of opioid dependence. Clin Pharmacokinet. 2005;44(7):661–80.
2. Lange WR, Fudala PJ, Dax EM, Johnson RE. Safety and side-effects of buprenorphine in the clinical management of heroin addiction. Drug Alcohol Depend. 1990;26(1):19–28.
3. Fareed A, et al. Safety and efficacy of long-term buprenorphine maintenance treatment. Addict Disord Their Treat. 2011;10(3):123–30.

4. Kakko, et al. Buprenorphine improved treatment retention in patients with heroin dependence. Lancet. 2003;361:662–8.
5. Kakko J, et al. A stepped care strategy using buprenorphine and methadone versus conventional methadone maintenance in heroin dependence: a randomized controlled trial. Am J Psychiatry. 2007;164:797–803.
6. Scherer R, et al. Complications related to thoracic epidural analgesia: a prospective study in 1071 surgical patients. Acta Anaesthesiol Scand. 1993;37(4):370–4.
7. Inagaki Y, et al. Mode and site of analgesic action of epidural buprenorphine in humans. Anesth Analg. 1996;83(3):530–6.
8. Celleno D, Capogna G. Spinal buprenorphine for postoperative analgesia after caesarean section. Acta Anaesthesiol Scand. 1989;33(3):236–8.
9. Matsumoto S, Mitsuhata H, Akiyama H, et al. The effect of subcutaneous administration of buprenorphine with patient controlled analgesia system for post-operative pain relief. Masui. 1994;43(11):1709–13 (The Japanese Journal of Anesthesiology, in Japanese).
10. Varrassi G, Marinangeli F, Ciccozzi A, et al. Intra-articular buprenorphine after knee arthroscopy. A randomized, prospective, double-blind study. Acta Anaesthesiol Scand. 1999;43(1):51–5.
11. Candido K, Winnie A, Ghaleb A, et al. Buprenorphine added to the local anesthetic for axillary brachial plexus block prolongs postoperative analgesia. Reg Anesth Pain Med. 2002;27(2): 162–7.
12. Karlsson M, Berggren AC. Efficacy and safety of low-dose transdermal buprenorphine patches (5, 10, and 20 microg/ h) versus prolonged-release tramadol tablets (75, 100, 150, and 200 mg) in patients with chronic osteoarthritis pain: a 12-week, randomized, open-label, controlled, parallel-group non inferiority study. Clin Ther. 2009;31:503–13.
13. Heit H, et al. Dear DEA. Pain Med. 2004;5:306–7.
14. Malinoff HL, et al. Sublingual buprenorphine is effective in the treatment of chronic pain syndrome. Am J Ther. 2005;12:379–84.
15. Budd K, Collett BJ. Old dog, new matrix. Br J Anaesth. 2003;90(6):722–4.
16. Alford D, Compton P, Samet J. Acute pain management for patients receiving maintenance methadone or buprenorphine therapy. Ann Intern Med. 2006;144(2):127–34.
17. Roberts D, Meyer-Witting M. High-dose buprenorphine: perioperative precautions and management strategies. Anaesth Intensive Care. 2005;33(1):17–25.
18. Book S, Myrick H, Malcolm R, et al. Buprenorphine for postoperative pain following general surgery in a buprenorphine-maintained patient. Am J Psychiatry. 2007;164(6):979.
19. Silverman S. Opioid induced hyperalgesia: clinical implications for the pain practitioner. Pain Physician. 2009;12:679–84.
20. Johnson RE, Fudala PJ, Payne R. Buprenorphine: considerations for pain management. J Pain Symptom Manage. 2005;29(3):297–326.

Chapter 24
Opioid-Sparing Drugs (Ketamine, Gabapentin, Pregabalin, and Clonidine)

Jasmina Perinpanayagam, Mohammed Jamil Abu-Asi, Sara Bustamante, and Sreekumar Kunnumpurath

Key Points

- Ketamine
- Physiological systems associated with effects of ketamine
- Gabapentin
- Pregabalin
- Clonidine
- Acute drug abuse
- Chronic drug abuse
- Approach to management
- Pharmacodynamics
- Pharmacokinetics

J. Perinpanayagam, M.B.B.S., B.Sc. (Hons.) (✉) • M.J. Abu-Asi, M.B.B.S., M.R.C.P.
Department of Anaesthetics, Epsom and St. Helier University Hospitals NHS,
Wryth Lane, Carshalton, Surrey SM5 1AA, UK
e-mail: jasmina16@doctors.org.uk; mohammed.abu-asi@doctors.org.uk

S. Bustamante, F.F.P.M.R.C.A., F.R.C.A.
S. Kunnumpurath, M.B.B.S., M.D., F.F.P.M.R.C.A., F.R.C.A., F.C.A.R.C.S.I.
Department of Anaesthetics and Pain Management, Epsom and St. Helier University
Hospitals NHS Trust, Wryth Lane, Carshalton, Surrey SM5 1AA, UK
e-mail: skunnumpurath@gmail.com; skunnumpurath@gmail.com

© Springer Science+Business Media New York 2015
A.D. Kaye et al. (eds.), *Substance Abuse*, DOI 10.1007/978-1-4939-1951-2_24

Ketamine

Background

Pain is defined by the international association for the study of pain (IASP) as "An unpleasant sensory and emotional experience associated with actual or potential tissue damage, or described in terms of such damage" [1] Analgesics are a group of medications which are used by almost every individual at some point in their life and as with any drug have a potential for abuse. Chronic pain patients pose a specific group of individuals who may be at greater risk of drug abuse as a result of their access to certain drugs as well as psychological state. There has been a gradual introduction of new analgesics into medical practice including drugs such as ketamine, gabapentin, pregabalin, and clonidine. Opioids continue to be the mainstay analgesics and the use of opioid sparing drugs has increased [2]. These changes in pain management have led to the need for clinicians to become more familiar with the signs and symptoms of their abuse and this chapter aims to highlight the important issues relating to the more commonly used opioid sparing analgesics. Substance use disorders are strongly associated with major causes of youth mortality [3] and the recent rise in the prevalence of recreational abuse of drugs such as ketamine means that it is the clinician's duty to be aware of their effects and treatment so appropriate management can be given.

Ketamine, a synthetic derivative of phencyclidine is a dissociative anaesthetic agent, which has been used for the induction of general anaesthesia since its development in 1962. It has become one of the fastest growing party drugs with over 125,000 users in the UK [4, 5] and as a result there has been an increase in the number of people presenting to medical professionals with complications due to ketamine abuse [5, 6] highlighting the need for clinicians to be aware of its consequences.

The pharmacological action of ketamine includes reduction of excitatory neurotransmitters such as glutamate by noncompetitive antagonism at NMDA receptors in the central nervous system. It also acts by reducing glutamate release at presynaptic neurones and has a complex interaction with MOP and KOP opioid receptors. Ketamine is cardiovascularly stable causing an increase in heart rate and also stimulates respiration, however, its use as an induction agent in general anaesthesia has gradually declined as a result of adverse psychological effects [7, 8] such as hallucinations, confusion and dissociation in certain patients. Ketamine is still commonly used in the prehospital setting, armed forces, paediatrics, chronic pain, and veterinary medicine.

Ketamine is classified as a class C drug under the Misuse of Drugs Act 2006 [9, 10] and its abuse has been growing recently so much that in 2008 it was shown to be the fastest growing "party drugs" amongst 16–24-year-olds [4]. It is used to produce a range of experiences from sedation, amnesia, and analgesia to hallucinations, confusion, and dissociation [7]. "K-hole" is the term used to describe the intense feeling where the user experiences detachment from their body or a near death experience [7, 9].

In medical practice Ketamine is administered as in intravenous agent, however, in the recreational scenario it is often taken nasally or orally (liquid or smoked) although there are many reports of intravenous and intramuscular injections too [7]. The effects of ketamine are dose dependent and can be classified into various physiological systems as follows [10, 11]:

Neurological

- Flashbacks
- Amnesia
- Dizziness
- Derealisation
- Loss of coordination
- Speech impairment
- Nystagmus
- Delirium (hallucinations or disorientation)
- Feeling invincible
- Aggressive/violent behaviour

Musculoskeletal

- Muscle twitching/rigidity
- Impaired motor function

Cardiorespiratory

- Tachycardia
- Hypertension
- Respiratory depression

Genitourinary

- Haematuria
- Dysuria
- Urgency
- Frequency
- UTIs/Cystitis

Gastrointestinal

- Nausea and vomiting
- Abdominal cramps

Death from Overdose

Individuals who abuse ketamine may present to healthcare providers with a range of clinical signs and symptoms or even as a result of social problems secondary to abuse, which may be acute or long term.

Acute Drug Abuse

In the acute setting ketamine commonly causes neurological features such as confusion, disorientation, amnesia drowsiness and loss of consciousness. In addition, there have been reports of patients presenting with anxiety, chest pain and palpitations [4, 9, 12–14] and even acute dystonic reactions [15], although the latter is a rarer complication. The majority of cases are managed with conservative and supportive care and patients can be discharged after a few hours [12, 14].

Physical signs that can occur with acute ketamine abuse include tachycardia, erythema, nystagmus, speech difficulty, hypertension and arrhythmias. Patients can present with anxiety, depression and feelings of invincibility; which can result in users embarking on a multitude of risk taking behaviours further adding to the list of adverse effects to abusers. Case reports have documented severe agitation and rhabdomyolysis as a result of ketamine abuse [11, 14, 16].

One of the more concerning features of acute ketamine abuse is the psychological state of the user following administration. This can often result in the user being unable to make decisions and loss of motor control, which when combined, can expose them to harm from other individuals and their environment [10].

Chronic Drug Abuse

Chronic use of ketamine has been reported to have significant effects on the urinary system with patients reporting symptoms of cystitis, dysuria, urgency and frequency [5, 9, 12]. The damage can be so severe that patients may require surgical intervention with reports of some individuals undergoing surgical removal of their bladder [9]. In a letter by Cottrell et al. in the BMJ there were reports of an increase in the number of patients presenting to urology services as a result of chronic ketamine use in South West England [6].

Other effects of chronic ketamine use include: abdominal pains known as "K-cramps" [8, 9, 17], biliary tract disease, hepatic dysfunction [8, 17, 18] episodic memory loss [13], and depression [9].

The management of ketamine-induced abdominal pain is again supportive and the key is to stress abstinence from ketamine to improve symptoms. Death is also a real possibility when consistently abusing ketamine.

Ketamine tolerance can develop over a short period of time for individuals who frequently abuse ketamine (daily use) and can result in withdrawal symptoms including nausea, diarrhoea, anxiety, laboured breathing, depression and schizophrenia type behaviour [10, 16].

In the long term there is clear evidence of damage to the urinary tract and bladder. Users may experience pain on urination and blood in the urine, which can lead to permanent bladder damage. Longer-term use can also lead to more persistent depression, lack of energy and anxiety [4].

Approach to Management

Unless clinicians are aware of the effects of ketamine signs and symptoms of ketamine abuse can easily be ignored or mistaken for alternative diagnoses, as they are widespread and nonspecific. A structured approach to history and examination are fundamental to making the diagnosis. Examination should include inspection of the nose to identify white residue, which will help confirm diagnosis.

All patients with the suspected diagnosis should have vital signs recorded, basic investigations; full blood count, urea and electrolytes, liver function tests and electrocardiograph. There is currently no specific investigation for ketamine overdose and again no specific antidote—management is purely supportive.

Gabapentin

Background

Gabapentin was initially developed for the treatment of epilepsy but has recently been increasingly used in the management of neuropathic pain disorders. It is an analogue of GABA and is another opioid sparing drug that has significant potential for abuse.

Gabapentin does not interact with GABA receptors but instead binds to the $\alpha2\delta$ subunit of voltage gated calcium channels resulting in a reduction of monoamine neurotransmitters such as glutamate. The use of the drug in the treatment of neuropathic pain relates to an upregulation of the $\alpha2\delta$ subunit in central sensitisation as a consequence of nerve damage.

Gabapentin has analgesic and anticonvulsive effects and it also produces psychoactive effects including; euphoria, improved sociability, feeling "high", relaxation and sense of calmness [19] which form the basis for its potential as a recreational drug of abuse. Toxic effects include dizziness, ataxia, nystagmus, somnolence, tremor, diplopia, nausea and vomiting, erectile dysfunction and weight gain.

Effects of gabapentin vary according to the demographics of the user, dose, previous experience, psychiatric history and expectations [19]. The particular population groups that have been identified as likely abusers include prison inmates, individuals with a history of drug abuse and in some patients using gabapentin as a treatment for alcohol withdrawal.

Acute Drug Abuse

Signs and symptoms of gabapentin overdose include double vision, slurred speech, drowsiness, lethargy and diarrhoea [20]. The immediate management involves supportive care and if indicated haemodialysis may be used to remove the drug from the patient's system although there are no documented reports of its use in cases of overdose.

Chronic Drug Abuse

Tolerance to gabapentin happens extremely rapidly with recreational use [21] with some patients having to double the dose to achieve the same effect after a few days.

Withdrawal symptoms following abrupt cessation of gabapentin include; sweating, pallor, irritability, agitation, anxiety, tachycardia, palpitations, confusion, disorientation, catatonia [21–23] and even one report of status epilepticus [24].

Approach to Management

Clinicians involved in prescribing gabapentin should take care to prevent and detect addiction and when taking patients off gabapentin the dosage should be gradually tapered, especially when taking high doses. There is no specific antidote for gabapentin overdose and the serious withdrawal effects have led patients to require hospitalisation [22] and as a result risks and benefits should be thoroughly considered prior to prescribing gabapentin.

Pregabalin

Background

Pregabalin was invented by medicinal chemist Richard Bruce Silverman at Northwestern University in the USA. It was designed as a more potent successor to gabapentin. Pregabalin is marketed by Pfizer under the trade name Lyrica®. In 2005 the FDA approved it use for adjunctive therapy in adults with partial onset seizures, management of postherpetic neuralgia and neuropathic pain associated with spinal cord injury and diabetic peripheral neuropathy, perioperative pain and the treatment of fibromyalgia [25]. In 2006 pregabalin had also been approved in the European Union and Russia (but not in USA) for treatment of generalised anxiety disorder as it appears to have anxiolytic effects similar to benzodiazepines [26, 27] The maximum dose of pregabalin depends on its indication but should not exceed 600 mg/day [28].

Clinical studies including 5,500 patients showed that euphoric effects were reported more frequently in pregabalin groups versus placebo (4 % versus 1 %, respectively) [29]. A clinical abuse liability study in 15 drug and alcohol abusers found that pregabalin and diazepam differentiated from placebo consistently and suggested that pregabalin had a potential for euphorigenic activity in susceptible populations [30]. Therefore, pregabalin was scheduled by the US Drug Enforcement Administration as a Schedule V drug, indicating that it had abuse potential [30]. In Canada, it was listed under schedule F, as a "prescription drug" [31].

Pregabalin is classified as a CNS depressant but its potential for abuse is less than the potential with benzodiazepines; additionally the euphoric effects of pregabalin disappear with prolonged use [32]. Although pregabalin appears to have low potential for abuse, certain populations may be more liable to abuse or misuse. Further psychopharmacological studies with pregabalin are needed, including assessing its abuse liability across a range of doses in sedative abusers, as well as testing the drug in combination with other CNS-active drugs and alcohol within the same subject population.

Pharmacodynamics

Pregabalin is an analogue of γ-aminobutyric acid, a major inhibitory neurotransmitter in the brain. It does not bind at γ-aminobutyric acid, benzodiazepine, or opioid receptors. Pregabalin binds to the $\alpha_2\delta$ (alpha-2-delta) subunit of the voltage-dependent calcium channel in the central nervous system. Pregabalin decreases the release of neurotransmitters including glutamate, norepinephrine, substance P and calcitonin gene-related peptide. Pregabalin neither binds directly nor augments $GABA_A$ currents or affects GABA metabolism. The half-life for pregabalin is 6.3 h.

Pharmacokinetics

Absorption: Pregabalin is rapidly absorbed when administered on an empty stomach, with peak plasma concentrations occurring within 1 h. Pregabalin oral bioavailability is estimated to be greater than or equal to 90 % and is independent of dose.

Distribution: Pregabalin has been shown to cross the blood–brain barrier in mice, rats, and monkeys. Pregabalin has been shown to cross the placenta in rats and is present in the milk of lactating rats. In humans, the volume of distribution of pregabalin for an orally administered dose is approximately 0.56 L/kg and is not bound to plasma proteins [33].

Metabolism: undergoes negligible metabolism in humans. The major metabolite is
N-methylpregabalin.

Excretion: eliminated from systemic circulation primarily by renal excretion as
unchanged drug.

Acute Drug Abuse

According to pregabalin users different dosages are associated with a vast range of
effects (online report):

- 200 mg: dizziness.
- 600 mg: stumbling, disorientation, increased physic and psychological awareness, difficulty to drive, slurred and broken speech, hearing and visual altera-
  tions/hallucinations, double and blurred vision, uninhibited behaviours,
  talkativeness, increased body energy, increased sexual performances.
- 900 m: strong feelings of drunkenness, difficulty to walk, alterations of colours
  perception, little euphoria.
- 1,200 mg: drowsiness, euphoria, entactogenic feelings, (feelings of empathy).
- >1,500 mg (to 5 g): uncontrollable drowsiness, frequent hallucinations, great
  euphoria, frequent dissociative events, behavioural inhibition, anxiety and necessity to move.

Acute overdosage may be manifested by somnolence, tachycardia and hypertonicity [34–36]. In one case series [37], sixty percent of patients presented to the ED
with seizures and 20 % required ICU admission. Plasma, serum or blood concentrations of pregabalin may be measured to monitor therapy or to confirm a diagnosis of
poisoning in hospitalised patients. There is no specific antidote. If the overdose was
recent elimination of any unabsorbed drug might be attempted by giving medications to induce vomiting or gastric pumping. Emergency staff should contact the
National Poisons Information Service/TOXBASE. As with all emergencies and
"ABCDE" approach should be adopted and early contact with specialist's help
should be sought if patients are clinically deteriorating.

Chronic Drug Abuse

Pregabalin may also cause withdrawal effects after long-term use if discontinued
abruptly. When prescribed for seizures, quitting "cold turkey" can increase the
strength of the seizures and possibly cause the seizures to reoccur. Withdrawal
symptoms include restlessness, insomnia, anxiety, headache, nausea, depression,
pain, hyperhidrosis and dizziness. Pregabalin should be reduced gradually when
finishing treatment.

Several renal failure patients developed myoclonus while receiving pregabalin,
apparently as a result of gradual accumulation of the drug [34–36].

Approach to Management

As with any CNS-active drug, carefully evaluate patients for history of drug abuse and observe them for signs of pregabalin misuse or abuse (e.g. development of tolerance, dose escalation, drug-seeking behaviour). Patients at a heightened level of risk, in terms of developing abuse or dependence with pregabalin, seem to be those who have had a prior history of substance use disorder. On this basis, clinicians should be mindful, in their therapeutic treatment of patients presenting to addiction services, of the potential for abuse/dependence in relation to pregabalin and the associated complex difficulties that may be encountered should such abuse/dependence develop.

Clonidine

Background

Clonidine has been investigated and prescribed first as an antihypertensive drug in the 1950s. It has found new uses later, including treatment of some types of neuropathic pain, opioid detoxification, sleep hyperhidrosis, and as veterinary anaesthetic drug. Clonidine is used to treat anxiety and panic disorder. It is also FDA approved to treat ADHD in an extended release form [38]. It is becoming a more accepted treatment for insomnia, as well as for relief of menopausal symptoms.

Clonidine also has several off-label uses, and has been prescribed to treat psychiatric disorders including stress, sleep disorders, and hyperarousal caused by post-traumatic stress disorder, borderline personality disorder, and other anxiety disorders [39–45]. Clonidine is also a mild sedative, and can be used as premedication before surgery or procedures [41].

Pharmacodynamics

Clonidine is a centrally acting α-adrenergic receptor agonist with more affinity for α_2 than α_1. It selectively stimulates α_2-receptors in the brain, which decreases peripheral vascular resistance, lowering blood pressure. It has specificity towards the presynaptic α_2-receptors in the vasomotor centre in the brainstem. This binding decreases presynaptic calcium levels, thus inhibiting the release of norepinephrine. The net effect is a decrease in sympathetic tone [42].

It has also been proposed that the antihypertensive effect of clonidine is due to agonism on the I_1-receptor (imidazoline receptor), which mediates the sympatho-inhibitory actions of imidazolines to lower blood pressure [43].

Pharmacokinetics [38]

Bioavailability: 75–85 % (immediate release), 89 % (extended release)
Protein binding: 20–40 %

Metabolism: Hepatic to inactive metabolites
Half-life: 12–16 h
Excretion: urine (72 %)

Acute Drug Abuse

Clonidine may cause lightheadedness, dry mouth, dizziness and constipation. Clonidine may also cause hypotension [44].

Clonidine also has peripheral α-agonist activity, which can lead to hypertension—especially when it is injected intravenously. This blood pressure increase is sometimes witnessed in cases of overdose in children. As clonidine is eliminated by the body, the peripheral effects wear off and its basic hypotensive effect becomes evident. Both the hypertensive and hypotensive effects can be harmful.

Chronic Drug Abuse

The high prevalence of illicit clonidine use by opiate-abusing individuals raises a number of clinical concerns. High costs for clonidine urinalysis assays make routine screening impractical. If clinicians are unaware of the concurrent use of clonidine by opiate-addicted individuals, they may not prescribe the appropriate treatment for management of opiate detoxification, overdose, or withdrawal. Pharmacologically, clonidine use can result in marked sedation. Abrupt cessation of clonidine use can produce rebound hypertension and other symptoms of withdrawal (e.g. nervousness, headache, tachycardia, sweating).

If clonidine is suddenly withdrawn the sympathetic nervous system will revert to producing high levels of epinephrine and norepinephrine, higher even than before treatment, causing rebound hypertension. Rebound hypertension can be avoided by slowly withdrawing treatment.

Clonidine is classed by the FDA as pregnancy category C. It is not known whether clonidine is harmful to an unborn baby. Additionally, clonidine can pass into breast milk and may harm a nursing baby. Therefore, caution is warranted in women who are pregnant, planning to become pregnant, or who are breastfeeding [45].

Approach to Management

As with any CNS-active drug, carefully evaluate patients for history of drug abuse and observe them for signs of clonidine misuse or abuse (e.g. development of tolerance, dose escalation, drug-seeking behaviour). Patients at a heightened level of risk, in terms of developing abuse or dependence with pregabalin, seem to be those who have had a prior history of substance use disorder.

References

1. IASP. Part III: pain terms, a current list with definitions and notes on usage. In: Merskey H, Bogduk N, editors. Classification of chronic pain, IASP Task Force on Taxonomy. 2nd ed. Seattle: IASP; 1994. p. 209–14.
2. Power I. An update on analgesics. Br J Anaesth. 2011;107(1):19–24.
3. Kaplan G, Ivanov I. Pharmacotherapy for substance abuse disorders in adolescence. Pediatr Clin North Am. 2011;58(1):243–58.
4. Ketamine [Internet]. 2013. http://www.bdp.org.uk/pages/druginfo-ketamine [cited 2013 Nov 10].
5. Rickman D. Ketamine reality [Internet]. 2010. http://www.theguardian.com/society/2010/apr/02/drugs-ketamine-bladder-problems-incontinence [updated 2010 Apr 1; cited 2013 Nov 16].
6. Cottrell AM, Athreeres R, Weinstock P, Warren K, Gillatt D. Urinary tract disease associated with chronic ketamine use. BMJ. 2008;336:973.
7. Lankenau SE, Clatts MC. Ketamine injection among high risk youth: preliminary findings from New York City. J Drug Issues. 2002;32(3):893–905.
8. Ng SH, Tse ML, Ng HW, Lau FL. Emergency department presentation of ketamine abusers in Hong Kong: a review of 233 cases. Hong Kong Med J. 2010;16:6–11.
9. Ketamine [Internet]. 2011. http://www.drugscope.org.uk/resources/drugsearch/drugsearch-pages/ketamine [Updated 2011 Nov; cited 2013 Nov 16].
10. Ketamine [Internet]. 2013. http://www.cesar.umd.edu/cesar/drugs/ketamine.asp [Updated 2013 Oct 29; cited 2013 Nov 10].
11. The Maryland Drug Early Warning System (DEWS). DEWS alert: ketamine. College Park: Centre for Substance Abuse Research (CESAR), University of Maryland; 1999. p. 22.
12. Yiu-Cheung C. Acute and chronic toxicity pattern in ketamine abusers in Hong Kong. J Med Toxicol. 2012;8(3):267–70.
13. Morgan CJ, Curran HV. Acute and chronic effects of ketamine upon human memory: a review. Psychopharmacology (Berl). 2006;188(4):408–24.
14. Weiner AL, Vieira L, McKay CA, Bayer MJ. Ketamine abusers presenting to the Emergency Department: a case series. J Emerg Med. 2006;18(4):447–51.
15. Fesler JM, Orban DJ. Dystonic reaction after ketamine abuse. Ann Emerg Med. 1982;11(12):673–5.
16. Ketamine abuse causes, statistics, addiction signs, symptoms and side effects. 2013. [Updated 2013 Aug 13; cited 2013 Nov 10].
17. Turkish A, Luo JJ, Lefkowitch JH. Ketamine abuse, biliary tract disease, and secondary sclerosing cholangitis. Hepatology. 2013;58:825–7.
18. Wood D, Cottrell A, Baker SC, Southgate J, Harris M, Fulford S, Woodhouse C, Gillatt D. Recreational ketamine: from pleasure to pain. BJU Int. 2011;107:1881–4.
19. Webb J. Gabapentin—another drug of misuse? BCPhA. 2008;17(3):12–3.
20. Neurontin [Internet]. 2013. http://www.rxlist.com/neurontin-drug/overdosage-contraindications.htm [updated 2013 Mar 6; cited 2013 Nov 16].
21. Hellwig TR, Hammerquist R, Termaat J. Withdrawal symptoms after gabapentin discontinuation. Am J Health Syst Pharm. 2010;67(11):910–2.
22. Gabapentin and pregabalin: abuse and addiction. Prescrire Int. 2012; 21(128):152–4.
23. Norton JW. Gabapentin withdrawal syndrome. Clin Neuropharmacol. 2001;24:245–6.
24. Barrueto F, Green J, Howland MA, Hoffman RS, Nelson LS. Gabapentin withdrawal presenting as status epilepticus. Clin Toxicol. 2002;40(7):925–8.
25. Pregabalin [Internet]. Pfizer to pay $2.3 billion to resolve criminal and civil health care liability relating to fraudulent marketing and the payment of kickbacks. 2013. http://www.stopmedicarefraud.gov/west.pdf [updated 2009 Oct 15; cited 2013 November 18].
26. Pregabalin [Internet]. Pfizer's Lyrica approved for the treatment of generalized anxiety disorder (GAD) in Europe. 2013. http://www.medicalnewstoday.com/releases/40404.php [updated 2006 Mar 28; cited 2013 Nov 18].
27. Bandelow B, Wedekind D, Leon T. Pregabalin for the treatment and generalized anxiety disorder: a novel pharmacologic intervention. Expert Rev Neurother. 2007;7(7):769–81.

28. Filipetto FA, Zipp CP, Coren JS. Potential for pregabalin abuse or diversion after past drug-seeking behavior. J Am Osteopath Assoc. 2010;110(10):605–7.
29. Lyrica [Internet]. Highlights of prescribing information. 2013. http://labeling.pfizer.com/ ShowLabeling.aspx?id=561 [updated 2011 June 1; cited 2013 Nov 16].
30. Lyrica [Internet]. Center for Drug Evaluation and Research, U.S. Food and Drug Administration. Medical review(s). 2013. http://www.fda.gov/downloads/drugs/drugsafety/ucm152825.pdf [updated 2012 June; cited 2013 Nov 16].
31. Pregabalin [Internet]. Drug product database online query. 2013. http://webprod3.hc-sc.gc.ca/ dpd-bdpp/index-eng.jsp [updated 2009; cited 2013 Nov 21].
32. Chalabianloo F, Schjøtt J. Pregabalin and its potential for abuse. J Norweg Med Assoc. 2009;129(3):186–7.
33. Pregabalin [Internet]. Summary of product characteristics. European Medicines Agency; 2013. http://www.ema.europa.eu/docs/en_GB/document_library/EPAR_Product_Information/ human/000546/WC500046602.pdf [updated 2013 Mar 6; cited 2013 Nov 16].
34. Murphy NG, Mosher L. Severe myoclonus from pregabalin (Lyrica) due to chronic renal insufficiency. Clin Toxicol. 2008;46:594.
35. Yoo L, Matalon D, Hoffman RS, Goldfarb DS. Treatment of pregabalin toxicity by hemodialysis in a patient with kidney failure. Am J Kidney Dis. 2009;54(6):1127–30.
36. Baselt RC. Disposition of toxic drugs and chemicals in man. 8th ed. Foster City: Biomedical Publications; 2008. p. 1296–7.
37. Millar J, Sadasivan S, Weatherup N, Lutton S. Lyrica nights-recreational pregabalin abuse in an urban emergency department. Emerg Med J. 2013;30:874.
38. Clonidine [Internet]. 2013. http://reference.medscape.com/drug/catapres-tts-clonidine-342382 [updated 2007 Dec 1; cited 2013 Nov 10].
39. Ziegenhorn A, Roepke S, Schommer N, Merkl A, Danker-Hopfe H, Perschel F, Heuser I, Anghelescu I, Lammers C. Clonidine improves hyperarousal in borderline personality disorder with or without comorbid posttraumatic stress disorder: a randomized, double-blind, placebo-controlled trial. J Clin Psychopharmacol. 2009;29(2):170–3.
40. Clonidine [Internet]. Understanding comorbid depression and anxiety. 2013. http://www.psy-chiatrictimes.com/articles/understanding-comorbid-depression-and-anxiety. [updated 2007 Dec 1; cited 2013 Nov 10].
41. Fazi L, Jantzen EC, Rose JB, Kurth CD, Watcha MF. A comparison of oral clonidine and oral midazolam as preanesthetic medications in the paediatric tonsillectomy patient. Anesth Analg. 2001;92(1):56–61.
42. Shen H. Illustrated pharmacology memory cards: pharmnemonics. Minireview; 2008. p. 12. Minireview; 1st edition (16 Feb 2007).
43. Reis DJ, Piletz JE. The imidazoline receptor in control of blood pressure by clonidine and allied drugs. Am J Physiol. 1997;273(5):1569–71.
44. Hossmann V, Maling TJ, Hamilton CA, Reid JL, Dollery CT. Sedative and cardiovascular effects of clonidine and nitrazepam. Clin Pharmacol Ther. 1980;28(2):167–76.
45. Clonidine [Internet]. Prescription marketed drugs. 2013. http://www.drugsdb.eu/drug.php?d= Clonidine&m=Physicians%20Total%20Care,%20Inc.&id=b65742b7-5db5-41cf-bf69-41700cdd2c59.xml [updated 2009 Aug; cited 2013 Nov 13].

Chapter 25
Substance Abuse Recovery Groups

Anjuli Desai and Frank John English Falco

Key Points

- Physical dependence
- Tolerance
- Addiction
- Pseudo addiction
- Signs of drug abuse on physical examination
- Specific Groups for Substance Abuse

Introduction

Substance abuse is a broad term encompassing tobacco, alcohol, marijuana, heroin, cocaine, methamphetamines, and narcotics, as well as more rare substances such as bath salts, which may be inhaled, smoked, injected, or swallowed in order to obtain a feeling of euphoria. Substance abuse is the number one cause of preventable illness and death in the United States. Every year, more than 500,000 deaths in the United States

A. Desai, M.D. (✉)
Department of Pain Medicine, Temple University Hospital,
3401 North Broad Street, Philadelphia, PA 21921, USA
e-mail: julidahiya@yahoo.com

F.J.E. Falco, M.D.
Mid Atlantic Spine and Pain Physicians, Newark, DE, USA

American Society of Interventional Pain Physicians, Paducah, KY, USA

Temple University Medical School, Philadelphia, PA, USA

Pain Medicine Fellowship Program, Temple University Hospital,
139 East Chestnut Hill Rd., 19713 Newark, DE, USA
e-mail: cssm01@aol.com

© Springer Science+Business Media New York 2015
A.D. Kaye et al. (eds.), *Substance Abuse*, DOI 10.1007/978-1-4939-1951-2_25

occur secondary to the abuse of alcohol, tobacco, or the other drugs listed above. Of all of these, alcohol is the most commonly abused psychoactive substance [1].

There are several aspects of medication use that patients and their treating clinicians should be familiar with when prescribing any medication. Below are general definitions of such concepts.

Physical Dependence: a physiologic state initiated by a sudden dose decrease or termination of opioid treatment which causes the patient to experience withdrawal symptoms.

Tolerance: a physiologic state created when a patient is treated with chronic opioids in which a higher dose may be needed to achieve the equivalent analgesic effect.

Addiction: a "neurobiological disease" with psychological, social, genetic, and environmental factors in which the patient may exhibit drug-seeking behaviors, diminished control over their drug use, cravings, compulsive behaviors, and repeated use despite negative consequences.

Pseudo addiction: an iatrogenic condition of abnormal patient behavior, often exhibited as exaggerated pain behavior, which develops as a direct result of inadequate pain management [1].

The healthcare professional's role with every patient population also includes proper screening to recognize substance abuse. If you are concerned that your patient may be abusing an illicit substance, there are certain signs that you can look for in their history, physical examination, and review of medical records. On clinical history, the patient may report that their medications were lost or stolen, or they may frequently request early refills or dose increases. Screening for drug and alcohol disorders can be incorporated into the healthcare professional's routine history taking, and can be supplemented with more objective tests such as urine drug screens or blood tests. When taking a history, it is important to remain empathetic, and use a direct approach to inquire about the amount and frequency of substance use. By doing so, the healthcare professional can obtain a sense of the severity of substance abuse, and thus tailor the treatment approach accordingly. The "CAGE" questionnaire was developed in 1970 by Dr. John A. Ewing to assess for alcoholism, but this general questionnaire can be applied to any illicit substance. The CAGE questionnaire is shown below:

1. Have you ever felt that you should cut down on your drinking or drug use?
2. Have people ever annoyed you by criticizing you're drinking or using drug?
3. Have you ever felt bad or guilty about your drinking or drug use?
4. Have you ever had a drink or used drugs first thing in the morning to steady your nerves, to get rid of a hangover or to get the day started?

A positive response to two or more of the above questions suggests the need for additional assessment for possible substance abuse [2].

On physical examination, the patient may have unkempt appearance, appear intoxicated or sedated, or exhibit evidence of drug use, such as track marks. Below are signs often seen on physical examination with the abuse of certain drugs:

Marijuana:

- Glassy, red eyes; loud talking, inappropriate laughter followed by sleepiness; loss of interest, motivation; weight gain; poor memory; paranoid thoughts.

Barbiturates and Benzodiazepines: e.g. alprazolam (Xanax), diazepam (Valium), clonazepam (Klonopin), gamma-hydroxybutyric acid (GHB)

- Contracted pupils; difficulty concentrating; poor judgment; sleepiness; lack of coordination; poor memory; slowed breathing, and decreased blood pressure.

Stimulants: e.g. cocaine, crystal methamphetamine, methylphenidate (Ritalin)

- Dilated pupils; hyperactivity; euphoria; irritability; anxiety; excessive talking followed by depression or excessive sleeping at odd times; weight loss; nasal congestion or dry oral mucosa; increased heart rate, blood pressure, and temperature.

Inhalants: e.g. glue, paint thinner, gasoline, cleaning fluid, household aerosols, vapors

- Watery eyes; impaired vision, memory and thought; secretions from the nose or rashes around the nose and mouth; headaches, nausea; drowsiness; poor muscle control; changes in appetite; anxiety; irritability.

Hallucinogens: e.g. lysergic acid diethylamide (LSD), phencyclidine (PCP)

- Hallucinations, reduced perception of reality (e.g. "hearing colors"), rapid heart rate, high blood pressure, tremors, flashbacks.

Club Drugs: e.g. ecstasy, rohypnol, ketamine

- Euphoria, reduced inhibitions, decreased coordination, poor judgment, poor memory, increased or decreased heart rate and blood pressure, drowsiness.

Opioid Analgesics: morphine, fentanyl, dilaudid, oxycodone, heroin* (discussed below)

- Sedation, depression, confusion, constipation, slowed breathing.

Heroin:

- Contracted pupils; no response of pupils to light; needle marks; sleeping at unusual times; sweating; vomiting; coughing, sniffling; twitching; loss of appetite [3].

Upon review of the patient's medical records, you may find evidence that they are obtaining their medications from multiple pharmacies or prescribers. A urine drug screen or oral swab can help to confirm inconsistent medication use, or the presence of illicit substances.

In order to effectively recognize or screen for possible substance abuse in your patient population, it is also essential to understand the demographics most often affected by substance abuse. Individuals between the ages of 18 and 25 are the most likely group to use illicit drugs, and the age that an adolescent begins to use alcohol and illicit drugs is a strong predictor of later alcohol and drug abuse issues. Typically, adolescents first use alcohol and tobacco, and then progress to marijuana and other illicit substances [1].

On the other end of the spectrum, the elderly are also prone to substance abuse, as they have a higher incidence of chronic painful physical conditions which may require the use of high-dose analgesic medications. Additionally, the elderly are more vulnerable to addiction secondary to depression, anxiety, and anger in regards to the aging process [1].

Once you have verified that your patient is abusing a substance, such as those mentioned above, you should review your medication contract and discuss alternative therapies. These may include nonnarcotic medications, physical and occupational therapy, acupuncture and massage, and modalities such as transcutaneous electrical stimulation (TENS) units. If the patient is not interested in pursuing these alternate therapies or discontinuing use of the illicit substance, you should discuss the various facilities and programs available for them to address their addiction and seek treatment.

If the patient is willing to discuss alternative treatment options, it may be beneficial to provide an explanation of what they should expect from a substance abuse facility.

There are numerous facilities available for patients. The Substance Abuse Facility Locator is a useful website used to locate alcohol and drug abuse treatment facilities around the country. The following website can be provided to the patient: http://findtreatment.samhsa.gov. The patient should also be made aware of the various types of groups available for substance abuse, with most of them being based on the type of illicit substance being abused. Below is a list of a few of the major groups available and a very brief overview of what they offer.

Specific Groups for Substance Abuse

Alcoholics Anonymous (AA) is a 12-step recovery group of men and women who share their experiences and strengths with each other with the common goal of quitting alcohol consumption. Membership to AA is free of charge, and is based on spirituality with no religious base. For more information, patients and healthcare professionals can visit www.aa.org [4].

Cocaine Anonymous (CA) is a 12-step recovery group for individuals who desire to stop using cocaine or other mind-altering substances. Membership in CA is free and there is no affiliated politics, religion, organization, or denomination. For more information, patients and healthcare professionals can visit www.ca.org [5].

Heroin Anonymous (HA) is a 12-step recovery group for individuals who desire to stop using heroin. Membership to HA is free of charge and there is no affiliated political, religious, or denominational base. For more information, patients and healthcare professionals can visit www.heroinanonymous.org [6].

Crystal Methamphetamine (CM) is another commonly abused substance. The Rehab International program is one of many available for CM abuse. The Rehab International program uses the Matrix Model to treat its patients. This model generally lasts 16 weeks, and involves various modalities of help. A CM abuser may work with a counselor to learn about addiction for part of the week, and then engage in group sessions with other CM abusers for the remainder of the week. During this time, he or she may be randomly drug tested to assess for a possible relapse, and if positive, he or she would be sent to the relapse prevention group. This model varies from others in that the CM abuser spends significant time in multiple types of groups. For more information, patients and healthcare professionals can visit http://rehab-international.org/crystal-meth-rehab-guide/ or www.crystalmeth.org [7, 8].

Marijuana Anonymous (MA) is a 12-step recovery group for individuals who desire to stop using marijuana. Membership to MA is free of charge and there is no affiliated political, religious or denominational base. For more information, patients and healthcare professionals can visit https://www.marijuana-anonymous.org/ [9].

Nicotine Anonymous is a 12-step recovery group for individuals who desire to stop using nicotine. Membership to Nicotine Anonymous is free of charge and there is no affiliated political, religious or denominational base. For more information, patients and healthcare professionals can visit http://www.nicotine-anonymous.org/ [10].

Narcotics Anonymous (NA) is a 12-step recovery group for individuals who desire to stop using any drugs or alcohol. Membership to NA is free of charge and there is no affiliated political, religious or denominational base. For more information, patients and healthcare professionals can visit http://www.na.org [11].

Pills Anonymous is another 12-step recovery group for individuals who desire to stop using pills or other mind-altering substances. Membership in Pills Anonymous is free and there is no affiliated politics, religion, organization, or denomination. For more information, patients and healthcare professionals can visit http://www.pillsanonymous.org/ [12].

Women for Sobriety (WFS) is a non-profit organization for women who strive to overcome alcoholism or addiction to other mind-altering substances. WFS has self-help groups which are based upon a Thirteen Statement Program which encourages emotional and spiritual growth. Membership to WFS is free and there is no affiliated politics, religion, organization, or denomination. For more information, patients and healthcare professionals can visit http://www.womenforsobriety.org [13].

Oftentimes, patients may relapse and present back to the healthcare professional seeking advice. With any chemical dependency, relapsing is the act of taking the first drink or using the first drug after a period of being intentionally clean and sober for a certain time period. Relapsing is often caused by a combination of factors, and the healthcare professional can watch for certain warning signs. Some of these warning signs include the patient reporting that they are spending more time with individuals that may be involved with substance abuse. Alternatively, they may report that they are isolating themselves by not attending their support group meetings. Other patients may present with a sense of overconfidence, stating that they no longer need support, and others may set unrealistic goals and feel overwhelmed. As a healthcare professional, it is essential to take notice of these early warning signs to help prevent relapse in this patient population.

References

1. http://healthsciences.utah.edu/utahaddictioncenter/healthcare_professionals/Training_Modules/module1.htm
2. Ewing JA. Detecting alcoholism: the CAGE questionnaire. JAMA. 1984;252(14):1905–7.
3. http://www.mayoclinic.com/health/drug-addiction/DS00183
4. http://www.aa.org
5. http://www.ca.org

6. http://www.heroinanonymous.org
7. http://rehab-international.org/crystal-meth-rehab-guide/
8. http://www.crystalmeth.org
9. https://www.marijuana-anonymous.org/
10. http://www.nicotine-anonymous.org/
11. http://www.na.org
12. http://www.pillsanonymous.org/
13. http://www.womenforsobriety.org

Chapter 26
Relaxation Techniques

Kareem Hubbard and Frank John English Falco

Key Points

- Relaxation techniques
- Autogenic training
- Hypnosis
- Guided imagery
- Meditation
- Yoga
- Progressive muscle relaxation

Relaxation techniques have been around as long as there has been stress in people's lives. When stressful situations present themselves whether one takes deep breaths to relax, meditates, or imagines a pleasant place or experience, these methods have been in existence since the beginning of time. Although these techniques, or training for relaxation, have been in existence it has only been recently that the western medical community has been accepting of them. Now that the greater medical community has gained acceptance of these relaxation techniques, many practitioners find it difficult to understand the utility and/or how to incorporate these methods into treatment plans. This chapter will help educate and guide medical practitioners

K. Hubbard, M.D. (✉)
Redwood Medical Center, 20439 Glasgow Dr., Saratoga, Pleasanton, CA 95070, USA
e-mail: khubbard@redwoodmedicalcenter.com

F.J.E. Falco, M.D.
Mid Atlantic Spine and Pain Physicians, Newark, DE, USA

American Society of Interventional Pain Physicians, Paducah, KY, USA

Temple University Medical School, Philadelphia, PA, USA

Pain Medicine Fellowship Program, Temple University Hospital,
139 East Chestnut Hill Road, 19713 Newark, DE, USA
e-mail: cssm01@aol.com

© Springer Science+Business Media New York 2015
A.D. Kaye et al. (eds.), *Substance Abuse*, DOI 10.1007/978-1-4939-1951-2_26

about relaxation techniques and how they can be implemented in one's treatment plans and goals.

Relaxation techniques have been used to relieve stress, improve concentration, improve performance, relieve anxiety, alleviate pain, and even help treat medical ailments. Relaxation techniques can be as simple as taking a quick moment to recite a quick chant or prayer. Techniques can also be as profound as setting an ambience with candles, music, fragrances, and performing choreographed maneuvers and positions. The overall goal of relaxation techniques is to help alter and improve one's emotional, psychological, physical, and physiological well-being.

Stress is known to be a precipitating factor in the development and progression of many psychological conditions and ailments. Not only that, but it is well documented that stress also can negatively affect one's existing medical conditions. From raising one's blood pressure to causing headaches, stress is definitely a factor in one's overall health whether it is physiological, physical, or mental health. Stress can cause individuals to act impulsively or out of character in an attempt to deal with their stressors. The majority of people engage in healthy outlets for stress. Though most people participate in a positive means to relieve their stress, a subset of the population do turn to alcohol and or substances of abuse as a means of coping with their stress. Many times these individuals site the quick release alcohol and drugs offer them to escape from their stress and daily problems. Though there are many contributing factors that lead to alcohol and substance abuse, stress is likely one of the main contributing factors that leads to the transition from recreational use to abuse.

One's ability to manage stress and or "triggers" is imperative for individuals suffering from alcohol or drug dependence. The "ability to control" ones stressors or triggers could make all the difference in the world for someone who is struggling to break free from the grips of substance abuse. Mastery of relaxation techniques can help one overcome stress to make rational decisions in the face of drug and/or alcohol relapse.

Among practitioners, one of the most under used adjunct treatment options for substance abuse is relaxation techniques. As mentioned previously, stress and coping behaviors have important implications for the initiation or progression of many major diseases [1]. Before any treatment plan is considered, individuals with issues of substance abuse should first be meticulously assessed. The underlying and physiological causes of substance abuse must be addressed, though it should be done so in more than a unilateral approach. Once clear understandings of the primary problems are established and basic medical issues addressed, the practitioners should begin to consider relaxation techniques.

Relaxation techniques provide further treatment modalities that a participant can use independently of the practitioner in the daily struggles of addiction. Relaxation techniques or mind-body therapy goals are to help one lower blood pressure, decrease heart rate, calm breathing, reduce muscle tension, and improve clarity of thinking. In the substance abuser, relaxation techniques can be used as a tool in one's arsenal to help manage their body as well as the cravings and the triggers that leads one to abuse.

Relaxation Techniques

Numerous relaxation techniques and combinations of techniques exist that one can use. Nowhere in the literature is there a rule or algorithm per se that one should use when suggesting relaxation techniques. The practitioner must assess which technique or techniques the substance abuser is open minded to and are effective for that particular individual. There are however, major types of relaxation techniques practitioners tend to refer to, highly recognized categories consist of hypnosis and imagery, yoga and meditation, and progressive muscle relaxing. All of these techniques closely parallel autogenic training, which consists of a mixture of physical relaxation and yoga. All types of practitioners can use these techniques, physicians, psychologists, counselors, physical, occupational, speech language pathologists, and even music therapists.

Relaxation training should be tailored to one's individual specifics. Not only should they be tailored to one's individual particular needs, but multiple modalities can and should be combined for optimal results. This relaxation "training" is often thought of as regimented automatic process for the participants; though in actuality these techniques can be implemented in numerous and various ways. One's relaxation process may include music, an image, or a trigger word. When this is the case, often plans are developed to help ensure the participant these tools, devices, or thoughts are readily accessible. The process of these relaxation techniques is not only tailored, but can be very personal to the participant. Relaxation techniques not only can be used to help medical ailments, but have been used for self-improvement and to help overcome phobias. There really are multiple applications to how relaxation techniques can be used in one's life.

Autogenic Training

Autogenic training is a relaxation technique developed by German psychiatrist Johannes Heinrich Schultz and first published in 1932. Autogenic training is very similar to hypnosis and guided imagery; autogenic training uses some of these principles to help achieve a state of relaxation. The technique involves daily sessions that last around 15 min, usually in the morning, at lunch time, and in the evening. During each session, the participant will repeat a set of visualizations that induce a state of relaxation.

Autogenic training has a strong emphasis on focusing on the central nervous system specifically, the sympathetic and parasympathetic nervous systems as a means to control one's emotions and anxiety level. Some of the effects of Autogenic Training is thought to restore the balance between the activity of the sympathetic (flight or fight) and the parasympathetic (rest and digest) branches of the autonomic nervous system. This has important health benefits, as the parasympathetic activity promotes digestion and bowel movements, lowers the blood pressure, slows the heart rate, and promotes the functions of the immune system. Autogenic training has been subject to clinical evaluation from its early days in Germany, and from the early 1980s worldwide. In 2002, a meta-analysis of 60 studies was published in *Applied Psychophysiology and Biofeedback* [2], finding significant positive effects of treatment when compared to normal over a number of diagnoses; these finding effects appear to be similar to best recommended rival therapies; and finding positive additional effects by patients, such as their perceived quality of life.

Hypnosis

Hypnosis is "a special psychological state with certain physiological attributes, resembling sleep only superficially and marked by a functioning of the individual at a level of awareness other than the ordinary conscious state." One theory suggests that hypnosis is a mental state while another theory links hypnosis to imaginative role-enactment [3–5].

A hypnotic procedure is used to encourage and evaluate responses to suggestions. Hypnosis typically involves an introduction to the procedure; this introduction is achieved through hypnotic induction. Hypnotic induction involves a series of preliminary instructions and suggestions [6]. During hypnotic induction, the subject is told that suggestions for imaginative experiences will be presented. The hypnotic induction is an extension of an individual's imagination, and the introduction may contain further elaborations to achieve such state. Although there are many different induction techniques, most include suggestions for relaxation, or instructions to imagine or think about pleasant experiences or feelings of well-being [7, 8]. The most common function of hypnosis is the ability of a trance to facilitate relaxation [7].

Persons under hypnosis are said to have a heightened level of focus and concentration with the ability to concentrate intensely on a specific thought or memory, while blocking out sources of distraction [9]. The hypnotic suggestions may be delivered by a hypnotist in the presence of the subject, or may be self-administered ("self-suggestion" or "autosuggestion"). While the participant is hypnotized, the mental health professional can suggest that they are experiencing changes in sensations, perceptions, thought, and even behavior all go which perceived as real.

A person under hypnosis experiences heightened suggestibility and focus accompanied by a sense of tranquility [10]. It could be said that hypnotic suggestion is explicitly intended to make use of the placebo effect. It is suggested that it explicitly makes use of the placebo effect because it is a method that openly makes use of suggestion and employs methods to amplify its effects [11, 12]. The writings of Freud and his collaborators suggest that gaining a greater understanding of the unconscious motivations of patients facilitates treatment goals [7]. These understandings of a patient's unconscious motivation help manage and direct treatment goals when one is being hypnotized.

Though hypnotism is suggested as a tool a healthcare professional can use to help promote relaxation, a person's ability to be hypnotized or hypnotic susceptibility should be measured. Though there are many hypnotic susceptibility scales one of the most recognized was developed by Andre Weitzenhoffer and Ernest R. Hilgard in 1959, the Stanford Scale of Hypnotic Susceptibility, it consists of 12 suggested test items following a standardized hypnotic eye-fixation induction script. This has become one of the most widely referenced research tools in the field of hypnosis. Whereas the older "depth scales" tried to infer the level of "hypnotic trance" based upon supposed observable signs, such as spontaneous amnesia, most subsequent scales measure the degree of observed or self-evaluated responsiveness to specific suggestion tests, such as direct suggestions of arm rigidity (catalepsy).

Most susceptibility scales convert numbers into an assessment of a person's susceptibility as "high," "medium," or "low." Approximately 80 % of the populations are medium, 10 % are high and 10 % are low. These "Hypnotizability" Scores are highly stable over a person's lifetime. Research by Dierdre Barrett has found that there are two distinct types of highly susceptible subjects, which she terms fantasizers and dissociaters. Fantasizers score high on absorption scales, find it easy to block out real-world stimuli without hypnosis, spend much time daydreaming, report imaginary companions as a child and grew up with parents who encouraged imaginary play. Dissociaters often have a history of childhood abuse or other trauma, learned to escape into numbness, and to forget unpleasant events. Their association to "daydreaming" was often going blank rather than vividly recalled fantasies. Both score equally high on formal scales of hypnotic susceptibility [13–15]. Individuals with dissociative identity disorder have the highest hypnotizability of any clinical group, followed by those with posttraumatic stress disorder [16].

Guided Imagery

Guided imagery is a technique used to aid individuals to use mental imagery to help with anything from their bodies to solving problems or reducing stress. Suggestions or "images" are given to an individual by the practitioner. The goal of the directed thought is to guide ones imagination toward a relaxed, focused state. The facilitator uses descriptive language to stimulate one's senses and imagination. This is achieved based on the concept that your mind, body, and senses are all interconnected. There are numerous ways to induce this state other than the use of descriptive words and images.

Music has been known as a powerful tool to enhance the imagery experience by making images more vivid and increasing absorption, or involvement in the imagery [17, 18]. In addition to making images more accessible and vivid, music-evoked images increase duration and quality [17, 19]. Reported benefits included getting in touch with emotions, increased insight, increased relaxation, and spiritual growth [20]. These are some of the same traits needed in managing substance abuse.

Meditation

Meditative practices are derived from traditions in both Eastern and Western cultures, many dating back centuries [21, 22]. Very similar types of meditation exercises are found in most of the world's different religions and cultures [21].

Christian meditation is found in written works throughout its history some dating back to the earliest Christian sects. Meditation practices are also found in Islam and Judaism [21]. Probably the most popular techniques of meditation in the Western world over the last half-century are the Buddhist and Indian forms, including various yoga forms. Though many dogmas of meditation are rooted in religion, there are many different techniques that often are independent of a religious belief system.

Cardoso et al. [23] have also suggested an operational definition of meditation based on several criteria. Their conceptualization requires a mediation technique to be a specific technique, which involves muscle relaxation, "logic relaxation" and produces a self-induced state involving an "anchoring" or self-focusing technique, in order to be considered meditation. Commonly used forms of meditation are: Mindfulness, Vipassana, Transcendental Meditation, Sahaja Yoga, Relaxation Response, Kundalini Yoga, and Meditative Prayer (Table 26.1) [24]. Relaxation techniques do not have to be strictly meditation. Relaxation techniques can be any mental activity or mental procedure that can produce positive emotional or physiologic response.

Yoga

Yoga has become a popular practice in the 1980s due to its link to not only heart and mental health benefits, but overall health benefits in general. Although yoga as we know it today is associated with exercise or a form of alternative medicine, the practice of yoga dates back to the mid-3rd millennium BCE (Before Common Era). Yoga in general is a term for the physical, mental, and spiritual practices or disciplines, which began in India with the objective to attain permanent peace. Its origins exist in the religious beliefs of Hindu, Buddhism, and Jainism.

In the 1980s, Dean Ornish M.D. connected yoga to heart health, legitimizing yoga as a purely physical system of health exercise outside of counter culture and religious denomination. There are many types of yoga (see Table 26.1), the form of yoga focusing on physical and mental strength building is known as Hatha yoga. Hatha yoga and alternate versions of the physical exercises in Hatha yoga have become popular as a kind of low-impact physical exercise, and are used for therapeutic purposes [25].

Some research says that regular yoga practice (at least once weekly) helps to decrease levels of depression significantly. Twice weekly yoga practice for months showed a significant decrease in levels of depression as well as levels of both state and trait anxiety [26]. Some studies also indicate that Hatha yoga has a significant effect on lowering levels of anxiety and accompanying stress. Hatha yoga encourages an increased awareness of breath, internal centering, relaxation, and meditation. These strategies helped participants experience significantly lower stress and anxiety levels in addition to higher quality of life scores [27].

Hatha yoga incorporates asanas, or the body positions, typically associated with the practice of yoga. Asana is now known as a term for various postures useful for

Table 26.1 Multidimensional description of meditation and yoga techniques

Techniques	Physical activity and goal	Mental activity and goal	Additional training content	Authentic	Relaxation response	Duration
Mindfulness meditation	Can be sitting, lying down, or walking	Thoughtless awareness	Varies	Yes	Yes	Varies
Transcendental meditation		Focus on mantra, return to mantra as thoughts stray	Varies	Yes	Yes	Usually suggested 15–20 min twice a day or more
Sahaja yoga	Sitting	Two parts: 1. Thoughtless awareness 2. Self-affirmations	Related to Kundalini tradition and Vipassana	Yes	Yes	Suggested 15 min twice daily
Kundalini yoga	Various combination of breathing patterns, mantras, eye postures, and hand and arm postures, usually sitting	Thoughtless awareness, expansion toward, transcendent states, amelioration of psychiatric symptoms and disorders	Purpose is to access higher levels of spiritual energy	Yes	Varies	Varies
Meditative prayer	Varies	Varies, can include imagery	Varies	Sometimes	Sometimes	Varies
Relaxation response	Sitting	Thoughtless awareness, but varies	None	Yes	Yes	10–20 min one or two times daily
Hatha yoga	Obtaining and maintaining different positions to build strength, flexibility, and balance. Also includes breathing exercises	Varies. Usually a relaxation component. Sometimes combined with more typical meditative techniques	Varies	Sometimes	Varies	Varies

restoring and maintaining a participant's well-being and improving the body's flex-ibility and vitality, with the goal of cultivating the ability to remain in seated medita-tion for extended periods. There have been numerous studies showing the practice of asana and yoga could possibly improve flexibility, strength, balance, reduce stress and anxiety, reduce symptoms of lower back pain, be beneficial for asthma and chronic obstructive pulmonary disease (COPD), increase energy and decrease fatigue, shorten labor and improve birth outcomes, improve physical health and quality of life measures in the elderly, improve diabetes management, reduce sleep disturbances, and reduce hypertension [28–33] With all the possible health benefits of practicing yoga including mental health improvement and stress relief, it is not a far reach for its use in substance abuse management.

Mindfulness based stress reduction (MBSR) programs include yoga as a mind-body technique to reduce stress. A study found that after 7 weeks the group treated with yoga reported significantly less mood disturbance and reduced stress compared to the control coup [34]. Substance abusers who have incorporated yoga into their lifestyle have shown similar positive results in their lives in general. Implementation of the Kundalini Yoga Lifestyle has shown to help substance abuse addicts increase their quality of life according to psychological questionnaires like the Behavior and Symptom Identification Scale and the Quality of Recovery Index [35]. The way that yoga is theorized to improve one's mental states is the increase of GABA levels in the brain. Regular yoga practice increases brain GABA levels and has been shown to improve mood and anxiety [36].

Yoga has reached its highest heights in 2013 when President Barack Obama spoke about yoga in a speech promoting active lifestyles, "Yoga has become a uni-versal language of spiritual exercise in the United States, crossing many lines of religion and culture,"… "Every day, millions of people practice yoga to improve their health and overall well-being."

Progressive Muscle Relaxation

Progressive Muscle Relaxation is a technique for learning to control the state and tension in one's muscles. The technique involves learning when each specific mus-cle group in the body is tense by tensing that muscle group and then letting it go. A patient starts to deliberately contract muscles and hold the tension; secondly they release all tension and focus on the sensation of relaxation.

Regular practice helps patients to recognize tension and to voluntarily relax affected muscles [37]. One has to learn the differences between one's own tensing and an external stress. These learning sessions are not exercises or self-hypnotism. These training sessions are started in a darkened room with the learner in a reclined position and eyes closed. The learner is told to relax, just let go. If the learner has any thoughts or physical distractions, just relax. If the participant is slow in learning how to let the tension go for a particular muscle group, that group is focused on in the next session. The learner is told to continue to practice the relaxation technique in their daily lives. It is not our natural response to relax when there is an external or internal stimulant. However, as in many other physical conditions that we have no control over, the body's best response would be: no response at all [38].

Conclusion

It is unclear, at this point, what are the dominant factors, which lead to substance abuse, whether it is primarily genetics, environment, internal, external, or social pressures more research needs to be done. Since it is more likely than not that substance abuse is due to multiple factors a multidisciplinary approach should be implemented with treatment regardless of the setting. In substance abuse management one must always treat the addiction acutely and manage any foreseeable medical issues.

Once the individual has been medically stabilized, willingness to rehabilitate should be assessed. Determination as to whether an individual is treated in an inpatient or outpatient setting is dictated by an individual's environment and peers. For the severely addicted or individuals with poor social structure, often an inpatient setting is first initially required to help maintain sobriety and rethinking. At this time, it should be explored which relaxation techniques or combination of techniques works best for that particular individual. Once the individual seems highly motivated with a good support structure and a sponsor a transition should take place from inpatient to outpatient treatment.

Treatment teams should be established early in the process and generally should include medical doctors, psychologists, physician assistants, and nurses. Treatment teams should be presumably led by a psychiatrist, though this is not mandated. Substance abuse like many other conditions is likely a multi-factorial cause. For that reason, despite the type of physician leading the treatment team their can and should be consultation from other specialties for management of comorbidities that may lead to relapse.

Once this has been established, relaxation techniques can and should be practiced and reinforced on a continuous basis to further incorporate them into individual's daily lifestyle. It is highly important that these relaxation practices become part of their lifestyle, for fighting substance abuse is a daily battle for most. It is also just as important to provide continuous medical and moral support to establish with the individual that they are not alone in their battle.

Dealing with the day to day struggles of life, it is important for recovering substance abusers to feel empowered over the power of addiction. Relaxation techniques can help provide an individual with one additional tool they can go to that can make the difference between continued sobrieties and relapse.

References

1. Sierpina V, Levine R, Astin J, Tan A. Use of mind-body therapies in psychiatry and family medicine faculty and residents: attitudes, barriers, and gender differences. Explore (NY). 2007;3:12.
2. Stetter F, Kupper S. Autogenic training: a meta-analysis of clinical outcome studies. Appl Psychophysiol Biofeedback. 2002;27(1):45–98.
3. Lynn S, Fassler O, Knox J. Hypnosis and the altered state debate: something more or nothing more? Contemp Hypn. 2005;22:39.
4. Coe W, Buckner L, Howard M, Kobayashi K. Hypnosis as role enactment: focus on a role specific skill. Am J Clin Hypn. 1972;15(1):41–5.
5. Lynn SJ, Rhue JW, editors. Theories of hypnosis: current models and perspectives. New York: Guilford; 1991.
6. New definition: hypnosis division 30 of the American Psychological Association.
7. Newmark TS, Bogacki DF. The use of relaxation, hypnosis, and imagery in sport psychiatry. Clin Sports Med. 2005;24(4):973–7.
8. Begel D, Burton RW. Sports psychiatry: theory and practice. New York: W. W. Norton & Company; 2000.
9. Segi S. Hypnosis for pain management, anxiety and behavioral disorders. Factiva. Retrieved December 7, 2012.
10. Brink TL. Psychology: a student friendly approach. Unit 5: perception; 2008, p. 88.
11. Kirsch I. Clinical hypnosis as a non-deceptive placebo: empirically derived techniques. Am J Clin Hypn. 1994;37(2):95–106.
12. Kirsch I. Clinical hypnosis as a non-deceptive placebo. In: Kirsch I, Capafons A, Cardeña-Buelna E, Amigó S, editors. Clinical hypnosis and self-regulation: cognitive-behavioral perspectives. Washington, DC: American Psychological Association; 1999. p. 211–25.
13. Barrett D. Deep trance subjects: a schema of two distinct subgroups. In: Kunzendorf R, editor. Imagery: recent developments. New York: Plenum; 1991. p. 101–12.
14. Barrett D. Fantasizers and dissociaters: an empirically based schema of two types of deep trance subjects. Psychol Rep. 1992;71(3 Pt 1):1011–4.
15. Barrett D. Fantasizers and dissociaters: two types of high hypnotizable, two imagery styles. In: Kuzendorf R, Spanos N, Wallace B, editors. Hypnosis and imagination. New York: Baywood; 1996.
16. Feuerstein G. The Shambhala guide to yoga. Boston: Shambhala; 1996. p. 26.
17. Quittner A, Glueckauf R. The facilitative effects of music on visual imagery: a multiple measures approach. J Ment Imagery. 1983;7:105–19.
18. Band JB. The influence of selected music and structured vs. unstructured inductions on mental imagery. Unpublished doctoral dissertation, University of South Carolina; 1996.
19. McKinney C, Tims F. Differential effects of selected classical music on the imagery of high versus low imagers: two studies. J Music Ther. 1995;32:22–45.
20. Burns D. The effects of the bonny method of guided imagery and music on the mood and life quality of cancer patients. J Music Ther. 2001;38:51–65.
21. West M, editor. The psychology of mediation. Oxford: Clarendon; 1987.
22. Manocha R. Why meditation? Aust Fam Physician. 2000;29:1135–8.
23. Cardosos R, de Souza E, Camano L, et al. Meditation in health: an operational definition. Brain Res Protocol. 2004;14:58–60.
24. Arias AJ, Steinberg K, Banga A, Trestman RL. Systematic review of the efficacy of meditation techniques as treatments for medical illness. J Altern Complement Med. 2006;12:817–32.
25. Ross A, Thomas S. The health benefits of yoga and exercise: a review of comparison studies. J Alternative Compl Med. 2010;16(1):3–12.
26. Javnbakht M, Hejazi Kenari R, Ghasemi M. Effects of yoga on depression and anxiety of women. Complement Ther Clin Pract. 2000;15(2):102–4.

27. Smith C, Hancook H, Blake-Mortimer J, Ecker K. Randomized comparative trial of yoga and relaxation to reduce stress and anxiety. Complement Ther Med. 2007;15(2):77–83.
28. Thomas RA. The health benefits of yoga and exercise: a review of comparison studies. J Altern Complement Med. 2010;16(1):3–12.
29. Hayes M, Chase S. Prescribing yoga. Prim Care. 2010;37(1):31–47.
30. Alexander GK, Taylor AG, Innes KE, Kulbok P, Selfe TK. Contextualizing the effects of yoga therapy on diabetes management: a review of the social determinants of physical activity. Fam Community Health. 2008;31(3):228–39.
31. Gooneratne NS. Complementary and alternative medicine for sleep disturbances in older adults. Clin Geriatr Med. 2008;24(1):121–38.
32. Silverberg DS. Non-pharmacological treatment of hypertension. J Hypertens Suppl. 1990;8(4): S21–6.
33. Labarthe D, Ayala C. Nondrug interventions in hypertension prevention and control. Cardiol Clin. 2002;20(2):249–63.
34. Smith K, Pukall C. An evidence based review of yoga as complementary intervention for patients with cancer. Psychooncology. 2009;18(5):465–75.
35. Khalsa SB, Khalsa GS, Khalsa HK, Khalsa MK. Evaluation of a residential Kundalini yoga lifestyle pilot program for addiction in India. J Ethn Subst Abuse. 2008;7(1):67–79.
36. Yoga's ability to improve mood and lessen anxiety is linked to increased levels of a critical brain chemical, research finds. Sciencedaily.com. 2010:11–12.
37. Deutsche Gesellschaft Für Allgeminmedizin (DEGAM). Leitlinie Nr. 13- Nachenschmerzen; 2009.
38. Craske M, Barlow D. Worry. New York: Oxford University Press; 2006. p. 53.

Chapter 27
Acupuncture as a Treatment for Substance Abuse in Pediatric Patients

Shu-Ming Wang

Key Points

- What is acupuncture?
- The rises and falls of acupuncture in history
- How does acupuncture work?
- What are the potential mechanisms of acupuncture for substance abuse?
- Acupuncture as treatment for substance abuse disorders
- Dose acupuncture work to treat drug addition?

Background

Adolescence is an important period of physical, psychological, cognitive, and social growth. However, it is also common for adolescence to experiment with substances as part of growing up [1]. Multiple surveys were conducted in a group of adolescences from in United States between 2002 and 2013. The results of these surveys consistently showing a significant and yet progressive increasing number of teens having abused illegal substance and/or nonmedical prescription pain medications despite of multiple task forces have been in place to prevent substance abused. Several risks factors, such as age of early exposure, victims of assault, witness violence familial substance abuse behavior, exposure to violence, compulsive obsessive disorder, depression, anxiety, and/or posttraumatic stress disorder, are linked to substance abuse in adolescences [2]. Teens who abuse substances frequently also suffering from other disorders. Thus when dealing with teens having drug addition or abuse substances, a comprehensive evaluation is necessary prior to prescribing treatment.

S.-M. Wang, M.D. (✉)
Department of Anesthesiology, St. Francis Hospital, Hartford, CT, USA
e-mail: smwang800@gmail.com

© Springer Science+Business Media New York 2015
A.D. Kaye et al. (eds.), *Substance Abuse*, DOI 10.1007/978-1-4939-1951-2_27

Moreover, a workable treatment strategy should be applied to achieve the desirable target in managing teens with drug addition problem. Both pharmacological interventions and several behavioral therapies have shown promising results in treating coexisting conditions among teenage drug abusers. Complementary and alternative treatments such as acupuncture, hypnosis, and meditation also have been used as a treatment and/or an adjunctive treatment for substance abuse as well as psychological illness in these clients [3–6]. The focus of this chapter is to discuss the use of acupuncture as a treatment or adjunctive treatments for addition and its effects.

What is Acupuncture?

Acupuncture is a collection of interventions that have been used to apply stimulation of area/points (acupuncture points) on the body [7]. The stimuli have evolved; they can be pressure, needling, cupping, moxibustion, injection of fluid/medication, electrical stimulation, laser, and most recently ultrasound. Acupuncture was first described in *The Yellow Emperor's Classic of Internal Medicine*, dating from about 100 BCE. Acupuncture was described as an organized system of diagnosis and treatment. The concept of meridians was well developed around that time but the locations of acupuncture were developed later. Acupuncture continued to develop and codify in tests over the subsequent centuries [8]. Gradually, acupuncture became one of the standard therapies used in China along with herbs. The discovery of Bronze statue indicated that acupuncture was taught and standardized in fifteen century [8]. *The Greatest Compendium of Acupuncture and Moxibustion,* which forms the basis of modern acupuncture, was published in Ming Dynasty. In it, a full description of 365 acupuncture points where needles and other stimuli can be applied to modify the flow of "Qi," i.e., vital energy. Chinese believe the vital energy "Qi" is the essence of life, which flows through channels (Meridians) in the body. The rhythmic flow of "Qi" determines the health condition of a person. When a person is ill, the rhythm of Qi disrupted. Acupuncture points are gateways to adjust the rhythm and flow of "Qi". Through application of stimuli at the acupuncture points, the rhythm and flow of Qi can be regulated and health can be restored.

The Rises and Falls of Acupuncture in History

Acupuncture was one of the oldest and standardized therapies, but through seventeenth century onwards, it was regarded as superstitious and irrational. Thus the practice was excluded from Imperial Medical Institute in 1822. The knowledge and skills of acupuncture were retained mainly through rural healers [8]. It is not until late 1966 acupuncture has regained its status as a medical therapy [9]. Chairman Mao revived Traditional Chinese Medicine including acupuncture mainly because a shortage of western trained physicians and health care providers to provide the much needed health care to the general public in China at that time. In 1972, Mr. Reston, a New York Time reporter, accompanying President Nixon to Beijing China. Unfortunately, Mr Reston suffered acute appendicitis and required emergency surgery. Postoperatively, he experienced significant abdomen discomfort. Amazingly, his discomfort was relieved by the insertion of acupuncture needles at elbow and knee as well as the application of moxa nearby the abdomen. As a result of Mr Reston's experience and article in New York Time [10], acupuncture was reintroduced to modern western medical community and has become a mainstream medical intervention. Over the last 4 decades, many clinical studies and scientific research have been conducted to explore the efficacy and underlying mechanism of acupuncture, e.g., the National institutes of Health has funded 200 million per year in acupuncture-related research [11]. To date, World Health Organization (WHO) has identified more than 40 clinical disorders that can benefit from acupuncture [12].

How Does Acupuncture Work?

The mechanism of acupuncture remains unclear; multiple studies suggest an intact nerve pathway that is essential for the effect of acupuncture [12–15]. In mid-1970s, scientist discovered different frequencies of electroacupuncture stimulations resulting in the release of different neurotransmitters [16]. Other studies suggested the involvement of connective tissue [17, 18]. The classic "de QI" sensation is defined as a sensation of soreness, aching, and numbness or distension experienced by patients receiving acupuncture. While the patient experiencing "de Qi" sensation, the acupuncture practitioners also experience "needle got caught (fish took the bait)" sensation. This "de Qi" sensation is found to be a phenomenon related to the fibroblasts entangling with acupuncture needle at the loose connective tissue level [17, 18]. One study shows that acupuncture can contribute to the biochemical balance in the central nervous system to maintain or restore homeostasis [19]. For example, the stimulation applied to stomach 36 acupuncture point can suppress hyperfunction (decreases motility of intestine) or stimulates hypofunction (increases motility of intestine). Although these phenomena may not be fully explained by neurohumoral theory, neurophysiological basis of acupuncture effect is still the most widely accepted theory by the scientific arena.

What are the Potential Mechanisms of Acupuncture for Substance Abuse?

The primary effect of acupuncture is to stimulate relaxation. In addition to reducing withdrawing symptoms, acupuncture provides a strong calming effect on substance abusers and substantially reduces drug craving. Clients describe the effects of acupuncture as allowing them to feel relaxed yet alert. Based on Dr. Smith, the feeling of relaxation induced by acupuncture is the essential benefit of treatment protocol [20].

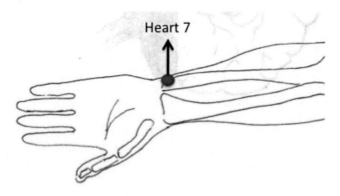

Fig. 27.1 The location of heart-7

Acupuncture is not like methadone maintenance treatment for drug abusers. Acupuncture affects the patient's state of mind during withdrawal, not the body's need for drug [20]. Using rat as model, scientists investigated the effect of acupuncture on anxiety-like behavior and corticotrophin-releasing factor and neuropeptide Y mRNA expression in the amygdala during nicotine withdrawal [21]. The researchers found that acupuncture at heart 7 (HT-7) attenuated anxiety-like behavior during nicotine withdrawal (Fig. 27.1). This anti-withdrawal effect of acupuncture is through the modulation of corticotropin release factor in the amygdala [21]. Zhao and colleague [22] showed acupuncture at HT-7 point significantly prevented a decrease of extracellular dopamine levels in nucleus accumbens during ethanol withdrawal and an increase in accumbal dopamine level related to ethanol challenge. The results of this study provide strong evidence that stimulations applied to HT-7 help normalize the dopamine level in the mesolimbic system following usage or abstentious of ethanol [22]. Utilized animal model, it seems the anti-withdrawal effect of acupuncture is mediated through neurotransmitters. To date, acupuncture is found to exert it's anti-addition/withdrawal effects via different regions of the brain in different types of addiction. Other studies suggested that differential involvement of GABA system in mediating behavioral and neurochemical effect of acupuncture in ethanol-withdrawn rats [23], β-endorphins, and serotonin are thought to be involved in the mechanisms of acupuncture as an adjunctive and/or treatment of drug addition [24].

Acupuncture as Treatment for Substance Abuse Disorders

Acupuncture as treatment for substance abusers was dated back to early 1970 [25]. While Dr. Wen, a neurosurgeon in Hong Kong, was researching the effects of acupuncture for postsurgical pain. He coincidently found that the application of electrical stimulation at the lung point of the external ear relieved opiate withdrawal symptoms. After learning the discovery from Dr. Wen, two detoxification centers in United States started utilizing acupuncture as a treatment for opioid addiction (Fig. 27.2).

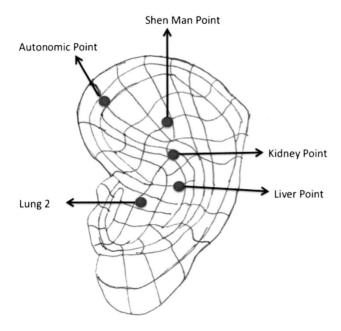

Fig. 27.2 The auricular acupuncture points used for detoxification

One Clinic is located in Bronx NYC, Lincoln Hospital, and another is located in Saint Francisco, Haight Ashbury Free Clinic. Lincoln hospital in New York incorporated the ear lung point with electrical stimulation as an adjunctive treatment for prolonged withdrawal symptoms after a 10-day methadone detoxification cycle in 1974. The protocol consisted of administering acupuncture twice per day in a group setting while tapering methadone doses. The clinicians found that there is reduction in opiate withdrawal symptoms and prolonger program retention [26]. Haight Ashbury Clinic, Saint Francisco, detoxification center was sponsored by funding from Mr. Bill Pone. The detoxification acupuncture treatment protocol at Haight Ashbury clinical was based on individual's signs and symptoms presented. Although early clinical trails and anecdotal reports supported the use of acupuncture a wide variety of randomized controlled clinical trails and outcome summaries of the effects of acupuncture as a detoxification treatment have been controversial [25, 27, 28]. Nevertheless, Dr. M. Smith established the National Acupuncture Detoxification Association (NADA) in 1985 [29]. NADA is a not-for-profit training and advocacy organization. It is funded by the annual membership and fee from trainees learning NADA protocol. The missions of NADA are several: To educate the public about acupuncture as a tool for recovery from drug and alcohol addiction, from trauma and other behavioral health issues; to train health care workers in using NADA detoxification protocol; to offer consultation to local organization in setting up or adapting treatment sites; to offer consultation to other health care advocates in promoting polices and legislation which increase the ability for clients accessing NADA-style treatment, and to distribute NADA-approved reference material and through the newsletter. The NADA protocol consists of 5 designated ear points in each auricle. These five auricular points are lung, shenmen, autonomic point, liver, and kidney. Clinicians trained through NADA learn to insert fine gauge, sterilized, one-time use stainless steel needles into the above five auricular points. Once these needles are in place, they will be kept in place for up to an hour while the patient is asked to stay quiet and relax. In addition, auricular acupuncture also has served as an adjunct to a comprehensive treatment program. The comprehensive treatment program offers the basic therapeutic elements of counseling, education, family involvement, and mutual support group involvement, as well as supportive general health care. The above approach is found to improve program retention rate and enhance the optimistic and cooperative attitude toward the process of recovery as well as reduce craving, anxiety, sleep disturbance, and the consumption of pharmaceuticals. Accordingly to NADA website that more than 2000 clinics worldwide since NADA training and treatments have taken root in many locations outside North American. Globally, more than 25,000 health workers have completed the NADA training. NADA detoxification protocol has been adapted to various setting including: Emergency Medicine/Disaster Relief, Addiction Treatment, Mental Health, Court Diversion, Prisons, Community health, Self-Help, and Peer Support Groups.

Dose Acupuncture Work to Treat Drug Addition?

To date, acupuncture is widely accepted around the world as a safe intervention for both adults and children by trained acupuncturists [30–32]. Acupuncture as a treatment for pain [33], asthma [34], arthritis [35], postoperative nausea and vomiting (PONV) [36], and post-stroke rehabilitation [37] have been investigated through clinical trails. Similarly, acupuncture as a treatment for substance abusers also has been investigated clinically. A 1989 study, published in Lancet, indicated that acupuncture was highly effective in treating alcoholism [38]. The alcoholic patients were divided into two groups: one group received the correct-point acupuncture and the other group received the no-specific points on the ear. The researcher found that the clients who received acupuncture at no-specific points on the ear (control group) had twice as many relapses in the 6 months following the intervention and the number of clients in the control group admitting to detoxification centers was well over twice that of treatment group clients [38]. However, many large meta-analyses and review article indicated that the effect of both true and sham acupuncture as a treatment for cocaine [39], alcohol [40], and opioid addiction [28] are very similar. Does this mean acupuncture is ineffective? The answer is no. First, acupuncture is an intervention that cannot be masked completely because no sham acupuncture is without eliciting somatosensation, e.g., "de Qi" sensation is a form of sensory response [41]. Second, the effect of acupuncture can be affected by the expectation [41, 42]. Although there is no direct evidence about the effect of acupuncture as treatment for addiction, Kong et al. [42] found that conditioning positive expectation can amplify acupuncture analgesia but only true acupuncture not sham acupuncture significantly inhibit the brain responses to calibrated pain stimuli. The researchers suggested that acupuncture stimulation may directly inhibit incoming noxious stimuli and expectation may work through the emotional circuit [42]. Furthermore, Harris et al. [43] showed both true and sham acupuncture treatment produce similar pain relief in fibromyalgia patients but the brain pathways of two effects were very different. Sham acupuncture evokes an increased release of endogenous opioids, whereas true acupuncture increases receptors affinity and/or number [43]. A recent meta-analysis indicates acupuncture combined with opioid receptor agonists can effectively be used to manage the withdrawal symptoms [44]. Another study conducted by D'Alberto [45] indicated that NADA protocol of five treatment points still offers the acupuncturists the best possible combination as a treatment of cocaine/crack abuse.

Summary

Drug and substance abuse is a significant problem among teenagers around the world. In spite of educational efforts to prevent teenager use and/or addict to substance, there is an increased number of substance abusers in adolescences over the last decade. In order to help teenage substance addict recovery, significant responses and funding are needed. The uniqueness of acupuncture as a treatment of drug addiction is in its simplicity, safe, relative low cost, patient/client oriented, and can be performed in a group therapy. Although the systematic reviews and western standard clinical trials has yet to prove acupuncture's efficacy as a treatment for addiction recovery, the benefit of acupuncture as a treatment for withdrawal or adjunct to pharmaceutical interventions are undeniable.

References

1. National Institute on Drug Abuse. Preventing drug use among children an adolescent: a research-based guide for parents, educators and community leaders. 2nd ed. United States Department of Health and Human Services. 2003. http://www.nida.nih.gov/pdf/preevntion/Redbook.pdf
2. Kilpatrick DG, Acierno R, Saunders B, Resnick HS, Best CL, Schurr PP. Risks factors for adolescent substance abuse and dependence data from a national sample. J Consult Clin Psychol. 2000;68(1):19–30.
3. Russell LC, Sharp B, Gilbertson B. Acupuncture for addicted patients with chronic histories of arrest: a pilot study of the consortium treatment center. J Subst Abuse Treat. 2000;19(2):199–205.
4. Janssen PA, Demorest LC, Whynot EM. Acupuncture for substance abuse treatment in the downtown eastside of Vancouver. J Urban Health. 2005;82(2):285–95.
5. Cui C-L, Wu L-Z, Luo W-F. Acupuncture for the treatment of drug addition. Neurochem Res. 2008;33(10):2013–22.

6. Meade CS, Lukas SE, McDonald LJ, Fitzmaurice GM, Eldridge JA, Merrill N, Weiss RD. A randomized trial of transcutaneous electric acupoint stimulations adjunctive treatment for opioid detoxification. J Subst Abuse Treat. 2010;38(1):12–21.

7. Wang SM, Harris R, Lin YC, Gan TJ. Acupuncture in 21st century anesthesia: is there a needle in the haystack? Anesth Analg. 2013;116(6):1356–9.

8. White A, Ernst E. A brief history of acupuncture. Rheumatology. 2004;43(5):662–3. doi:10.1093/rheumatology/keg005.

9. Atwood K. "Acupuncture anaesthesia": a proclamation from chairman Mao (Part IV). 2009. http://www.sciencebasedmedicine.org/index.php/acupuncture-anesthesia-a-proclamation-from-chairman-mao-part-iv/

10. Kwong-Robbins C. Traditional Chinese medicine: a clinical guide to acupuncture. US Pharmacist a Jobson Publication; 2005;28. post 5/15/03. http://legacy.uspharmacist.com/index.asp?show=article8page=8_1072.htm

11. Salzber S. Does NIH recommend acupuncture? Fobes. 2011. http://www.forbes.com/sites/stevensalzber/2011/08/14/does-nih-recommend-acupuncture/

12. World Health Organization. Acupuncture: review and analysis of reports on controlled clinical trial. WHO Library Cataloguing-in-publication Data. Geneva: World Health Organization 2003, p. 87. http://apps.who.int/medicinedocs/en/d/Js4926e/

13. Cho ZH, Hwang SC, Wong EK, Son YD, Kang CK, Park TS, Bai SJ, Kim YB, Lee YB, Sung KK, Lee BH, Shepp LA, Min KT. Neural substrates, experimental evidences and functional hypothesis of acupuncture mechanism. Acta Neurol Scand. 2006;113(6):370–7.

14. Zhao ZQ. Neural mechanism underlying acupuncture analgesia. Prog Neurobiol. 2008;85(4):355–75. doi:10.1016/j.pneurobio.2008.05.004. Epub 2008 Jun 5.

15. Napadow V, Ahn A, Longhurst J, Lao L, Stener-Victorin E, Harris R, Langevin HM. The status and future of acupuncture mechanism research. J Altern Complement Med. 2008;14(7):861–9. doi:10.1089/acm.2008.SAR-3.

16. Han JS. Acupuncture and endorphin. Neurosci Lett. 2004;361(1-3):258–61.

17. Langevin HM, Churchill DL, Cipolla M. Mechanism signaling through connective tissue: a mechanism for the therapeutic effect of acupuncture. FASEB J. 2001;15(12):2275–82.

18. Langevin HM, Yandow JA. Relationship of acupuncture points and meridians to connective tissue plan. Anat Rec. 2002;269:257–65.

19. Zukauskas G, Dapsys K. Bioelectrical homeostasis as a component of acupuncture mechanism. Acupunct Electrother Res. 1991;16(3–4):117–26.

20. Smith M, McKenna B. The integration of acupuncture into existing chemical dependency treatment programs. 21st International Institute on Drug Prevention and Treatment of Drug Dependence. Prague, Czech Republic, June 7; 1994. p. 3.

21. Chae Y, Yeom M, Han J-H, Park H-J, Hahm D_H, Shin I, Lee H-S, Lee H. Effect of acupuncture on anxiety-like behavior during nicotine withdraw and relevant mechanism. Neurosci Lett. 2008;430(2):98–102.

22. Zhao RJ, Yoon SS, Lee BH, Kwon YK, Kim KJ, Shim I, Choi KH, Kim MR, Golden GT, Yang CH. Acupuncture normalizes the release of accumbal dopamine during the withdrawal period and after the ethanol challenge chronic ethanol-treated rats. Neurosci Lett. 2006;395(1):28–32. Epub 2005 Nov 10.

23. Lee BH, Zhao RJ, Moon JY, Yoon SS, Kim JA, An H, Kwon YK, Hwang M, Choi SH, Shim I, Kim BH, Yang CH. Differential involvement of GABA system in mediating behavioral and neurochemical effect of acupuncture in ethanol-withdrawn rats. Neurosci Lett. 2008;443(3):213–7. Epub 2008 Jul 31.

24. Scott S, Scott WN. A biochemical hypothesis for effectiveness of acupuncture in the treatment of substance abuse: acupuncture and the reward cascade. Am J Acupunct. 1997;15(2):121. http://acupuncturejournal.com/AJASple2.html

25. Clement-Jones V, Lowry PJ, Mcloughlin L, Besser GM, Rees LH, Wen HL. Acupuncture in heroin addicts: changes in Met-enkephalin and β-endophin in blood and cerebrospinal fluid. Lancet. 1979;2(8139):380–3.

26. Spray JR, Jones SM. The use of acupuncture in drug addiction treatment. News Brief. 1995. http://www.ndsn.org/sept95/guest.html
27. Ter Riet G, Kleijnen J, Knipschild P. A meta-analysis of studies into the effect of acupuncture on addiction. Br J Gen Pract. 1990;40(338):379–82. http://www.ncbi.nlm.nih.gov/pmc/articles/PMC1371348/
28. Jordan JB. Acupuncture treatment for opiate addiction: a systematic review. J Subst Abuse Treat. 2006;30(4):309–14.
29. The NADA Protocol. Acupuncture Today. http://www.acupuncturetoday.com/abc/nadaprotocol.php
30. Lao L, Hamilton GR, Fu J, Berman BM. Is acupuncture safe? A systematic review of case reports. Altern Ther Health Med. 2003;9(1):72–83.
31. Yamashita H, Tsukayama H, White AR, Tanno Y, Sugishita C, Ernst E. Systematic review of adverse events following acupuncture: the Japanese literature. Complement Ther Med. 2001;9(2):98–104.
32. Jindal V, Ge A, Mansky PJ. Safety and efficacy of acupuncture in children a review of the evidence. J Pediatr Hematol Oncol. 2008;30:431–42.
33. Wang SM, Kain ZN, White PF. Acupuncture analgesia: II. Clinical considerations. Anesth Analg. 2008;106:611–21.
34. Chu KA, Wu YC, Ting YM, Wang HC, Lu JY. Acupuncture therapy results in immediately bronchodilating effect in asthma patients. J Chin Med Assoc. 2007;70(7):265–8.
35. Berman BM, Lao L, Langenberg P, Lee W, Gilpin AMK, Hochberg MC. Effectiveness of acupuncture as adjunctive therapy on osteoarthritis of the knee: a randomized, controlled trial. Ann Intern Med. 2004;141(12):901–10.
36. Lee A, Done MI. Stimulation of the wrist acupuncture point P6 for preventing postoperative nausea and vomiting. Cochrane Database Syst Rev. 2009;2:CD003281. doi:10.1002/14651858. CD003281.pub3.
37. Sällström S, Kjendahi A, Østen PE, Stanghelle JK, Borchgrevink CF. Acupuncture in the treatment of stroke patients in the subacute stage. A randomized control study. Complement Ther Med. 1996;4(3):193–7. doi:10.1016/S0965-2299(96)80009-4.
38. Bullock ML, Culliton PD, Olander RT. Controlled trial of acupuncture for severe recidivist alcoholism. Lancet. 1989;1(8652):1435–9.
39. Margolin A, Kleber HD, Avants K, Konetal J, Gawin F, Stark E, Sorensen J, Midkiff E, Well E, Jackson R, Bullock M, Culiton PD, Boles S, Vaughan R. Acupuncture for treatment of cocaine addition a randomized controlled trial. JAMA. 2002;287(1):55–63.
40. Trümpler F, Oez S, Stähli P, Brenner HD, Jüni P. Acupuncture for alcohol withdrawal a randomized controlled trial. Alcohol Alcohol. 2003;38(4):369–75.
41. Han JS. Acupuncture analgesia: areas of consensus and controversy. Pain. 2011;152(3 Suppl):S41–8. doi:10.1016/j.pain.2010.10.012.
42. Kong J, Kaptchuk TJ, Polich G, Kirsch I, Vangel M, Zyloney C, Rosen B, Gollub RL. An fMRI study on the interaction and dissociation between expectation of pain relief and acupuncture treatment. Neuroimage. 2009;47(3):1066–76.
43. Harris RE, Zubieta JK, Scott DJ, Napadow V, Gracely RH, Clauw DJ. Traditional Chinese acupuncture and placebo(sham) acupuncture are differentiated by their effects on mu-opioid receptors (MORs). Neuroimage. 2009;47:2077–85. doi:10.1016/j.neuroimage.2009.05.087. Epub 2009 Jun 6.
44. Liu TT, Shi J, Epstein DH, Bao Y-P, Lin L. A meta-analysis of acupuncture combined with opioid receptor agonists for treatment of opiate-withdrawal symptoms. Cell Mol Neurobiol. 2009;29(4):449–54. doi:10.1007/s10571-008-9336-4. Epub 2008 Dec 25.
45. D'Alberto A. Auricular acupuncture in the treatment of cocaine/crack abuse: a review of efficacy, the use of the national acupuncture detoxification association protocol, and the selection of sham points. J Altern Complement Med. 2004;10(6):985–1000.

Chapter 28
Neurostimulation and Drug Abuse

Maria Teresa Gudin

Key Points

- Addiction and cerebral physiology
- Neurostimulation and drug abuse
- Brain stimulation
- Transcranial magnetic stimulation (TMS)
- Transcranial direct current stimulation (tDCS)
- Vagus nerve stimulation
- Deep brain stimulation (DBS)
- Role of acupuncture in addiction
- Acupuncture and intensified negative effects of drug abuse
- Acupuncture and endogenous opioid system
- Acupuncture and the positive reinforcement effects of addictive drugs
- Inhibition of dopamine release by acupuncture
- Acupuncture, electroacupuncture, and transcutaneous electric stimulation (TENS)

Introduction

Addiction to substances such as alcohol or drugs is a disease. The road to addiction usually begins with the voluntary use of one or more controlled substances such as narcotics, barbiturates, methamphetamine, alcohol, and nicotine. With time and the widespread use of controlled substances, the voluntary ability to refrain from taking these substances is compromised because of the effects of prolonged use on brain

M.T. Gudin, M.D. (✉)
Department of Anesthesiology, Getafe University Hospital,
Marques de Valdecilla 13, Madrid 28002, Spain
e-mail: mtgudin@gmail.com

© Springer Science+Business Media New York 2015
A.D. Kaye et al. (eds.), *Substance Abuse*, DOI 10.1007/978-1-4939-1951-2_28

function and behavior. Substance addiction is usually characterized by compulsive desire for the substance, and the search and use of the substance that persists, even knowing its negative consequences.

Compulsive or casual drug abuse can be seen as a behavior that is maintained by its consequences; when they reinforce a form of behavior with a pleasant effect (positive reinforcement) or end with any adverse situation for the individual (negative reinforcement), as is the relief of pain or anxiety. The secondary social reinforcement is independent of the pharmacological effects of the drug and can play an important role.

Although substance abuse and alcoholism cannot be cured, they can be treated. With treatment, many addicts can stop abusing a particular substance. However, treatment is not always effective. Many recovered addicts are persistently unable to resist either the desire to take the substance or the withdrawal symptoms.

Addiction and Cerebral Physiology

Addictions are associated with changes in brain activation patterns [1]. It is thought that disorders related to substance abuse are due to imbalances of certain brain neurological systems, possibly multilevel. The repeated use of substances can change the balance between neurotransmitters and induce long-term changes in brain excitability. For example, the mesolimbic dopaminergic system is strongly associated with stimulants and cocaine. The locus coeruleus is strongly associated with opiate dependence. The basal ganglia are strongly associated with compulsive behavior.

The mesolimbic dopaminergic system originates in the ventral tegmental area (VTA) and is projected to regions including the accumbens nucleus and prefrontal cortex. The neurobiological substrate for self-administration of all addictive drugs affects the dopaminergic system in the nucleus accumbens (NAcc), a primitive structure that is one of the most important brain pleasure centers [2]. Dopaminergic VTA pulses modulate the activity of neurons in the NAcc. These dopaminergic terminals from the VTA are the sites of action of highly addictive drugs such as cocaine and amphetamine, which cause an increase in dopamine release in the NAcc. In addition to cocaine and amphetamine, it has been observed that almost all recreational drugs (heroin, morphine, nicotine) are capable of increasing, by various mechanisms, dopamine levels in the NAcc. It is thought that dopamine is responsible for the exhilarating rush that reinforces the desire to take substances in drug addicts and plays an important role in the development of drug addiction. These drugs of abuse induce changes in brain levels of dopamine that are associated with feelings of well-being and pleasure and they provide positive reinforcement contributing to continued drug abuse [2]. Moreover the repeated administration of drugs causes increased release of dopamine in the brain. Conversely, withdrawal of chronic administration of substances results in decreased dopamine release in the NAcc. As many studies suggest, dopamine depletion induced by drugs in the mesolimbic system may be the mechanism responsible for the dysphoria and anhedonia that accompany drug abstinence and may also contribute to the intense desire for the drug that addicts experience.

Neurostimulation and Drug Abuse

In recent years, new techniques of neurostimulation able to modify the activity of brain circuits have been developed and are being explored in the treatment of addictions. The most important are the Transcranial Magnetic Stimulation (TMS), the Transcranial Direct Current Stimulation (tDCS), Vagus Nerve Stimulation (VNS), and Deep Brain Stimulation (DBS) [1].

Moreover, clinical trials are underway to determine the clinical efficacy of acupuncture in the treatment of drug addiction. Little is known about the basic mechanism of acupuncture in the treatment of drug addiction. The neurochemical data show that acupuncture directly or indirectly affects the mesolimbic dopaminergic system. There are very few studies with the aim of determining effectiveness of the acupuncture mechanism. Studies in rats have shown that acupuncture attenuates the rewarding effects induced by addictive drugs [2].

Brain Stimulation

Transcranial Magnetic Stimulation (TMS)

TMS is based on inducing a short and strong electrical current in a coil placed on the scalp [3]. The rapid change of current induces a transient magnetic pulse of high intensity that penetrates the scalp, skull, and underlying meninges crust generating an electric field which can depolarize cortical neurons under the coil (Fig. 28.1).

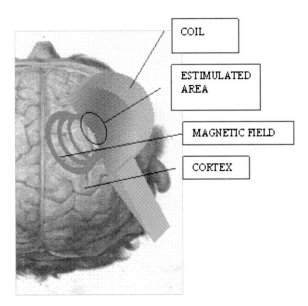

Fig. 28.1 Transcranial magnetic stimulation (TMS)

TMS can be used both to stimulate and to disrupt neural activity in specific cortical regions. It can modify cortical excitability in a reversible, focal, noninvasive, and relatively painless way. These pulses can also be repetitive and the technique is called repetitive Transcranial Magnetic Stimulation (rTMS). This embodiment in which the TMS is applied repetitively is able to modulate the brain activity, in the brain region affected, beyond the duration of the stimulation itself.

In the field of addiction and substance abuse, TMS seems able to increase the release of mesolimbic dopamine during withdrawal of heroin and cocaine in animals [4]. In another study in rats that were chronic cocaine consumers, the TMS decreased their substance-seeking behavior. There have been controlled studies in which the TMS has been shown to be effective in helping patients to reduce the consumption of tobacco [5].

Transcranial Direct Current Stimulation (tDCS)

tDCS consists of applying an electric field of low intensity at the surface of the skull through electrodes that can modulate the cortical activity with little discomfort (Fig. 28.2). It has been shown that tDCS administered in the dorsolateral prefrontal cortex (DLPFC) in populations with drug dependence reduces consumption and the intense desire for substance use.

Vagus Nerve Stimulation

VNS involves connecting an electrode around the vagus nerve and transmitting electrical impulses of low frequency originating on a device that is implanted in the chest (Fig. 28.3). It could reduce heroin-seeking behavior in rats dependent on this substance, suggesting the possibility that it might be useful in human addicts [6].

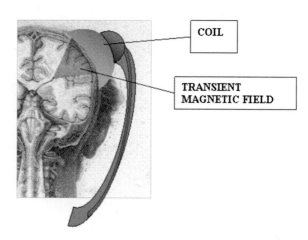

COIL

TRANSIENT MAGNETIC FIELD

Fig. 28.2 Electrical current in the coil creates a transient magnetic field and results in electrical impulses in neurons in cortex under the coil

Fig. 28.3 Vagus nerve
stimulation

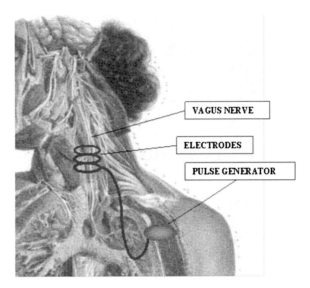

Deep Brain Stimulation (DBS)

DBS is an invasive and reversible technique introduced in recent times for the treatment of neurological and psychiatric diseases.

It is a technique of localized and invasive brain stimulation, with the advantage that it is reversible, unlike ablative surgery, and its parameters are adjustable from the outside.

It consists of an intracerebral implant via stereotactic surgery, of intracerebral electrodes, which will be permanently connected to a neurostimulator. This is what generates the pulses, and it is implanted in an intraabdominal or infraclavicular area.

Regarding the possibility of using the DBS in substance addiction, it is a technique that could be useful since the addictive disease is caused by a fault in a particular well-known and well-described circuit, which is the reward system. The reward system has two main areas, which are the VTA and the NAcc, which have connections with the prefrontal cortex and the limbic region, and could be therapeutic targets of the DBS.

There is reference to a case of spontaneous resolution of previous addictive behavior in a patient treated for neurological and psychiatric diseases [7]. There have also been encouraging studies in animals, as well as tests of its use in isolated cases of particularly refractory patients [8].

Role of Acupuncture in Addiction

The discovery of the central endorphin system was an important step in understanding the analgesic effect of acupuncture. The endorphin neurons in the hypothalamus project to the dorsal raphe nucleus and periaqueductal gray matter of the mesencephalon and today are known to be mainly responsible for producing the analgesic effect of acupuncture. Furthermore, neurotransmitters as serotonin, catecholamines, and GABA (γ-aminobutyric acid that plays a role in regulating neuronal excitability throughout the nervous system), have been linked to the analgesic effects produced by acupuncture [9].

Acupuncture and Intensified Negative Effects of Drug Abuse

Chronic exposure to drugs can cause a "syndrome of deficiency in the reward system" due to dysfunction of the basal dopaminergic reward system of the brain. Serotonin is believed to play a mediator role in the efficacy of acupuncture in treating withdrawal. Acupuncture may have a role in normalizing dopamine release via serotonergic neurons in the hypothalamus. It could help normalize neuronal activation and thus reverse the withdrawal symptoms. Studies using animal models have provided evidence that acupuncture may have a role in reducing the negative reinforcing effects of the drug.

A theoretical model on possible interactions between the endogenous opioid reward system and the release of dopamine in the NAcc has been proposed. This model explains the possible bidirectional effects of acupuncture on dopamine release in the NAcc.

In the positive reinforcement: (a) active acupuncture treatment with the GABA-B receptor in dopaminergic cell bodies resulting in decreased dopamine release in the NAcc via inhibition of dopaminergic neurons, (b) acupuncture activates presynaptic opioid μ in the NAcc through dynorphin neurons and results in decreased dopamine release in the NAcc.

In the negative reinforcement, encephalitic acupuncture stimulates neurons in the hypothalamus, so that the methionine-encephalin released in VTA interacts with opioid-μ receptors to inhibit GABAergic interneurons of the VTA, inducing a disinhibition of the dopaminergic neurons and, thus, finally increasing dopamine release on NAcc (Fig. 28.4).

Acupuncture and Endogenous Opioid System

Experimental studies have investigated the effect of electroacupuncture in the endogenous opioid system. Electroacupuncture is a form of acupuncture where a small electric current is passed between pairs of acupuncture needles. These studies have used animal models and have provided evidence that low-frequency electroacupuncture can activate enkephalinergic neurons and beta-endorphinergics in the arcuate nucleus of the hypothalamus. Accordingly, it seems reasonable that electroacupuncture can help increase dopamine release through δ opioid receptors in the NAcc and the μ receptors in the VTA. There is also important neurochemical evidence that acupuncture treatment directly affects the mesolimbic dopaminergic system. Low-frequency electroacupuncture facilitates release of endorphins and enkephalins β in the central nervous system (CNS), while high-frequency

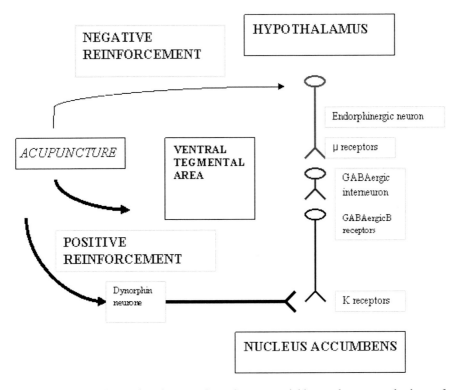

Fig. 28.4 Possible interactions between the endogenous opioid reward system and release of dopamine in the nucleus accumbens

electroacupuncture causes increased release of dynorphin. It would therefore be expected that low-frequency electroacupuncture has a leading role in attenuating withdrawal activating β endorphin and enkephalinergic neurons. However, high-frequency electroacupuncture is more effective in suppressing the withdrawal syndrome compared with low-frequency electroacupuncture. The low-frequency electroacupuncture appears to have a key role in mitigating the motivational aspects of drug withdrawal while high-frequency electroacupuncture appears to be more effective in reducing the symptoms of withdrawal.

Acupuncture and the Positive Reinforcement Effects of Addictive Drugs

Studies in rats have shown that acupuncture attenuates the rewarding effects induced by addictive drugs. Electroacupuncture increases the release of dynorphin that interacts with the brain κ receptor. Dynorphin results in decreased dopamine release in the NAcc via the action of the opioid κ receptor localized on presynaptic dopaminergic nerve terminals in the region.

Inhibition of Dopamine Release by Acupuncture

The increase in dopamine transmission in the NAcc induced by all addictive drugs has long been associated with addictive behaviors. Therefore, decreased behavior due to acupuncture may be mediated by the attenuation of dopamine release and neuronal activity in the NAcc.

Acupuncture, Electroacupuncture, and Transcutaneous Electric Stimulation (TENS)

Several studies have shown that manipulation with needles stimulates nerve impulses that are transmitted through the CNS afferent nerve fibers. The physiological effect of acupuncture (antinociceptive effect) can be readily blocked by local anesthetic injection deep at that point or through the nerve trunk. If the nerve activation causes the transmission of signals from acupuncture, similar effects can be induced by the manipulated needle or directly by electrical impulses through needles at the point or even by electrodes on the surface of the skin at the point, which causes a current to pass through the underlying tissue and produces the sensation of the electrical impulse (numbness and myalgia). The analgesic effects induced by acupuncture (via needle) and by transcutaneous stimulation (through electrodes in the skin) have been compared in an experiment performed on rats. No significant difference in analgesic efficacy between the two paths was found. So, it does not matter the way in which electrical stimulation is done, whether through needles or through electrodes.

References

1. Feil JZ. Brain stimulation in the study and treatment of addiction. Neurosci Biobehav Rev. 2010;34:559–754.
2. Erhardt A, Sillaber I, Welt T, Muller MB, Singewald N, Keck Me. Repetitive Transcranial Magnetic Stimulation increases the release of dopamine in the Nucleus Accumbens shell of morphine-sensitized rats during abstinence. Neuropsychopharm. 2004;29:2074–80.
3. Liu H, Liu Y, Lai M, Zhu H, Sun A, Zhou W. Vagus nerve stimulation inhibits heroin-seeking behavior induced by heroin priming or heroin-associated cues in rats. Neurosci Lett. 2011;494:70–4.
4. Garcia-Toro M, Gili M, Roca M. [New neurostimulation techniques in addictions]. Adicciones. 2011;23(4):273–6.
5. Yang CH, Lee BH, Sohn SH. Possible mechanism underlying the effectiveness of acupuncture in the treatment of drug addiction. Evid Based Complement Alternat Med. 2008;5(3):257–66.
6. Zheng Z, Guo RJ, Helme RD, Muir A, Da Costa C, Xue CC. The effect of electroacupuncture on opioid-like medication consumption by chronic pain patients: a pilot randomized controlled trial. Eur J Pain. 2008;12:671–6.

7. Kuhn J, Lenartz D, Huff W, Lee S, Koulousakis A, Klosterkoetter J, et al. Remission of alcohol dependency following deep brain stimulation of the nucleus accumbens: valuable therapeutic implications? J Neurol Neurosurg Psychiatry. 2007;78:1152–3.
8. Kuhn J, Moller M, Bogerts B, Mann K, Grundler TO. Deep brain stimulation for the treatment of addiction. Addiction. 2011;106:1536–7.
9. Amiaz R, Levy D, Vainiger D, Grunhaus L, Zangen A. Repeated high-frequency transcranial magnetic stimulation over the dorsolateral prefrontal cortex reduces cigarette craving and consumption. Addiction. 2009;104:653–60.

Chapter 29
Hypnosis for Substance Abuse

Sumit Gulati, Yashwin Agnelo D'Costa, Lara Zador, and Sreekumar Kunnumpurath

Key Points

- History
- Definition
- Phenomena of hypnosis
- Neurophysiology
- Substance abuse
- Psychological therapies for substance abuse
- Hypnosis for substance abuse
- Smoking
- Alcohol
- Other substance abuse
- Self-hypnosis

S. Gulati, M.D., F.R.C.A., F.F.P.M.R.C.A. (✉)
Department of Pain Medicine, The Walton Centre NHS Foundation Trust,
Lower Lane, Fazakerley, Liverpool L9 7LJ, UK
e-mail: drsumitgulati@gmail.com

Y.A. D'Costa, M.B.B.S., M.D. (Anaesthesiology)
Department of Anesthetics, St. Helier Hospital, Wrythe Lane, Carshalton, Surrey SM5 1AA, UK
e-mail: yashwind@doctors.org.uk; yashwind@hotmail.co.uk

L. Zador, M.D.
Department of Anesthesia, Yale New Haven Hospital, 27 Hubinger Street, New Haven,
CT 06511, USA
e-mail: lara.zador@yale.edu

S. Kunnumpurath, M.B.B.S., M.D., F.F.P.M.R.C.A., F.R.C.A., F.C.A.R.C.S.I.
Department of Anesthetics and Pain Management, Epsom and St. Helier University Hospitals
NHS Trust, Wrythe Lane, Carshalton SM5 1AA, UK
e-mail: skunnumpurath@gmail.com

© Springer Science+Business Media New York 2015
A.D. Kaye et al. (eds.), *Substance Abuse*, DOI 10.1007/978-1-4939-1951-2_29

- Steps commonly used for self-hypnosis
- Group hypnosis
- Pain and hypnosis

History

Hypnosis as a therapy is unique and has an interesting history dating back to ancient Egypt. It has transformed over the years and yet has an intrigue about it that makes it poorly understood. This is because of lack of knowledge about its neurophysiological basis, patchy evidence base, lack of scientific basis, cultural correlates, and a complementary medicine image. However it is no different from other such things like Placebo, Fibromyalgia, depression whose neurobiology is only partially understood. Several groups have staked a claim as its practitioners ranging from "Healers" to early scientists like Mesmer and Freud and more recently psychologists, behavioral therapists, physicians, and researchers.

Hypnosis has been practiced in varied forms over the centuries and different names have been given to it. From early references in ancient Egyptian and Ebers Papers (one of the oldest human writings known, dated 300 BC), scientific basis of Hypnosis started to be experimented with over 200 years ago. Franz Mesmer, a Viennese physician proposed "Animal Magnetism" and achieved successful cure for several conditions. In 1784, a Royal commission could not find evidence of animal magnetism, and it fell into disrepute.

The term hypnosis was coined in 1841 by James Braid, a Manchester surgeon, who believed that a psychological state similar to sleep accounted for the phenomena observed. The use of hypnosis by the French neurologist Charcot, and by Breuer and Freud in the 1880s extended its use to the treatment of neurotic disorders broadly referred to as "hysterical." Interest in the clinical application of hypnosis developed rapidly throughout the nineteenth century. The early twentieth century saw a temporary lessening of interest in internal psychological processes such as hypnosis followed by renewed scientific interest from the middle of twentieth century. The late twentieth and twenty-first centuries had increasingly started looking at the neurophysiology and scientific principles as well outcomes through controlled trials and meta-analysis [1].

Hypnosis has been used for many psychological and medical problems and literature exists for its use in the treatment of chronic addiction [2], cancer pain, childbirth, irritable bowel syndrome [3], depression, anxiety, stress, eating disorders, addiction, smoking cessation, wound healing, and asthma [4].

Unlike psychoanalysis or cognitive behavior therapy, hypnosis is a facilitator of therapy and not a therapy itself. It allows a person to enter a relaxed and altered state of consciousness where messages of personal change and healing can be seeded. There is however, little consensus about how hypnotherapy might induce these effects. It is also recognized that treatment success could be influenced by other factors such as the transference relationship between patient and therapist and the hypnotizability of subjects [5].

Definition

While there are many definitions of hypnosis, the most widely accepted is that proposed by the British Medical Association in (BMA) in 1955 and in 1982.

Hypnosis is a temporary condition of altered perception in the subject which may be induced by another person and in which a variety of phenomena may appear spontaneously or in response to verbal or other stimuli. These phenomena include alterations in consciousness and memory, increased susceptibility to suggestion, and production in the subject of responses and ideas unfamiliar to him in his normal state of mind. Further phenomena such as anaesthesia, paralysis and the rigidity of muscles, and vasomotor changes can be produced and removed in the hypnotic state.

Phenomena of Hypnosis

A variety of phenomena accompany the hypnotic state, which may be induced on the instruction of a therapist or self-induced by the subject [1]. The extent that the phenomena are experienced and observed depends upon the depth of the hypnotic state, which is a characteristic of the subject and commonly referred to as hypnotizability or hypnotic susceptibility.

During the hypnotic process the focus of attention is narrowed and shifted towards an internal cognitive focus. This leads to a reduction in awareness of the sensory input requiring a response. There is a relative reduction in arousal of sensory and response systems of the central nervous system,

- Reduction in critical thinking, reality testing, and tolerance of reality distortion
- Heightened imagery vividness or reality
- Volitional changes and alterations in voluntary muscle activity
- Alterations in involuntary muscles, organs, and glands
- Alterations in perceptions
- Distortions of memory
- Heightening of expectations and motivations
- Increased reality acceptance of fantasy experiences

Neurophysiology

With the advent of neuroimaging techniques such as functional Magnetic Resonance Imaging (fMRI), positron emission tomography (PET), single photon emission computer tomography (SPECT), the mysteries of consciousness, and its altered state are being unraveled. There is evidence that hypnotic phenomena selectively involve cortical and subcortical processing. At a neurophysiological level, highly hypnotizable subjects often demonstrate greater EEG hemispheric asymmetries in hypnotic and nonhypnotic conditions.

Derbyshire et al. [6], for example, showed that the same suggestions to increase or decrease fibromyalgia pain using fMRI produced greater changes in activation in pain-related brain areas when participants were hypnotized compared to when they were not. Relatively little is known from a cognitive neuroscience perspective about the underlying processes involved in hypnotic experience in the absence of suggestion—so-called "neutral hypnosis." Using PET, Rainville et al. [7] compared a no-hypnosis baseline condition with a hypnosis condition that produced a co-ordinated pattern of activity involving brainstem, thalamus, anterior cingulate cortex, right inferior frontal gyrus, and right inferior parietal lobule. Preliminary sets of findings are indicative of a distinct "default mode" or neural signature associated with hypnosis together with increases in mental absorption and reduction in spontaneous conceptual thought commonly reported by hypnotized individuals [8].

Substance Abuse

The problem of substance abuse plagues the modern world and although major strides have been made in stopping this through public health initiatives, its successful treatment for individual patients is often challenging.

The World Health Report 2002 [9] indicated that 8.9 % of the total burden of disease comes from the use of psychoactive substances. The report showed that tobacco accounted for 4.1 %, alcohol 4 %, and illicit drugs 0.8 % of the burden of disease in 2000. UNODC estimates that there are 25 million problem drug users in the world, of whom 15.6 million are problem opioid users and 11.1 million problem heroin users (approximately 0.3 % of the global population).

Psychological Therapies for Substance Abuse

World Health Organization published its guidelines for Psychosocially Assisted Pharmacological Treatment of Opioid Dependence in 2009 [10]. It suggests that determinants and the problematic consequences of drug dependence may be biological, physiological or social, and usually these interact. The authors concluded that psychosocial treatments offered in addition to pharmacological detoxification treatments are effective in terms of completion of treatment, use of opiate, participants abstinent at follow-up and clinical attendance.

Clinicians and health providers should choose which psychosocial intervention to offer to opioid-dependent patients, based on research evidence, how appropriate a method is to the patient's individual situation, how acceptable it is to the patient, whether trained staff are available, and cultural appropriateness. However, providing medications without offering any psychosocial assistance fails to recognize the complex nature of opioid dependence, loses the opportunity to provide optimal interventions, requires treatment staff to go against their clinical inclination to respond to the total needs of their patients. Treatment services should aim to offer onsite, integrated, comprehensive psychosocial support to every patient [10].

Behavioral treatments as part of psychological therapy for substance abuse have been established and provide a framework for allowing hypnosis to be used in shaping and reinforcing new behaviors while extinguishing undesired behaviors.

Hypnosis for Substance Abuse

Hypnosis is becoming increasingly popular for helping patients with Substance Abuse problems because it focuses on the individual's "subconscious" mental state rather than the more logical "conscious" level. In the "hypnotic" state patients are more relaxed and receptive to new ideas or suggestions. The "subconscious" mental state is more receptive to new thoughts and easily programmable to support the individual's desire to kick whatever habit they have become addicted to. Hypnotherapy, which is therapy imparted with aid of hypnosis, is different because the counselling sessions focus on the person's "subconscious" mental state. This approach to modifying the fundamental beliefs or thought patterns and, ultimately behaviors, through hypnosis has great promise for this group of patients.

In his article in Alcohol Quarterly in 1991, Miller eloquently summarised the context of hypnotherapy and suggestion for Recovering Addicted Patient [11]. Suggestion is a very powerful healing tool in the mind–body healing process. Suggesting that changing the behavior is possible, desirable and rewarding to the conscious and unconscious is an important message to communicate to the patient. Hypnosis can be helpful in changing an individual's belief system, controlling physiological responses, and in personality reintegration. It is easier to substitute a positive behavior for a negative one, rather than to attempt to extinguish a behavior type. It is important to reduce the issues down to manageable parts. If you are going to climb a mountain, it is important not to be overwhelmed by its size, but to think of it in manageable "legs."

He considers it important for patients to be internally motivated to change for their own welfare, rather than change for some external force such as a family member, legal reasons, employer, or friend. And therefore he promotes the concept of patient being the "Captain of the ship" with the therapist being merely the "navigator".

Detoxification First

Patient should be detoxified of the alcohol or drug before any meaningful hypnotherapy can be commenced. Hypnosis should not be used when patients are intoxicated. After detoxification, the first hypnotherapy session should be scheduled as soon as possible to be supportive to the patient in maintaining a physically drug-free state.

Direct Induction

A preinduction interview should be conducted before a direct induction. It should include a personal and social history encompassing, school or occupational adjustment, family constellation, family history of drug abuse, past and present health. Questions about psychological and physiologic manifestations can be asked through a questionnaire. The subsequent trance experience should be "future paced" with post-hypnotic suggestions, suggestions to safeguard against any unpleasant "side effects," cues, and anchors.

He emphasises rational use of confrontational approach only to "break down denial." As this approach can, in turn, reinforce denial and resistance. Confrontations should be balanced with permissive and supportive techniques, which serve to maintain rapport, provide support, and caring. The utilization approach is especially effective in working with resistant patients. That is acknowledging, accepting their reality and utilizing it to initiate change.

Destabilizing the System

Addicted and compulsive patients have a tendency to adhere rigidly to their ritualist behaviors. For example, those addicted to alcohol will tell you they continue to use the same "hangouts," bars and clubs and the same routes to and from those locations.

Once the system has been destabilized, a variety of hypnotherapy techniques may be utilized. Metaphors, embedded metaphors, paradoxes, contingency suggestions, stories, antidotes, age regress, future pacing time, reframing, and homework assignments may be used to transform the behavior.

Smoking

There are various studies which reported favorable outcome with treatment of tobacco habituation. Hypnotherapy has been claimed to have a greater effect on 6-month quit rates than other interventions or no treatment. Various modes of hypnotherapy are used to help people quit smoking [12–14].

Some methods include:

- Weakening people's desire
- Strengthening their will to quit
- Help them concentrate on a quit program

Hypnotherapy could be as effective as counseling, although there is no good research evidence of this claim [12].

Alcohol

There are several reports of successful hypnotherapy for individual alcohol addiction and abuse. Group interaction psychotherapy of simultaneously hypnotized patients is a new therapy trialled to treat alcoholism [15]. Group therapy sessions were lively and productive, noticeably more so than in the waking state. Sessions were terminated by a short free dreaming period, followed by awakening without amnesia.

Advantages of group interaction psychotherapy include:

– Economy of staff time
– Facilitation of awareness and communication
– Effective use of patient initiative [16, 17; personal communication Lassoff, 1970]

Other Substance Abuse

Hypnotherapy may be significantly effective as a treatment for withdrawing patients from methadone maintenance and enabling them to continue a drug-free life. A high percentage of subjects remained abstinent for 6 months after treatment. This result suggests that withdrawal might be a realistic treatment goal for those patients who have stabilized their addiction and are ready to regain their self-control [18–21].

Self-Hypnosis

Self-hypnosis is used extensively in modern hypnotherapy. It can take the form of hypnosis carried out by means of a learned routine. Hypnosis allows one to gain from deep potential present in them.

Hypnosis may help in:

– Pain management
– Anxiety
– Depression
– Sleep disorders
– Obesity
– Asthma
– Skin conditions
– It can improve concentration, recall, enhance problem solving, alleviate headaches, and even improve one's control of emotions

Steps Commonly Used for Self-Hypnosis

Step 1: *Motivation*: Without this motivation or dire need, the individual will find it difficult to practice self-hypnosis.

Step 2: *Relaxation*: The individual must be thoroughly relaxed and must set aside time to perform this act. Additionally, distractions should be eliminated as full attention is needed.

Step 3: *Concentration*: the individual needs to concentrate completely as energy is generated each time the mind focuses on a single image.

Step 4: *Directing*: This is an option used only when the individual wants to work on a specific goal. The individual must direct his concentration on visualizing the desired result.

Group Hypnosis

Group hypnosis is an interaction between individuals and the hypnotherapy practitioner. Everyone will be able to respond to the same anchors or keywords that will be given during the session. The hypnotherapist interviews each and every person in the group and then develops what words he or she will use so that there is no confusion during the hypnosis session.

There are benefits to group hypnosis compared to individual sessions. For one, there is the security of not being all by yourself. You can also save money by dividing the cost of the therapy session which is less expensive than what you would have to pay if you undergo a one-on-one session [22].

Pain and Hypnosis

Hypnotherapy for pain management can either be used alongside prescribed medication or alone. Hypnotherapy has been used by many to manage numerous instances of pain:

– Irritable bowel syndrome
– Sciatica
– Spinal stenosis
– Burns
– Joint pain
– Neck pain
– A variety of other injuries and illnesses

The basic premise of hypnotherapy is to change the way individuals perceive pain messages in order to reduce the intensity of what they are feeling. This can be achieved using a number of techniques which may either be used alone or in combination depending on your individual circumstances. Commonly employed certain hypnotherapy techniques are:

– Suggestion hypnotherapy
– Analytical hypnotherapy
– Visualization

Some practitioners may also use Neurolinguistic Programming (NLP) and psychotherapy to enhance their treatment. Many hypnotherapists will also include self-hypnosis [23–26].

References

1. Burrows GD, Stanley RO, editors. Introduction to clinical hypnosis and the hypnotic phenomena. International handbook of clinical hypnosis. New York: Wiley; 2001.
2. Hartman B. The use of hypnosis in the treatment of drug addiction. J Natl Med Assoc. 1972;64:35–8.
3. Whorwell PJ. Use of hypnotherapy in gastrointestinal disease. Br J Hosp Med. 1991;45(1): 27–9.
4. Morrison JB. Chronic asthma and improvement with relaxation induced by hypnotherapy. J R Soc Med. 1988;81(12):701–4.
5. Perry C, Gelfand R, Marcovitch P. The relevance of hypnotic susceptibility in the clinical context. J Abnorm Psychol. 1979;88(5):592–603.
6. Derbyshire SW, Whalley MG, Oakley DA. Fibromyalgia pain and its modulation by hypnotic and non-hypnotic suggestion: an fMRI analysis. Eur J Pain. 2009;13(5):542–50.
7. Rainville P, Hofbauer RK, Bushnell MC, Duncan GH, Price DD. Hypnosis modulates activity in brain structures involved in the regulation of consciousness. J Cogn Neurosci. 2002;14(6):887–901.
8. Oakley DA, Halligan PW. Hypnotic suggestion and cognitive neuroscience. Trends Cogn Sci. 2009;13:264–70.
9. Neuroscience of psychoactive substance abuse and dependence. World Health Organization. 2004. http://www.who.int/substance_abuse/publications/en/Neuroscience.pdf
10. World Health Organization. Guidelines for the psychosocially assisted pharmacological treatment of opioid dependence; 2009.
11. Miller Jr WA. Using hypnotherapy in communicating with the recovering addicted patient. Alcohol Treat Q. 1991;8:1–18.
12. Barkley RA, Hastings JE, Jackson Jr TL. The effects of rapid smoking and hypnosis in the treatment of smoking behavior. Int J Clin Exp Hypn. 1977;25(1):7–17.
13. Carmody TP, Duncan C, Simon JA, Solkowitz S, Huggins J, Lee S, Delucchi K. Hypnosis for smoking cessation: a randomized trial. Nicotine Tob Res. 2008;10(5):811–8.
14. von Dedenroth TE. The use of hypnosis in 1000 cases of "tobaccomaniacs". Am J Clin Hypn. 1968;10(3):194–7.
15. Beahrs JO, Hill MM. Treatment of alcoholism by group-interaction psychotherapy under hypnosis. Am J Clin Hypn. 1971;14:60–2.
16. Langen D. Modern hypnotic treatment of various forms of addiction, in particular alcoholism. Br J Addict Alcohol Other Drugs. 1967;62(1):77–81.
17. Smith-Moorhouse PM. Hypnosis in the treatment of alcoholism. Br J Addict Alcohol Other Drugs. 1969;64(1):47–55.
18. Manganiello AJ. A comparative study of hypnotherapy and psychotherapy in the treatment of methadone addicts. Am J Clin Hypn. 1984;26(4):273–9.
19. Senay EE. IDAP—five year results. Proceedings of the 5th national conference on methadone treatment. New York: National Association for the Prevention of Addiction to Narcotics; 1973.
20. Shaprio D, Zifferblatt S. Reducing methadone dosage in drug addiction. Am Psychol. 1976;31(7):519–32.
21. Yaffe G, et al. Physical symptoms complaints of patients on methadone maintenance. Proceedings from the 5th national conference of methadone treatment. New York: National Association for the Prevention of Addiction to Narcotics; 1973.

22. Panyard C, Wolf K. The use of systematic desensitization in an outpatient drug treatment center. Psychother Theory Res Pract. 1974;11:329–30.
23. Truman L. Hypnosis may help cure girl of drug habit. San Diego: Copely News Service; 1971.
24. Woody RH, Schauble PG. Desensitization of fear by video tapes. J Clin Psychol. 1969;25(1):102–3.
25. Glick B. Conditioning therapy with phobic patients: success and failure. Am J Psychother. 1970;24:91–101.
26. Glick B. Some limiting factors in reciprocal inhibition therapy. Psychiatr Q. 1969;44:223–9.

Chapter 30
Postoperative Pain Control
in Drug Abusing Patients

Clifford Gevirtz, Nalini Vadivelu, and Alan David Kaye

Key Points

- Methadone
- Buprenorphine
- Liposomal bupivacaine
- Gabapentinoids
- New vistas in postoperative management

Opioid addiction is a complex and difficult-to-treat illness [1]. The terms addict and addiction, derive from the Latin legal term addictus which describes someone who has surrendered to a debt holder for indefinite servitude until their debt is paid. While not a slave, the addictus was expected to toil long and hard until, if ever, the debt was paid. Clearly, the metaphor is of the drug enslaving the addict and the obligation is incumbent upon the medical profession to enable the addict to pay his or her debt in a compassionate manner.

Drug abusers are notoriously demanding and uncooperative. The first consideration should be the realization that their endogenous opiate system doesn't work and that conventional demand only PCA will not be very effective at meeting their needs.

C. Gevirtz, M.D., M.P.H. (✉)
LSU New Orleans Health Sciences Center, 627 West Street, Harrison, NY 10528, USA
e-mail: cliffgevirtzmd@yahoo.com

N. Vadivelu, M.D.
Department of Anesthesiology, Yale University, 333 Cedar Street, New Haven, CT 06520, USA
e-mail: nalinivg@gmail.com

A.D. Kaye, M.D., M.B.A., M.D., Ph.D.
Departments of Anesthesiology and Pharmacology, Louisiana State University
Health Sciences Center, Louisiana State University Interim Hospital,
and Ochsner Kenner Hospital, New Orleans, LA, USA
e-mail: alankaye44@hotmail.com

© Springer Science+Business Media New York 2015
A.D. Kaye et al. (eds.), *Substance Abuse*, DOI 10.1007/978-1-4939-1951-2_30

Alternative therapeutic approaches are needed here:

The options for postoperative pain control in drug abusing patients include opiates such as methadone, the partial agonist buprenorphine, local anesthetics, low-dose ketamine, and the gabapentinoids.

Methadone

Methadone for the Treatment of Pain

Though the prescription of methadone for addiction treatment is restricted to those with a special license, all physicians able to prescribe schedule II medications can issue prescriptions for methadone for analgesia. It can be used for the treatment of acute postoperative pain as well as chronic pain. It is an NMDA antagonist and this property along with its long half-life makes it particularly useful in the treatment of long-term persistent neuropathic pain. Animal studies have shown that about 40 % of pain relief from methadone is via non-opioid mechanisms most likely the NMDA receptor, while 60 % of pain relief from methadone is via the opioid receptor and can be reversed with naloxone [2]. Other classes of medications for the treatment of chronic pain such as gabapentin, tricyclic antidepressants, and serotonin norepinephrine reuptake inhibitors can be combined with methadone to increase efficacy. Methadone has been shown to decrease postoperative opioid requirements for pain [3].

Methadone has been found to significantly reduce postoperative pain as well as decrease the consumption of opioids in studies by Gottschalk et al. [3] where methadone given as a single bolus of 0.2 mg/kg reduced pain by almost 50 % as compared to patients treated with sufentanil 48 h after surgery at 0.25 mcg/kg/h after a bolus load of 0.75 mcg/kg of sufentanil and reduced the intravenous patient-controlled analgesia used for postoperative pain. Steady state achievement with methadone can take up to 3–5 days due to its long half-life for ranging from 8 h to over 2 days. Methadone is usually prescribed every 8 h for pain since the analgesic effect of methadone is shorter than that of morphine and lasting for about 6–8 h.

Significant tolerance is often seen in patients with past history of opioid abuse and these patients may require much higher doses of opioids for analgesic control [4, 5]. It is important to recognize that some patients may be so tolerant of the opiates as to require heroin doses. Methadone has been used in patients with a past history of opioid abuse and in patients with opioid tolerance for the treatment of pain, especially when they present from a methadone maintenance program. It is important to clarify the current dose the patient is receiving as well as notifying the program that the patient is receiving anesthetic medications as these may show up on subsequent urine toxicology tests and the patient might be labeled as using abusing drugs that were in fact administered therapeutically. Though Methadone is a powerful analgesic and its long half-life can lead to difficulty with titration when used for the treatment of pain. It is important for physicians prescribing methadone to be aware of its unique properties to avoid serious risks including cardiac arrhythmias, respiratory depression, and death. Prior to starting Methadone, an electrocardiogram is indicated and patients with a prolonged QT should not receive this drug for concern of sudden death via Torsades de Pointes.

Buprenorphine

While there is limited published data involving patients on buprenorphine who present for procedures or surgery requiring anesthesia, case reports have offered suggestions for the management of postoperative pain.

The successful management of post-cesarean section pain in two patients maintained on buprenorphine was achieved using intravenous morphine patient-controlled analgesia (PCA) and oral oxycodone at markedly elevated doses [6]. In both cases the patients were able to continue buprenorphine therapy throughout their hospital stay. Each was able to achieve acceptable levels of pain control with a total dose of 180 mg per day of morphine. When switched to oral medications, one patient was able to achieve pain relief with 60 mg per day of oxycodone and 6 g of acetaminophen; however, the second patient required 600 mg of ibuprofen every 8 h in addition to this regimen.

Supplemental doses of sublingual buprenorphine have been used to control postoperative pain in patients who are already maintained on buprenorphine [7]. Recommendations have been proposed for the control of acute pain in the patient maintained on buprenorphine by using shorter acting opioid analgesics in addition to the maintenance dose of buprenorphine and titrating to effective pain control [8]. By dividing the buprenorphine-maintenance dose over the course of 24 h and relying on the analgesic properties of buprenorphine, replacing the buprenorphine with methadone and then adding another opioid analgesic, or replacing the buprenorphine with another opioid analgesic altogether, adequate pain relief can be achieved in the acute setting. Whichever method is chosen, patients maintained on buprenorphine usually require much higher doses of opioid agonists to achieve adequate pain relief.

Options for Pain Control in Buprenorphine-Maintenance Patients

Some patients on buprenorphine may desire to avoid opioids, if at all possible, because of the risk of re-starting opiate addiction. The use of regional anesthetics, NSAIDs, gabapentinoids (vide infra) may be helpful in avoiding the use of opiates. High-dose buprenorphine used for opioid substitution has a long half-life, which combines with its strong affinity for the mu-opioid receptor and slow receptor dissociation to account for the long duration of action of the drug [9].

Studies have demonstrated that the opioid-blocking action of buprenorphine can persist for several days following discontinuation of the medication, which would make conventional pain therapy difficult or impossible. In one study of male subjects with a recent history of opioid addiction, sublingual buprenorphine, at a dose of 8 mg daily for 1 week, blocked the subjective and respiratory depressant effects of hydromorphone 4 mg intramuscularly for up to 5 days following discontinuation of the buprenorphine [10].

Because buprenorphine is a partial agonist, patients maintained on this drug have a significantly increased tolerance for opioids and may require extremely high doses to achieve analgesia. This affinity of buprenorphine for mu-receptors is so high that it has been reportedly used to reverse heroin overdose [10]. There are no controlled trials that demonstrate the extent to which required doses of opioid agonists administered to patients maintained on buprenorphine are increased. One option for treatment of acute pain is to increase the dose of buprenorphine itself in order to achieve pain relief, though there is a ceiling effect and, if analgesia is not achieved, other options need to be considered.

Liposomal Bupivacaine

An important approach to postoperative pain relief in these patients is the use of local anesthetics. A new approach is the use of liposomal bupivacaine (LBup). The first use of liposomal bupivacaine was reported by Boogaerts et al. [11] for acute postoperative pain. They studied 26 ASA physical status II and III patients who had undergone major surgery (abdominal, vascular, urologic, thoracic, orthopedic). After completion of the operation, the patients were divided into two groups to receive 1 of 2 bupivacaine preparations epidurally for postsurgical pain:

- Group 1 ($n=12$) received plain 0.5 % bupivacaine with 1:200,000 epinephrine
- Group 2 ($n=14$) received liposomal 0.5 % bupivacaine

The following observations were made: onset and quality of analgesia, quality of motor block according to the Bromage scale, and sympathetic block. Onset time of sensory block averaged 15 min in both groups. Pain relief durations were 3.2 ± 0.4 h with plain bupivacaine and 6.25 ± 1.13 h with the liposomal preparation ($p < 0.05$). In the liposomal bupivacaine group, no motor block was recorded. Low sympathetic block occurred in all patients. Analgesia in a subset of patients following abdominal aortic surgery increased from 2.4 ± 0.35 h to 10.6 ± 1.4 h by encapsulation of bupivacaine ($p < 0.01$). There was no neurotoxicity or cardiotoxicity in any of the patients. The authors concluded that the liposomal formulation of bupivacaine increased duration of analgesia without motor block or adverse side effects.

Pharmacokinetics

LBup (Exparel, Pacira Pharmaceuticals) exhibits dose-proportional pharmacokinetics [12], following single-dose administration in the setting of wound infiltration, at a dose of up to 532 mg. LBup contains a small amount (3 %) of extra-liposomal bupivacaine to allow for faster onset, similar to regular infiltration with non-liposomal bupivacaine. LBup demonstrates slow and prolonged duration of action. At on-label doses of up to 266 mg, there is an initial peak within 1 h of administration and a later peak at 10–36 h. At doses up to 532 mg, the duration of action extends to 72 h. The Cmax of the 266 mg dose is similar to the 100 mg dose and never exceeds 40 % of the toxic level. At a dose of 532 mg, the Cmax is 935 ng/mL, which is less than half the experimental 2,000 ng/mL toxic level for demonstrating central nervous system and cardiovascular effects. No QTc interval changes have been observed at therapeutic dose levels.

Distribution

After bupivacaine has been released from the liposome, its distribution characteristics are identical to subcutaneously injected bupivacaine.

Metabolism

Bupivacaine is metabolized in the liver by conjugation with glucuronic acid. The liposomal stroma is a lipid that is broken down by fatty acid metabolism.

There are physicochemical incompatibilities between LBup and certain other drugs (e.g. lidocaine). Direct contact of LBup with these drugs results in a rapid increase in free (unencapsulated) bupivacaine, altering LBup characteristics, and potentially affecting the safety and efficacy of LBup. Therefore, admixing LBup with other drugs prior to administration is not advised. The administration of LBup may follow the administration of lidocaine after a delay of 20 min or more.

Other key warnings include:

- Bupivacaine, when injected immediately before LBup, may change the pharmacokinetic and/or physicochemical properties of the drugs when the milligram dose of bupivacaine HCl solution exceeds 50 % of the LBup dose.
- When a topical antiseptic such as povidone iodine (e.g., Betadine®) is applied, the site should be allowed to dry before LBup is administered into the surgical site. LBup should not be allowed to come into contact with antiseptics such as povidone iodine or chlorhexidine in solution. Different formulations of bupivacaine are not bioequivalent to LBup even if the milligram dosage is the same. Therefore, it is not possible to convert dosing from any other formulations of bupivacaine to LBup and vice versa.

Special Populations

LBup has not been studied in patients younger than 18 years of age, pregnant patients, or patients who are nursing. No overall differences in safety or efficacy have been detected in patients over 65 years of age.

Hepatic Failure

Patients with moderate to severe liver disease are at greater risk of developing toxic plasma concentrations. An increase in Cmax of up to 60 % has been observed in liver-failure patients, so caution is advised.

Renal Insufficiency

Bupivacine is substantially excreted by the kidneys. The risk of toxicity increases significantly in renal failure patients.

Chondrolysis

Intra-articular infusions of local anesthetics following arthroscopic and other surgical procedures is an off-label use, and there have been numerous postmarketing reports of chondrolysis in patients receiving such infusions. The majority of reported cases of chondrolysis have involved the shoulder joint; cases of glenohumeral chondrolysis have been described in pediatric patients and adult patients following intra-articular infusions of local anesthetics with and without epinephrine for periods of 48–72 h. The time of onset of symptoms, such as joint pain, stiffness, and loss of motion, can be variable, but may begin as early as the second month after surgery. Currently, there is no effective treatment for chondrolysis; patients who have experienced chondrolysis have required additional diagnostic and therapeutic procedures. Some required arthroplasty or shoulder replacement.

LBup has not been evaluated for the following uses and, therefore, at this time, is not recommended by the manufacturer for these types of analgesia or routes of administration:

- Epidural
- Intrathecal
- Major regional blocks (brachial or lumbar-sacral plexus blocks)
- Sympathetic ganglion block
- Intravascular (Bier block) or intra-articular use

Drug Interactions

LBup can be administered undiluted or diluted up to 0.89 mg/mL (i.e., 1:14 dilution by volume) with preservative-free normal (0.9 %) sterile saline for injection. LBup must not be diluted with water or other hypotonic agents, as it will result in disruption of the liposomal particles.

Candiotti [12] reviewed the use of LBup in two pivotal, multicenter, randomized placebo-controlled, double-blind, parallel-group trials in 189 adults undergoing soft-tissue surgery (hemorrhoidectomy) and 193 adults undergoing orthopedic surgery (bunionectomy).

Among patients undergoing hemorrhoidectomy, liposomal bupivacaine significantly reduced cumulative pain scores for up to 72 h (primary end point) as measured by the area under the curve of pain scores on the numeric rating scale ($p < 0.0001$). The formulation also reduced overall opioid consumption ($p \leq 0.0006$), increased the proportion of patients who did not receive opioids ($p < 0.0008$), delayed time to first opioid by more than 13 h ($p < 0.0001$), and was associated with significantly higher rates of patient satisfaction ($p = 0.0007$), compared with placebo.

Similarly, in patients undergoing bunionectomy, liposomal bupivacaine significantly reduced total consumption of rescue opioids ($p = 0.0077$) and cumulative pain scores as measured by the area under the curve of pain scores on the numeric rating scale ($p = 0.0005$) during the first 24 postsurgical hours (primary end point) relative to placebo.

Furthermore, liposomal bupivacaine also significantly delayed the time to first use of opioid rescue ($p < 0.0001$) and increased the proportion of patients requiring no rescue opioid treatment ($p \leq 0.0404$) compared with placebo. The most common adverse events with liposomal bupivacaine were nausea, vomiting, and constipation. No adverse effects on the QTc interval or cardiac safety signal have been detected in the clinical trial development program ($n = 823$ patients) when liposomal bupivacaine was infiltrated into the surgical site. Candiotti concluded that the beneficial effects of liposomal bupivacaine on postsurgical pain management and opioid use, significantly reducing both, are likely to translate into improved clinical and economic outcomes.

Marcet et al. [13] studied the use of LBup in gastrointestinal surgery patients who are at high risk for opioid-related adverse events. They assessed the impact of an opioid-sparing multimodal analgesia regimen with liposome bupivacaine, compared with the standard-of-care intravenous (IV) opioid-based, PCA on postsurgical opioid use and health economic outcomes in patients undergoing ileostomy reversal.

In an open-label, multicenter study, sequential cohorts of patients undergoing ileostomy reversal received IV opioid PCA (first cohort); or multimodal analgesia including a single intraoperative administration of liposome bupivacaine (second cohort).

Rescue analgesia was available to all patients. Primary outcome measures were postsurgical opioid use, hospital length of stay, and hospitalization costs. Incidence of opioid-related adverse events was also assessed.

The authors enrolled 27 patients who underwent ileostomy reversal, and did not meet any intraoperative exclusion criteria; 16 received liposome bupivacaine-based multimodal analgesia and 11 received the standard IV opioid PCA regimen. The multimodal regimen was associated with significant reductions in opioid use compared with the IV opioid PCA regimen (mean, 20 mg vs. 112 mg; median, 6 mg vs. 48 mg, respectively; $p < 0.01$), postsurgical length of stay (median, 3.0 days vs. 5.1 days, respectively; $p < 0.001$), and hospitalization costs (geometric mean, \$6,482 vs. \$9,282, respectively; $p = 0.01$). They concluded that a liposome bupivacaine-based multimodal analgesic regimen resulted in statistically significant and clinically meaningful reductions in opioid consumption, shorter length of stay, and lower inpatient costs than an IV opioid-based analgesic regimen.

LBup is an important addition to our armamentarium in dealing with these patients, it allows for prolonged somatic block. Further research is needed before its use can be expanded to other routes of administration.

Gabapentinoids

In a recent meta-analysis, Schmidt et al. [14] reviewed over 100 clinical trials examining the use of gabapentin perioperatively to reduce postoperative pain and a smaller number examining the efficacy of pregabalin. They concluded that the perioperative use of gabapentinoids reduces early postoperative pain and opioid use.

While most studies have utilized a dose administered 1–2 h prior to surgery, measurements of plasma and CSF levels suggest that administration up to 8 h earlier may be needed to allow the medication to exert its full opioid-sparing, pain-relieving, and pain preventing effects.

The optimum dosing of gabapentin is still uncertain, but best estimates are approximately 22 mg/kg or approximately 1,500 mg/70 kg adult with normal renal function preoperatively and 600 mg TID postoperatively. Similarly with pregabalin, the optimum dose is unclear, but 4.3 mg/kg or approximately 300 mg in a 70 kg adult and then 150 mg BID postoperatively.

New Vistas in Postoperative Management

A number of innovative low-dose sub-anesthetic ketamine infusion protocols have been established for patients with substance abuse and drug dependence issues for pain management in the postoperative setting. These protocols vary and typically they provide ketamine infusions at 60–120 mcg/kg/h (which is equal to 0.06–0.12 mg/kg/h) over a 4-h period. No additional narcotics, sedative or central nervous system depressants are given unless authorized by the Acute Pain Service or Palliative Care Service. Assessment of respiratory rate, heart rate, blood pressure, sedation, analgesia, adverse psychological manifestations and/or muscle stiffness will result in notification to the primary team and re-evaluation of dosing regimen.

Conclusion

In addition to pain control, management of anxiety, psychological states, and hemodynamic control are all factors to be considered to provide optimum treatment for the drug-dependent and -addicted patient in the perioperative setting.

Management of acute pain in patients with drug addiction and drug-dependent patients is truly a challenge. Opioids are the mainstay for the control of acute pain. In the drug-addicted and drug-dependent patients, other therapeutic options include alternative routes of administration of local anesthetic, ketamine infusion, and/or can be combined with the use of regional anesthesia. The perioperative healthcare provider should be cognizant of any methadone maintenance programs the patient might be enrolled in or the use of buprenorphine for the treatment of drug dependence in order to best treat the patient. For pain control in addition to opioids, peripheral nerve blocks, intrathecal or epidural techniques are increasingly being employed for the treatment of pain in the perioperative setting in these patients along with newer sub-anesthetic (low-dose) ketamine regimens.

In well-supervised settings, patients have benefitted with the use of intravenous patient-controlled analgesia, including the use of basal rate settings. A team-oriented multimodal approach could be the best route to control pain in the perioperative setting in the drug-dependent and drug-addicted patient. In drug-addicted and drug-dependent patients with chronic pain, in addition to opioids, non-opiate medications such as anti-depressants, anticonvulsants, and anti-inflammatory medications can be beneficial.

References

1. Jaffe JH, Jaffe AB. Opioid related disorders. In: Sadock BJ, Sadock VA, editors. Comprehensive textbook of psychiatry. 7th ed. New York: Lippincott Williams and Wilkins; 2000. p. 1038–63.
2. Sotgiu ML, Valente M, Storchi R, Caramenti G, Biella GE. Cooperative N-methyl-D-aspartate (NMDA) receptor antagonism and mu-opioid receptor agonism mediate the methadone inhibition of the spinal neuron pain-related hyperactivity in a rat model of neuropathic pain. Pharmacol Res. 2009;60(4):284–90.
3. Gottschalk A, Durieux ME, Nemergut EC. Intraoperative methadone improves postoperative pain control in patients undergoing complex spine surgery. Anesth Analg. 2011;112(1): 218–23.
4. Umbricht A, Hoover DR, Tucker MJ, Leslie JM, Chaisson RE, Preston KL. Opioid detoxification with buprenorphine, clonidine, or methadone in hospitalized heroin-dependent patients with HIV infection. Drug Alcohol Depend. 2003;69(3):263–72.
5. Hughes JR, Bickel WK, Higgins ST. Buprenorphine for pain relief in a patient with drug abuse. Am J Drug Alcohol Abuse. 1991;17(4):451–5.
6. Jones HE, Johnson RE, Milio L. Post-cesarean pain management of patients maintained on methadone or buprenorphine. Am J Addict. 2006;15(3):258–9.
7. Book SW, Myrick H, Malcolm R, Strain EC. Buprenorphine for postoperative pain following general surgery in a buprenorphine-maintained patient. Am J Psychiatry. 2007;164:979.
8. Alford DP, Compton P, Samet JH. Acute pain management for patients receiving maintenance methadone or buprenorphine therapy. Ann Intern Med. 2006;144(2):127–34.
9. Robert DM, Meyer-Witting M. High-dose buprenorphine: perioperative precautions and management strategies. Anaesth Intensive Care. 2005;33:17–25.
10. Schuh KJ, Walsh SL, Stitzerr ML. Onset, magnitude and duration of opioid blockade produced by buprenorphine and naltrexone in humans. Psychopharmacology (Berl). 1999;145:162–74.
11. Boogaerts ND, Lafont AG. Declercq epidural administration of liposome associated bupivacaine for the management of postsurgical pain: a first study. J Clin Anesth. 1994;6:315–20.
12. Candiotti K. Liposomal bupivacaine: an innovative nonopioid local analgesic for the management of postsurgical pain. Pharmacotherapy. 2012;32(9 Suppl):19S–26S. doi:10.1002/j.1875-9114.2012.01183.x.
13. Marcet JE, Nfonsam VN, Larach S. An extended pain relief trial utilizing the infiltration of a long-acting Multivesicular liposome formulation of bupivacaine, EXPAREL (IMPROVE): a Phase IV health economic trial in adult patients undergoing ileostomy reversal. J Pain Res. 2013;6:549–55. doi:10.2147/JPR.S46467.
14. Schmidt PC, Ruchelli G, Mackey SC, Carroll IR. Perioperative gabapentinoids. Anesthesiology. 2013;119:1215–21.

Chapter 31
Management of the Drug Abusing Patient in the ICU

Ranjit Deshpande, Jhaodi Gong, Ryan Chadha, and Ala Haddadin

Key Points

- Opioid abuse
- Clonidine–naltrexone detoxification
- Benzodiazepine abuse and withdrawal
- Flumazenil for benzodiazepine reversal
- Synthetic cathinone ("Bath Salts") abuse
- Phencyclidine (PCP)
- Lysergic acid diethylamide (LSD)
- Bromo-DragonFLY
- Alcohol abuse and withdrawal
- Nicotine abuse and withdrawal
- Stimulant abuse and withdrawal

Opioid Abuse

Pathophysiology of Opioid Abuse and Withdrawal

The dopaminergic mesolimbic system originates in the ventral tegmental nucleus with a projection to the nucleus accumbens and plays a critical role in mediating effects of opioid. The opioid receptors include mu, kappa, sigma, delta, and epsilon.

R. Deshpande, M.B.B.S. (✉) • J. Gong, M.D. • A. Haddadin, M.D.
Department of Anesthesiology, Yale University School of Medicine,
333 Cedars Street, New Haven, CT 06510, USA
e-mail: ranjit.deshpande@yale.edu

R. Chadha, M.D.
Department of Anesthesiology, Yale University School of Medicine,
Yale-New Haven Hospital, New Haven, CT, USA

© Springer Science+Business Media New York 2015
A.D. Kaye et al. (eds.), *Substance Abuse*, DOI 10.1007/978-1-4939-1951-2_31

Opioid-induced activation of mu and sigma receptors increases the activity of the dopaminergic mesolimbic system releasing dopamine into the nucleus accumbens, which produces feelings of euphoria and well-being. Stimulation of the kappa receptors decreases activity of the mesolimbic system, resulting in dysphoria.

Enzymatic inhibition at the mu receptors in the locus ceruleus leads to a decrease in norepinephrine production. However, chronic use of opioids leads to increased enzymatic activity at the mu receptors, thereby resulting in normal or higher levels of norepinephrine. Following opioid deprivation, there is loss of inhibitory effect on enzyme activity. The excess norepinephrine released leads to symptoms such as muscle cramps, diarrhea, anxiety, and tremors.

Signs and Symptoms of Opioid Abuse/Intoxication

Opioid users can develop tolerance, as well as psychological and physical dependence to opioids when they take them over an extended period of time. Signs and symptoms of opioid abuse include analgesia, sedation, euphoria, respiratory depression, nausea, vomiting, itching or flushed skin, constipation, slurred speech, confusion, and poor judgment. Miosis is not universally present with intoxication; normal or enlarged pupils have been documented. The most easily recognized abnormality in cases of opioid overdose is a decline in respiration culminating in apnea. Respirations are characteristically slow and shallow.

Management

Diagnosis is mainly clinical. The triad of respiratory rate <12 breaths /min, miosis and circumstantial evidence of opioid use have a sensitivity of 92 % and a specificity of 76 % for opioid overdose. Urine toxicology screen can detect morphine-related products like morphine, codeine, and heroin up to 2 days after single use.

Opioid-related disorders that require medical management include opioid overdose, opioid intoxication, and opioid withdrawal.

For opioid intoxication, general supportive measures include assessment and assurance of patent airway, ventilatory support if needed, assessment and support of cardiac function along with intravenous hydration. Opioid-intoxicated patients require frequent vital sign and cardiopulmonary monitoring until opioids are cleared from the patient's system. If necessary, naloxone, a specific opiate antagonist, can be administered intravenously or subcutaneously to rapidly reverse the respiratory depression and sedation caused by opioid intoxication.

For opioid overdose patients who present with stupor and have respiratory rates of 12 breaths per minute or less, ventilation should be provided with a bag-valve mask. Chin-lift and jaw-thrust maneuvers should be performed to ensure clear airway without obstruction. Naloxone is effective in treating acute opioid overdose and is first-line treatment. Patients who are intoxicated by long-acting or extended-release opioid formulations with recurrent respiratory depression may require naloxone infusion or endotracheal intubation and admission to intensive care unit [1, 2].

Signs and Symptoms of Opioid Withdrawal

The time to onset of opioid withdrawal symptoms depends on the half-life of the drug abused. For example, withdrawal symptoms usually start 4–6 h after last heroin usage, but up to 36 h after last methadone exposure [3].

Early physical symptoms of withdrawal include muscle aches, lacrimation, insomnia, rhinorrhea, sweating, and yawning. Late physical symptoms of withdrawal include abdominal cramping, diarrhea, dilated pupils, piloerection (also known as goose bumps or "gooseflesh"), nausea, and vomiting. In addition, mild tachycardia and/or hypertension are often signs associated with opioid withdrawal. Psychological symptoms include agitation, anxiety, dysphoria, craving for opioids, restlessness, insomnia, and fatigue. Opioid withdrawal symptoms are not life threatening in otherwise healthy individuals. However, they can cause remarkable discomfort which frequently leads to a relapse to drug use [4].

The severity of opioid withdrawal varies with the dose and duration of drug use. Although physical withdrawal symptoms generally resolve by 5–10 days, psychological withdrawal symptoms may last weeks to months.

Management of Opioid Withdrawal

Treatment of opioid withdrawal involves supportive care and medications. Mild to moderate opioid withdrawal does not usually require specific treatment expect general supportive care. However, patients and families should be reassured that patient's withdrawal symptoms are under close monitor and taken seriously with supportive care.

The American Psychiatric Association (APA) guideline identified the following three treatment modalities to be effective strategies for managing opioid dependence and withdrawal [5].

Opioid Substitution Therapy

It is important that methadone or buprenorphine should not be given to an opioid-dependent patient until withdrawal symptoms appear. Maintenance therapy with methadone or buprenorphine followed by a gradual taper is appropriate for use in patients who have a history of dependence lasting more than 1 year [6]. Methadone replacement therapy became the first treatment modality for opioid dependence, and its use became widely available in the late 1960s [7]. One treatment strategy is to stabilize opioid-dependent patient with methadone initially given in 5 mg increments up to a total of 10–20 mg over the first 24 h then gradually decrease the methadone dose by tapering 20 % a day for inpatients, leading to a 1- to 2-week procedure.

Buprenorphine, a high-affinity, partial agonist at the opioid receptor, is a newer treatment modality that became available since the year 2000. Buprenorphine has been shown to work better than other medications for treating withdrawal from opiates, and it can shorten the length of detoxification. It may also be used for long-term maintenance like methadone. Buprenorphine and buprenorphine–naloxone (Suboxone) were approved by the US FDA as a pharmacotherapy for opioid dependence in 2002 [8]. The usual dose of buprenorphine–naloxone to treat opioid withdrawal symptoms should start with a dose of 8 mg and can increase up to 24 mg daily.

One limitation to the use of buprenorphine in the treatment of opioid dependence in the ICU is its sublingual administration and lack of effect with opioids for pain control because of buprenorphine's higher affinity to opioid receptor.

Abrupt Opioid Discontinuation

Some drug treatment programs have widely advertised treatments for opiate withdrawal called detox under anesthesia or rapid opiate detox first described by Loimer et al. in 1988 [9]. The rapid opiate detoxification programs involve placing patients under anesthesia and injecting large doses of opiate-blocking drugs (i.e., naloxone), hoping to speed up the return the body to normal opioid system function. In some cases, such program may reduce the intensity of symptoms. Evidence is lacking that these programs actually reduce the time spent in withdrawal and there have been several deaths associated with these procedures, particularly when performed in out of hospital settings. Additionally, because opiate withdrawal produces vomiting, and vomiting during anesthesia significantly increases risk of death, many specialists think the risks of this procedure significantly outweigh the potential (and unproven) benefits. Research remains to be done to determine long-term outcomes.

Clonidine–Naltrexone Detoxification

Clonidine is generally considered a safe, non-narcotic medication and is being used to help patient in withdrawal from opioids. It is a centrally acting alpha-2 adrenergic agonist and works to minimize the noradrenergic hyperactivity seen in opioid withdrawal [6, 10]. Typical doses used to treat opioid withdrawal range between 0.1 and 0.3 mg orally up to every 6 h.

One advantage of clonidine is its lack of tolerance or dependence which is in contrast to naltrexone [6]. In fact, some clinicians will rapidly withdraw patients from opioids using a combination of clonidine and naltrexone by pretreatment with clonidine to avoid some of the abrupt withdrawal symptoms caused by naltrexone. However, the use of clonidine in opioid withdrawal is limited due to its orthostatic hypotension and sedative side effects.

Benzodiazepine Abuse and Withdrawal

Pathophysiology of Benzodiazepine Abuse and Withdrawal

Benzodiazepines exert their action by potentiating the activity of GABA. Benzodiazepines bind to a specific receptor on the GABA A receptor complex, which facilitates opening of the chloride channel resulting in membrane hyperpolarization and inhibition of cellular excitation.

Chronic ingestion of benzodiazepines leads to conformational changes in the GABA receptor, which ultimately reduce the receptor's affinity for the agent and result in decreased GABA activity. This decreased activity manifests as tolerance to the agent. When benzodiazepines are no longer present or present at lower concentrations, this decreased GABA receptor activity has less inhibition of excitatory neurotransmitters, and thus, there is a pro-excitatory state seen in benzodiazepine withdrawal.

Signs and Symptoms of Benzodiazepine Abuse

Benzodiazepines abuse is partially related to their widespread availability. They can be chronically abused or, as seen more commonly in hospital emergency departments, intentionally or accidentally taken in overdose. Death and serious illness rarely result from benzodiazepine abuse alone; however, they are frequently taken with either alcohol or other medications. This combination of benzodiazepines and alcohol can be extremely dangerous.

Signs and symptoms of acute toxicity or overdose may include drowsiness, confusion, dizziness, blurred vision, weakness, blurred speech, lack of coordination, difficulty breathing, even coma.

Signs of chronic drug abuse can be very nonspecific and include changes in appearance and behavior that affect relationships and work performance. Chronic abuse of benzodiazepines can lead to the symptoms that mimic many of the indications for using them in the first place such as insomnia, anorexia, headaches, and weakness.

Management of benzodiazepine abuse/intoxication: benzodiazepine overdose can be easily diagnosed by urine toxicology screen, the possibility of emergency department administration should be excluded in agitated and combative patients. Whether the presence of benzodiazepine is from emergency department or chronic usage needs to be clarified by looking through charts and astute history-taking.

Treatment of acute benzodiazepine intoxication usually depends on type and quantity of drug taken. If the drugs were taken within the previous 1–2 h, gastric lavage can be considered. If the patient comes to the emergency department within 4 h of taking drugs, a single dose of activated charcoal is recommended to prevent absorption of the medication.

Flumazenil, a specific benzodiazepine antagonist, can be administered in emergency. However, flumazenil is only indicated for reversal of benzodiazepine overdose during procedures or acute intoxication in benzodiazepine naive patient as it can precipitate withdrawal and seizures in chronic benzodiazepine abusers. It is also contraindicated in patients receiving benzodiazepine for life-threatening conditions (e.g., status epilepticus). In the critical care setting, caution should be exercised in head trauma, history of seizures, and chronic alcoholism. Flumazenil may not reverse amnesia.

Flumazenil for Benzodiazepine Reversal

Rarely patient may require titration up to total dose of 5 mg. If no response after 5 min, sedation appears unlikely to be secondary to benzodiazepines [11].

The treatment of chronic abuse in ICU setting should be primarily supportive to prevent withdrawal and detoxification is not usually initiated until acute ICU issues resolve.

Signs and Symptoms of Benzodiazepine Withdrawal

Patients who are physically dependent on short-acting anxiolytic benzodiazepines may experience what is known as interdose withdrawal, which occurs between doses when the previous dose wears off. This can lead to symptoms such as rebound anxiety between doses and craving for the next dose of short-acting benzodiazepines.

Withdrawal symptoms can occur while on a stable dose of benzodiazepines due to the "tolerance withdrawal" phenomenon, where the body experiences "withdrawal effects" while weaning off benzodiazepines. Patients crave for the drug leading to dosage escalation.

Symptoms commonly seen in patients undergoing benzodiazepine withdrawal are characterized by severe sleep disturbance, irritability, increased anxiety, panic attacks, hand tremor, sweating, difficulty in concentration, confusion and cognitive difficulty, memory problems, dry retching and nausea, weight loss, palpitations, headache, muscular pain and stiffness, a host of perceptual changes, hallucinations, seizures, psychosis, and suicide. These symptoms are notable for their fluctuations in severity from day to day or week by week instead of steadily decreasing in a straightforward linear manner.

The acute benzodiazepine withdrawal syndrome generally lasts for about 2 months but clinically significant withdrawal symptoms may persist, although gradually declining, for many months or even several years.

The severity and length of the withdrawal syndrome is likely determined by various factors including rate of tapering, length of use of benzodiazepines and dosage size and possibly genetic factors. For example, some people experience little or no withdrawal when stopping long-term benzodiazepine usage. It is not known for sure why there is such a variation between patients but recent research in animals suggests that withdrawal from sedative hypnotic drugs may be influenced by a genetic component.

On the other hand, an abrupt discontinuation of benzodiazepines may result in a more serious and very unpleasant withdrawal syndrome that may additionally result in convulsions, which may result in death.

Management of Benzodiazepine Withdrawal

Benzodiazepine withdrawal follows the same treatment protocol as for alcohol withdrawal. A long-acting benzodiazepine is more effective than short-acting preparations in suppressing withdrawal symptoms and in producing a gradual and smooth transition to the abstinent state. In general, greater patient compliance and lower morbidity can be expected with the use of the longer-acting benzodiazepines, since withdrawal symptoms are less intense.

A taper over 8–12 weeks or longer may be indicated in patients who have been taking benzodiazepines for several years. The rate of taper can be adjusted according to patient tolerance. The maximum suggested rate of taper is a reduction in dosage of approximately 25 % per quarter of the withdrawal period (e.g., 25 % per week for 1 month).

The use of carbamazepine has also been suggested to be effective in the treatment of benzodiazepine withdrawal. However, the medication must be administered for at least 2 week before gradually tapered [12].

Synthetic Cathinone ("Bath Salts") Abuse

Pathophysiology of Synthetic Cathinone Abuse

Synthetic cathinones are the synthetic derivatives of the natural cathinone, a psychoactive compounds present in Catha edulis (khat). At least 12 different types of synthetic cathinones have been described. However, mephedrone and 3,4-methylendioxypyrovalerone (MDPV) are most commonly used. These drugs stimulate the release and inhibit the reuptake of norepinephrine, serotonin, and dopamine [13]. Bath salt, plant food, vanilla sky, and ivory wave are some common street names of these agents.

Signs and Symptoms of Synthetic Cathinone Abuse

Due to the similarity to amphetamines, people who have taken the synthetic cathinones can show signs of sympathomimetic toxidrome including agitation, psychosis, significant tachycardia, hypertension, and seizures. Furthermore, hyperthermia and hyponatremia can present in these patients. Duration of effects depend on the method of use, lasting up to 4 h after ingestion. These agents are not detected in routine urine toxicology screens.

Other signs and symptoms that may appear after taking synthetic cathinones are chest pain, ST segment changes, palpitations, myocarditis, anxiety, confusion, drowsiness, headache, hyperreflexia, myoclonus, dystonia, paresthesia, dizziness, tremors, parkinsonism, depression, panic attacks, seizures, hyperthermia, and rhabdomyolysis.

Management of Synthetic Cathinone Abuse

Treatment for patients intoxicated with synthetic cathinones is centered on supportive care. Hydration with intravenous fluids should be initiated along with measures to actively cool patients if they are hyperthermic.

It is critical to control agitation as rhabdomyolysis and cardiovascular collapse from excitatory delirium can occur. While stimuli reduction may be of benefit, benzodiazepines, such as lorazepam or diazepam, should be the first-line agents in trying to sedate these patients and manage seizures.

When benzodiazepines do not have the desired effect, antipsychotics such as haloperidol can be an effective alternative to treat agitation, aggression, or psychosis in conjunction with benzodiazepines.

Sometimes, physical restraints may be needed to prevent these patients from hurting themselves or others. While treating these patients, it is important to keep in mind that severely agitated patients are at risk for sudden death.

In the events of hypertension, in addition to benzodiazepines, further control of blood pressure can be achieved with alpha-adrenergic receptor antagonist, i.e., doxazosin. If the patient presents with coronary ischemia, routine protocol treatment with nitroglycerine, morphine, and antiplatelet drugs should be considered. However, beta-blocker is contraindicated which may worsen hypertension and coronary vasoconstriction. Treatment of hypotensive episodes should be with a direct acting vasopressor, e.g., phenylephrine.

Several other conditions can mimic the sympathomimetic excess seen with synthetic cathinones toxicity. Antimuscarinic toxidrome, sedative-hypnotic withdrawal states, neuroleptic malignant syndrome, serotonin syndrome, infectious etiologies (i.e., meningitis), endocrine abnormalities (i.e., thyroid storm), and intracranial hemorrhage could all present similarly and should be considered and ruled out.

Signs and Symptoms of Synthetic Cathinone Withdrawal

Currently there is no focused research on the addiction potential or withdrawal syndromes related to synthetic cathinones. A survey of 1,500 mephedrone users found that over 50 % consider it to be addictive [14]. Users describe strong cravings to repeat or increase doses after taking mephedrone. However, a physical withdrawal syndrome has not been reported although users report feelings of depression and anxiety at the end of use.

Phencyclidine (PCP)

Phencyclidine (PCP) also known as Angel Dust, KJ (kristal joint), Ashy Larry, illy, or wet, is a recreational dissociative drug. PCP works primarily as an NMDA receptor antagonist, which blocks the activity of the NMDA receptor and, like most anti-glutamatergic hallucinogens.

PCP's effects are unpredictable which typically last for several hours even to days. PCP users often report feeling of detachment from reality, including distortions of space, time, and body image. Some may experience hallucinations, panic, and fear, while others may report feelings of invulnerability and exaggerated strength. Repeated use of PCP can result in addiction, and recent research suggests that repeated or prolonged use of PCP can cause withdrawal syndrome such as memory loss and depression that may persist for as long as a year after a chronic user stops taking PCP.

To prevent self-injury, a common form of PCP-induced morbidity and mortality, the patient must be safely restrained, initially physically, and then chemically. An IV line must be inserted and blood drawn for electrolytes, glucose, BUN, and creatinine concentrations as well as for volume repletion and electrolyte supplementation because hyperthermia increases fluid loss from sweat. Chemical treatment can be successfully accomplished with benzodiazepines such as diazepam, administered in titrated doses of up to 10 mg intravenously every 5–10 min until agitation is controlled [15].

Lysergic Acid Diethylamide (LSD)

LSD (lysergic acid diethylamide) is one of the major drugs making up the hallucinogen class. LSD affects a large number of the G protein-coupled receptors, including all dopamine receptors and all adrenergic receptor subtypes. The psychedelic effects of LSD are attributed to its strong agonist effects at 5HT2A receptors. Exactly how this produces the drug's effects is unknown, but it is thought that it works by increasing glutamate release in the cerebral cortex and therefore excitation in this area, specifically in layers IV and V.

The effects of LSD are unpredictable. Usually, the user feels the first effects of the drug 30–90 min after taking it. The physical effects include dilated pupils, higher body temperature, increased heart rate and blood pressure, sweating, loss of appetite, sleeplessness, dry mouth, and tremors. Sensations and feelings change much more dramatically than the physical signs. The user may feel several different emotions at once or swing rapidly from one emotion to another. If taken in a large enough dosage, the drug produces delusions and visual hallucinations. Sensations may seem to "cross over," giving the user the feeling of hearing colors and seeing sounds. These changes can be frightening and can cause panic.

Users refer to their experience with LSD as a "trip" and to acute adverse reactions as a "bad trip" such as severe, terrifying thoughts and feelings, fear of losing control, fear of insanity and death, and despair while using LSD.

Some fatal accidents have occurred during states of LSD intoxication. Many LSD users also experience "flashbacks," recurrence of certain aspects of a person's experience, without the user having taken the drug again. Bad trips and flashbacks are only part of the risks of LSD use. LSD users may manifest relatively long-lasting psychoses, such as schizophrenia or severe depression.

Most users of LSD voluntarily decrease or stop its use over time. LSD is not considered an addictive drug since it does not produce compulsive drug-seeking behavior. However, like many of the addictive drugs, LSD produces tolerance, so some users who take the drug repeatedly must take progressively higher doses to achieve the state of intoxication that they have previously achieved. This is an extremely dangerous practice, given the unpredictability of the drug.

Bromo-DragonFLY

Bromo-DragonFLY is the name for another synthetic amphetamine modified from the common phenylethylamine structure. The name comes from the molecular structure that resembles a dragonfly. The hallucinogenic effect of Bromo-DragonFLY is mediated by its agonist activity at the 5-HT_{2A} serotonin receptor. Bromo-DragonFLY also has a high binding affinity for the 5-HT_{2B} and 5-HT_{2C} serotonin receptors.

Bromo-DragonFLY is considered an extremely potent hallucinogen, only slightly less potent than LSD with a very narrow safe dosing window. It has a much longer duration of action than LSD and can last for up to 2–3 days following a single large dose, with a slow onset of action that can take up to 6 h before the effect is felt [16].

Due to both adrenergic and serotonergic activity, the risk of cardiovascular toxicity is quite high. Confusion, heart problems, hallucinations, seizures, and even death have been reported from the consumption of DragonFLY. Moreover, many of the individuals who have suffered from its use were first time users.

Management

Because there is no specific antidote for PCP, LSD, and Bromo-DragonFLY, the treatment of patients intoxicated with these drugs mostly consists of supportive care—controlling breathing, circulation, and body temperature—and, in the early stages, treating psychiatric symptoms. Benzodiazepines, such as lorazepam, are the drugs of choice to control agitation and seizures when present. Typical antipsychotics such as phenothiazines and haloperidol have been used to control psychotic symptoms. But antipsychotic medications may produce many undesirable side effects, such as dystonia, and their use is therefore no longer preferred.

Alcohol Abuse and Withdrawal

Alcoholism is a common entity seen by the ICU clinician, as their patient population is commonly status post trauma and/or homeless, both of which are risk factors. Patients who present to the critical care setting intoxicated are at a higher risk of alcohol withdrawal. To assess a critically ill patient's risk of developing withdrawal, it is important to determine if this individual is classified as alcohol dependent (Table 31.1). An important consideration is prior episodes of alcohol withdrawal while being treaded for an alcohol related disorder [17].

Pathophysiology of Alcohol Intoxication and Alcohol Withdrawal

Signs and symptoms of alcohol intoxication are due to the depressant effects of alcohol on GABA receptors leading to NMDA receptor upregulation. Alcohol withdrawal results due to the lack of opposition to the NMDA receptors.

Table 31.1 Checklist of DSM-IV-TR criteria for alcohol abuse disorders

Criteria for alcohol abuse
The patients' drinking has repeatedly caused or contributed to one or more of the following adverse consequences in the past 12 months:
Risk of bodily harm (i.e., drinking and driving, operating machinery, or swimming)
Problems with relationships (family or friends)
Interference with home, work, or school role obligations
Arrests or other legal problems
Criteria for alcohol dependence
The patient has had three or more of the following behavioral or physiological consequences in the past 12 months:
Behavioral consequences (loss of control or preoccupation)
Has repeatedly exceeded drinking limits
Has not been able to cut down or stop (repeated failed attempts)
Has continued drinking despite recurrent physical or psychological problems
Has spent a lot of time drinking (or anticipating or recovering from drinking)
Has spent less time on activities that had been important or pleasurable
Physiological consequences
Has shown tolerance (needed to drink a lot more to get the same effect)
Has had signs of withdrawal (tremors, sweating, nausea, or insomnia when trying to quit or cut down)

The criteria are based on the Diagnostic and Statistical Manual of Mental Disorders, 4th edition, text revision (DSM-IV-TR). A patient who meets the criteria for both abuse and dependence is considered to have dependence, the more severe disorder. The table is adapted from the DSM-IV-TR and information from the National Institute on Alcohol Abuse and Alcoholism (modified from Friedmann [34])

Clinical Features of Alcohol Withdrawal Syndrome

The clinical course of alcohol withdrawal is traditionally divided into four stages.

- *Stage I or autonomic hyperactivity* (6–8 h of reduction in alcohol use). The patient may display tremulousness, nervousness, and nausea, but maintain a clear sensorium [18, 19].
- *Stage II* (24–48 h). The patient may display worsening agitation and alcoholic hallucinations, usually tactile in nature [18, 19].
- *Stage III or neuronal hyperexcitability* (6–48 h from last alcoholic ingestion). The patient presents with tonic-clonic seizures.
- Stage IV or Delirium Tremens (DTs) (48–96 h from last alcoholic ingestion). This is classified by exaggerated sympathetic activity, psychomotor agitation, and delirium [20, 21]. As many as 5 % patients suffering from alcohol withdrawal suffer from DTs. It is associated with a 5–15 % mortality rate and death is often caused by arrhythmias or respiratory collapse (Table 31.2) [18–20].

The Clinical Institute Withdrawal Assessment of Alcohol Scale (CIWA) is scoring system established for assessing the severity and progression of alcohol withdrawal syndrome. A score of less than 10 reflects mild AWS, 10–18 moderate

Table 31.2 Diagnostic criteria for alcohol withdrawal

1. Cessation of (or reduction in) alcohol use that has been heavy and prolonged
2. Two (or more) of the following developing within several hours to a few days after criterion A
(a) Autonomic hyperactivity (e.g., sweating or pulse rate >100/min)
(b) Increased hand tremor
(c) Insomnia
(d) Nausea or vomiting
(e) Transient visual, tactile, or auditory hallucinations or illusions
(f) Psychomotor agitation
(g) Anxiety
(h) Grand mal seizures
3. The symptoms in criterion B cause clinically significant distress or impairment in social, occupational, or other important areas of functioning
4. The symptoms are not due to a general medical condition and are not accounted for by another medical disorder. Specify if with perceptual disturbances. This specifier may be noted in the rare instance when hallucinations with intact reality testing or auditory, or tactile illusions occur in the absence of a delirium. Intact reality means that the person knows that the hallucinations are induced by the substance and do not represent external reality. When hallucinations occur in the absence of intact reality testing, a diagnosis of substance-induced psychomotor disorder, with hallucinations, should be considered.

Based on the Diagnostic and Statistical Manual of Mental Disorders, 4th edition, text revision (DSM-IV-TR). Modified from Carlson et al. [18]

to severe, and greater than 20 is severe. Studies have shown that an initial CIWA 15–18 are associated with a greater risk of complications [19]. The score should be calculated on admission, and should be reassessed hourly to look for signs of progression. Patients with score of 20 or greater should be transferred to ICU for management, with the goal of reducing the score to 10 or less in the next 24 h [19].

Management of Alcohol Withdrawal Syndrome in the ICU

The key to managing a patient with intoxication and withdrawal are symptom control, preventing progression, and treatment of coexisting comorbidities [22]. A toxicology screen should be performed in all intoxicated patients as it is important to rule out other potential substance involvement. Early treatment suppresses significant manifestations of withdrawal and prevents progression to DTs [20]. Treatment includes continuous vital monitoring, aggressive hydration, electrolyte correction, and multivitamin administration. Respiratory support with endotracheal intubation may be necessary in the setting of altered mental status or seizure. IV thiamine and dextrose should also be administered for the prevention of Wernicke's encephalopathy [18, 19].

Benzodiazepines are the gold standard of treatment of alcohol withdrawal. No one benzodiazepine is superior for the management for alcohol withdrawal. Benzodiazepines with a longer duration of action like valium and chlordiazepoxide have shown to be efficacious in preventing alcoholic seizures and delirium tremens [20]. The dose of benzodiazepine is variable, and adjustment must be done based on symptom severity [19].

Dosing and duration of therapy with benzodiazepines has been a controversial topic among clinicians. In studies comparing symptom-triggered therapy versus fixed dose therapy, it had been shown that fixed dosing has a longer duration of *treatment* and a larger volume of benzodiazepine administered [20]. As a result, using the CIWA-Ar as a guide, most institutions have initiated symptoms triggered protocols for the treatment of alcohol withdrawal. However this approach has not been validated for the ICU [23]. ICU-based studies comparing protocol and symptom-triggered therapies have shown that protocol-driven therapy is associated with less benzodiazepine use and lower complication rates of intubation and excessive sedation, while symptom-triggered therapy was associated with higher doses of benzodiazepines, but a significant decrease in mechanical ventilation [17]. For severe cases of withdrawal in the ICU, some studies have recommended a titrated infusion of benzodiazepines for patients requiring high doses of benzodiazepines [18]. However, it has been shown that patients treated with bolus IV medications had a much decreased ICU length of stay as well as less need for mechanical ventilation when compared to patients on infusion therapies [21].

A number of therapies have been shown to be good adjuvants to benzodiazepines. Haloperidol is effective at reducing tremulousness and anxiety associated with withdrawal, but is less effective in reducing delirium. Haloperidol increases seizure threshold and has been shown to increase mortality when not used in conjunction with benzodiazepines [19, 23]. Beta-adrenergic antagonists are useful in treating autonomic symptoms, but do not reduce the incidence of seizures [22, 23]. Carbamazepine has been used in Europe extensively and has shown to be effective in treating mild to moderate symptoms of alcohol withdrawal and seizures in animal studies, but very few studies have been performed in humans. In addition, it does not treat delirium.

The alpha-2 agonists Clonidine and Dexmedetomidine have been found to be effective in managing alcohol withdrawal in critically ill patients when used along with benzodiazepines. They help control agitation and autonomic hyperactivity, while maintaining respirations. It has also allowed for much lower doses of benzodiazepines to be administered to patients in acute alcohol withdrawal. However both agents fail to control delirium or seizures [21]. Propofol has also been used successfully in cases of benzodiazepine-resistant AWS, but whether or not it simply provides general anesthesia with little effect on neurotransmission is to be determined.

Nicotine Abuse and Withdrawal

Pathophysiology

Nicotine stimulates nicotinic cholinergic receptors, which subsequently release dopamine into the ventral tegmental area of the midbrain and the shell of the nucleus accumbens.

Symptoms and Management of Nicotine Withdrawal

The traditional symptoms of nicotine withdrawal include irritability, anxiety, tension, difficulty concentrating, decreased heart rate, GI disturbances, frequent urination, and difficulty sleeping [24]. More importantly, in the ICU setting, it can manifest as agitation, delirium, and pulling at lines and catheters [25]. The symptoms peak in the first 24–36 h, with a gradual decrease in severity in 3–4 days [26] Critical illness can heighten the effect of withdrawal symptoms [25].

Management of nicotine withdrawal for ICU physician begins with the clinician being able to identify nicotine withdrawal. This usually starts with getting a complete history. Scales like the Fagerstrom Test for Nicotine Dependence and the Nicotine Dependence Syndrome Scale can be used to assess for signs of nicotine dependence, which leads to a higher risk of withdrawal [27]. Studies have shown nicotine replacement therapy as an effective treatment for the symptoms of withdrawal [25, 26].

Stimulant Abuse and Withdrawal

Characteristics and Pathophysiology

Two of the most commonly abused stimulants are cocaine and amphetamines. Cocaine has a high lipid solubility, resulting in rapid distribution in and out of the central nervous system. This results in blockade of dopamine, norepinephrine, and serotonin reuptake [28]. Amphetamines, like crystal methamphetamine and designer amphetamines like "ecstacy" (3,4-methylenedioxymethamphetamine) resemble epinephrine and dopamine in structure, and block reuptake of neurotransmitters similarly to cocaine [28]. Drugs structurally similar to amphetamines include propylhexedrine, khat, cathinone, and methcathinone [29].

Symptoms of Stimulant Intoxication and Withdrawal in the ICU

Suspicion of stimulant intoxication should be increased for patients who present with symptoms of increased alertness, lower anxiety, and a generalized feeling of euphoria. Binge stimulant users may present acutely psychotic with paranoia and delusions, but rarely with hallucinations [30]. Severe systemic symptoms can also be observed. Specifically, cocaine intoxication can present with acute myocardial ischemia secondary to vasospasm, as well as seizures, while amphetamine intoxication can potentially result in hyperpyrexia with resulting rhabdomyolysis and hyponatremia [28].

Cessation of stimulant use results in a three-phase pattern: crash, withdrawal, and extinction. The crash is the extreme exhaustion that follows active use, and manifests initially with intense depression, agitation, and anxiety, followed by prolonged hypersomnolence and hyperphagia. Withdrawal symptoms are decreased energy, minimal interest, and limited ability to experience pleasure. Withdrawal symptoms peak at 12–96 h, and craving for stimulant will continue beyond that period. The phase of extinction is when the deconditioning for cravings is no longer present [30].

Chronic use of cocaine or amphetamine does not produce physical dependence as seen with alcohol, but its users develop tolerance to its euphoric effects, with resulting psychological dependence and escalating use. These patients are at a high risk of withdrawal. Cocaine or amphetamine withdrawal is defined by depressed mood and any two of the following: fatigue, vivid dreams, sleep disturbances, increased appetite, psychomotor retardation, or agitation [31].

Management of Stimulant Intoxication and Withdrawal

Management of stimulant intoxication insures maintenance of a patent airway, monitoring respiratory status, and avoidance of excessive sympathetic stimulation. Psychosis, hyperthermia, seizures, and cardiovascular excitation can be treated

Table 31.3 Therapies for symptomatic treatment in patients with stimulant overdose and withdrawal

Agitation	Benzodiazepines (usually adequate for the cardiovascular manifestations)
	Diazepam 10 mg (or equivalent) IV, repeat rapidly until the patient is calm (cumulative dose may be as high as 100 mg of diazepam)
Seizures	Benzodiazepines
	Barbiturates
	Propofol
Hyperthermia	External cooling
	Control agitation rapidly
Gastric decontamination and elimination	Activated charcoal for recent oral ingestions
Hypertension	Control agitation first
	α-Adrenergic receptor antagonist (phentolamine)
	Vasodilator (nitroprusside, nitroglycerine, or possibly nicardipine)
Delirium or hallucinations with abnormal vital signs	If agitated: Benzodiazepines
Delirium or hallucinations with normal vital signs	Consider risk/benefit of haloperidol or droperidol

Modified from Chang et al. [29]

with benzodiazepine administration and calcium channel blockers. The use of beta-blockers in cocaine-induced acute coronary syndrome is controversial, as there is a concern of precipitating vasospasm. However, labetalol and carvedilol has been shown to be effective is treatment of cocaine toxicity [32, 33]. Management of common complications of amphetamine intoxication can be seen in Table 31.3 [29]. Withdrawal symptoms, while protracted in time course and uncomfortable for the patient, are rarely life threatening. They are traditionally treated with supportive measures. However, in this withdrawal period, chronic stimulant abuser usually feel a dependence on the drug to prevent them from feeling ill, and intense cravings occur. Studies have looked into potential pharmacotherapy to help these symptoms. Use of the dopamine agonist bromocriptine has been shown to be effective for cocaine users in some trials. A recent study has shown amineptine and mirtazepine to be ineffective in managing symptoms of amphetamine withdrawal [31].

References

1. Hoffmann JR, Schriger DL, Luo JS. The empiric use of naloxone in patients with altered mental status: a reappraisal. Ann Emerg Med. 1991;20:246–52.
2. Nelsen J, Marraffa J, Jones L, Grant W. Management considerations follow overdoses of modified-release morphine preparations. World J Emerg Med. 2010;1:75–6.

3. Jaffe JH. Drug addiction and drug abuse. In: Gilman AG, Rall TW, Nies AS, et al., editors. Goodman and Gilman's the pharmacological basis of therapeutics. 8th ed. New York: Pergamon Press; 1990. p. 522–73.
4. O'Connor PG, Kosten TR, Stine SM. Management of opioid intoxication and withdrawal. In: Graham AW, Schultz TK, Mayo-Smith MF, et al., editors. Principles of addiction medicine. 3rd ed. Chevy Chase: American Society of Addiction Medicine; 2003. p. 651–68.
5. American Psychiatric Association. Practice guideline for the treatment of patients with substance use disorders. 2nd ed. Washington, DC: American Psychiatric Association; 2006.
6. Fiellin DA, O'Connor PG. Office-based treatment of opioid-dependent patients. New Engl J Med. 2002;347(11):817–23.
7. Gouldin WM, Kennedy DT, Small RE. Methadone: history and recommendations for use in analgesia. Am Pain Soc Bull. 2000;10(5):1–11.
8. Fiellin DA, O'Connor PG. New federal initiatives to enhance the medical treatment of opioid dependence. Ann Intern Med. 2002;137(8):688–92.
9. Loimer N, Schmid R, Presslich O, et al. Naloxone treatment for opiate withdrawal syndrome. Br J Psychiatry. 1988;153:851–2.
10. Amass L, Ling W, Freese TE, et al. Bringing buprenorphine–naloxone detoxification to community treatment providers: the NIDA clinical trials network field experience. Am J Addict. 2004;13 Suppl 1:S42–66.
11. http://reference.medscape.com/drug/romazicon-flumazenil-343731
12. Kosten TR, O'Connor PG. Management of drug and alcohol withdrawal. N Engl J Med. 2003;348(18):1786–95.
13. Mas-Morey P, Visser MHM, Winkelmolen L, et al. Clinical toxicology and management of intoxications with synthetic cathinones ("Bath Salts"). J Pharm Pract. 2013;26(4):353–7. doi:10.1177/0897190012465949.
14. Carhart-Harris RL, et al. A web-based survey on mephedrone. Drug Alcohol Depend. 2011;118(1):19–22. doi:10.1016/j.drugalcdep.2011.02.011.
15. Nelson L, Lewin N, Howland MR, Hoffman R, Goldfrank L, Flomenbaum N, editors. Goldfrank's toxicologic emergencies. 9th ed. New York: McGraw-Hill Professional; 2010.
16. http://www.erowid.org/chemicals/bromo_dragonfly/bromo_dragonfly_dose.shtml
17. Awissi D, Lebrun G, Coursin DB, Riker RR, Skrobik Y. Alcohol withdrawal and delirium tremens in the critically ill: a systemic review and commentary. Intensive Care Med. 2013;39(1):16–30. doi:10.1007/s00134-012-2758-y [Epub 27 Nov 2012].
18. Carlson RW, Kumar NN, Wong-Mckinstry E, et al. Alcohol withdrawal syndrome. Crit Care Clin. 2012;28(4):549–85. doi:10.1016/j.ccc.2012.07.004. Review.
19. Al-Sanouri I, Dikin M, Soubani AO. Critical care aspects of alcohol abuse. South Med J. 2005;98(3):372–81.
20. Tetrault, J, O'Connor PG. Substance abuse and withdrawal in the critical care setting. Crit Care Clin. 2008;24(4):767–88, viii. doi:10.1016/j.ccc.2008.05.005
21. Corfee F. Alcohol withdrawal in the critical care unit. Aust Crit Care. 2011;24(2):110–6. doi:10.1016/j.aucc.2010.08.005 [Epub 25 Sep 2010].
22. Jenkins DH. Substance abuse and withdrawal in the intensive care unit. Surg Clin North Am. 2000;80(3):1033–53.
23. Sarff M, Gold JA. Alcohol withdrawal syndromes in the intensive care unit. Crit Care Med. 2010;38(9 Suppl):S494–501. doi:10.1097/CCM.0b013e3181ec5412.
24. Honisett TD. Nicotine replacement therapy for smokers admitted to intensive care. Intensive Crit Care Nurs. 2001;17(6):318–21.
25. Lucidarme O, Seguin A, Daubin C, et al. Nicotine withdrawal and agitation in ventilated critically ill patients. Crit Care. 2010;14(2):R58. doi:10.1186/cc8954 [Epub 9 Apr 2010].
26. Padula C, Willey C. Tobacco withdrawal in CCU patients. Dimens Crit Care Nurs. 1993;12(6):305–12.
27. Shiffman S, Waters A, Hickcox M. The nicotine dependence syndrome scale: a multidimensional measure of nicotine dependence. Nicotine Tob Res. 2004;6(2):327–48.
28. Wong G, Irwin MG. Poisoning with ilicit substances: toxicology for the anaesthetist. Anaesthesia. 2013;68 Suppl 1:117–24. doi:10.1111/anae.12053.

29. Chang W. Amphetamines. In: Nelson L, Lewin N, Howland MR, Hoffman R, Goldfrank L, Flomenbaum N, editors. Goldfrank's toxicologic emergencies. 9th ed. New York: McGraw-Hill Professional; 2010.
30. Gawin F, Ellinwood Jr EH. Cocaine and other stimulants. N Engl J Med. 1988;318(18):1173–82.
31. Shoptaw SJ, Kao U, Heinzerling K, Ling W. Treatment for amphetamine withdrawal (review). Cochrane Database Syst Rev. 2009;2:CD003021. doi:10.1002/14651858.CD003021.pub2.
32. Hoskins MH, Leleiko RM, Ramos JJ, Sola S, Caneer PM, Khan BV. Effects of labetalol on hemodynamic parameters and soluble biomarkers of inflammation in acute coronary syndrome in patients with active cocaine use. J Cardiovasc Pharmacol Ther. 2010;15(1):47–52. doi:10.1177/1074248409358409.
33. Damodaran S. Cocaine and beta-blockers: the paradigm. Eur J Intern Med. 2010;21(2):84–6. doi:10.1016/j.ejim.2009.11.010 [Epub 16 Dec 2009].
34. Friedmann PD. Alcohol use in adults. N Engl J Med. 2013;368(17):1655–6. doi:10.1056/NEJMc1302445.

Chapter 32
Chronic Pain Patients and Substance Abuse

Rahul Rastogi, Narendren Narayanasamy, and Paul Sraow

Key Points

- Silent epidemics: chronic pain and substance abuse
- Terminology
- Managing pain patients within the pain/substance abuse interface
- Screening
- Screening tools
- Abuse-deterrent drug formulations
- Managing patients—specific groups
- Opioid withdrawal and detoxification

Introduction

The physical and mental states of human beings are governed by lifetime experiences and biopsychosocial makeup. They reinforce each other, and sometimes lead to maladaptive states, such as chronic pain, addiction, and so on. Pain and addiction are

R. Rastogi, M.D. (✉)
Department of Anesthesiology, Washington University School of Medicine,
23 Bon Price Terrace, St. Louis, MO 63132, USA
e-mail: rastogir@anest.wustl.edu

N. Narayanasamy, M.D.
Department of Anesthesiology, Washington University School of Medicine,
1127 Terrace Drive, St. Louis, MO 63117, USA
e-mail: dr_narendren@yahoo.com

P. Sraow, M.D., M.S.
Spine & Sports Rehabilitation Institute, 2600 E. Southern Avenue, STE I-1,
Tempe AZ 85282, USA
e-mail: ssriarizona@gmail.com

© Springer Science+Business Media New York 2015
A.D. Kaye et al. (eds.), *Substance Abuse*, DOI 10.1007/978-1-4939-1951-2_32

altered biopsychosocial experiences that are both subjective in nature and interact with one another. This interface of pain and addiction has brought about serious public health problems. It also poses ethical and healthcare dilemmas through the conflicting goals of managing pain states: pain relief, i.e. beneficence, and "do no harm", i.e. nonmaleficence [1]. With the rise of medicinal management for chronic pain over the last two decades, addiction has become more prevalent, significantly increasing the risk of morbidity and mortality in this patient population. It is the responsibility of healthcare providers to utilize all the multimodal tools in their armamentarium to provide effective pain relief without unintentionally facilitating substance abuse.

Silent Epidemics: Chronic Pain and Drug Abuse

Pain practitioners simultaneously deal with two significant public health problems, chronic pain and drug abuse. "Chronic pain" is widespread and results in significant bio-socio-economic burden. Almost a third of the US adult population, i.e. over 100 million people suffer from chronic pain [2, 3], costing more than $600 billion annually in healthcare and loss of productivity costs [4]. Chronic pain alone was responsible for 21 % emergency room visits in the United States and almost 25 % of missed workdays [5]. Early and effective pain control is essential to decrease suffering, improve function, and facilitate earlier return to work.

Among other analgesics, opioids are commonly used for managing pain. Their use has substantially grown over the last 10–15 years as a result of guideline changes, newer formulations, and increased awareness to management protocols [6]. Hence, healthcare providers should be able to recognize substance abuse among chronic pain patients due to the inherent abuse potential of opioids. "Drug abuse", i.e. illicit drug use has steadily increased for decades and has now reached a plateau over the last 2–3 years. In 2011, 8.7 % of the total American population aged 12 and over, i.e. 22.5 million Americans, had used an illicit drug in the prior 30 days, which was similar to rate in 2009 [6]. These endemic proportions account for an estimated annual cost of $193 billion in healthcare, criminal justice, and lost productivity [7]. There has been a gradual increase in emergency room (ER) utilization for health issues related to non-medical prescription drug use, as reflected by 1.1 million total ER visits in 2009 alone [8].

Although Marijuana remains the first agent of choice for illicit use [9], there is increasing prescription drug abuse year after year, which ranks second among the most commonly abused agents [6]. Among the US population of 12 years and older, 6.1 million Americans (2.7 % population) used psychotherapeutics for non-medical reasons, while 4.5 million (1.7 % population) Americans were non-medical users of analgesics [9].

"Co-Existence of Chronic pain and Drug Abuse" studies have found relatively lower drug abuse rates in chronic pain patient populations treated with a controlled substance than earlier thought. The prevalence rate of this coexistence varied from 3 to 48 % [10]. Data for chronic pain patients taking a controlled substance suggested the presence of aberrant drug behavior in 12 % patients, while 3 % were found to develop established drug abuse [11]. On the other hand, studies have shown an increased incidence of chronic pain in substance abusers, i.e. 37 % of patients in a methadone maintenance program reported chronic pain, while 24 % patients in short-term inpatient drug abuse treatment programs reported chronic pain problems [12].

Opioids, being a front-line agent for pain management with a high abuse liability are the most commonly abused prescription agents [8]. Hydrocodone, oxycodone, along with methadone, are the three most common individual opioid agents [6]. With a 400 % increase in prescription opioids, there has been a parallel six fold increase in drug abuse-related health problems. These include a fourfold increase in opioid overdose and a threefold increase in deaths from prescription drug overdoses between 1999 and 2008 [13]. A staggering three-fourth of these deaths were reported as opioid overdoses [13]. To put this in perspective, illicit opioid overdose deaths have surpassed total traffic-related deaths [14]. The risk of drug abuse-related mortality is significantly increased with higher opioid doses and concurrent use of other abused drugs. Polysubstance abuse is a common practice among illicit drug users, with tobacco and alcohol as the commonest agents used in conjunction with another drug. This can be illustrated by the data that showed 34 % of patients in a methadone maintenance program and 51 % in a short-term drug rehabilitation who were admitted for alcohol addiction also abused other agents [11].

Besides the drug abuse-related healthcare issues, there is criminal aspect as well, i.e. drug diversion. Doctor shopping, prescription fraud, and theft are the leading causes of diversion. Almost 70 % of abusers obtain drugs from a friend or relative by borrowing, buying, or stealing [6].

Terminology

There are many terms that are used to describe abnormal drug usage, i.e. dependence, tolerance, misuse, addiction, etc. These terms are often used interchangeably, and sometimes inappropriately.

1. *Physical dependence*: The body's physiologic neuronal response to a specific chemical agent due to prolonged exposure. It is characteristically manifested by "withdrawal symptoms" upon rapid de-escalation or abrupt discontinuation of that specific drug or after administration of drug-specific antagonist.
2. *Tolerance*: The body's physiologic response after repetitive use of drug characterized by the need of increase in dosing of that specific drug to maintain the same effect.
3. *Addiction*: A chronic neurobiological disease state manifested by a pattern of behavior of craving and compulsive use of drug despite resultant self-biopsychosocial harm. This behavior continues to persist even after discontinuation of drug.
4. *Pseudo addiction*: An inappropriate drug-seeking behavior in order to achieve better symptom control reflecting under treatment. This behavior resolves upon symptom relief.

5. *Substance misuse*: Use of prescribed medications for other medical reasons than which it is prescribed for.
6. *Substance abuse*: Use of any drug (prescription or illicit) for non-medical purposes.
7. *Aberrant drug behavior*: Behaviors suggesting drug abuse. These include prescription alteration, borrowing/stealing drugs from others, selling drugs, obtaining prescriptions from multiple providers simultaneously, multiple reports of loss of prescription and drug, using non-prescribed route of drug administration, and obtaining drugs illegally.
8. *Substance use disorder*: A broad umbrella term proposed through psychiatric literature that incorporates the above-mentioned issues.

Managing Pain Patients Within the Pain/Substance Abuse Interface

It is challenging for pain practitioners to achieve a balance between safe and effective pain management, while preventing drug abuse and diversion. This interface creates several patient scenarios and each requires specific attention in management of their pain. These scenarios include:

1. Chronic pain management in patients with

   (a) Low aberrant drug abuse behaviors/risk

      • With no history of drug misuse/abuse
      • With past history of drug misuse/abuse

   (b) Moderate aberrant drug abuse behaviors/risk

      • With no history of drug misuse/abuse
      • With past history of drug misuse/abuse
      • With current drug misuse/abuse

   (c) High aberrant drug abuse behaviors/risk

      • With past history of drug abuse
      • With current drug abuse

2. Acute pain management in patients with

   (a) No history of drug abuse/misuse
   (b) Past history of drug abuse/misuse

      • Remote history
      • Recent, but in recovery
      • Currently in drug maintenance rehabilitation program

   (c) Current drug abuse

Prescription drug abuse is the leading cause of death within substance use disorders. Prescription opioids are the most abused class of medications in the United States [15]. It is vital for healthcare providers to understand the associated risk when an opioid is an option to choose for their pain management. Healthcare providers should utilize all tools to improve identification and/or prevent drug abuse/diversion, while practicing safe and effective medicine. This requires comprehensive initial assessment and drug abuse risk stratification, while maintaining judicial use of resources. The frequency and extent of assessment, monitoring, and resource utilization should be proportional to drug abuse risk stratification, i.e. high-risk patients need more frequent and random urine/blood screening as well as more frequent follow up [16].

Several strategies have been suggested to reach this goal, which help develop individualized management plans for specific patients.

1. Comprehensive clinical history, with emphasis on drug history
2. Psychosocial screening interview
3. Drug risk stratification

    (a) Aberrant behavior screening tools

4. Drug adherence/maintenance

    (a) Screening tools: including screening questionnaires, urinary drug screens

5. Practice support tools—including controlled-substance (i.e. opioid) therapy drug agreement, Risk Evaluation & Mitigation Strategies (REMS), Prescription Drug-Monitoring Programs (PDMPs).

Screening

Every doctor–patient interaction should begin with understanding the patient's problem and background. A detailed clinical history is an essential first step, and should include alcohol, tobacco, prescription, and illicit drug use histories. A psychological screening interview can also be very useful in the evaluation of a patient before introducing any opioids in their treatment regimen (Table 32.1).

When the risk of drug abuse can be stratified, it facilitates developing individualized management plans. Risk stratification divides patients into low, moderate, or high-risk categories. In addition to a detailed history, aberrant behavior screening tools used for risk stratifications include:

1. Urinary Drug Screen—prior to initiating opioid therapies
2. The Screener and Opioid Assessment for Patients with Pain Revised (SOAPP-R)—a validated patient-administered screening tool which contains 24 items designed specifically to stratify the risk of drug abuse in patients with chronic pain. A score of 18 or more reflects risk for opioid abuse. It has sensitivity of 80 % with specificity of 52 % [17].

Table 32.1 Screening of pain patients for drug abuse risk

When considering a controlled-substance in the treatment plan	
Initial risk stratification	Treatment adherence
Comprehensive clinical history	Repeat comprehensive clinical history
Comprehensive medicinal/drug history	Medicinal history
Psychological screening interview	
Aberrant Risk Behavior Assessment Tools	Random urine drug screen (UDS)
Pre-opioid urinary drug screen (UDS)	Aberrant Risk Behavior Assessment Tools
Screener & Opioid Assessment for Patient with Pain (SOAPP-R)	The Current Opioid Misuse Measure (COMM)
Opioid Risk Tool (ORT)	The Pain Medication Questionnaire (PMQ)
Practice support tools	The Pain Assessment and Documentation Tool (PADT)
Prescription Drug-Monitoring Program (PDMP)	Practice support tools
Controlled-Substance Agreement	Prescription Drug-Monitoring Program (PDMP)
Risk Evaluation and Mitigation Strategies (REMS)	Risk Evaluation and Mitigation strategies (REMS)

3. The Opioid Risk Tool (ORT)—another validated 5-item opioid abuse risk tool, administered by the clinician to assess the risk of opioid abuse in pain patients. A score of 4–7 suggests moderate risk, while 8 or more suggests high risk for opioid abuse [17].

These screening tools only reflect the risk of drug abuse, but do not necessitate opioid abstinence. The decision of prescribing opioids depends upon the physician and the patient's individual clinical scenario. Once opioids are initiated and continued in treating a patient's pain, it important to continue appropriate compliance monitoring. Repetitive clinical histories during each visit play a vital role. Several aberrant behavior screening and practice supporting tools have been suggested, including:

1. Random and frequent Urinary Drug Screens
2. Aberrant Behavior Screening tools

   - The Current Opioid Misuse Measure (COMM): a self-administered 17-item validated tool for pain patients with current opioid use to measure ongoing aberrant drug behavior. It should be applied repeatedly during continuation of opioids as a part of an ongoing treatment regimen. Increasing scores correlate with increasing aberrant drug behavior for opioid misuse [17].
   - The Pain Medication Questionnaire (PMQ): a self-administered 26-item questionnaire validated for measuring the progress of chronic pain patients with ongoing opioid usage. Higher scores correlate with increased risk for opioid abuse [17].
   - The Pain Assessment and Documentation Tool (PADT): a clinician administered 41-item questionnaire assessing various pain dimensions and outcomes in long-term opioid usage [17].

3. Practice support tools: Opioid therapy agreements, REMS, PDMPs, abuse-deterrent drug formulations, etc.

There are several screening tools that have been compared. One study showed their efficacies as SOAPP-R>ORT>PMQ>COMM individually, while SOAPP-R with psychological interview had the best sensitivity when utilized in conjunction [18].

Screening Tools

Drug Abuse Risk Factors

There are several parts of a patient's comprehensive history that may suggest drug abuse risk, and identified risk factors require close attention (Table 32.2) [19].

Aberrant Drug Behaviors

During a comprehensive patient evaluation, it is necessary to recognize behaviors, which can reflect the risk of drug abuse or ongoing use. Certain behaviors are more or less predictive of drug misuse (Table 32.3) [20].

Urinary Drug Screens (UDS)

Urine drug screens are used to reveal illicit drugs use, stratify drug-misuse risk, and monitor treatment adherence. They are used randomly and the frequency of use depends on the level of risk and/or changes in patient behavior during treatment.

Table 32.2 Risk factors for drug misuse

Biological	Psychological	Social
Young age	Current/past polysubstance use	Poor social support
Male gender	Illicit drugs	Previous/current history of
Family history of polysubstance abuse	Alcohol	Criminal activity
Exaggeration of pain, beyond extent of injury	Tobacco	DUIs
	Psychological comorbidities	Frequent contact with high risk
	Depression	Situations/places/events
	Severe anxiety	Personnel
	Psychiatric disorders	Decrease functioning at
	History of	Family
	Thrill seeking behaviors	Society
	Preadolescent sexual abuse	Workplace/school

Table 32.3 Aberrant drug behaviors [20]

	Probably less predictive	Probably predictive
Symptoms/signs	Symptom exaggeration	Intoxicated appearance
	Repetitive requests for higher doses	Altered behavior at work, family, or society
Compliance	1–2 occasion of self-dose increase	Several occasions of self-dose increase
		Resisting to get old medical records
		Resisting for urine or blood drug screens
		Noncompliance in appointment for
		Regular, nonprescription-related visits
		Multidisciplinary appointments
Prescription	Drug misuse	Dose prescription forgery
	Trying to get from other practitioners (openly)	Frequent prescription/drug losses
		Trying to get drugs from
		Several providers (doctor shopping)
		Non-medical sources
		Borrowing or stealing drugs from others
		Buying from street (drug dealers, etc.)
Drugs	Requesting specific drug	Selling prescribed drug
	Drug hoarding from periods of lesser pain	Using non-prescribed route of drug administration
		Tampering with drug formulations
		Injection oral formulation
		Snorting oral formulation
Concurrent usage	Tobacco	Alcohol
		Illicit drugs

This information can also be helpful in emergency rooms or within the workplace. However, these tests may not be sufficient for drug-misuse monitoring as they use fixed concentration cut-off levels. Thus can detect recent use or higher drug concentrations, but may miss lower concentrations. Information provided to the clinician may be further limited as most tests only detect a particular class of drugs, and not individual drugs of that class. There is also the possibility of cross-reactivity among different drugs. Furthermore, they do not provide information respective to a patient's variable dosing of medications.

There are two commonly used methods used for Urine Drug Screening: Qualitative Immunoassay and Analytical (Qualitative & Quantitative) Mass Spectrometry [21].

The basis of Qualitative immunoassay UDS is a specific antibody reaction to a particular drug. Rapid "point of care" (POC) evaluations of urine among pain patients monitor treatment adherence, and this is an immunoassay qualitative UDS model. Several POC models such as "UDS cups" or "UDS sticks" are available, and are designed to detect various illicit drugs including some specific drugs, i.e. opioids. By using lower cut-off concentration levels in POC UDS, sensitivity of drug detection is increased and this may be more clinically relevant. Depending on the situation, these samples can be sent out for further confirmative and even quantitative analysis to designated labs.

Analytical mass spectroscopy utilizes the separation of drug molecules based on their mass and fragmentation pattern through chromatography in order to identify a specific drug molecule, and also isotopic dilution analysis to quantify the drug in urine sample. This method is considered the gold standard for UDS [21]. Not only is drug presence or absence determined through direct drug molecule or metabolite identification, but also the status of the urine sample — adulterated or non-adulterated. There are two chromatographic models available: liquid chromatography–mass spectroscopy or gas chromatography–mass spectroscopy. Liquid chromatography–mass spectroscopy has advantages in that it requires only a very small amount of urine, identifies many more drugs in one test run, and has a faster run time to allow more rapid results to clinicians.

UDS use should be individualized depending on clinical history, comorbid conditions, and drug-misuse risk stratification. The limitations of a particular UDS should be kept in mind while making interpretations from the results. The patient's medicinal history helps in making these inferences (Table 32.4). Various specialty societies recommended the random use of UDS, as studies have shown they can identify high-risk drug abuse, even in the absence of aberrant drug behavior [21].

Controlled-Substance (Opioid) Therapy Agreement

It is common and good clinical practice, to clearly outline the roles and expectations between patients, and healthcare providers in regards to the use and compliance of prescribed controlled substances. One commonly used tool to help establish this understanding is a "Controlled-Substance Agreement" [22]. This is a mutual consent between a patient and healthcare provider/clinic to educate them clearly about

Table 32.4 How to use urinary drug screens

• Should be individualized
• Used randomly
• Should be used as initial evaluation tool for drug-risk stratification
• Should be used on the basis of risk strata:
– *Minimal Risk:* Initial visit, random use, should be used twice a year for treatment adherence monitoring
– *Possible Risk*: Initial visit, random use, more frequent use, i.e. 4–5 times per year or every refill
• Used upon any addition of new drug
• Used upon any new aberrant behavior change
• Confirm test results quantitatively
• Upon positive UDS (i.e. presence of non-prescribed drug, absence of prescribed drug) — Interact with patient for possible discontinuation of opioids, or to establish stricter monitoring including UDS, etc.

their roles, expectations, and possible actions upon noncompliance. These agreements can be quite different among practitioners, but should all incorporate the following statements and conditions [22]:

1. Patients should only:

   (a) use medication(s) as prescribed
   (b) receive scripts for controlled medication(s) only from one physician
   (c) use only one pharmacy to fill those medication(s)

2. Patient should agree to:

   (a) taper off a medication upon no improvement of quality of life or function as directed by the physician
   (b) participate in multidisciplinary aspects of treatment including physical therapy, psycho/behavioral therapies, etc.
   (c) give periodic urine or blood samples for screening

3. Patient is responsible for:

   (a) the safe custody of medication(s)
   (b) maintaining regular appointments

4. Patient fully understands:

   (a) they will not get prescription refills early
   (b) medication(s) will not be replaced if lost/stolen
   (c) upon noncompliance, medication(s) will be discontinued

The purpose of Controlled-Substance Agreement is to promote the patient's education, their compliance, and to ultimately improve outcomes including decreased morbidity and mortality.

Prescription Drug-Monitoring Programs (PDMP)

With the rise in availability and use of more controlled drugs for the management of pain, there has also been a rise in prescription drug abuse and associated mortality. A federal initiative in 2007 suggested that each state should establish and operate a statewide electronic prescription drug-monitoring program (PDMPs) [23]. These programs should monitor drugs prescription in real-time, and should also be accessible to healthcare providers when prescribing controlled substances as part of their treatment plans. PDMPs can not only improve medical care through prescription drug monitoring (i.e. drug interactions, aberrant drug behavior, doctor shopping, etc.), but can also be used as investigative tools to prevent or address drug misuse and diversion.

Except for the state of Missouri, all US states and territories have PDMPs either up and running or in the process of being established. Studies from early PDMP states showed improved medical outcomes and better utilization of opioids.

Table 32.5 Elements of Risk Evaluation and Mitigation Strategy (REMS)

1	A patient package insert – medication guide	Highlighting patient safety information, implemented through the pharmacist with each prescription refill
2	A communication plan for healthcare providers	Tools and materials for healthcare provider education regarding safe prescribing and use of medications i.e. CMEs, letters to practitioners
3	Elements to assure safe use (ETASU)	Dispensing drugs through specific registered pharmacies
		Provider's education and certification for safe prescribing of drugs
		Enrollment of patients, pharmacies, physicians in central registry program
4	An implementation plan for ETASU	An implementation plan for ETASU
		Monitoring of implementation
5	Timetable for submission of assessments	Assess and submit by 18 months, 3 years, and 7 years after or an otherwise specified timetable upon initial approval for REMS by FDA

CME Continuing Medical Education, *ETASU* Elements to assure safe use, *FDA* Federal Drug Administration

Adjustment of opioid treatment regimens resulted in 61 % patients being prescribed less opioid, while 39 % were prescribed higher opioid doses within their treatment regimens [24]. Although different states collect different data points and allow different authorities to get access, PDMPs have significant potential to improve outcomes upon full utilization. Furthermore, PDMPs are becoming increasingly more interactive between states that can further improve their effectiveness.

Risk Evaluation and Mitigation Strategy (REMS)

Various drugs have been approved for clinical use when their benefits outweigh the risks, but still certain medications continue to carry relatively higher risks. The Food and Drug Administration (FDA) recommends/mandates a strategy to ensure the continued benefits outweighing the risks of a specific drug or biological product. This is termed as the "Risk Evaluation and Mitigation Strategy (REMS)" [25]. The FDA requires REMS for several drugs, and various opioids are in this list [26]. REMS has several elements (Table 32.5) all which are not necessarily required for each drug, and the FDA determines these elements for each specific drug.

Upon the finding of new safety information, the FDA reviews drug status for REMS requirements again to ensure that the benefits of the drug outweigh its risks.

Abuse-Deterrent Drug Formulations (ADF)

Pain is an eternal biopsychosocial and socioeconomic problem. It is of prime importance to manage pain early and effectively. Opioids are commonly used to achieve this. With increasing acceptance of opioids for the management of chronic pain, there has been a significant rise in their availability and utilization in the last decade. Likewise, there has been an increase in drug abuse-related mortality, which has surpassed motor vehicle accidents as the leading cause of death [14]. Opioids are the most common agents used illicitly, with hydrocodone and oxycodone leading the pack [15]. Drug abusers show three patterns of drug use and aberrant drug behaviors:

1. Taking medications faster than prescribed for the prescribed indication, i.e. taking more pills
2. Taking medications illicitly

    (a) using medication faster than prescribed for non-prescribed indications
    (b) mixing controlled medications with other non-prescribed controlled substances, i.e. controlled medications with alcohol or other drugs

3. Illicit use of the drug by manipulative formulations or unapproved alternate routes of administration other than prescribed, i.e. crushing slow release matrix formulations to achieve high concentrations instantly, crushing drug to snort or smoke, crushing, and/or dissolving drugs to inject intravenously

The purpose of these behaviors is to achieve a euphoric state by releasing a high amount of medication at once or delivering a high dose faster. This results in a higher drug concentration (C_{max}) in shorter time (T_{max}). All three aberrant drug behavior patterns are troubling, but the latter two can be life threatening. Drug formulations with the lowest abuse liabilities (C_{max}/T_{max} ratio) should be utilized to prevent or deter drug abuse. Pharmaceutical companies continue developing formulations of opioids with lower abuse liabilities that are difficult and cumbersome to abuse. These formulations are termed as "Abuse-Deterrent Opioids" [27].

Abuse-deterrent formulations are being developed using various pharmacologic engineering processes and they can be categorized broadly into four categories (Table 23.6) [27]:

Table 23.6 Abuse-deterrent technologies [27]

Physical barrier	To avoid destruction or make it difficult to extract an active drug	Oxycontin (new)—resists crushing
		Exalgo (hydromorphone ER)
		Remoxy (oxycodone CR)—resists dissolution/snorting
Aversion	Noxious agents are added to produce an unpleasant sensation upon use through non-prescribed routes of delivery	Acurox (oxycodone + niacin)
Agonist/ antagonist combinations	Addition of an antagonist to reduce euphoric effects or cause withdrawal symptoms upon tampering of the drug	Embeda (morphine + naltrexone)
		Suboxone (buprenorphine + naloxone)
Prodrug	Non-active drug that can only be activated in the presence of gastrointestinal enzymatic milieu	KP511 (hydromorphone prodrug)

1. *Physical barriers*: Abuse of a drug can be deterred by:
   (a) physically making the tablet difficult to crush
   (b) a chemical barrier that makes extraction of medication difficult, i.e. upon trying to dissolve with a solvent, it becomes a thick gel, deterring injection

2. *Aversion technology*: Another substance is added with the drug that creates an unpleasant sensation when used in alternate unapproved routes of administration, i.e. snorting. Commonly used aversive agents include niacin, capsaicin, ipecac, etc.

3. *Agonist/antagonist combinations*: Addition of insulated antagonists, i.e. naltrexone, naloxone, with opioids to prevent the euphoric effect of the opioid or to cause an unpleasant withdrawal effect when the otherwise insulated antagonist is released due to manipulation of the drug.

4. *Pro Drug*: A prodrug is an agent that requires enzymatic cleavage or activation in gastrointestinal tract to become an active opioid, thus preventing alternate routes of drug administration.

Some formulations are under development combining two deterrent technologies resulting in even lower abuse liability ADFs. Although ADFs are still in very early stages, there has been no evidence that ADFs will completely stop drug abuse, and ADFs have not yet been shown to decrease the prevalence of drug abuse. Despite this, the use of ADFs can be a good practice to at least attempt to deter drug abuse and promote safer management.

Managing Patients: Specific Groups

Managing Pain in High Abuse Risk Patients

In addition to comprehensive initial assessments, patients with chronic pain and "high drug abuse risk" stratification require more frequent ongoing assessments and increased resource utilization to deliver safe and effective analgesia [28]. Closer monitoring is necessary to prevent abuse and diversion. "Resources" comprise of tools for risk stratification, screening, monitoring, and various aspects of healthcare and judicial systems, including manpower (Table 32.7).

Managing Acute Pain in the Setting of Substance Abuse

Substance abusers also suffer from other health problems requiring certain interventions leading to acute pain that needs to be managed early and effectively. While managing their acute pain needs, practitioners should be aware about their potential risk of reactivation of their addiction issues. For acute pain management these patients fall into three clinical scenarios: Past substance abuser, Patient in Substance abuse maintenance rehab and current active substance abuser (Table 32.8) [29].

Table 32.7 Managing pain in high-abuse risk patients

More assessment	More resources	More monitoring
Detailed initial assessment	Maximize concurrent treatments	More frequent follow-up
Frequent follow-up assessment	Physical rehabilitation	Screening questionnaires for aberrant drug behaviors
More consultation, as needed	Adjuvant analgesics	
Detailed previous history	Psychological therapies	Strict prescribing
Verification of history	Active recovery program	Fewer excuses
Chart reviews	Controlled-Substance Agreement	Supervised dosing
Collateral information	One prescriber	Pill counting on each visit
Supportive networks	One pharmacy	Frequent, but random urine or blood drug screen
Frequent assessment of function	No replacement of	
Detailed medicinal history	"Lost" scripts	Frequent utilization of PDMP
Past medications	"Lost" medications	
Response to medications	No early refills	
Attention to side effects	Prescribing pattern	
Drug-misuse risk stratification	Shorter dispensing intervals	
Initial Urinary Drug Screen	No phone refills	
Risk assessment tools	More education	
	For patients	
	For family members	
	For providers i.e. REMS	

PDMP prescription drug-monitoring programs, *REMS* Risk Evaluation and Mitigation Strategies

Table 32.8 Managing acute pain with history of substance abuse in in-patient setting

Assessment	In-patient management	Discharge
A. Patient recovered from a Substance Abuse Disorder		
Detailed initial assessment	Maximize concurrent treatments	Drug abuse risk stratification
Frequent assessment	Physical rehabilitation	Pre-discharge urine drug screen
More consultation, as needed	Adjuvant analgesics	Education
Pain, addiction, psychiatry	Psychological therapies	Discharge plan
Detailed previous history	Regional anesthetic modalities	Monitoring
Verification of history	More education	Close follow ups
Chart reviews	For patients	Weaning of opioids
Collateral information	For family members	Maximizing adjuvant therapy
Supportive network	Medication choice	Appropriate screening
Frequent assessment of function	Avoid partial-agonist opioid	Aberrant drug behavior

(continued)

Table 32.8 (continued)

Assessment	In-patient management	Discharge
Detailed medicinal history	Choose low abuse-potential drug formulations	Adherence to prescribed drug
Past medications	Develop a plan to avoid relapse or a therapeutic plan upon relapse	
Response to medications		
Attention to side effects		
B. Patient in a Substance Abuse Maintenance Rehabilitation Program		
In addition to "A" above	*In addition to "A" above*	*In addition to "A" above*
Consult—addiction specialists	Continue maintenance drug	Follow up with their maintenance program
Confirm	i.e. Methadone	
Drug	Maximize adjuvants	
Methadone	For buprenorphine/naltrexone	
Buprenorphine	Discontinue 48 h before elective procedure	
Naltrexone	Watch for withdrawal	
Doses from	Upon resumption, titrate up slowly	
Maintenance program		
Prescribing physician		
C. Patient with current substance abuse		
In addition to "A" above	*In addition to "A" above*	*In addition to "A" above*
Confirm drug and frequency of abuse	Emphasis on non-opioid multimodal management	Clear discharge plan
Assess abuse related co-morbidities	Maximize adjuvants	Avoid outpatient opioids
	Use opioids judiciously	May choose abuse-deterrent formulations
Consult—addiction specialist	Use IV opioids i.e. PCA	
		Short, limited quantity scripts
Consult—psychiatry/ psychologist	May consider abuse-deterrent formulations	Close follow-up, i.e. weekly visits
	Avoid agonist–antagonist formulations	Weaning protocols
		Maximize adjuvant therapy
		Follow-up with addiction specialist
		Clear monitoring
		Compliance with follow-up appointments
		Frequent assessment and abuse risk stratification
Attention for withdrawal		Frequent and random use of screening tools i.e. UDS, PDMP

PCA patient-controlled analgesia, *PDMP* prescription drug-monitoring programs, *UDS* urinary drug screening

Opioid Withdrawal and Detoxification

Physical dependence of opioids could develop as early as within 7 days of exposure to typically several weeks to months of opioid use. This physical dependence predisposes to opioid withdrawal syndrome upon abrupt/rapid discontinuation of opioid, administration of a partial-agonist (i.e. buprenorphine), and/or administering of opioid antagonist (i.e. naloxone, naltrexone). Short-acting substances tend to have a higher potential for a withdrawal compared to long-acting agents, while longer-acting substances tend to have a longer, but less intense withdrawal duration [30].

Acute opioid withdrawal involves multiple systems and often demonstrates predictable patterns. Understanding these clinical manifestations and patterns are essential to make an early diagnosis to prevent any catastrophe. The relevant clinical characteristics of opioid withdrawal symptoms [30] are:

1. Increased pain, irritability, anxiety, restlessness, and myalgias often reported in the back and legs are some of the first subjective complaints.
2. Piloerection and fever are associated with more severe withdrawal, but less commonly seen as patients usually retake the substance before these symptoms appear.
3. Symptoms of anxiety, dysphoria, anhedonia, and insomnia may persist during a less acute phase lasting for weeks to months.
4. Drug craving may be seen throughout, and is likely responsible for relapse during attempted abstinence.

The American Psychiatry Association has defined the DSM V criteria in order to make the diagnosis of opioid withdrawal (Table 32.9) [30].

Table 32.9 Criteria for opioid withdrawal [30]

1. Presence of either of the following:
(a) Cessation of (or reduction in) opioid use that has been heavy and prolonged (i.e. several weeks or longer)
(b) Administration of an opioid antagonist after a period of opioid use
2. Three (or more) of the following, developing within minutes to several days after Criterion A:
(a) Dysphoric mood
(b) Nausea or vomiting
(c) Muscle aches
(d) Lacrimation or rhinorrhea
(e) Pupillary dilation, piloerection, or sweating
(f) Diarrhea
(g) Yawning
(h) Fever
(i) Insomnia
3. The signs or symptoms in Criterion B cause clinically significant distress or impairment in social, occupational, or other important areas of functioning
4. The signs or symptoms are not attributable to another medical condition and are not better explained by another mental disorder, including intoxication or withdrawal from another substance

Throughout its course, opioid withdrawal can be both subjectively and objectively measured. The Subjective Opiate Withdrawal Scale (SOWS) and the Objective Opiate Withdrawal Scale (OOWS) are valid and reliable indicators of severity over a wide range of signs and symptoms [31, 32]. The SOWS contains 16 symptoms whose intensity the patient rates on a scale of 0 (not at all) to 4 (extremely). The OOWS contains 13 physically observable signs, rated present or absent, based on a timed period of observation of the patient by a healthcare provider. These scales can be useful for clinicians to not only measure withdrawal severity, but also to monitor patient progress throughout a planned and structured detoxification course.

Detoxification [33]

Detoxification, or monitored withdrawal, usually involves gradual tapering or discontinuing a substance in a dependent individual. The goal is to achieve this safely, while attempting to mitigate the unpleasant effects of the withdrawal syndrome.

Opioid detoxification in an outpatient setting is the preferred method, but patients with polysubstance abuse, complex/unstable medical condition, associated psychiatric disorders, prior failed outpatient detoxification, and noncompliance to treatment will need inpatient detoxifications. Due to their long-acting properties, methadone or Suboxone (buprenorphine–naloxone) are commonly used in outpatient settings. Overall patient treatment retention and total cost [34] is better for methadone, while patient satisfaction [36], convenience [34], and less likelihood of elicit drug [36] usage is better with Suboxone treatment group (Table 32.10). Inpatient anesthesia assistance in rapid opioid withdrawal to minimize undesirable effects of withdrawal i.e. Ultra-Rapid detoxification, is used as a last resort secondary to its increased risk

Table 32.10 Characteristics of methadone and buprenorphine/naloxone

Characteristics	Methadone	Buprenorphine/naloxone (Suboxone)
Receptor affinity	Opioid agonist	Partial opioid receptor agonist
Composition	Racemic mixture of methadone	Abuse-deterrent formulation 4:1 ratio—buprenorphine:naloxone
Half-life	Long 8–59 h	
Initial effect	Takes up to 10 days	May precipitate withdrawal in very early phase
Additional adverse effects	QT_c interval prolongation and torsades de pointes	Less risk of respiratory depression from its "ceiling effect"
Screening needed	ECG screening at regular interval	Regular clinical monitoring
Dose delivery	Supervised	Unsupervised
Treatment retention	Better then Suboxone	Good
Satisfaction and convenience	Good	Better than methadone
Cost	Better than Suboxone, secondary to cost of medication	Comparable, but better than other detoxification strategies

Table 32.11 Opioid detoxification strategies

Setting	Patient with	Method	
Outpatient	Single agent	Long-acting opioid	Step 1: Calculate total daily dose of the long-acting opioid that does not produce withdrawal
			Step 2: Taper the total requirement by 10 % every 3–7 days
		Short-acting opioid	Step 1: Choose a long-acting pure-opioid agonist[a,b]
			Step 2: Calculate total daily dose of short-acting opioid used that does not produce withdrawal
			Step 3: Equi-analgesic conversion to a long-acting opioid of choice[c]
			Step 4: Taper the total requirement by 10 % every 3–7 days
	Multiple agents	Step 1: Choose a long-acting pure-opioid agonist[a,b]	
		Step 2: Calculate total daily dose of opioid used that does not produce withdrawal	
		Step 3: Equi-analgesic conversion to single long-acting opioid of choice[c]	
		Step 4: Taper the total requirement by 10 % every 3–7	
In-patient	Same as outpatient		
	Ultra-rapid	Step 1. Comprehensive medical assessment	
		Step 2. Patient heavily sedated or under general anesthesia with continuous monitoring	
		Step 3. Discontinue opioid and treated with opioid antagonists[d]	
		Step 4. Treat associated adverse symptoms with adjuvants[e]	

[a]Increasing dosing intervals of short-acting opioid may result in repetitive period of withdrawal and thus high risk of relapse
[b]Sustained-Release Oxycodone, Sustained-Release Morphine, methadone, buprenorphine–naloxone (Suboxone)
[c]Upon conversion of opioid reductions for cross-tolerance should be done
[d]Naloxone, naltrexone, etc.
[e]Clonidine for adrenergic overactivity, benzodiazepines for anxiety, muscle relaxants for myalgias

of serious adverse events and lack of additional over all benefit [37]. If inpatient detoxification is required, an addiction specialist/psychologist consultation is needed along with social worker involvement for discharge plan.

Different strategies exist in order to achieve opioid detoxification i.e. increasing dosing interval, tapering down of doses, or both. Patients could be on a single agent or multiple agents, and short-acting and long-acting opioids. A conservative approach to formulate a detoxification plan is shown in Table 32.11.

Conclusion

Opioids are a double-edged sword and chronic pain state is a never-ending war. Healthcare practices across the country are faced with increasing morbidity and mortality related to the use of opioids and substance abuse, which has an overall negative impact on the socioeconomic burden of this country. Further, diversion, stealing, and illegal acquisition of opioids take a toll on crime and law enforcement. All this is expected to have a staggering growth with changes in healthcare policies that would allow more patients to have access to health care in combination with new government policies such as liberalization of Marijuana Prohibition Laws across the Unites States of America. Hence, it is absolutely essential for healthcare providers to understand the use and abuse potential of opioids, sufficiently equip, and certify themselves in order to perform and conduct opioid detoxification and maintenance programs, and also develop prudent practices to detect, control, and curb the menace of substance abuse in this society.

References

1. Geppert C. To help and not to harm: ethical issues in the treatment of chronic pain in patients with substance use disorders. In Clark MR, Treisman GJ, editors. Pain and depression. An interdisciplinary patient-centered approach. Adv Psychosom Med. Karger: Basel; 2004;25: 151–71.
2. Tsang A, Von Korff M, Lee S, et al. Common chronic pain conditions in developed and developing countries: gender and age differences and comorbidity with depression-anxiety disorders. J Pain. 2008;9(10):883–91.
3. Johannes CB, Le TK, Zhou X, Johnston JA, Dworkin RH. The prevalence of chronic pain in United States adults: results of an Internet-based survey. J Pain. 2010;11(11):1230–9.
4. Institute of Medicine Report from the Committee on Advancing Pain Research, Care, and Education. Relieving pain in America, a blueprint for transforming prevention, care, education and research. The National Academies Press; 2011.
5. Stewart WF, Ricci JA, Chee E, Morganstein D. Lost productive work time costs from health conditions in the United States: results from the American Productivity Audit. J Occup Environ Med. 2003;45(12):1234–46.
6. Results from the 2010 National Survey on Drug Use and Health: Summary of National Findings. http://www.oas.samhsa.gov/NSDUH/2k10NSDUH/2k10Results.pdf. Accessed Nov 2013.
7. The Economic Impact of Illicit Drug Use on American Society. National Drug Intelligence Center. Washington, DC: United States Department of Justice; April 2011. http://www.simeoneassociates.com/assets/pdfs/SAI_Assessment1.pdf. Accessed Nov 2013.
8. Substance Abuse and Mental Health Services Administration. Center for Behavioral Health Statistics and Quality. Drug abuse warning network, 2009: national estimates of drug-related emergency department visits; 2009. http://www.samhsa.gov/data/2k11/dawn/2k9dawned/html/dawn2k9ed.htm. Accessed Nov 2013.
9. Substance Abuse and Mental Health Services Administration. Results from the 2011 National Survey on drug use and health: summary of national findings, NSDUH series H-44, HHS Publication No. SMA 12-4713. Rockville: Substance Abuse and Mental Health Services Administration; 2012. http://www.samhsa.gov/data/NSDUH/2k11Results/NSDUHresults2011.pdf. Accessed Nov 2013.
10. Heimer R, Dasgupta N, Irwin KS, Kinzly M, Harvey AP, Givens A, Grau LE. Chronic pain, addiction severity, and misuse of opioids in Cumberland County, Maine. Addict Behav. 2011;37:346–9.
11. Fishbain DA, Cole B, Lewis J, Rosomoff HL, Rosomoff RS. What percentage of chronic non-malignant pain patients exposed to chronic opioid analgesic therapy develop abuse/addiction and/or aberrant drug-related behaviors? A structured evidence-based review. Pain Med. 2008;9(4):444–59.

12. Rosenblum A, Joseph H, Fong C. Prevalence and characteristics of chronic pain among chemically dependent patients in methadone maintenance and residential treatment facilities. JAMA. 2003;289:2370–8.

13. Centers for Disease Control and Prevention. Vital signs: overdoses of prescription opioid pain relievers—United States, 1999–2008. MMWR Morb Mortal Wkly Rep. 2011;60(43): 1487–92.

14. Warner M, Chen LH, Makuc DM, Anderson RN, Miniño AM. Drug poisoning deaths in the United States, 1980–2008. NCHS Data Brief # 81. December 2011.

15. http://www.cdc.gov/nchs/data/databriefs/db81.pdf. Accessed Nov 2013.

16. Topics in brief: prescription drug abuse—December 2011: a research update from the National Institute on Drug Abuse. http://www.drugabuse.gov/publications/topics-in-brief/prescription-drug-abuse. Accessed Nov 2013.

17. Gourlay D, Heit H, Almahrezi A. Universal precautions in pain medicine: a rational approach to the treatment of chronic pain. Pain Med. 2005;6(2):107–12.

18. Jamison RN, Serraillier J, Michna E. Assessment and treatment of abuse risk in opioid prescribing for chronic pain. Pain Res Treat. 2011;2011. Article ID 941808.

19. Moore TM, et al. A comparison of common screening methods for predicting aberrant behavior among patients receiving opioids for chronic pain management. Pain Med. 2009;10:1426–33.

20. Katz NP, Adamd EH, Benneyan JC, Birnbaum HG, Budman SH, Buzzeo RW, Carr DB, Cicero TJ, Gourlay D, Inciardi JA, Joranson DE, Kesslick J, Land SD. Foundations of opioid risk management. Clin J Pain. 2007;23:103–18.

21. Portenoy RK. Chronic opioid therapy in non-malignant pain. J Pain Symptom Manage. 1990;5:S46–62.

22. Owen GT, Burton AW, Schade CM, Passik S. Urine drug testing: current recommendations and best practices. Pain Physician. 2012;15:ES119–33.

23. Hariharan J, Lamb GC, Neuner JM. Long-term opioid contract use for chronic pain management in primary care practice. A five year experience. J Gen Intern Med. 2007;22(4):485–90.

24. Finklea KM, Bagalman E, Sacco LN. Prescription drug monitoring programs. http://ccc.healthcaredistribution.org/gov_affairs/pdf_misc/2012-08-20-crs_report.pdf. Accessed Nov 2013.

25. Baehren DF, Marco CA, Droz DE, Sinha S, Callan EM, Akpunonu P. A statewide prescription monitoring program affects emergency department prescribing behaviors. Ann Emerg Med. 2010;56(1):19–23.

26. Guidance for industry format and content of proposed Risk Evaluation and Mitigation Strategies (REMS), REMS assessments, and proposed REMS modifications. http://www.fda.gov/downloads/Drugs/Guidances/UCM184128.pdf. Accessed Nov 2013.

27. Extended-release (ER) and long-acting (LA) opioid analgesics risk evaluation and mitigation strategy (REMS). http://www.fda.gov/downloads/drugs/drugsafety/postmarketdrugsafetyinformationforpatientsandproviders/ucm311290.pdf. Accessed Nov 2013.

28. Raffa RB, Pergolizzi Jr JV, Muñiz E, Taylor Jr R, Pergolizzi J. Designing opioids that deter abuse. Pain Res Treat. 2012;2012 [Epub 8 Nov 2012].

29. Laroche F, Rostaing S, Aubrun F, Perrot S. Pain management in heroin and cocaine users. Joint Bone Spine. 2012;79:446–50.

30. Passik SD, Kirsh KL. The interface between pain and drug abuse and the evolution of strategies to optimize pain management while minimizing drug abuse. Exp Clin Psychopharmacol. 2008;16(5):400–4.

31. American Psychiatric Association. Diagnostic and statistical manual of mental health disorders: DSM-5. 5th ed. Washington, DC: American Psychiatric Publishing; 2013.

32. Handelsman L, Cochrane KJ, Aronson MJ, Ness R, Rubinstein KJ, Kanof PD. Two new rating scales for opiate withdrawal. Am J Drug Alcohol Abuse. 1987;13(3):293–308.

33. Plunkett A, Kuehn D, Lenart M, Wilkinson I. Opioid maintenance, weaning and detoxification techniques: where we have been, where we are now and what the future holds. Pain Manage. 2013;3:277–84.

34. Jones ES, Moore BA, Sindelar JL, O'Connor PG, Schottenfeld RS, Fiellin DA. Cost analysis of clinic and office-based treatment of opioid dependence: results with methadone and buprenorphine in clinically stable patients. Drug Alcohol Depend. 2009;99(1–3):132–40.
35. Barry DT, Moore BA, Pantalon MV, Chawarski MC, Sillivan LE, O'Connor PG, Schottenfeld RS, Feillin DA. Patient satisfaction with primary care office-based buprinorphine/naloxone treatment. J Gen Intern Med. 2007;22(2):242–5.
36. Fischer G, Gombas W, Eder H, Jagsch R, Paternell A, Stuhlinger G, Pezawas L, Aschauer HN, Kasper S. Buprenorphine versus methadone for treatment of opioid dependence. Addiction. 1999;94(9):1337–7.
37. Gowing L, Ali R, White JM. Opioid antagonists under heavy sedation or anaesthesia for opioid withdrawal. Cochrane Database Syst Rev. 2010;1, CD002022.

Chapter 33
Management of Acute Pain

Michael Alan Fishman and Donna-Ann M. Thomas

Key Points

- Implications of substances abused on acute pain management
- Altered perceptions and pain tolerance
- Approach to the patient
- Multimodal acute pain management
- Opioid-induced hyperalgesia
- Management of the patient receiving opioid addiction maintenance therapy

Introduction

The management of acute pain in the opioid-tolerant patient is a growing challenge as the incidence of licit and illicit opioid use has tripled since 1998 [1, 2]. Providers are frequently faced with clinical and ethical dilemmas surrounding the safe and effective management of acute pain in these patients. Accompanying comorbid substance abuse, mental illness, behavioral issues, and social concerns further complicate treatment.

Cognizance of the great potential for abuse and diversion of prescription opioids should underlie therapeutic decision-making, as legally prescribed drugs make up the majority of abused opioids in the United States [2]. The United States (US) accounted for 56 % of global morphine and 81 % of global oxycodone consumption

M.A. Fishman, M.D., M.B.A. (✉)
Department of Anesthesiology, Perioperative and Pain Medicine, Stanford University
School of Medicine, Palo Alto, CA, USA
e-mail: fishman4@pain.stanford.edu

D.-A.M. Thomas, M.D.
Department of Anesthesiology, Yale University School of Medicine, New Haven, CT, USA
e-mail: fishman4@pain.standford.edu; donna.thomas@yale.edu

© Springer Science+Business Media New York 2015
A.D. Kaye et al. (eds.), *Substance Abuse*, DOI 10.1007/978-1-4939-1951-2_33

in 2009 [1]. More than half of nonmedical pain reliever users report obtaining the drug from friends or relatives with bona fide prescriptions [2]. Two million Americans reported using prescription drugs for nonmedical purposes for the first time in 2010—more than 5,000 a day [3]. Serious adverse events occur when prescription opioids are used as directed, and abuse only serves to magnify and compound these ill effects. One hundred Americans die from drug overdoses every day, and the majority of these deaths are attributable to prescription opioids [3]. The US Food and Drug Administration responded to this opioid epidemic with increased regulation and mandates for risk mitigation strategies, including development of diversion-resistant formulations for extended-release (ER) opioids [4]. As the prevalence of opioid abuse and misuse continues to rise, clinicians are more frequently faced with the challenge of managing acute pain in this patient population.

Principles of acute pain management in opioid-tolerant patients focus on attaining adequate analgesia via a multimodal approach while being vigilant of the surrounding psychosocial and medicolegal issues. A holistic therapeutic approach should be employed with clear and sustainable exit and entry strategies, with longitudinal follow-up whenever possible.

This chapter will discuss strategies to provide safe and effective pain management in patients with comorbid substance abuse disorders, no matter what the stage of treatment is. This will include treatment recommendations for the active substance abuser, the former addict, and patients receiving opioid substitution therapy. The phenomena of opioid tolerance and opioid-induced hyperalgesia (OIH) and their treatment will be reviewed.

Implications of Substances Abused on Acute Pain Management

Substances of abuse have been extensively discussed in section "Approach to the Patient" of this text. Though users typically have a preference for one particular drug of abuse, polysubstance use and abuse is the reality. Patients who present with acute pain and concurrent opioid abuse present a particular conundrum, as opioids remain the cornerstone of acute pain management in the inpatient and outpatient setting [5].

There is no consensus as to the optimum use of opioids in the management of acute pain in the actively abusing or recovering patient, however, it is generally agreed that opioids can be used effectively in this population [1, 5–10]. Employing opioids and other drugs of abuse for pain treatment in this population is fraught with pitfalls. These patients exist on a precarious continuum, with life-threatening abstinence syndromes on one side and life-threatening adverse effects associated with overdosing on the other. There is high interindividual variability in responses to treatment, and dangerous adverse effects may be more likely to occur, especially if patients overestimate their usage history for secondary gain. The clinician should also always be mindful of the potential for surreptitious street drug use in both the inpatient and outpatient settings.

Altered Perceptions and Pain Tolerance

Pain is a common reason for substance abusing patients to seek care, and it is not surprising that traumatic injury is a leading cause of hospital admission in this population [11, 12]. Managing an opioid-tolerant or pain-intolerant individual with an acute traumatic injury can be challenging. This is especially true when acute pain commingles with any of the host of comorbidities and aberrant behaviors associated with this population, including: acute intoxication or withdrawal, altered mental status or mood, and generally distasteful comportment.

Caring for the agitated, intoxicated trauma patient in the acute care setting is a prime example of this type of encounter. However, no matter how unsavory the presentation, stigmatizing these patients as "addicts" or "junkies" who overestimate their pain for secondary gain only further complicates care by underestimating and inadequately treating their pain [12, 13]. Underutilization of opioids not only leads to uncontrolled pain, but may also precipitate withdrawal syndromes [13].

Opioid-tolerant patients require higher doses to achieve an analgesic effect. There is also evidence indicating that patients actively using opiates or cocaine have lower pain tolerance than users in recovery. Compton subjected active and recovered opiate and cocaine users to a cold-pressor test to assess their pain thresholds [14]. Active users had significantly lower pain tolerance than former users in recovery, with opioid users exhibiting lower pain tolerance than cocaine users [14]. It is imperative that providers recognize that these patients receive a diminished analgesic effect from opioids and likely have decreased pain tolerance when assessing analgesic requirements. Neighbor et al. found that substance abuse patients presenting to the emergency department reported significantly more severe pain and more chronically painful conditions than the general population [15]. The mechanism and extent of injury will not always be proportional to the pain response in the context of a milieu of substance abuse, mental illness, psychosocial stress, and other comorbidities.

Approach to the patient

> May I never see in the patient anything but a fellow creature in pain.
>
> —Moses Maimonides (1135–1204) [16]

Approaching the active or recovering substance abuse patient in the acute setting requires that the provider be gentle but firm, establish rapport, and set common goals from the outset. There may be times when extreme pain requires that the provider quickly "put out the fire." This may serve as a catalyst to create trust and gain

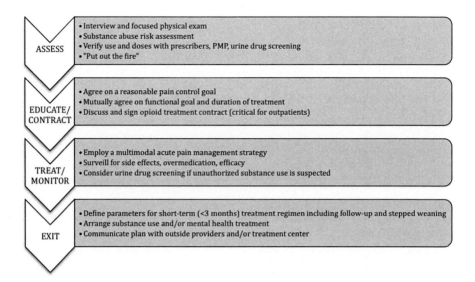

ASSESS
- Interview and focused physical exam
- Substance abuse risk assessment
- Verify use and doses with prescribers, PMP, urine drug screening
- "Put out the fire"

EDUCATE/ CONTRACT
- Agree on a reasonable pain control goal
- Mutually agree on functional goal and duration of treatment
- Discuss and sign opioid treatment contract (critical for outpatients)

TREAT/ MONITOR
- Employ a multimodal acute pain management strategy
- Surveill for side effects, overmedication, efficacy
- Consider urine drug screening if unauthorized substance use is suspected

EXIT
- Define parameters for short-term (<3 months) treatment regimen including follow-up and stepped weaning
- Arrange substance use and/or mental health treatment
- Communicate plan with outside providers and/or treatment center

Fig. 33.1 Approach to managing acute pain in the substance abuse patient

the patient's confidence so as to facilitate obtaining an accurate history and develop a mutually agreeable and realistic set of pain management goals and strategies. It is critical that this set of goals and the overall strategy is uniform amongst the different stakeholders, as discussed in section "Multimodal Acute Pain Management": The Multidisciplinary Approach to Treatment (Fig. 33.1).

Interview

The purpose of the interview is to establish a relationship as well as to obtain an accurate history to identify substance use and abuse patients. Candor is essential for the clinician in this regard, and it is helpful to remind the patient that this information will only be used to assist in their care and in no way will their openness be incriminating. It can be helpful to share with the patient that your intention is to provide adequate analgesia, prevent withdrawal, and assist with psychosocial issues. Reassure them that this cannot be accomplished without accurate information and their drug use history or dependence will not preclude adequate pain relief.

Identification of the opioid-tolerant patient is the first step. Looks may be deceiving, and the provider should never prejudge patients based on their appearance. All patients should be questioned about their licit and illicit substance use habits beginning with alcohol and tobacco and moving on to other substances. Instead of asking the patient if they use illicit drugs, it is helpful to employ the nonspecific colloquialism "do you get high at all?" to evoke a candid response. Follow-up questions should focus on ascertaining the patient's use and abuse patterns, history of legal problems, history of addiction treatment, and family history of substance abuse. Patients should be pointedly asked about a history of withdrawal syndromes. A full discussion of screening and assessment in the inpatient and outpatient setting can be found in the section: "Altered Perceptions and Pain Tolerance."

Verify

Doses of prescribed substances should be confirmed, either with the prescribing physician, dispensing pharmacy, or addiction treatment center. Urine drug screening can be used to confirm which substances, if any, the patient is actively using. Prescription Monitoring Programs (PMPs) are in place in 42 states and are used to monitor statewide controlled substance dispensation. Most states permit pharmacists and prescribers to query the state PMP database for patients under their care. PMP reports are useful tools to verify dosages, identify suspicious prescription patterns (i.e., doctor shopping), and identify the patient's other prescribers. The patient does not need to consent to, or be informed of, a PMP query since PMP reporting by pharmacies is mandatory and not discretionary. Additionally, consulting other prescribers is permitted within the HIPAA definition of treatment and also does not need to be disclosed to the patient unless required by state law. More information about PMPs in the United States and state-by-state regulations can be found at PMPAlliance.org.

Titrate

Caution must be used when restarting a patient's home dosage, even after verification. This is especially true with high-dose prescriptions, as it is common for patients to divert their medications. More than half of nonmedical pain reliever users report obtaining the drug from friends or relatives with bona fide prescriptions [2]. Starting patients on doses they are unaccustomed to can result in dangerous respiratory depression and possibly death. High-dose opioid replacement should be administered in divided doses using instant release (IR) formulations. Extended-release (ER) formulations should only be restarted once IR tolerability has been confirmed. Patients receiving high-dose opioids should be monitored for respiratory depression using, at minimum, continuous pulse oximetry. End tidal carbon dioxide monitoring is another useful tool, and should be employed if available. Resuscitation equipment and qualified first responders must be readily available.

Assessment

Pain is the only core vital sign that is subjectively measured, and it is important that these assessments be used contextually to guide therapy. Acute pain scores in substance users tend to be consistently higher when compared to non-users [17]. In a retrospective review of acute pain service patients, Rapp et al. found that chronic pain and opioid consuming patients reported higher pain scores than controls despite using more opioids and anxiolytics [17]. This may be attributed to a combination of coexisting baseline chronic pain, reduced effect of acute pain treatment, and to pain intolerance in this population [14]. It is not unusual to find this type of patient sitting placid in bed reporting a pain score of 10/10. When questioned further, they may consider this their baseline and either tolerable or unrelated to the acute injury. A reasonable pain score goal should be discussed openly with the patient and their nurse and agreed upon by all parties. Once agreed to, this should become a part of the patient's record and should be an integral part of the clinician and staff's transfer of care. A frank discussion should be had explaining that a pain score of 0/10 is not a reasonable or realistic goal.

Given the highly subjective nature of the numerical rating scale, it is useful to employ dynamic pain scores to better describe the functional impact of pain (i.e., during deep breathing, coughing, incentive spirometry, and ambulation). Since many pain complaints may be present, it is helpful to have the patient identify the relative contribution of each one as a percentage (i.e., 10 % elbow pain, 80 % rib pain, 10 % back pain). This allows the patient and provider to design a pain management strategy that prioritizes their major complaint(s).

Monitoring

It behooves the provider to review the patient's vital signs and appearance from afar as these can provide clues as to the adequacy of analgesia, overmedication, and signs of withdrawal. It is not uncommon for the patient's countenance and presentation to change when a member of the care team enters the room.

Side Effects

Patients who regularly consume opioids generally experience fewer side effects, such as nausea, pruritus, and respiratory depression than opioid-naïve patients [1, 17]. However, Rapp et al. found that 50 % of opioid-tolerant patients using patient-controlled analgesia (PCA) experienced moderate or severe sedation as compared to 19 % of opioid-naïve controls [17]. Monitoring of level of sedation and respiratory rate should be standard in patients receiving opioids. Many institutions require that patients with obstructive sleep apnea (OSA) who are receiving high-dose or continuous opioids be in a continuously monitored setting.

Discharge Planning

No plan is complete without an exit strategy, and this is particularly true when treating acute pain in the substance abuse population. The goal of discharge is to provide adequate short-term analgesia while maintaining a strict end-titration schedule for opioids and other habit-forming prescriptions. It is the authors' opinion that end-titration should occur optimally within 4–12 weeks of discharge and be coupled with outpatient addiction treatment whenever possible.

For inpatients, a great deal of multidisciplinary resources can be leveraged for discharge planning, including social work, addiction psychiatry, inpatient or outpatient drug treatment centers, the patient's primary care physician (if they have one), and responsible loved ones as discussed extensively in the section "Multimodal Acute Pain Management."

For an outpatient, the exit strategy is more challenging as it puts the provider in the unenviable position of weighing the altruistic desire to treat pain with the ethical and medicolegal consequences of prescribing opioids to a high-risk patient. In this circumstance the provider may have to prescribe a few days' supply of opioids and maintain close follow-up. An opioid treatment agreement with this patient should stipulate that to obtain further prescriptions the patient must subject themselves to urine toxicology studies and actively seek addiction treatment.

Multimodal Acute Pain Management

The foundation of modern acute pain management is based on the concept of multimodal analgesia, which is recommended in the 2012 American Society of Anesthesiologists' guidelines on acute pain management [18]. This approach relies on the synergistic use of several different analgesics acting with different mechanisms on discrete sites in the nervous system to attain adequate analgesia. Though opioids remain a core therapeutic, multimodal treatment has been shown to be opioid sparing [19]. Employing a multimodal approach is particularly important in the opioid-tolerant population who enjoy a diminished analgesic effect from these medications as a result of misuse and abuse.

Tissue injury elicits a complex psychoneurohumoral response that can be best addressed using a combination of peripheral- and central-acting agents to specifically target each of the four elements of the pain pathway: transduction, transmission, perception, and modulation. While a complete discussion of the pathophysiology of pain is beyond the scope of this text, a basic primer is included to provide context for developing a multimodal analgesic strategy.

The Pathophysiology of Pain

Transduction is the process by which peripheral injury (i.e., trauma, thermal, caustic, surgical) is translated into an electrical impulse by nociceptive afferents at the site of injury. The primary afferents involved in nociception are myelinated A-delta nociceptors and unmyelinated C-nociceptors. A-delta nociceptors fire in response to thermal and mechanical stimuli, and the rapidly (~10 m per second) conducted impulse is responsible for the sharp sensation of acute pain. C-nociceptors mount a slower (1 m per second) response to thermal, mechanical, and chemical injury and are responsible for the sensation of dull, throbbing pain. When the noxious impulse exceeds the threshold potential of the nociceptors, it is transmitted via peripheral nerves to synapse with second-order neurons in the dorsal root ganglion of the spinal cord. There are many connections that occur at the level of the spinal cord. Interneurons connecting sensory and motor neurons can activate local reflex arcs (i.e., withdrawing from heat). Impulses may ascend via the spinothalamic tract to the thalamus and thereafter to other portions of the brain that are organized and interpreted in the conscious patient as the subjective experience of pain. Descending inhibitory modulation that dampens the pain sensation can also occur, especially in times of stress (i.e., being chased by a saber-toothed tiger), excitement (i.e., playing in the Super Bowl) or after conditioning (i.e., meditation) [20–24].

Analgesic Ladder

The World Health Organization introduced the concept of the analgesic ladder for the treatment of cancer pain in 1986 [25]. Despite their initial oncologic scope, the basic tenets of this approach can be broadly applied to developing a multimodal treatment strategy for acute pain. The general principle of the analgesic ladder is that aggressiveness of therapy should be commensurate with the degree of pain. That is, mild pain should be treated with nonsteroidal anti-inflammatory drugs (NSAIDs), moderate pain with NSAIDs and weak opioids, and severe pain with NSAIDs and strong opioids. Non-opioid adjuvants (i.e., gabanoids, antidepressants, anxiolytics, muscle relaxants) should be used whenever indicated. The use of intravenous lidocaine, ketamine, and regional or neuraxial techniques should be considered in the treatment of severe pain unless contraindicated. A detailed discussion of regional anesthesia can be found in Chap. 27.

Individualized Approach

The analgesic ladder serves as a framework for developing a pain management plan for each patient, yet it is not universal. A tailored approach to the patient and to the etiology of the acute pain, while concurrently managing the coexisting mental

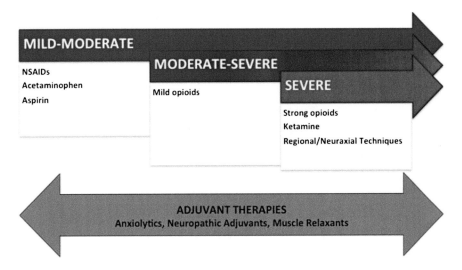

Fig. 33.2 The analgesic ladder. Therapy should be tailored to degree of pain in an additive approach. Adjuvant therapies should be used whenever appropriate to address specific symptomatology (i.e., muscle spasm, neuropathy, anxiety) contributing the pain experience

health and substance abuse disorders present (Fig. 33.2). In the short-term, frequent manipulations that warrant inpatient management may be necessary, and may require consultation with an expert in acute pain management. Most large institutions have the infrastructure to support this with dedicated inpatient acute pain management teams. In the community, consultation with the nearest pain management expert may be warranted, whether it is an anesthesiologist, neurologist, or psychiatrist. The individualized approach should employ a combination of agents to target each level of the pain pathway, from the site of injury to the cortex [19].

NSAIDs, COX-2 Inhibitors, and Acetaminophen

NSAIDs inhibit the cyclooxygenases (COX), preventing the conversion of arachidonic acid to prostaglandins centrally and peripherally. Peripheral injury incites a local inflammatory response with release of a host of mediators from damaged cells (e.g., bradykinin, cytokines, prostaglandins, substance P). Prostaglandins (particularly PGE_2 and thromboxane) sensitize nerves at the site of injury, facilitating nociceptive transmission and effectively decreasing the local pain threshold. Early treatment with NSAIDs can attenuate the local inflammatory response, reduce sensitization of the wound, and reduce the transduction of the noxious stimulus [19]. The 2012 American Society of Anesthesiologists (ASA) guidelines on acute pain management state that "unless contraindicated, all patients should receive around-the-clock regimen of NSAIDs, COX-2 inhibitors, or acetaminophen" [18].

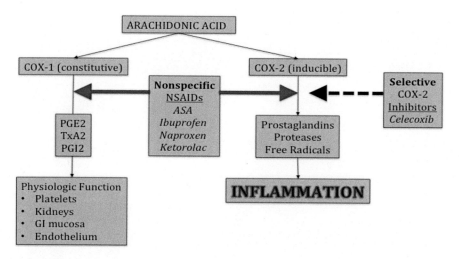

Fig. 33.3 Simplified action of nonsteroidal anti-inflammatory drugs (NSAIDs). The nonspecific NSAIDs include a variety of over-the-counter (OTC) formulations, including aspirin (ASA), ibuprofen, naproxen, and others. Ketorolac is a commonly used parenteral NSAID. Celecoxib is the only selective COX-2 inhibitor approved for use in the United States

Cyclooxygenase has at least two main isoforms, COX-1 and COX-2, which have different physiologic functions. COX-1 is constitutively expressed and plays a role in a host of processes. The major adverse effects associated with NSAID use are directly related to inhibition of COX-1's constitutive functions, among which are platelet aggregation, renal blood flow regulation, and gastric mucosal protection [26]. These bear the risks of bleeding, kidney injury, and gastric ulceration, respectively. As such, NSAIDs are contraindicated in patients with a history of peptic ulcer disease, bleeding diatheses, or renal impairment. Patients should be monitored for development of any of these side effects, and therapy should be discontinued if any emerge.

Ketorolac is the parenteral NSAID of choice and is an effective and potent analgesic, and has been shown to be opioid sparing in postoperative patients (Fig. 33.3) [19]. However, its side effect profile mirrors its clinical efficacy and as such its use is typically limited to 5 days of therapy. Despite its opioid-sparing COX-2 expression is induced in the setting of acute injury and is involved in pain, fever, and inflammation. Selective COX-2 inhibitors were developed with the intent of achieving anti-inflammatory effects at the site of injury while minimizing the aforementioned adverse effects associated with COX-1. This is particularly of concern given that patients with acute injury are often also at risk for renal injury and bleeding in the setting of recent trauma. Though experts advocate the use of selective COX-2 inhibitors such as celecoxib in the treatment of acute pain, there is little data to suggest they reduce the incidence of opioid-related side effects [19].

Local Anesthetics

Local anesthetics can be used in a variety of formats (i.e., topical, local infiltration, perineural, epidural, intrathecal) to deliver analgesia or anesthesia in the acute setting. A complete discussion of these techniques as they pertain to surgical pain can be found in Chap. 27.

Regional and neuraxial anesthesia and analgesia are well integrated into the perioperative environment, and can also be a valuable tool outside the operating room. Regional techniques can be used to rapidly provide analgesia to patients in whom the administration of systemic analgesia poses a significant risk. Trauma patients are at risk for "hypoanalgesia" due to hemodynamic instability, respiratory distress, and a frequent medical need to serially assess mental status that precludes the use of systemic analgesics [27].

Peripheral nerve blocks (PNBs) are an excellent and safe choice for controlling pain in the upper and lower extremities. There are few cardiopulmonary side effects, and perineural blockade has been shown to reduce opioid consumption and opioid-related side effects. This is particularly important in our substance abuse patients who have baseline opioid requirements and experience a diminished analgesic effect from additional opioid administration. There is no tolerance to modern local anesthetics, and the commonly used local anesthetics have no abuse potential (other than cocaine, of course) [28]. Local anesthetic toxicity is one of the few significant potential side effects of these techniques. Another potential consequence is analgesia that is so potent it may mask life- or limb-threatening compartment syndromes [27]. PNBs are not appropriate for all patients; a trained provider should determine the appropriateness of employing regional techniques.

Thoracic paravertebral blocks are an excellent modality for controlling pain secondary to trauma of the thorax. This selective block provides unilateral analgesia comparable to epidural analgesia without the hemodynamic effects associated with the latter. Patients requiring bilateral analgesia can be treated with either bilateral paravertebral blocks or a thoracic epidural if hemodynamics allow. Patients with more than three or four rib fractures benefit most from regional analgesia [27]. Pulmonary splinting is the natural reaction to injury of the chest and underlying lung, leading first to atelectasis and eventually to pneumonia and respiratory failure requiring intubation and mechanical ventilation. Adequate analgesia is critical to recovery in these patients, as it facilitates the deep breathing and coughing necessary to avoid the aforementioned downward spiral of pulmonary complications.

The administration of local anesthetics by a number of routes should be considered in all patients in whom it is suspected systemic analgesics may have diminished effect. Regional and neuraxial techniques are safe and provide excellent analgesia at minimal risk when used in appropriate patients. Consultation with a trained provider to determine patient eligibility should be obtained at the earliest possible time point to derive maximal benefit. Contraindications to regional techniques include infection at the site, systemic infection, and coagulopathy.

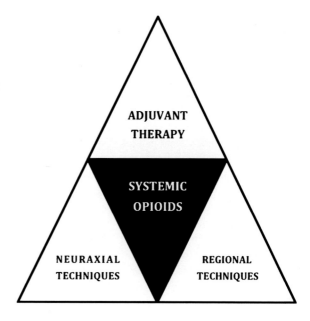

Fig. 33.4 Opioids are the cornerstone of acute pain management. Multimodal analgesia incorporates a variety of medications and techniques to achieve synergy

Opioids

Opioids remain the mainstay of moderate–severe pain management in all patients, even in opioid-tolerant patients (Fig. 33.4). All appropriate non-opioid adjuvants should be used to minimize or even obviate the need for opioids. Earlier in the chapter we discussed the importance of eliciting an accurate dosage and usage history. This baseline requirement should be prescribed regularly with the patient's home medication or an equianalgesic substitute [13]. Long-acting formulations should initially be replaced with frequent equipotent doses of short-acting drugs to test the veracity of the patient's reported tolerance and use. Additional opioids should be administered to achieve adequate analgesia for the patient's pain complaint, unless limited by the development of side effects. Keep in mind that there is great variability in opioid requirements among opioid-tolerant patients, and careful attention must be used to avoid the development of dangerous adverse effects from overdose.

Parenteral and oral formulations can be used in concert when appropriate to address background and breakthrough pain. Initially, the use of PCA with a continuous background infusion has been successfully used to titrate opioids in this patient population [13]. There is inherent safety in using PCA, as it requires the patient to be awake and have the wherewithal to use the system to obtain a bolus dose. Some PCA systems have integrated capnography that prevents bolus dose administration if the respiratory rate is below a set value. Frequent assessments and adjustments of PCA dosing are oftentimes required to achieve adequate analgesia. While labor-intensive, these frequent reassessments allow for more interactions between patient and provider and may help to galvanize a cooperative relationship with a mutual goal of pain control. Opioid-tolerant patients have been shown to require more frequent PCA adjustments and longer care by an acute pain service than opioid-naïve controls [1].

Opioid rotation exploits the incomplete cross-tolerance amongst opioids to provide analgesia to patients accustomed to a particular opioid. This technique has been used successfully in the palliative care population to provide excellent analgesia while minimizing adverse effects [1]. First, determine the daily dose of the current opioid and use an equivalence table to determine the equianalgesic dose of a different opioid. This calculated dose should then be reduced by 30–50 % at first to account for incomplete cross-tolerance. Opioid conversion is not an exact science and there is a wide variability amongst published conversion tables—when in doubt, err on the side of caution and use lower doses more frequently.

NMDA Antagonists

Ketamine was previously discussed in Chap. 26. It is a non-opioid phencyclidine derivative that antagonizes the N-methyl-D-aspartate (NMDA) receptor, which has been linked to central sensitization and nociceptive pain transmission [19]. Ketamine is frequently used as an analgesic adjunct, and has been shown to improve analgesia and reduce opioid requirements in both opioid-naïve and -tolerant patients [1]. The authors routinely use ketamine in clinical practice for inpatients as a continuous infusion at doses of 0.1–0.5 mg/kg/h. Therapy with ketamine should be discontinued if the patient develops dysphoria and/or unpleasant hallucinations, however these do not commonly develop during low-dose infusion. Ketamine should be discontinued once steady state pain control has been achieved and the patient is being transitioned to oral analgesics. There is some data to suggest that the analgesic effects of ketamine are durable and last much longer than the pharmacokinetics of the drug would suggest—up to weeks after administration [1].

Methadone was discussed in detail in Chap. 26. The authors frequently use methadone as a background opioid in opioid-tolerant patients, especially if there is a neuropathic component to the pain complaint. Methadone is a mu-opioid agonist that also has weak NMDA activity that may account for its efficacy in opioid-tolerant patients. Parenteral methadone should be used cautiously, and only by experienced individuals. The long half-life of the drug (~27 h) should be considered when making dose adjustments, as serum levels will continue to rise for several days before reaching steady state. Serial ECG monitoring must be employed to screen for prolongation of the QTc, which occurs in a dose-dependent manner. This may portend development of malignant arrhythmias including torsades de pointes, especially in patients receiving other QTc-prolonging medications.

Neuropathic Adjuvants

Gabapentin and pregabalin are anticonvulsant medications with a shared mechanism of action that are also used for neuropathic pain. These drugs bind the $\alpha 2\delta$ subunit of voltage-gated calcium channels in the central nervous system [19].

Opioid-Induced Hyperalgesia

OIH is an adverse effect of opioid administration in which patients exposed to opioids can develop a paradoxical increased sensitivity to pain. Pathognomonic signs include hyperesthesia, allodynia, and worsening pain despite escalating opioid doses [29]. OIH is difficult to diagnose insofar as it resembles tolerance at its early stages and has been linked to acute and chronic exposure to different types of opioids in a multitude of patients, from healthy controls to substance abuse patients [29].

The mechanism underlying OIH is complex and hypothesized to result from central sensitization of pronociceptive pathways in the setting of a reduced threshold for nociceptive response [29, 30]. Glutaminergic spinal NMDA receptors have been implicated in the central sensitization process associated with OIH, in which receptor activation results in a surplus of pronociceptive excitation [30].

Practically, OIH is a diagnosis of exclusion. It can be distinguished from opioid tolerance by demonstrating an improvement in pain control after downtitration of opioids [30]. Treatment of OIH focuses on withdrawing the offending agents and utilizing NMDA antagonists (i.e., ketamine, methadone) and other adjuncts (i.e., clonidine, dexmedetomidine) [29]. Therapy for the underlying pain complaint should be accomplished using a multimodal, opioid-sparing approach as described above. Consultation with a pain or addiction specialist should be strongly considered if possible.

Management of the Patient Receiving Opioid Addiction Maintenance Therapy

The opioid agonists methadone and buprenorphine are commonly used as a component of addiction therapy. Opioid maintenance therapy (OMT) has been shown to reduce illicit drug use, improve treatment compliance, and curb criminal behavior [9]. As OMT is becoming more prevalent, the clinician is being more frequently challenged to treat acute pain complaints in OMT patients. As previously mentioned, these patients will have diminished pain tolerance and altered pain perception [17]. Providers may also be unwilling to treat these patients with opioids, a phenomenon known as "opiophobia" [9]. This places the patient at risk for uncontrolled acute pain, which is an independent risk factor for the development of chronic pain. Successful management of patients receiving OMT is a challenge, but not an insurmountable one.

Alford et al. describe four common misconceptions of health providers when treating patients receiving OMT [9]:

1. OMT provides analgesia
2. The use of opioids for pain control may cause an addiction relapse
3. The addition of opioid analgesics to OMT will result in serious adverse effects
4. The patient's pain complaint may be due to drug-seeking behavior

OMT should be considered analogous to medical therapy for other chronic diseases such as hypertension or COPD—it provides maintenance therapy for the disease state that is sufficient at baseline but requires supplementation in the setting of an exacerbation. From a pharmacodynamic and pharmacokinetic standpoint, the duration of analgesia of buprenorphine and methadone (4–8 h) is significantly shorter than their ability to suppress opioid withdrawal (24–48 h) [9]. Patients who have been on OMT for long periods of time may derive little or no analgesia from their baseline dose due to tolerance.

Acute pain in OMT patients should be treated in a multimodal fashion as described above, with the caveat that they will require higher and more frequent doses of opioids. The little analgesic benefit that these patients do derive from OMT with methadone or buprenorphine can be improved by splitting the administration of their typical OMT twice daily [31]. The authors sometimes increase this dose by 25 % and administer it every 8 h to further improve analgesia. Short-acting opioids are added in a regularly scheduled and PRN dosing schedule or PCA to achieve analgesia as well as to curtail patient's feelings of being treated as a "junkie" or "addict."

Early communication with the patient's OMT provider is essential to developing a reasonable and durable exit strategy for discharge. Continuing methadone at an increased dose and frequency and/or continuing a short-acting opioid should be considered in patients who have demonstrated compliance with their OMT provider. The provider must be cautious with patients who have a history of continued illicit drug use while on OMT, as they may not be trustworthy with additional methadone or other opioids. If their pain cannot be controlled without additional opioids, inpatient treatment may be required until resolution of the acute pain state.

References

1. Huxtable CA, Roberts LJ, Somogyi AA, MacIntyre PE. Acute pain management in opioid-tolerant patients: a growing challenge. Anaesth Intensive Care. 2011;39(5):804–23.
2. Substance Abuse and Mental Health Services Administration Public Health Service. U.S. Results from the 2010 national survey on drug use and health: summary of national findings. NSDUH Series H-41, HHS 2011; Publication No. (SMA) 11-4658.
3. National Center for Injury Prevention and Control. Policy impact: prescription painkiller overdoses. Centers for Disease Control Nov 2011. http://www.cdc.gov/HomeandRecreationalSafety/pdf/PolicyImpact-PrescriptionPainkillerOD.pdf
4. Liscinsky M. FDA introduces new safety measures for extended-release and long-acting opioid medications. 2012. http://www.fda.gov/NewsEvents/Newsroom/PressAnnouncements/ucm310870.htm. Accessed 3 Jan 2013.
5. Markowitz JD, Francis EM, Gonzales-Nolas C. Managing acute and chronic pain in a substance abuse treatment program for the addicted individual early in recovery: a current controversy. J Psychoactive Drugs. 2010;42(2):193–8.
6. Krashin D, Murinova N, Ballantyne J. Management of pain with comorbid substance abuse. Curr Psychiatry Rep. 2012;14(5):462–8.
7. Manchikanti L, Helm 2nd S, Fellows B, Janata JW, Pampati V, Grider JS, et al. Opioid epidemic in the United States. Pain Physician. 2012;15(3 Suppl):ES9–38.
8. Mackenzie JW. Acute pain management for opioid dependent patients. Anaesthesia. 2006;61(9):907–8.

9. Alford DP, Compton P, Samet JH. Acute pain management for patients receiving maintenance methadone or buprenorphine therapy. Ann Intern Med. 2006;144(2):127–34.

10. Gandhi K, Heitz JW, Viscusi ER. Challenges in acute pain management. Anesthesiol Clin. 2011;29(2):291–309.

11. Palepu A, Tyndall MW, Leon H, Muller J, O'Shaughnessy MV, Schechter MT, et al. Hospital utilization and costs in a cohort of injection drug users. CMAJ. 2001;165(4):415–20.

12. Blay N, Glover S, Bothe J, Lee S, Lamont F. Substance users' perspective of pain management in the acute care environment. Contemp Nurse. 2012;42(2):289–97.

13. Mehta V, Langford RM. Acute pain management for opioid dependent patients. Anaesthesia. 2006;61(3):269–76.

14. Compton MA. Cold-pressor pain tolerance in opiate and cocaine abusers: correlates of drug type and use status. J Pain Symptom Manage. 1994;9(7):462–73.

15. Neighbor ML, Dance TR, Hawk M, Kohn MA. Heightened pain perception in illicit substance-using patients in the ED: implications for management. Am J Emerg Med. 2011;29(1):50–6.

16. Tan S, Yeow M. Moses Maimonidies (1135-1204): Rabbi, Philosopher, Physician. Singapore Med J. 2002;43(11):551–3.

17. Rapp SE, Ready LB, Nessly ML. Acute pain management in patients with prior opioid consumption: a case-controlled retrospective review. Pain. 1995;61(2):195–201.

18. American Society of Anesthesiologists Task Force on Acute Pain Management. Practice guidelines for acute pain management in the perioperative setting: an updated report by the American Society of Anesthesiologists Task Force on Acute Pain Management. Anesthesiology. 2012;116(2):248–73.

19. Buvanendran A, Kroin JS. Multimodal analgesia for controlling acute postoperative pain. Curr Opin Anaesthesiol. 2009;22(5):588–93.

20. Carr DB, Goudas LC. Acute pain. Lancet. 1999;353(9169):2051–8.

21. Besson JM. The neurobiology of pain. Lancet. 1999;353(9164):1610–5.

22. Brennan TJ. Pathophysiology of postoperative pain. Pain. 2011;152(3 Suppl):S33–40.

23. Hurley RW, Wu CL. Acute postoperative pain. In: Miller RD, Eriksson LI, Fleisher LA, Wiener-Kronish JP, Young WL, editors. Miller's anesthesia. 7th ed. Philadelphia: Churchill Livingstone; 2009. p. 2757–81.

24. Fu D, Froicu D, Sinatra R. Anatomic and physiologic principles of pain. In: Vadivelu N, Urman RD, Hines RL, editors. Essentials of pain management. Springer: New York; 2011. p. 31–44.

25. Ventafridda V, Saita L, Ripamonti C, De Conno F. WHO guidelines for the use of analgesics in cancer pain. Int J Tissue React. 1985;7(1):93–6.

26. Slevin K, Ballantyne J. Management of acute postoperative pain. In: Longnecker DE, Brown DL, Newman MF, Zapol WM, editors. Anesthesiology. 2nd ed. New York: McGraw-Hill Professional; 2012.

27. De Buck F, Devroe S, Missant C, Van de Velde M. Regional anesthesia outside the operating room: indications and techniques. Curr Opin Anaesthesiol. 2012;25(4):501–7.

28. Kettner SC, Willschke H, Marhofer P. Does regional anaesthesia really improve outcome? Br J Anaesth. 2011;107 Suppl 1:90–5.

29. Low Y, Clarke CF, Huh BK. Opioid-induced hyperalgesia: a review of epidemiology, mechanisms and management. Singapore Med J. 2012;53(5):357–60.

30. Crofford LJ. Adverse effects of chronic opioid therapy for chronic musculoskeletal pain. Nat Rev Rheumatol. 2010;6(4):191–7.

31. Murnion B. Management of opioid substitution therapy during medical intervention. Intern Med J. 2012;42(3):242–6.

Chapter 34
Pediatric Drug Use, Misuse, and Abuse

Shu-Ming Wang

Key Points

- Substance abuse in children and adolescents
- Statistics
- Risks factors, mass media, and cultural influences
- Responsibility of parents, school, and healthcare providers

Overview

Substance addiction is a chronic disease with genetic, environmental, and behavioral factors that contribute to its cause, manifestations, and natural history. It is a condition characterized by an overwhelming desire to continue taking a drug/substance to which one has become habituated through repeated consumption [1]. Tobacco, alcohol, over-the-counter drugs, prescription drug, and illicit drugs are considered to have great potential being misused and abused. Use of these drugs may lead to criminal penalty in addition to possible physical, social, and psychological harm [2]. Although with prevention the use of illicit drugs declined, legal substances such as tobacco and alcohol remain to be the common substances of addiction and cause substantial morbidity and mortality and significant economic cost. For example, smoking cigarettes and cigarette related problems have caused more than 400,000 deaths yearly in the United States [3–5]. There are approximately 80,000 deaths attributable to excessive alcohol use each year in the United States and it is the 3rd leading life-related cause of death for the nation [6]. In 2009, about 10.4 million young people between age 12 and 20 drank more than "just a few

S.-M. Wang, M.D. (✉)
Department of Anesthesiology, St. Francis Hospital, 114 Wood Land Street,
Hartford, CT 06105, USA
e-mail: smwang800@gmail.com

© Springer Science+Business Media New York 2015
A.D. Kaye et al. (eds.), *Substance Abuse*, DOI 10.1007/978-1-4939-1951-2_34

sips" of alcohol and underage drinking has contributed to 5,000 deaths in people younger than age 21 [7]. The total costs of drug abuse and addiction (i.e. tobacco, alcohol, and illegal drugs) reaches $524 billion per year. Illicit drugs alone account for 181 billion I health care, productivity loss, crime and incarceration, and drug enforcement [8]. Epidemiological studies have shown that the substance addition in adults is closely related to the childhood experience [9]. Studies suggest that the younger an individual is at the onset of substance use, the greater the likelihood that a substance use disorder will develop and continue to adulthood. In fact, more than 50 % of adults with current diagnosis of substance use disorders started before age 18, and 50 % of those began before age 15 [10].

Substance Abuse in Children and Adolescents

Adolescence is a progression of human development period. It is a transitional stage of physical and psychological development that occurs from puberty to legal adulthood. Not only the physical growth but also cognitive development mark the period of adolescent. Our human brain is not fully developed by the time a person reaches puberty. In ages 10 to 25, the brain undergoes changes in the cortex where are important processes of cognitive and emotional information that have important implications for behavior development. Adolescence is the stage of life in which the individual's thoughts start taking more of an abstract from and allow the individual to think and reason in a wider perspective. Through experience, and changing social demands, there is a rapid cognitive growth. This is also a period adolescents are undertaking risk and experiment. More importantly, this is a period adolescents increase self-consciousness and place special emphasis on peers' approval. There may be evolutionary benefits that an increased propensity for risk-taking in adolescence is important for them to have the motivation or confidence necessary to make changes in society from child to adulthood. Adolescence is the time when teenagers are seeking for personal identity and have a desire to feel important in their peer groups and enjoy social acceptance and attention. Moreover the cognitive developments in early adolescence result in greater self-awareness, greater awareness of others and their thoughts and judgments, the ability to think about abstract, future possibilities, and the ability to consider multiple possibilities at once. Environment also plays a huge role in adolescence identity development. Several factors attribute to the developing social identity of an adolescent from commitment, to coping devices, to social media. It is important to remember that adolescence is a sensitive period in the development process, and exposure to the wrong things at that time can have a major affect on future decisions [11]. In the past, it is thought that child from a more privileged upbringing is exposed to more opportunities and better situations in general. An adolescent from an inner city or a crime-driven neighborhood is more likely to be exposed to an environment that can be detrimental to their development. However, recent studies have showed that many children in affluent environments (middle or upper social economic classes) actually have abuse substances such as prescription, nonprescription drugs [12].

In 1998, the adverse childhood experiences (ACE) study showed more than half of the responders reported at least one, and one-fourth reported greater than two categories of childhood substance exposures [13]. There is strong correlation between the number of categories of childhood exposure and each of the adult health risk behaviors and diseases that were studied. The study also showed that when comparing a person who had experienced four or more categories of childhood exposure and those who did not, there were 4- to 12-fold increased health risks for alcoholism, drug abuse, depression, and suicide attempt and a two to fourfold increase in smoking, poor self-rated health and reckless sexual pattern and sexually transmitted diseases. The number of categories of adverse childhood exposures showed graded relationship to the presence of adult diseases including ischemic heart disease, cancer, chronic lung disease, skeletal fractures, and liver disease. Substance abuse/ addiction have caused substantial morbidity and mortality and it has significant negative impacts on the individual, the society, and the economy. As a result, adolescent substance abuse has been one of the major national health foci for decades [14].

Common substances used and abused are as following: legal substance i.e. alcohol and cigarettes; recreation and club drug; over-the-counter drugs; prescription drugs and combination of them. They can be stimulants (amphetamine, cocaine); inhalants (solvents, nitrous oxide); hallucination [MDMA (3,4,-methylenedioxy-N-methylamphetamine), LSD, Mescaline], sedative/hypnotics [GHB (gamma-hydroxybutyric acid), rophynol, benzodiazepines, alcohol]; miscellaneous (marijuana, ketamine, dextromethorphan) [15]. It is not surprising that many youth were polysubstance users. Study has shown about 15 % of adolescents had positive results on the CRAFFT screen after adjustment for demographic factors. Statistical modeling estimated that 11.3 % of all responders had problematic use, 7.1 % had abuse, and 3.2 % had dependence. Substance use is associated with the leading causes of death among US teenagers: unintentional injuries, homicides, and suicides [16]. Knight and colleagues at Harvard medical School and Children's Hospital Boston, administered a substance abuse screening test consisting of six questions focused on the use of alcohol or other drugs and risky behavior to 2,133 adolescents age 12 to 18 who received outpatient medical care from March 2003 to August 2005. The sample consisted of 56.3 % female participants and 48.6 % non-Hispanic whites. Most of teens engaged in substance usage were from middle-class and upper middle-class families. In total, 43.5 % reported any use of alcohol or other drugs and 24.1 % reported impaired driving risk during their lifetimes at the time of survey.

Statistics

According to National Drug Statistic 2012 Report [17], the rate of current illicit drug use varied by age. Among all participants between age 12 and 17 in 2011, the rate increased from 3.3 % at age 12 or 13 to 9.2 % at age 14 or 15 to 17.2 % at ages 16 or 17. Among 18- to 20-year-olds, the rate of illicit drug used increases to 23.8 %. The rate of current use of a tobacco product was significantly decreased among 12 to 17 years old from 15.2 % in 2002 to 10.0 % in 2011. Current Alcohol use was

2.5 % among persons aged 12 or 14. 11.3 % of persons aged 14 or 15, 25.3 % of 16- or 17-year-old. 46.8 % of 18 to 20 years. Rate of binge alcohol use in 2011 were 1.1 % among 12 or 13 years old, 5.7 % among 14 or 15 years old, 15 % among 16 or 17 years old, 31.2 % among 18 to 20 years old. The only encouraging news is that the rate of binge drinking has declined in 2011 as compare to 2010 among 15 or 15 years old. Regardless of different survey studies, the percentages of youth who use cocaine, inhalant, alcohol, and cigarette in the past month decreases between 2001 and 2011. In the prevalence of past year misuse of pain killers/narcotics other than heroin has deceased from 7.2 to 5.9 % between 2006 and 2011.

Risks Factors, Mass Media, and Cultural Influences

Many risk factors have been linked to the tendency of substance abuse [18]. These factors are: 1. A family history of substance abuse or mood disorder-substance use by a family member is associated with higher rates of substance use in adolescents. 2. Household disruption and lack of parental supervision are associated with risk behavior and substance use. 3. Low academic achievement/or academic aspirations. 4. Untreated attention /hyperactivity disorder. 5. Perceived peer acceptance of substance use and substance use in peers. The rapid emergence of social media and the power of advertising have significant influence on children and adolescents' tendency of trying out substances i.e. tobacco, alcohol, and prescription medications. A meta-analysis of 51 separate studies revealed that exposure to tobacco marketing and advertising more than double the risk of a teenager beginning to smoke. Following cigarette smoking, six billion is spent annually on alcohol advertisement and promotion [19]. Hanewinkel et al. [20] have found that the specificity of the relationship between tobacco marketing and youth smoking is being associated with smoking behavior and intentions to smoke. The researchers suggest that as a content-related effect of tobacco advertisements. Similar to tobacco, the alcohol industry spent $1.7 billion in media advertising in 2009. Many alcohol advertisements are placed in different types of media that are popular among adolescents [21, 22]. Moreover, a sample of 9- to 10-year-old children found that they could identify the Budweiser frogs nearly as frequently as they could Bugs Bunny [23]. A South Dakota study conducted on more than 3,500 9th graders, nearly 90 % of them recognized the Budweiser ferret ad [24]. Many studies have revealed that exposure to alcohol advertising results in more positive beliefs about drinking that is predictive of drinking during early adolescence and young adults [25–28]. Estimate more than four billions per year of prescription drugs advertisement, and almost 50 % of physicians reported that majority of their patients requested the advertisement [29, 30]. Through these advertisements, children and adolescents get the idea that there is always a drug to cure any illness and a drug for every occasion. The advertisements of condom, contraceptive pills, and emergency contraception somehow suggest to children and adolescents that sexual activities should be part of their lives [31]. Making the matter worse, smoking, alcohol drinking, and substances usage have been a "normal" part of the film and TV series [32–35]. Simultaneously, media have actively reported many celebrities going in and out of substance rehabilitation programs and substances may fuel the creativities. For example, on "60 minutes" Lady Gaga admits to heavy drug use to Anderson Cooper on Feb 13, 2011. Story said that superstar lady Gaga relies on alcohol and drugs to "fuel" her songwriting, admitting she drank a lot of whiskey and smoked "a lot of weed" in creative process and she owed much of her success to her voice. Although she insisted that she was not urging her young fans to follow her bad example, public stating substances use to enhance the creativities certainly did not help her young fans. Career successfulness, creativities, and artistry somehow closely tie to both legal and illegally substances use. These media reports clearly did not send a strong message to children and teenagers to stay away from substance use.

Responsibility of Parents, School, and Healthcare Providers

Early "just say no" program has decreased the use of illegal substances but in exchange there is substantial increase of the legal substance such as alcohol and cigarettes as well as prescription drugs among teenagers of United States. Parents, teachers/school, and healthcare providers should team up to prevent children and teenagers using substance. Research has shown that parents can have significant influence on their kids. There are several ways parents can build a positive relationship with their kids and start talking to them about drugs i.e. tobacco, alcohol and prescription, and illegal drugs. (1) To establish and maintain good communications between parents and their kids, e.g. asking questions about their day, include them in making decision and value their thoughts and inputs. (2) Get involved in their children's lives, e.g. spending time doing something their children want to do every day, support their children's activities, and help them manage problems by asking what is wrong and offer help when they seem upset. (3) Make clear rule and enforce them consistently. (4) Parents should serve as a positive role model for their children. (5) Help their children to choose friends wisely. (6) Talk to their children about drugs. For details, please refer to http://www.ncpc.org/topics/drug-abuse/alcohol-tobacco-and-other-drugs. In school, teachers should create a positive classroom environment-drug education is most effective when students feel comfortable sharing their ideas and asking a lot of questions. Always listen to verbal and non-verbal communications without interruption, not making any judgment or giving advice. At the same time, teachers should also give age-appropriate messages and talking to their students about various drugs and their related side effects and dependence. Teacher should teach their student how to choose supportive friends who are drug free and who will continue helping them to remain drug free. Pediatricians are at the unique position in assisting their patients and families with substance prevention, detection, and treatments. Studies show that adolescents and their parents want clinicians to address risk-taking behaviors and prevention [36–38]. Adolescents see physicians as credible sources of health information [39]. In a survey of high school students, 80–90 % of adolescent respondents indicated that they would find it helpful to talk with a physician about sexual matters and 75 % stated that they would trust a physician to keep their questions confidential [40]. American Academy of Pediatrics has established the guidelines for preventive services. Pediatricians should include discussions of substance abuse as part of routine health care and incorporate substance abuse prevention into daily practice, and identify young people at risk of substance abuse as well as conducting screening test, intervention and treatment as needed [41].

Summary

Addiction is a complex disease that no single factor can predict who will become an addict thus far age of first use, genetic predisposition, and environment are the main risk factors. Addiction is a developmental disease that usually begins in adolescence or even childhood when the brain is undergoing major changes. It is important to recognize that fact that the most serious, costly, and widespread adolescent health problems such as use of alcohol, tobacco, other drugs, and risk involvement behaviors are potentially preventable. Prevention of drug use and abuse in children and adolescents should be everyone's responsibility.

References

1. Drug Abuse, Addiction, and the Brain. http://www.webmd.com/mental-health/drug-abuse-addiction
2. Mosby's Medical, Nursing & Allied Healthy Dictionary. 6th ed. Drug abuse definition P, 552 Nursing Diagnoses; 2002. p. 2109.
3. Strasburger VC. The council on communications, and media. children, adolescents, substance abuse and the. Pediatrics. 2010;126:791–9.
4. Center for Disease Control and Prevention. National Center for Chronic Disease Prevention and Health Promotion, Office on Smoking and Health, Department of Health and Human Service. Smoking and tobacco use fact sheet. Health effects of cigarette smoking. Updated January 2008. http://www.cdc.gov/tobacco/data_statistics/fact_sheets/health_effects/effects_cig_smoking/
5. Center for Disease Control and Prevention. National Center for Chronic Disease Prevention and Health Promotion, Office on Smoking and Health, Department of Health and Human Service. Tobacco use: targeting the nation's leading killer-t a glance. 2011. http://www.cdc.gov/chronicdisease/resources/publications/aag/osh.htm
6. Mokdad AH, Marks JS, Stroup DF, Gerberding JL. Actual causes of death in the United States 2000. JAMA. 2004;29(10):1238–45.
7. Underage Drinking. National Institutes on Alcohol Abuse and Alcoholism. http://www.niaaa.nih.gov/alcohol-health/special-populations-co-occurring-disorders/underage-drinking
8. National Institutes on Drug Abuse The Science of Drug Abuse & Addiction. Addiction science: from molecular to managed care. Last updated 2008. http://www.drugabuse.gov/publications/addiction-science
9. White HR, Widom CS. Three potential mediators of the effects of child abuse and neglect on adulthood substance use among women. J Stud Alcohol Drugs. 2008;69(3):337–47.

10. Chassin L, Pitts SC, Prost J. Binge drinking trajectories from adolescence to emerging adulthood in a high-risk sample: predictors and substance abuse outcomes. J Consult Clin Psychol. 2002;70(1):67–78. Fe.
11. Christle D, Viner R. Adolescent development. BMJ. 2005;330(7486):301–4.
12. Economic and social consequences of drug abuse and illicit trafficking. www.unodc.org/pdf/technical_series_1998-01-01_1.pdf
13. Adverse Childhood experiences (ACE) study. Centers for Disease Control and Prevention. http://wwwcdc.gov/ace
14. Physician Leadership on National Drug Policy. Adolescent substance abuse: a public health priority in position paper on adolescent drug policy August 2012 published by PLNDP National Office Project Office Center for Alcohol and Addiction Studies. http://www.plndp.org/Resources/adolescent.pdf
15. Substance Abuse WebMD Mental health Center. http://www.webmd.com/mental-health/substance-abuse
16. Knight J, Roberts T, Gabrielli J, Van Hook S. Adolescent alcohol and substance use and abuse. Performing prevention service: a bright future handbook. http://brightfutures.aap.org/pdfs/Preventive%20Services%20PDFs/Screening.PDF
17. Results from the 2012 National Survey on Drug Use and Health: summary of national findings and detailed tables. substance abuse and mental health service administration data, outcomes and quality. http://www.samhsa.gov/data/NSDUH/2012SummNatFindDetTables/index.aspx
18. Weinberg NZ. Risk factors for adolescent substance abuse. J Learn Disabil. 2001;34(4):343–51.
19. Wellman RJ, Sugarman DB, Difranza JR, Winickoff JP. The extent to which tobacco marketing and tobacco used in films contribute to children's use of tobacco: a meta-analysis. Arch Pediatr Adolesc Med. 2006;160(12):1285–96.
20. Hanewinkel R, Isensee B, Sargent JD, Morgensten M. Cigarette advertising and adolescent smoking. Am J Prev Med. 2010;38(4):359–66. doi:10.1016/j.amepre.2009.12.036.
21. Wilcox GB, Gangaharbatta H. What's issued? Does beer advertising affect consumption in the United States? Int J Advert. 2006;25(1):35–50.
22. Moreno MA, Furtner F, Rivara FP. Media influence on adolescent alcohol use. Arch Pediatr Adolesc Med. 2011;165(7):680. doi:10.1001/archpediatrics.2011.121.
23. Leiber L. Commercial and character slogan recall by children aged 9 to 11 years: Budweiser frogs versus bugs bunny. Berkeley: Center on Alcohol Advertisement; 1996.
24. Collin RL, Ellickson PL, MacCaffrey DF, Hambarsoomians K. Saturated in beer awareness of beer advertising in late childhood and adolescence. J Adolesc Health. 2005;37(1):29–36.
25. Grube J, Wallack L. Television beer advertising and drinking knowledge, beliefs, and intentions among schoolchildren. Am J Public Health. 1994;84(2):254–9. http://www.ncbi.nlm.nih.gov/pmc/articles/PMC1614998/.
26. Stacy AW, Zogg JB, Unger JB, Dent CW. Exposure to televised alcohol ads and subsequent adolescent alcohol use. Am J Health Behav. 2004;28(6):498–509.
27. Ellickson PH, Collins RL, Hambarsoomians K, Mc Caffrey DF. Does alcohol advertising promote adolescent drinking? Results from a longitudinal assessment. Addiction. 2005;100(2):235–46.
28. Austin EW, Chen MJ, Grube JW. How does alcohol advertising influence underage drinking? The role of desirability, identification and skepticism. J Adolesc Health. 2006;38(4):376–84.
29. Rosenthal MB, Berndt ER, frank RG, Donohue JM, Epstein AM. Promotion of prescription drugs to consumers. N Engl J Med. 2002;346(7):498–505. doi:10.1056/NEJMsa012075.
30. Spurgeon D. Doctor feet the pressure from direct to consumer advertising. WJM. 2000;172(1):60. http://www.ncbi.nlm.nih.gov/pmc/articles/PMC1070749/.
31. Strasburger VC. Adolescents, sex, and the media: ooooo, baby. Baby—a Q&A. Adolesc Med Clin. 2005;l16(2):269–88.
32. Christenson PG, Henriksen L, Roberts DF. Substance use in popular prime-time television. Washington, DC: Office of National Policy Control; 2000. http://library.stmarytx.edu/acadlib/edocs/supptt.pdf

33. Shields DL, Carol J, Balbach ED, McGee S. Hollywood on tobacco how the entertainment industry understands tobacco portrayal. Tob Control. 1999;8(4):378–86. http://www.ncbi.nlm.nih.gov/pmc/articles/PMC1759741/.
34. Glantz SA, Titus K, Mitchell S, Potansky J, Kaufmann RB. Smoking in top-grossing movie-United States. 1991-2009. MMWR Morb Mortal Wkly Rep. 2010;59(32):1014–7. http://www.medscape.com/viewarticle/727552.
35. Davis RM, Gilpin EA, Loken B, Viswanath K, Wakefield MA. The role of the media in promoting and reducing tobacco use NG tobacco control monograph no 19. Washington DC: US Department of Health and Human Service; 2008. http://cancercontrol.cancer.gov/brp/tcrb/monographs/19/m19_complete.pdf
36. Alcohol, Tobacco, and Other Drugs: Grade 4-5. http://www.ncpc.org/topics/by-audience/law-enforcement/teaching-children/activities-and-lesson-plans/alcohol-tobacco-and-other-drugs-grades-4-5/?searchterm=alcohol%20tobacco%20and%20other%20drugs
37. Substance Abuse Resources. https://www.hanleycenter.org/substance-abuse-prevention/substance-abuse-resources
38. Millstein SG. A view of health from the adolescent's perspective. In: Millstein SG, Peterson AC, Nightingale EO, editors. Promoting the health of adolescents. New York: Oxford University Press; 1993. p. 97–118.
39. Schuster MA, Bell RM, Petersen LP, Kanouse DE. Communication between adolescents and physicians about sexual behavior and risk prevention. Arch Pediatr Adolesc Med. 1996;150(9):906–13.
40. Public Health Service US. Clinician's handbook of preventive: put prevention into practice. 2nd ed. Alexandria: International Medical Publishing; 1998.
41. Kulig JW, Committee on Substance Abuse. Tobacco, alcohol and other drugs: the role of the pediatrician in prevention, identification, and management of substance abuse. Pediatrics. 2005;115(3):816–21. http://pediatrics.aappublications.org/content/115/3/816.full.

Chapter 35
Pregnancy and Substance Abuse

Gulshan Doulatram, Tilak D. Raj, and Ranganathan Govindaraj

Key Points

- All pregnant women must be screened early in pregnancy for substance abuse. Measures of screening include history, self-report, screening questionnaires, and toxicology screens.
- A toxicology screen, even with its limitations, represents the objective standard to detect substance abuse. Hair screens may be able to detect use in the past few months and urine screens may reflect more recent use.
- Women who are known to be positive for substance abuse need to be counseled early in pregnancy. Compliance with abstinence can be increased with a gentle, flexible approach emphasizing the deleterious effects on the fetus.
- Assessment and management of pregnant women is challenging due to the presence of multiple drugs including licit substances such as alcohol and tobacco, nutritional deficiencies, low socioeconomic conditions, and fear and humiliation.
- Amphetamine use is increasing in women compared to cocaine. Amphetamines cause significant maternal and neonatal effects including intrauterine growth retardation and preterm labor, and do not have specific antidotes for overdose or withdrawal.
- All pregnant women should be counseled about cessation of smoking, alcohol, and caffeine (licit substances) use. Nicotine replacement therapy should be considered. Adequate education of the ill effects of alcohol should be explained to the mother, including FAS, as alcohol is the number one cause of preventable birth defects.
- Cocaine exposure during pregnancy is associated with significant maternal and fetal mortality and morbidity.

G. Doulatram, M.D. (✉) • R. Govindaraj, M.D., F.R.C.A.
Department of Anesthesiology, University of Texas Medical Branch,
301 University Boulevard, Galveston, TX 77555-0591, USA
e-mail: gdoulatr@utmb.edu

T.D. Raj, M.D., M.R.C.P., F.R.C.A.
Department of Anesthesiology, Oklahoma University Health Sciences
Center/OU Medical Center, Oklahoma City, OK 73104, USA

© Springer Science+Business Media New York 2015
A.D. Kaye et al. (eds.), *Substance Abuse*, DOI 10.1007/978-1-4939-1951-2_35

- Complete detoxification from heroin and opioids is ideal, but, if not possible, opioid maintenance programs with methadone or buprenorphine should be implemented early to avoid relapse. Neonatal abstinence syndrome will develop in an infant chronically exposed to maternal opioids, hence early assessment and management of the infant is crucial.

Introduction

Substance abuse in pregnancy is a significant public health crisis causing increased morbidity in two individuals, the mother and the fetus [1]. Pregnant substance abusers often fail to get prenatal care due to ignorance, fear, and lack of resources including strong support systems. Substance abusers could also have other coexisting infectious diseases such as HIV, hepatitis, nutritional deficiencies, and sexually transmitted diseases, which add to the list of complications seen in the pregnant mother and the fetus [2]. Detection of individual substances remains a challenge despite the implementation of screening questionnaires and toxicology testing of urine, hair, and meconium [3]. Many female substance abusers in the child-bearing age may not realize it when they become pregnant, hence exposing the fetus to high levels of the abused substance and thereby increasing the risk of perinatal and fetal complications [4]. Even after appropriate detection, the management of these patients throughout pregnancy could remain a challenge. Barriers on the part of the physician, lack of information in the form of well-developed guidelines for treatment, psychosocial and socioeconomic factors such as domestic violence and poor prenatal care, are all established reasons why successful treatment of this entity eludes most practitioners. Antenatal education and counseling is essential to successfully treat this high-risk population. Abused substances have unique pharmacological effects both on the maternal and fetal systems. An understanding of these effects is essential for implementing effective management in the antepartum, peripartum, and postpartum stages of pregnancy. Effective pain management in the opioid-dependent individual requires an understanding of the interaction of maintenance therapies with medications used in the peripartum period [5]. Infants exhibiting effects of withdrawal including neonatal abstinence syndrome need to be monitored closely. Breastfeeding concerns are valid and guidelines vary depending on the drug of abuse. Finally, it is a well-established fact that most substances cause long-term behavioral and psychological problems extending well past infancy into early childhood and in some cases adulthood as well.

Epidemiology

Substance abuse during pregnancy is a challenging medical entity for healthcare providers including primary care physicians, obstetricians, anesthesiologists, pain physicians and addiction medicine specialists [6]. One third of individuals who suffer from substance abuse are women of child-bearing age, which prefaces the scope

Table 35.1 Substance abuse among pregnant vs. nonpregnant women

	Pregnant women (%)	Nonpregnant women (%)
Illicit drug use	4.4	10.9
Alcohol use	10.8	54.7
Binge drinking	3.7	24.6
Cigarette use	16.3	26.7

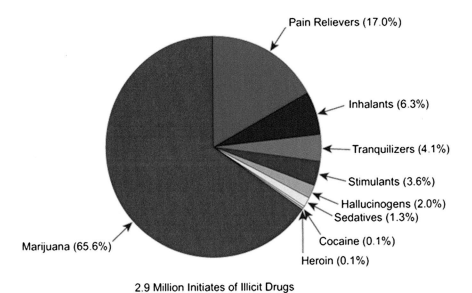

2.9 Million Initiates of Illicit Drugs

Fig. 35.1 Pie chart showing that of all the drugs, marijuana is the most commonly abused drug, followed by amphetamines and opiates [7]. Data from http://www.oas.samhsa.gov/nhsda.htm

and magnitude of this world wide problem (Table 35.1). In the United States, the Substance Abuse and Mental Health Services Administration reports the prevalence of substance abuse in pregnant women between the ages of 15–44 years. Current illegal drug use among pregnant women is stable from 2007–2008 (5.1 %) to 2009–2010 (4.4 %). These rates are lower than those for nonpregnant women of the same age (4.4 % vs. 10.9 % in nonpregnant women). However the prevalence is highest for those aged 15–17 years compared to 26–44 years. Of all the drugs, marijuana is the most commonly abused drug, followed by amphetamines and opiates (Fig. 35.1). The prevalence ranges from 4 to 17 % depending upon the substance abused. A survey done on pregnant women showed that about 10 % of them had used alcohol, 18 % had smoke cigarettes, and 4 % used an illicit substance in the prior month [7]. Actual figures are predicted to be much higher due to a high degree of underreporting. Prevalence in many countries around the world including United Kingdom, Brazil, and Australia is around 11 %, emphasizing that substance abuse in young women is a global crisis. The incidence of analgesic use alone, including prescribed and non-prescribed drugs, is 39.6 % and 62.3 % respectively, a figure much higher than other substances. These figures translate to 200,000–400,000

Table 35.2 Summary of effects of prenatal drug exposure

	Nicotine	Alcohol	Marijuana	Opiates	Cocaine	Methamphetamine
Short-term effects/birth outcome						
Fetal growth	+	+++	−	+	+	+
Anomalies	NCE	+++	−	−	−	−
Withdrawal	−		−	+++	−	Ψ
Neurobehavior	+	+	+	+	+	+
Long-term effects						
Growth	NCE	+++	−	−	NCE	Ψ
Behavior	+	+++	+	+	+	Ψ
Cognition	+	+++	+	NCE	+	Ψ
Language	+	+	−	Ψ	+	Ψ

infants born each year who have been exposed to prenatal drugs [8]. Drug use is reported to be as high as 15–30 % in the low income groups, younger age at pregnancy, ethnic minority groups, and patients with less education [9]. There also appears to be a genetic susceptibility to substance abuse, which will improve screening of patients [10].

Smoking and alcohol (licit substances) are associated with well-defined problems, including growth retardation with nicotine and cranio-facial and mental retardation seen with fetal alcohol syndrome [11]. Cocaine is associated with low birth weight and IUGR consistently. Substance abuse is closely linked to stress, smoking, and late or no prenatal (care which has also been shown to independently cause adverse birth outcomes) (Table 35.2) [12, 13]. The ongoing cost of medical care of mothers with substance abuse and their babies is huge. As an example, the costs of neonatal care for infants born to mothers who smoke is $700 per patient and this increases to $5,110 in those exposed to cocaine. The cost of substance abuse in Canada in the perinatal population, including healthcare costs and loss of productivity, was estimated to be 40 billion in 2002.

Definition of Substance Abuse

Substance abuse can simply be defined as a pattern of harmful use of any substance for mood-altering purposes. According to DSM-V guide, abused substances include ten separate classes of drugs: alcohol, caffeine, cannabis, hallucinogens (with separate categories for phencyclidine [or similarly acting arylcyclohexylamines] and other hallucinogens), inhalants, opioids, sedatives, hypnotics, and anxiolytics; stimulants (amphetamine-type substances, cocaine, and other stimulants), tobacco, and other (or unknown) substances [14]. Although the pharmacological mechanism may be different, the underlying feature with these substances is excess use resulting in direct activation of the brain reward center (high). The diagnosis of substance use disorder is based on a pathological pattern of behavior related to use of the substance. The eleven criteria according to DSM-V can be grouped under four headings, which include *impaired control, social impairment, risky use,* and *pharmacological criterion*

I. Impaired Control (criteria 1–4)

1. The individual may take the substance in larger amounts or over a longer period than was originally intended.
2. The individual may express a persistent desire to cut down or regulate substance use and may report multiple unsuccessful efforts to decrease or discontinue use.
3. The individual may spend a great deal of time obtaining the substance, using the substance, or recovering from its effects. In severe cases, virtually all of the person's daily activities revolve around the substance.
4. Craving is manifested by an intense desire or urge for the drug that may occur at any time but is more likely when in an environment where the drug previously was obtained or used.

II. Social Impairment (criteria 5–7)

5. Recurrent substance use may result in a failure to fulfill major role obligations at work, school, or home.
6. The individual may continue substance use despite having persistent or recurrent social or interpersonal problems caused or exacerbated by the effects of the substance.
7. Important social, occupational, or recreational activities may be given up or reduced because of substance use.

III. Risky Use (criteria 8–9)

8. May take the form of recurrent substance use in situations in which it is physically hazardous.
9. The individual may continue substance use despite knowledge of having a persistent or recurrent physical or psychological problem that is likely to have been caused or exacerbated by the substance.

IV. Pharmacological Criteria (criteria 10–11)

10. *Tolerance* is signaled by requiring a markedly increased dose of the substance to achieve the desired effect or a markedly reduced effect when the usual dose is consumed.
11. *Withdrawal* is a syndrome that occurs when blood or tissue concentrations of a substance decline in an individual who had maintained prolonged heavy use of the substance. This makes further consumption by the individual likely to relieve symptoms of withdrawal. Withdrawal symptoms vary greatly depending on the substance classes and there are separate criteria for withdrawal for the different classes.

Assessment of Substance Abuse in Pregnant Women

It is not uncommon for pregnant women to deny substance abuse on direct questioning. In fact, 66 % of parturients who tested positive for cocaine on urine toxicology denied using it at admission [15]. It is the responsibility of every practice to make sure that all pregnant and postpartum women are screened for substance abuse. Screening improves identification of substance abusing parturients, and by doing so early in pregnancy, treatment and preventive services can be made readily available thus reducing risk for the pregnancy and the child [16]. All pregnant women, regardless of socioeconomic status, should be asked about past and current substance use, including alcohol, tobacco, and illicit and prescribed drugs (Table 35.3). The diagnosis of substance abuse in pregnancy is made by a combination of clinical intuition, interview methodology, and lab testing.

Risk factors that require further assessment [17] before urine toxicology screen include:

- History of physical abuse or neglect
- Preterm labor
- Intimate partner violence
- Intrauterine Growth Restriction (IUGR)
- Mental illness
- Previous unexplained fetal demise
- Previous child with fetal alcohol
- Hypertensive episodes effects or syndrome or alcohol-related birth defects
- Stroke or heart attack related birth defects

Table 35.3 TWEAK and T-ACE questionnaires

TWEAK
T Tolerance
W Have friends or relatives complained about your drinking? (**W**orried)
E Eye-opener
A Has a friend or family member ever told you about things you said or did while you were drinking that you could not remember? (**A**mnesia or black-out)
K Cut down
Scoring: T: 2 points if >3 drinks; W, E, A, K: 1 point for each yes answer
A total score of 3 or more points indicates patient is at-risk drinking
T-ACE
T How many drinks does it take to make you feel high? (**T**olerance)
A Have people annoyed you by criticizing your drinking?
C Have you felt you ought to cut down on your drinking?
E Have you ever had a drink first thing in the morning to steady your nerves or get rid of a hangover? (**E**ye-opener)
Scoring: T: 2 points if >3 drinks; A, C, E: 1 point each for yes answer
A total of 2 or more points indicates patient is likely to have an alcohol problem

- Severe mood swings
- Fetal distress
- History of repeated spontaneous
- Placenta Abruption abortions

Certain risk factors that should raise the index of suspicion for substance abuse in the parturient include lack of prenatal care, inappropriate behavior like somnolence and disorientation, physical signs of substance abuse, smell of alcohol or chemicals, and recent history of substance abuse or treatment [18]. Certain behavior patterns and physical signs indicate the possibility of substance abuse and the need for laboratory testing. Suspicious behaviors include sedation/inebriation, euphoria, agitation, aggressive/violent behavior, paranoia, depression, irritability, prescription drug seeking, suicidal ideations or attempts, psychosis or memory loss. The first hints may be physical signs such as dilated or constricted pupils, nystagmus, tremors, track marks, abscesses, nose bleeds, eroded nasal mucosa, tachycardia, hypertension, raised body temperature, gum disease or severe teeth decay, malnutrition, and or weight loss [17].

As the substance abuser is prone to complications it is important that the healthcare provider be alert to certain laboratory (macrocytic anemia, elevated GGT, bilirubin, Hepatitis C) or medical history clues which might indicate the possibility of substance abuse (Table 35.4). Medical history clues would include frequent hospitalizations, gunshot or knife wounds, unusual infections (endocarditis, cellulitis), hepatitis, cirrhosis, pancreatitis or frequent falls and unexplained bruising.

There is no optimal screening tool for identifying substance abuse in pregnancy. Interviewing the pregnant woman with an open-ended, non-judgmental questioning

Table 35.4 Assessment for substance-related disorders [1]

Complete drug history
Name of drug, amount, frequency, duration, route(s), last use, injection drug use, sharing needles/paraphernalia, withdrawal symptoms
Consequences of substance use
Medical, social, personal, previous treatment programs, mutual aid programs (i.e., AA)
Medical history
HIV, Hepatitis B and C, STIs, chronic medical conditions (i.e., chronic pain), medications
Psychiatric history
Eating disorders, sexual/physical abuse, mood and anxiety disorders
Obstetrical history
Cycle regularity, LMP, past obstetrical outcomes and complications
Social history
Family situation (partner and number of children), custody status, housing situation, legal status (current charges and court dates), finances, nutrition, child protection agency involvement, child safety concerns
FIFE
Feelings, **i**mpressions/ideas, **f**unctioning, **e**xpectations about pregnancy and drug use

AA alcoholics anonymous, *STI* sexually transmitted diseases, *LMP* last menstrual period is more likely to elicit disclosure of perinatal substance abuse. Recently, physical, sexual, and emotional abuse has been identified as precursors to substance abuse in women; hence, domestic violence should be screened for. The T-ACE, TWEAK, and CAGE questionnaires should help in screening for alcohol use [19, 20].

CAGE (**C**ut down, **A**nnoyed by criticism, **G**uilty about drinking, **E**ye-opener) primarily targets heavy alcoholic drinking in men [21]. The T-ACE and TWEAK have been validated as reliable screening tools in obstetric practice but again, target primarily heavy drinkers and do not identify light drinkers or users of illicit drugs. The 4Ps [22] and 4Ps plus [23, 24] screen for a range of substances and can detect pregnant women with low levels of alcohol or drug use but have low to moderate specificity [25].

Other screening tools available include *NET* (Normal drinker, Eye-opener, Tolerance) which does not identify early stage drinkers or illicit substance users *PRO* (Prenatal Risk Overview), *AUDIT* (Alcohol Use Disorders Identification Test), and *SASSI* (Substance Abuse Subtle Screening Inventory).

The *PRO* is a 10–15 min structured interview, which addresses 13 psychosocial risk domains including home, social, and relationship status including physical and sexual abuse and drug and alcohol use [26]. It has been validated using Structured Clinical Interview for DSM-IV (SCID) in pregnant women [27].

AUDIT was developed by the World Health Organization (WHO) as a simple method of screening for excessive drinking (Table 35.5). Its reliability has been

Table 35.5 AUDIT (Alcohol Use Disorders Identification Test) developed by the WHO (World Health Organization) as a simple method of screening for excessive drinking [28, 29]

Specimen	Advantages	Limitations
Urine	Detection of diverse group of illicit substances (except volatile alcohols)	Underrepresents most illicit drug use
	Specimen and test readily available	Significant false-positive rate for phencyclidine (PCP)
	Short turnaround time (30 min at point of care: 2 h for laboratory specimens)	Narrow detection window compared with that for meconium and hair
	More sensitive (compared with meconium and hair) for cannabis	
Blood	Most commonly used for volatile alcohols (can detect other illicit substances)	Narrow detection window compared with that for urine, meconium, and hair
	Specimen and test readily available	
Meconium	Highly sensitive (compared with urine testing) for cocaine and opioids	Specimen may not be readily available
	Wide detection window	Low sensitivity for detecting Cannabinoids
	No false-positive results for cocaine	
Hair	Highly sensitive test for detecting cocaine (three times that of urine) and opioids	Multiple hairs required, harvested close to scalp
	Wide detection window (reflects chronic cumulative use)	Environmental contamination may cause false-positive result
	Samples can be stored at room temperature	Low sensitivity for detecting tetrahydrocannabinol
	Samples can be analyzed remote from collection	
Umbilical cord blood	Comparable to meconium with more rapid results	Specimen not available before delivery

validated in many studies [28, 29]. One study found a high prevalence of alcohol consumption in pregnant adolescents and various risk factors were identified [30].

SASSI is a brief self-report, easily administered psychological screening measure that is available in separate versions for adults and adolescents. Both versions are designed to identify individuals who have a high probability of having a substance use disorder, including both substance abuse and substance dependence, with an overall accuracy above 90 % [31]. SASSI was found to be a more effective clinical tool for identifying substance abuse and more cost effective than toxicology screening in pregnancy [32]. Alcohol abuse which is missed by toxicology and self-report is detected by the SASSI hence minimizing the need for toxicology screening of prenatal patients [33]. If the woman acknowledges substance use, a more complete assessment is then recommended.

Toxicology Testing

Drug toxicology testing determines the presence of a drug, but is not recommended for universal screening because of its numerous limitations. It may be useful as a follow up to a positive interview screen or the presence of risk factors. The benefits of lab testing include the confirmation of the presence of single or multiple drugs and the determination if the newborn is at risk for withdrawal. Detection also facilitates early intervention, which includes treatment of maternal and neonatal withdrawal, counseling and referral for treatment (Table 35.6).

The evaluation of in utero exposure to drugs of abuse has been achieved by testing biological matrices coming from the fetus or newborn (meconium, fetal hair, cord blood, neonatal urine), pregnant or nursing mother (hair, blood, oral fluid, sweat, urine, breast milk) or from both the fetus and the mother (placenta and amniotic fluid) [34].

Table 35.6 Drug toxicology laboratory testing

Drug	Analyte	Detection window
Tobacco	Cotinine	19 h (urine T1/2)
	Nicotine	2 h (urine T1/2)
Cocaine	Cocaine	3–6 h
	Benzoylecgonine	1–2 days, if used IV; 2–3 days if used intranasally
Amphetamines	Amphetamine	1–3 days
	Methamphetamine	60 h, if smoked
Methylenedioxymethamphetamine (MDMA, ecstasy)	MDMA	1–3 days
Marijuana (cannabis)	Tetrahydrocannabinol (THC)	10 h, if smoked
	THCCOOH	Up to 25 days
Lysergic acid diethylamine (LSD)	LSD	24 h
	2-Oxo-30H-LSD	96 h
Heroin	6-Acetyl morphine	2–4.5 h, if used IV
	Morphine	19–35 h

Both liquid and gas chromatography–mass spectrometry have been used for assays of drugs or metabolites on these matrices.

Placenta: Fatty acid ethyl esters (FAEFs) detected in neonatal matrices are produced by the fetus from ethanol that has been transferred from the mother, reflecting true fetal exposure to ethanol in utero. In newborns prenatally exposed to arecoline (principal alkaloid of the sliced nut of the areca palm) and suffering adverse birth outcomes, the analyte was found in the placenta [35].

Amniotic fluid: This has not gained popularity because it is invasive, difficult to obtain and can be harmful to the fetus. The presence of drugs in this fluid indicates exposure during the early fetal life [36].

Meconium: Meconium is the neonate's first several bowel movements, and can be collected between 1 and 5 days after birth. Its analysis allows detection of maternal drug use during the last 20 weeks of gestation providing information on chronic fetal drug exposure [36]. The wide window for sample collection is an advantage in newborns presenting with signs of withdrawal or impairment of physical or mental development to determine intrauterine drug exposure.

Neonatal hair: This is a sensitive biological marker that can define cumulative exposure to drugs during the last trimester of intra-uterine life. The detection window for neonatal hair is smaller than for meconium but has the advantage of being available for as long as 4–5 months of postnatal life [36, 37]. For extraction and analysis, 20–50 mg of hair is needed which may not be available in a newborn.

Neonatal urine: The major disadvantage of neonatal urinalysis is the narrow time window of drug detection reflecting drug use only a few days prior to delivery. This may produce false-negative results depending on time of last ingestion of the drug by the mother and the time after birth the sample was collected.

Cord blood: As with maternal blood measuring, drug and metabolite levels in cord blood indicates fetal exposure hours or days prior to collection. Recently, umbilical cord tissue was proposed as an alternative to meconium drug testing [38]. This was validated by comparison with meconium testing, and can be advantageous because passage of meconium might be delayed, especially in premature infants.

Maternal hair: This is considered the gold standard to assess chronic maternal drug use in pregnancy because hair collection is relatively noninvasive, a large quantity can be collected, and information on early use during pregnancy is possible. It is also more sensitive than urine testing [34]. As with all maternal matrices, maternal hair testing gives a direct estimate of maternal exposure to drugs but only an indirect estimate of those reaching the fetus. Hair cosmetics can interfere with testing [39].

Maternal urine: As in the case of neonatal urine, the detection window is extremely short. However, the advantages include ease of collection, and availability at all times with no limitations in collected volume. Currently, maternal urinalysis (Table 35.6) for illicit drugs is used to monitor drug use in pregnancy [40]. For cost-effective drug screening, maternal urine should be collected at the time of admission for labor [41].

Maternal blood and oral fluid: Maternal blood was one of the first matrices analyzed to detect drug use during pregnancy and fetal drug exposure [34]. Drug concentrations are related to intake a few days or hours before blood sampling thus disclosing recent consumption. Maternal blood testing is invasive and not well accepted by the subjects. For these reasons the practical applications of this method for monitoring drug use are limited [36].

Oral fluid (saliva) collection is less invasive and more cost effective than blood, and, hence is gaining popularity as an alternative medium. Similar to blood, saliva testing detects acute consumption in the hours prior to collection and repetitive sampling may be needed to verify a suspected abuser. This limitation prevents extensive use of oral fluid testing.

Maternal sweat: Sweat testing is relatively noninvasive, and the window of detection is somewhat wider than urine testing. Sweat is collected by a patch that can be worn up to a week. Drugs tend to accumulate in the patch and do not undergo degradation [42]. A potential application would be in the weekly monitoring of maternal consumption in cases of proven or suspected addiction. Despite this, maternal sweat has never been used to determine fetal exposure to drugs.

Amphetamines

Amphetamines are synthetic neurostimulants that cause increased wakefulness and decreased fatigue and appetite [43]. It has been reported that 5 % of pregnant women use methamphetamines and 24 % women admitted to hospitals related to substance abuse were due to amphetamines. Five percent of adults suffering from attention deficit hyperactivity disorder may need amphetamines in the treatment plan [44]. Amphetamine use has increased exponentially over the last few years compared to cocaine (partly due to increased accessibility) and is now second only to marijuana as the most commonly abused drug.

Pharmacology: Amphetamines exert their effects through the modulation of dopamine, serotonin, and norepinephrine, all of which are involved in the reward pathways [45]. They also produce intense CNS stimulation. Amphetamines, methylamphetamines, and methylenedioxymethamphetamines (MDMA) are slowly metabolized, causing sustained elevations of neurotransmitters such as serotonin and norepinephrine. They reach the central nervous system easily after oral, inhaled, or intravenous injection. The effects of these substances are felt within 5–20 min after ingestion. These drugs have a long half-life further prolonging their euphoric effects. Amphetamines and their metabolites can be detected in the urine for several days after use. Methylamphetamine, also known as crystal meth, is more potent than amphetamine and is usually smoked.

Systemic effects: Amphetamines cause release of catecholamines, which results in alertness, feelings of well-being, suppression of appetite, and euphoria. Similar to cocaine intoxication, some of the cardiovascular systemic effects include hypertension, arrhythmias, and tachycardia. Anxiety, hypotension, and somnolence occur with chronic use of amphetamines due to depletion of catecholamines

Effects on the mother and fetus: Amphetamines can cross the placenta quite easily and are found at high levels in the amniotic fluid and umbilical cord. They can increase the risk of placental hemorrhage, placental abruption, and uterine contractions mediated by serotonin, increasing the incidence of preterm labor [46]. They also accumulate in the fetal lungs, kidney, liver, brain, and heart. In fact, levels of amphetamines in the amniotic fluid correlate well with fetal brain exposure. Neonates show lethargy, somnolence and decreased feeding, similar to amphetamine withdrawal.

Amphetamine use may also cause the following in the fetus:

- Intrauterine growth retardation
- Prematurity
- Congenital malformations such as cardiac anomalies, cleft lip and palate and biliary atresia, cerebral lesions
- Withdrawal symptoms in the fetus
- Neurobehavioral and cognitive deficits
- Low birth weight

A meta-analysis of ten studies confirmed the association of amphetamine use with low birth weights, preterm labor, and small for gestational age [44]. Data for congenital disorders is scant and unsubstantiated. Amphetamines have been implicated in uterine vasoconstriction and decreased uterine blood flow, both of which can cause growth retardation. The effects of amphetamines are dose and time dependent. As is the case with most substances of abuse, it is often difficult to attribute these maternal and fetal effects entirely to amphetamine use due to coexisting conditions such as tobacco, alcohol and other drug abuse, poor socioeconomic status, sexually transmitted diseases, poor access to prenatal care and nutrition [43]. Long-term behavioral effects such as aggression have been demonstrated in children who were exposed to amphetamines prenatally and have been found to correlate well with low levels of serotonin and dopamine transporters.

Perinatal management: There is no specific drug therapy for the amphetamine addicted mother; hence it is imperative that full psychological support is available to encourage complete cessation of use. When this is not feasible, reduction in use, good antenatal care, adequate nutritional support and treatment of any associated psychiatric conditions could be realistic goals. Amphetamine users do not tend to remain compliant in treatment programs, as they may not consider the drug to have deleterious effects. Reinforcement based programs are more effective in improving outcomes [47]. Breastfeeding in infants of mothers using amphetamines is usually not encouraged due to infant restlessness and somnolence.

Pharmacotherapy: There is no specific antidote for amphetamine withdrawal akin to opioid-dependent patients in the mother and the fetus [43]. Supportive therapy is the best approach to these patients. Phenobarbitone in the presence of seizures is advocated in the neonate. Most neonates do not suffer from severe symptoms and do not require treatment beyond the first week. Amphetamine withdrawal in the pregnant woman causes profound fatigue, somnolence, depression, agitation, severe anxiety, and suicidal ideation. Symptoms of withdrawal may be exaggerated if there is concomitant abuse of other substances. Amphetamine can cause tolerance and dependence as well. Drugs that have been used to treat withdrawal include modafinil, bupropion, fluoxetine, and imipramine. Success of these therapies has been restricted to highly motivated patients, which may be only a small subset of the affected mothers. Amphetamine overdose manifests as hypertension, arrhythmias, hyperpyrexia, and seizures. Cooling, anticonvulsants and antihypertensive agents can be used to control symptoms.

Caffeine

Although the exact prevalence of caffeine use during pregnancy is unknown, a high percentage of women drink caffeinated beverages.

Pharmacology: Caffeine from various sources such as coffee, tea, and soft drinks is absorbed easily from the gastrointestinal system and can reach significant blood levels. The half-life of caffeine increases exponentially during pregnancy, causing high plasma levels and placental transfer. Abuse is defined as the daily consumption of 500–600 mg of caffeine. Caffeine causes CNS stimulation through the release of norepinephrine, dopamine, and serotonin and decreased levels of adenosine.

Systemic effects: Increased heart rate and blood pressure are due to sympathomimetic effects of caffeine. Other effects include alertness, decreased fatigue, improved mood, and diuresis.

Caffeine is known to be addictive and can cause physical dependence. Caffeine withdrawal can cause headache, fatigue, and anxiety. Signs and symptoms are not consistent and can occur to varying degrees depending on the amount of caffeine ingested and duration of use.

Effects on pregnancy and fetus: The general consensus is that the upper limit for caffeine exposure is 300 mg/day [48]. Moderate doses have not been shown to have deleterious effects on the mother and the fetus, however high doses may cause growth deficits, teratogenic effects, and possibly infertility [49]. Consumption of large amounts of caffeine has been associated with miscarriage [50]. Low to moderate amounts may actually be beneficial. These include a lower risk of developing diabetes in the infant and less neurological injury in animals after hypoxia [51].

Perinatal management: Pregnant mothers are advised to stop or reduce the amount of coffee consumption during pregnancy. Withdrawal headache promptly responds to caffeine; however behavior modifications may be necessary in mothers who report a high caffeine use.

Alcohol

Alcohol is very commonly abused in pregnancy because it is legal and permissible in several cultures. According to 2012 National Survey on Drug Abuse, the incidence of alcohol use in pregnancy is as high as 7.8 % [52]. About 1 % of women report heavy drinking, which is defined as one or more drinks a day for a woman. Binge drinking, which is consuming more than four drinks at one time occurs in 11.9 % of pregnant mothers and about 80,000 babies are born annually to a mother who reported heavy drinking throughout pregnancy. A safe limit of alcohol has not been identified; hence women who desire pregnancy or are pregnant should be counseled to stop alcohol completely. Screening women for alcohol use has been well studied and effective in the pregnant population (See Screening section).

Pharmacology: Alcohol is absorbed through the small intestine and is metabolized by alcohol and acetaldehyde dehydrogenase to form acetaldehyde and reduced form of nicotinamide adenine dinucleotide (NADH). Alcohol crosses the placenta easily and acts as a direct teratogen to the fetus. Alcohol depresses the central nervous system, leading to hypnosis and death in large doses. Normal fetal neurodevelopment requires neuronal cell to cell adhesion [53]. Alcohol disrupts this process by its effects on cell adhesion molecules. Alcohol also causes neuronal cell apoptosis by increasing reactive oxygen species and cytochrome production, affecting both mitochondrial and cytoplasmic DNA. Decreased oxygen delivery to the fetus occurs by vasoconstriction produced by alcohol associated decreased nitric oxide levels. The facial abnormalities are thought to be due to apoptosis of cranial neural crest cells. Neurotransmitter levels, such as serotonin, have been implicated to cause neuropsychiatric effects of FASD.

Systemic effects: In the mother, alcohol acts as a CNS depressant, having a direct toxic effect on neurons. Chronic alcoholics will present with brain atrophy, difficulties with learning, memory and information processing and Wernicke-Korsakoff syndrome in severe cases. Alcoholics also will have other problems such as cirrhosis, pancreatitis, gastritis, pneumonia, and cardiomyopathy.

Effects on the fetus and mother: Fetal alcohol syndrome (FAS) is the leading cause of preventable birth defects in the United States (US Dept of Health), causing physical, mental, and behavioral impairment. The incidence of FAS is 0.5 and 2 cases per 1,000 births. The prevalence is 20 times higher in chronic alcoholics compared to the general population [54, 55]. The impact of FAS is astronomical, with reports that lifetime cost for an individual with FAS is two million dollars. Extent of the damage in the fetus varies according to the dose, frequency, and timing of alcohol use. Some studies have shown that low or moderate doses of alcohol do not cause deleterious effects; however, the long-term effects are poorly understood. Alcohol consumed during critical gestational periods causes more significant neurological and behavioral problems. Developing neurons are more vulnerable to intermittent high exposure to alcohol in the first trimester, hence pregnant women and women of child-bearing age desiring pregnancy should avoid binge drinking.

The degree of damage to the fetus will depend on other factors, such as maternal health, nutrition, smoking and other drug use, and maternal and fetal genetics. Women of low socioeconomic status are more likely to develop complications related to alcohol use partly due to poor nutritional status and associated abuse of other substances such as nicotine or illicit drugs.

A separate disorder called fetal alcohol spectrum disorder (FASD) includes all the effects associated with alcohol use, and is three times more common than FAS. The incidence of FASD is 9.1 in 1,000 births. FASD includes all mental, physical, behavioral, and learning problems in the fetus of a woman who drank any amount or type of alcohol.

Diagnostic criteria were developed by the Institute of medicine (IOM) to identify and treat FASD. In the 1990s, a diagnostic system called the 4 Digit Diagnostic Code was introduced to increase diagnostic reliability of FASD. Due to its ambiguity, revised IOM criteria were developed and now exist with a focus on a multidisciplinary team approach and institution of a differential diagnosis approach in FASD [56]. Similar consortiums have been implemented in different countries, underscoring the importance and application of a unified diagnostic approach across cultures and geographic map lines [11].

1. Fetal Alcohol Syndrome (FAS) has the following criteria

   - Prenatal alcohol exposure (PAE)
   - Dysmorphic facial characteristics such as smooth philtrum, thin upper lip, and short palpebral fissures
   - Prenatal and postnatal growth deficiency in height or weight ($\leq$10th percentile);
   - CNS dysfunction, including structural, neurological, and/or functional brain abnormalities such as microcephaly, mental retardation, and attention deficit disorder

2. Partial FAS has one or two facial abnormalities
3. Alcohol-related birth defects (ARBD)
4. Alcohol-related neurodevelopment disorders (ARND)

Diagnosis of FASD

1. Maternal biomarkers—Carbohydrate deficient transferrin, F-glutamyltransferase, mean corpuscular volume, and hemoglobin-associated acetaldehyde may suggest an increased risk of FASD.
2. Second-trimester prenatal ultrasound—Symmetric intrauterine growth retardation; organ defects, cardiac or renal anomalies; defects of skeletal bones or ribs
3. Fatty acid ethyl esters (FAEEs)—These are fat-soluble metabolites of alcohol formed via a nonoxidative pathway. They can be used to quantify alcohol use in chronic alcoholics and binge drinkers. Maternal hair and newborn meconium analysis for FAEEs can be used to detect illicit drug use by mothers [53].

Treatment of FASD: Treatment of FASD can begin prenatally to prevent the progressive effects of alcohol on the fetal brain. Antioxidants such as superoxide dismutase, Vitamin C, Vitamin E, and green tea extract have been used in animals to prevent the damage to neurons done by free radicals. Serotonin agonists such as buspirone and ipsaspiron have also been used. In the postnatal period, therapy should aim at managing neuropsychological impairment. Providing a stable family environment, effective substance abuse treatment for the mother, and long-term neurobehavioral programs are essential [57].

Alcohol can cause other effects on the mother and the fetus apart from FASD. There is a higher incidence of placental abruption, antepartum hemorrhage, preterm delivery, and intrauterine growth retardation in mothers with heavy alcohol use. The incidence of spontaneous abortions and stillbirths is higher in women who consume more than three drinks in a day.

Perinatal Management

1. Inpatient detoxification program to achieve abstinence as quickly as possible.
2. Counseling to the mother, explaining the entire spectrum of disorders in the fetus.
3. Psychosocial intervention throughout pregnancy to avoid relapse. There is a high degree of noncompliance with therapy, making it imperative to screen and monitor these patients throughout pregnancy [58].
4. Disulfiram, naltrexone, acamprosate, topiramate, baclofen, and ondansetron have been used in alcohol dependence. Most of the drugs have pregnancy category B or C labeling, and hence may not be useful in the pregnant mother. Naltrexone has been shown to show good tolerability with very few side-effects in pregnant women although we need more studies to substantiate this.
5. Postpartum addiction treatment and follow up

Symptoms and treatment of alcohol withdrawal: In heavy drinkers, symptoms of withdrawal can occur 6–48 h after cessation of alcohol use. These include nausea and vomiting, tachycardia, hypertension, tremors, hallucinations, and agitation. Delirium tremens is a more severe presentation of withdrawal. It is associated with the usual signs of withdrawal as mentioned above and autonomic instability, arrhythmias, and seizures.

Treatment of Alcohol withdrawal includes all of the following:

1. Benzodiazepines—Although this is a standard treatment in alcohol withdrawal, its use in pregnancy warrants some caution. It is contraindicated in the first trimester due to studies showing some association with cleft palate and lips. Use in the third trimester may cause perinatal problems such as floppy infant syndrome.
2. Monitoring hydration status and hemodynamics
3. Correction of electrolyte abnormalities
4. Thiamine (100 mg orally every day for 3 days) and folic acid (5 mg orally once a day)
5. Alpha adrenergic agonists such as clonidine may be effective in controlling the sympathetic surge associated with withdrawal.

Hallucinogens

Lysergic acid diethylamide (LSD), phencyclidine (PCP), psilocybin, and mescaline are classified as hallucinogens. The prevalence of their use is unknown in pregnancy but they are not frequently abused drugs.

Pharmacology: Hallucinogens work as partial agonist or agonist and antagonist at serotonin, dopamine, and adrenergic receptors [59]. The effects are very similar to those caused by amphetamines and cocaine but to a lesser extent. These drugs can be ingested orally or smoked, but in some cases, like ketamine, they can be used intravenously as well. LSD can evoke auditory, visual, and tactile hallucinations by its serotonergic effects [60]. These effects occur within minutes of ingestion and can last for a few hours. Psilocybin is seen in wild mushrooms (magic mushroom) and has similar pharmacokinetics but is less potent than LSD. Phencyclidine is not used currently; however ketamine, a derivative of PCP is used as an anesthetic and can be abused. Ketamine is an *N*-methyl D-aspartate receptor antagonist that reduces brain glutathione levels, which has been implicated in the neuropsychiatric symptoms. Mescaline is ingested orally and can cause visual hallucinations for several hours.

Effects on mother and fetus: Fetal growth restriction, premature labor, and neonatal withdrawal syndrome can occur with exposure to hallucinogens.

Systemic effects: Hypertension, tachycardia, and hyperthermia can occur due to activation of the sympathetic nervous system. These adrenergic effects are not as severe as seen with cocaine, although some reports of coronary vasospasm with myocardial ischemia have been reported. PCP can cause seizures, catatonia, and intracerebral hemorrhage, especially with high doses. Hallucinogens can cause extreme anxiety and panic attacks, and can trigger psychiatric disorders, sometimes leading to accidental deaths. Ketamine is known to trigger psychotic symptoms similar to schizophrenia [60].

Perinatal management: There is no specific therapy for hallucinogen use or withdrawal [45]. Supportive therapy to treat the systemic effects may be appropriate. Early detecting and counseling is indicated in affected mothers to avoid fetal abnormalities. Hypertension from ketamine use may mimic preeclampsia and should be recognized early.

Nicotine

Pharmacology: There are more than 4,000 chemicals in tobacco smoke, including nicotine, carbon monoxide, and cyanide [61]. Tobacco may be smoked (most common), chewed, or sniffed. Nicotine, the principal chemical, produces its effect through both the central and peripheral nicotinic (acetylcholine) receptors. It causes release of catecholamines, and also produces peripheral autonomic effects. Nicotine has actions in many systems; GABAergic, noradrenergic, and serotonergic nuclei mediate nicotine addiction effects. Thus, nicotine addiction is affected by the action of the drug through many systems. Nicotine's effect is immediate, and it is metabolized rapidly in the liver, kidney, and lungs with cotinine as the major metabolic product, which is excreted in the urine. The half-life is a few hours, and the duration is shortened with heavy use.

Carbon monoxide, another product in tobacco smoke, competitively binds to hemoglobin to produce carboxyhemoglobin, thereby decreasing the oxygen-carrying capacity of blood. It also shifts the oxygen-hemoglobin dissociation curve to the left (increasing affinity). The carboxyhemoglobin concentration varies from 3 to 15 %, depending on usage.

Systemic effects: Peripherally, nicotine acutely increases sympathetic tone and, therefore, heart rate, blood pressure, and myocardial work. It also causes neurotransmitter release in different areas of the brain producing euphoria, alertness, and eventually dependence. Increased carboxyhemoglobin in smokers is thought to impair wound healing. In the lungs, it changes the volume and composition of mucus, increases airway irritability, and decreases mucociliary clearance. Chronic use leads to atherosclerosis, chronic bronchitis, and chronic obstructive pulmonary disease [62].

Tobacco is addictive, and withdrawal symptoms include cravings, irritability, headache, cough, and insomnia.

Effects on mother and fetus: Nicotine, because of its low molecular weight, readily crosses the placenta. Smoking decreases fetal oxygenation because of increased maternal carboxyhemoglobin concentrations and reduced uteroplacental perfusion. Smoking during pregnancy is a public health problem and can cause numerous adverse effects, including: spontaneous abortion, intrauterine growth restriction, placenta previa and placental abruption, premature rupture of membranes, preterm labor, low birth weight, perinatal mortality, and ectopic pregnancy [63]. Infant mortality was 40 % higher in babies born to pregnant women who smoked.

Children born to mothers who smoked during pregnancy have an increased risk of asthma, infantile colic and childhood obesity. Infants born to mothers who used smokeless tobacco during pregnancy have a higher nicotine exposure, low birth weight, and shortened gestational age compared to those born to mothers that smoked [64]. Secondhand smoke increases the risk of low birth weight by 20 % [65].

Perinatal management: Cessation of smoking, prevention of relapse, and prevention of secondhand smoke exposure are important intervention strategies during pregnancy. Quitting smoking before 15 weeks provides the greatest benefit although quitting at any point is beneficial. Smoking cessation before the third trimester almost eliminates low birth weight risk [66]. Almost 70 % of smokers visit a physician each year; a few see their dentists and other healthcare personnel including pain practitioners. A physician's advice to quit is an important motivator. Hence the 2008 guideline update is designed to spur clinicians and healthcare personnel to intervene effectively.

The first step in treating tobacco users is to identify them. Patients who are willing to try quitting will benefit from a brief '5 As' intervention' session [67].

Ask about tobacco use—enquire and document tobacco use status for every patient visit.

Advise to quit—in a clear and personalized manner advise the patient who smokes to quit, providing information about the risks of continued smoking to the pregnancy and the baby.

Assess willingness to quit.

Assist in quit attempt—by providing pregnancy-specific materials and information on support groups and smokers quit line.

Arrange follow up—to track the progress of the quit attempt, support and reinforce a successful quit attempt.

Women who are not ready to quit will benefit from repeated motivational approaches by their healthcare providers at follow up visits. More than 50 % of women who quit smoking during pregnancy return to it within a year, which underlines the importance of repeated enquiry into their continued abstinence and encouragement to stay off smoking at every healthcare appointment [68].

Pharmacotherapy: There is not enough evidence to support the use of nicotine replacement products during pregnancy or postpartum. Trials evaluating their efficacy have been stopped, either because of ineffectiveness or adverse effects [69–71]. Drugs used in smoking cessation in the nonpregnant population include varenicline [72], which acts on brain nicotine receptors, and bupropion, which is an antidepressant [73]. There is insufficient evidence on the safety and efficacy of these drugs in pregnancy and lactation. Both drugs now carry product warnings mandated by the Food and Drug Administration about the risk of psychiatric symptoms and suicide associations with their use [74].

Cocaine

Cocaine is commonly abused during pregnancy, with a reported incidence of usage in 4.6 million females resulting in 750,000 cocaine exposed births every year [75]. Ninety percent of the female cocaine abusers are in child-bearing age. "The crack baby epidemic" occurred in the 1980s, and the incidence has since decreased, although it continues to be a significant preventable health crisis. Cocaine abuse is commonly associated with concomitant abuse of alcohol, cigarettes and illicit drugs, sexually transmitted diseases and poor socioeconomic status, all of which worsen maternal and fetal outcomes.

Pharmacology: Cocaine, an alkaloid (benzoylmethylecgonine) derived from leaves of *Erythroxylon coca* plant in South America, was first used in medicine as a local anesthetic. The pure alkalinized form of cocaine called "crack" is abused most frequently [76]. Cocaine blocks the reuptake of sympathomimetic amines such as norepinephrine, dopamine, and serotonin. Sustained increase in norepinephrine causes hypertension and cardiac arrhythmias. Increased levels of dopamine in the limbic system and cortex cause the euphoric effects of cocaine leading to a "high" and reinforcement of addictive behavior. Cocaine is associated with withdrawal, usually manifested by fatigue and depression attributed to depletion of catecholamines. It has a very rapid onset of action; smoked cocaine acts within seconds, peaking at 5 min, and dissipating in 15 min. The intravenous formulation lasts for 60 min, whereas the intranasal and oral form peaks in 20 min and last for 90–180 min. Cocaine is metabolized by hepatic and plasma cholinesterase to form water-soluble inactive metabolites. Liver disease and pregnancy potentiate the systemic effects of cocaine. Combined use of cocaine and alcohol produces cocaethylene as a metabolite which has been shown to increase the risk of cardiac complications [77]. Cocaine metabolites are present for 72 h after consumption and form the basis for maternal screening [78].

Systemic effects: Acute cocaine use causes hypertension, tachycardia, arrhythmias, myocardial ischemia, and infarction [79]. Acute coronary vasospasm, thrombosis, and myocardial depression have also been seen [80]. In high doses, cocaine can cause hypotension and cardiovascular collapse due to inhibition of sodium channels. When smoked, cocaine causes thermal pharyngeal damage and pneumonitis. Some patients develop "crack lung," manifested by pulmonary edema, dyspnea, hypoxia, fever, hemoptysis, and respiratory failure. The vasoconstrictive effects of cocaine in CNS can lead to strokes and cerebrovascular incidents [81]. CNS excitation can lead to migraine headaches, seizures, hallucinations, and euphoria. Cocaine causes hyperthermia which can lead to adverse fetal outcomes such as prematurity, low birth weight and rarely fetal death, and also cause delirium in the mother [82].

Effects on fetus and pregnancy: The pregnant population is more sensitive to the cardiovascular effects of cocaine compared to the nonpregnant cohorts [83]. Some of the acute cardiovascular complications related to cocaine abuse include malignant hypertension, tachyarrhythmias, aortic dissection, cardiomyopathy, myocardial ischemia, and myocardial infarction [84]. Hepatic rupture, cerebral ischemia, and death have also been seen [85]. Cocaine-induced coronary syndrome has been described in patients with severe preeclampsia and acute myocardial infarction. The pregnant cocaine abuser also fails to seek timely prenatal care, which poses a challenge in the management of acute events related to cocaine abuse.

Cocaine crosses the placenta easily due to its low molecular weight, lipid solubility, and low ionization, reaching high concentrations in the fetus and causing severe vasoconstriction of uterine vessels [45]. Cocaine is present in the placenta and fetal tissues long after maternal exposure has ended, suggesting that even occasional use (especially in the first trimester) can have long-term effects. Cocaine metabolites accumulate in amniotic fluid and placental membranes which increase the duration of exposure to the fetus.

The increased levels of maternal catecholamines from cocaine exposure can cause increased uterine contractility, constriction of placental vessels, and decreased blood flow to the uterus, leading to spontaneous abortion, miscarriages, and still births [12, 86]. Cocaine associated vasospasm causes hypoxia to the placenta leading to placental abruption. The increased uterine contractility induced by the action of cocaine on b_2 receptors causes premature rupture of membranes, preterm labor, uterine rupture, and preterm delivery. Cocaine also causes low birth weight and intrauterine growth retardation (IUGR) due to constriction of uterine blood vessels and decreased perfusion of the placenta [87]. Poor maternal and fetal nutrition and associated drug abuse are other factors contributing to IUGR. Furthermore, uteroplacental insufficiency causes fetal hypoxia and acidosis, both of which cause adverse fetal outcomes [88]. Congenital malformations involving the cardiovascular and CNS systems have been seen in infants exposed to cocaine [87].

Cardiac effects on the fetus: Most of the evidence for cardiac effects of cocaine comes from well-established animal studies and human cases. Cocaine causes apoptosis, left ventricular remodeling, and increased sensitivity to ischemia/reperfusion injury in rat models [89]. Infants exposed to cocaine have a higher incidence of congenital cardiovascular malformations and intracardiac conduction abnormalities. Even in the absence of obvious cardiac defects, there is an increased incidence of hypertension and heart disease in adulthood with intrauterine cocaine exposure, suggesting that cocaine might cause epigenetic changes in utero which then translate into long-term changes. The emotional response to stress is enhanced in individuals who have been exposed to cocaine prenatally, as seen by increased salivary cortisol levels, elevated heart rate, and an abnormal anxiety and anger response [90].

CNS effects on the fetus: CNS malformations occur in 10 % of cocaine exposed pregnancies compared to controls [91]. Microcephaly is seen due to intracranial vasoconstriction [92]. Cocaine mediated vasoconstriction also causes bowel infarction, atresia, limb defects, and genitourinary abnormalities [93]. Cocaine also causes subtle neurobehavioral and cognitive difficulties extending into adulthood [94]. Infants exposed to cocaine are more alert and difficult to calm, and exhibit autonomic instability, suggesting autonomic nervous system involvement, as well [95]. Cocaine use in the mother affects parenting behavior and leads to neglect with decreased sensitivity to olfactory, auditory, and tactile cues, causing disengagement and lack of joy with infant interaction.

Perinatal Management: Serial monthly ultrasounds to assess both fetal and maternal well-being should be considered. Screening and treatment of other sexually transmitted diseases is important to improve maternal outcomes. Supportive care is the best approach for the mother and fetus exposed to cocaine in the perinatal period. There is no specific antidote for cocaine. Hallucinations, hypertension, seizures, hyperreflexia, fever, dilated pupils, tachycardia, proteinuria, and edema are signs of acute intoxication in the mother, and require symptomatic treatment with antipsychotics, anticonvulsants, and antihypertensives. The pulmonary symptoms of cocaine respond to steroids, though respiratory failure may require mechanical ventilation. Hypertension, proteinuria, and edema associated with cocaine use may mimic pregnancy-induced hypertension, and require a detailed history and toxicology screen to differentiate.

Withdrawal from cocaine is not life threatening, and causes a range of psychological symptoms and cravings. Mood symptoms of depression and irritability can be treated with benzodiazepines [96]. Extreme psychosis and hallucinations are treated with antipsychotics.

The infant exposed to cocaine has an increased incidence of CNS symptoms, such as tremors, high-pitched cry, irritability, alertness, and autonomic instability. Withdrawal in the infant is less common due to the persistence of cocaine metabolites in the urine for a week [93]. Due to strong association of cocaine abuse and fetal neglect, a strong supportive program is essential to provide optimum care to the infant [97].

Pharmacotherapy: Non-pharmacological measures have been successful in the treatment of the cocaine abusing parturient. They include cognitive-behavioral therapies, a community reinforcement approach seeking safety, and motivational interviewing (MI). One particularly promising approach is voucher based contingency management (CM) where financial incentives are offered to women to abstain from cocaine use. Although the program is expensive, the long-term benefits of mitigating costs related to the care of the cocaine abusing mother and the baby make it a viable option [98, 99].

Antidepressants such as serotonin reuptake inhibitors, methylphenidate, and tricyclic antidepressants can be used prophylactically to treat depressive symptoms associated with cocaine withdrawal. Drugs such as disulfiram, bromocriptine, propranolol, topiramate, and vigabatrin have been used to reduce the craving mediated by dopamine receptor dysfunction. Pure and partial dopamine agonists can be useful as a maintenance therapy, whereas dopamine antagonists can be used to reduce the addiction potential. Disulfiram is found to be very effective, especially if there is concomitant alcohol abuse. Antagonists and agonists at the glutamate receptor such as memantine, modafinil, and dextromethorphan can decrease the use of cocaine. Other medications, which potentiate the GABA neurotransmitter, such as lamotrigine, baclofen, and gabapentin, are also being investigated for cocaine abuse. However, the use of these medications has not been substantiated with larger double blinded trials and cannot be labeled as evidence based practice [100]. These drugs are classified as category C for use in the parturient; hence, risks and benefits must be considered and discussed with patients prior to their use.

There have been several approaches to develop active and passive cocaine vaccines. Active anti-cocaine vaccines have been developed by tagging cocaine analogs to large proteins (BSA, keyhole limpet hemocyanin [KLH], and cholera toxin) [101–103]. These vaccines increase anti-cocaine antibodies and suppress cocaine-induced central effects. Another approach includes use of a cocaine analog covalently linked to a disrupted serotype 5 human adenovirus [104]. The only cocaine vaccine so far used in Phase 1 and 2 human trials was made by covalently linking succinylnorcocaine (SNC) to cholera B protein (rCTB), adsorbed onto aluminum hydroxide adjuvant [105]. The vaccine was associated with adequate antibody levels in 38 % and decreased cocaine use in 53 %. However, the antibody levels decreased after 16 weeks, suggesting a transient effect.

Passive anti-cocaine vaccines are made by injecting exogenously produced cocaine-binding antibodies. Experimental animal studies have shown that high levels of anti-cocaine antibodies can sequester circulating cocaine in the peripheral circulation and promote its breakdown by naturally occurring plasma cholinesterases before the drug enters the brain, thus decreasing cocaine-induced central effects [106, 107]. These monoclonal antibodies usually have a short half-life and must be given repetitively, which is neither practical nor inexpensive. A newer gene transfer approach was used to deliver the genetic code for an anti-cocaine monoclonal antibody using an adenovirus-associated vector (AAV) [108]. This vector generates cocaine specific antibodies for 24 weeks, leading to persistent immunity against cocaine in animal models. The antibodies also bind to cocaethylene, a metabolite produced from the use of cocaine and alcohol, hence making it useful in a patient who abuses both [109]. Human studies with this vaccine are still pending.

Cocaine use in pregnancy is fraught with acute and long-term complications in the mother and fetus. Screening and timely non-pharmacological and pharmacological interventions will help to improve outcomes.

Opioids

Abuse of heroin and prescription opioids is quite common in pregnant women. 0.1 % of pregnant women have used heroin in the prior 30 days. One percent of pregnant women use opioid prescription medication for nonmedical indications [110, 111]. Genetic factors, easy access to opioids, psychosocial stressors in life, weak parental bonding, and posttraumatic stress disorder increase the risk of drug abuse [45, 112, 113].

Heroin addiction is associated with low socioeconomic status, concomitant substance abuse, presence of hepatitis B, hepatitis C and HIV [114]. Addicted mothers generally don't seek antenatal care and, in most cases, are not aware of their pregnancy in the early stages secondary to the amenorrhea and irregular menstruation caused by the opioid [115]. They have inadequate weight gain, bad hygiene, and erratic behavior.

Pharmacology: Opium is derived from a Greek word for "juice" and the juice of the poppy has 20 distinct alkaloids [116]. The term "narcotic" is derived from the Greek word for stupor and is traditionally used to refer to potent morphine-like analgesics with the potential to produce physical dependence. Opioids refer to all exogenous substances (natural, synthetic, or semisynthetic) that bind to opioid receptors. The common opioid receptors are mu, kappa, and delta 27 [117, 118]. They can be pure agonists or partial agonists. Heroin, morphine, codeine, fentanyl, meperidine, hydromorphone, and oxymorphone are pure agonists. Buprenorphine and pentazocine are partial agonists. They have high affinity for the opioid receptors but they are less efficacious so they have a ceiling effect. Naloxone and Naltrexone are pure antagonists. The endogenous opiates are enkephalins, endorphins, dynorphins, and nociceptins. The opioids vary slightly in their chemical structure; hence have different pharmacokinetic and pharmacodynamics characteristics [117, 118].

The opioid receptors are present throughout the brain with the highest density in areas modulating pain and reward (e.g., thalamus, amygdala, anterior cingulated cortex, and striatum). Activation of mu opioid receptors blocks GABA-mediated tonic inhibition of dopaminergic neurons in the ventral tegmental area [119]. It initiates a cascade of effects in different regions of the brain that are related to reward and repeated use [120, 121]. Heroin is a synthetic opioid; chemically it is diacetyl morphine and pharmacologically known as diamorphine. It is known by several street names including H, smack, horse brown, and black tar. It was first synthesized by C.R. Alder Wright in 1874 by adding two acetyl groups to the molecule found in the opium poppy. Heroin is the most rapidly acting opioid and is highly addictive [110]. Most prescription opioids have significant abuse potential [122].

Opioids can be administered through different routes. Heroin is commonly administered by intravenous, intramuscular, subcutaneous, oral, rectal, and intradermal (skin popping) routes. It can also be smoked and inhaled because of its low boiling point. The effects of the opioids are similar, but depending on the route of administration, differ in onset and duration of action and degree of euphoria [123]. In the United States, heroin is not prescribed for human use, and is available only for research purposes. In the United Kingdom, heroin is used in the treatment of acute postoperative pain and in palliative care. Methadone and buprenorphine are the standard opioid replacement drugs for heroin addicts. Recently, naltrexone is gaining popularity in the treatment of opioid addiction [124].

Systemic effects: Opioids produce generalized depression of the central nervous system. In high doses, they can cause respiratory arrest and death. Repeated use can cause physical dependence and tolerance, which can lead to drug seeking behavior [123]. Abrupt discontinuation of the drug leads to withdrawal symptoms, which, in short acting drugs like heroin, occur as early as 4–6 h or, in long acting drugs like methadone, after 24–36 h [5]. The incidence of relapse is high in opioid addiction because of the craving for the drug.

Maternal effects: Pregnant heroin addicts are prone to abruption placentae, preterm labor, and intrauterine passage of meconium, intrauterine growth retardation/low birth weight and higher neonatal mortality [125].

Fetal effects: Heroin freely crosses the placenta. Opioid use during pregnancy, especially in the first trimester, is associated with a small increase in birth defects [126–130]. Heroin withdrawal in the mother may not be dangerous; however fetal death can occur due to acute abstinence [131]. Prenatal heroin exposure causes neonatal abstinence syndrome (NAS) in babies born to opioid addicted mothers and mothers on opioid replacement therapy with methadone or buprenorphine.

Neonatal abstinence syndrome (NAS): Opioid replacement therapy in maternal addiction has improved the outcome of both mother and the baby, but the risk for the neonate to develop NAS still persists. The incidence of NAS in babies born to the opioid-abusing parturient ranges from 48 to 94 % [132]. It occurs as early as 24–72 h after delivery, and can last up to 10 days (depending on the opioid used, severity of the drug dependence in the mother and the rapidity of fetal metabolism).

In the case of methadone, NAS appears late, lasts longer and is more severe than with other opioids [133]. Buprenorphine related NAS develops within 12–48 h, peaks at 72–96 h, and resolves by 7 days [134].

Diagnosis is based on history of opioid use during the prenatal period and by the appearance of behavioral and physiological signs and symptoms in the neonate due to increased activity of the central and autonomic nervous systems [132]. Clinical features include irritability, high-pitched cry, vomiting, diarrhea, hyper tonicity, tremor, tachypnea, and, in severe cases, seizures [133]. Some neonates fail to thrive due to poorly coordinated sucking reflexes, causing feeding problems. All infants born to mothers who are addicted or on replacement therapy should be monitored for NAS [125].

Treatment of NAS: Supportive therapy is adequate in mild case of NAS. Swaddling associated with breastfeeding contributes to bonding between mother and infant as well as providing immunity to the infant. Severe cases will require pharmacological treatment with drugs like morphine, tincture of opium, barbiturates, and benzodiazepines. When NAS is recognized and treated properly, it does not cause any long-term effects on the child. Regular sleep, feeding, and weight gain indicate successful treatment of NAS.

Treatment of opioid and heroin addiction in pregnancy: Early identification of opioid abuse in pregnant women will improve both maternal and fetal outcomes [100]. All pregnant patients should be screened for illicit drug and alcohol abuse as recommended by the ACOG [111]. A thorough history and physical examination will assist in the diagnosis of drug use. Patients are prone to develop skin tracks, skin-popping abscesses, cellulitis, epidural abscess, and endocarditis. Diagnosis can be confirmed using urine drug screen or by testing body fluids. Once the diagnosis is confirmed, therapy should be started aggressively

Although methadone is the first drug of choice, buprenorphine and naltrexone have also been used in the treatment of heroin addicts [125]. Opioid maintenance therapy helps to prevent the withdrawal effects and reduces craving. Abdominal cramps, nausea, insomnia, irritability, and anxiety are the common withdrawal symptoms. The dosage of methadone should be titrated until the withdrawal symptoms disappear. Regular methadone supplementation to the pregnant addicted female through a comprehensive program with counseling, nutritional education, family therapy, and psychosocial therapy plays an important role in preventing relapse. Use of opioid replacement therapy will also reduce the incidence of criminal and anti-social behavior among opioid abusers.

Methadone: Methadone, a synthetic mu opioid receptor agonist exhibits stereoisomerism. The levo form has analgesic effects and the dextro form has NMDA antagonist activity [117, 118]. Methadone is available as a racemic mixture of both dextro and levo forms. Methadone is distributed widely throughout the body with extensive tissue reservoirs that release unchanged methadone back into the blood. During pregnancy, the methadone requirements increase due to increased fluid volume, a larger tissue reservoir, and altered opioid metabolism by the placenta and the fetus [135]. Hence, women often experience symptoms of withdrawal in later stages of pregnancy.

Methadone is relatively safe [136], but deaths have occurred due to respiratory depression when the patient is not adequately monitored [137] and when sedative medications like benzodiazepines are administered concomitantly [138]. It can also prolong the Q-Tc interval and cause cardiac arrhythmias [139].

NAS and small for gestational age babies are the main concerns in a pregnant mother on Methadone Maintenance Therapy. Previously, low dose therapy was thought to improve outcomes; this has been challenged more recently [131]. The effects of methadone on long-term cognitive and behavioral functions are controversial; one long-term follow up study of 27 children who had been exposed to methadone in utero found no cognitive impairment in the preschool years [140].

Buprenorphine: Buprenorphine is a semi-synthetic, highly lipophilic, thebaine derivative. It is 25 to 50 times more potent than morphine with partial agonist activity at mu, delta, and kappa opioid receptors. It is poorly absorbed when administered orally due to its extensive first pass metabolism, and is administered sublingually to increase its bioavailability [141]. Subdermal implants that deliver buprenorphine for 6 months can be used to treat opiate addiction. Buprenorphine is extensively protein-bound, mostly to globulin and distributed to various tissues. Plasma levels are achieved within 1–3 h after sublingual administration, and the elimination half-life is approximately 37 h following once daily dosing. Buprenorphine is metabolized to norbuprenorphine, which is an active metabolite and a weak partial agonist, and eliminated after glucuronidation in the kidneys [142].

The safety profile of buprenorphine is similar to or better than methadone due to its minimal adverse events [143]. Buprenorphine can cause respiratory depression because it has a higher receptor affinity compared to pure agonists. It has poor efficacy, and exhibits a ceiling effect whereby increasing dosage will not produce increased agonistic effects [144]. Deaths have been reported when buprenorphine was administered as injections along with other sedatives like benzodiazepines [145]. Buprenorphine is available as a hydrochloride (subutex) and in combination with naloxone in a ratio of 4:1 (suboxone) [146].

Buprenorphine cannot be used with pure agonists as it will induce withdrawal by displacing the pure agonist from the receptor. It has the ability to both precipitate withdrawal and treat withdrawal symptoms simultaneously because of its partial agonist activity and its high affinity to opioid receptors [145]. These properties make it useful in the treatment of opiate dependence [117, 147, 148]. Buprenorphine should not be administered for 12 h to patients on short acting opioids and for 24 h to those on long acting opioids.

Buprenorphine readily crosses the placenta and accumulates in the fetus. Exposure to buprenorphine has been linked to sudden infant death syndrome, behavioral problems, ADHD and anxiety. However, evidence for this is conflicting, with some studies showing that opiates can contribute to delayed cognitive development and behavioral problems [149–151], while other studies have found no association between prenatal exposure to opiates and mental performance in early childhood [152]. Use of buprenorphine in the antenatal period has not demonstrated a significant difference in the survival rates of the newborn. Children of mothers treated with buprenorphine have shown normal growth compared to the methadone treated mothers. There have been indications of better pregnancy outcomes in buprenorphine-treated mothers when the medication was started prior to conception.

Methadone vs. Buprenorphine in pregnancy: Methadone is the drug of choice in the management of the opioid-dependent woman. While methadone does carry the risk of triggering NAS, adequate monitoring and treatment by the neonatal care givers will reduce this risk significantly.

Goals of a Methadone Maintenance Therapy Program (MMTP) include reducing craving, blocking euphoria, and preventing the pregnant mother from experiencing withdrawal, which may prevent spontaneous abortion in first trimester of the pregnancy and premature labor in the last trimester of pregnancy. Methadone maintenance provides a "steady state" of opiate levels, thus reducing the risk of withdrawal in the infant. Methadone can be taken orally, lacks impurities, costs less, and can be carefully regulated. Methadone dispensing allows the engagement of the woman in a treatment program, providing daily contact with a healthcare provider.

Detoxification from methadone is generally not recommended during pregnancy. Detoxification can be attempted if necessary during the second trimester when the pregnancy is stable. A thorough assessment is important to determine whether a woman is an appropriate candidate for medically supervised withdrawal because it frequently results in relapse of opiate use.

Methadone and buprenorphine are secreted in breast milk, but the levels are generally too low to affect the baby [153]. Breast feeding is not contraindicated when the mother is on opioid replacement therapy, except when the mother is HIV positive [131, 154]. Studies have found minimal transmission of methadone in breast milk, regardless of the maternal dose [155].

Maternal Opioid Treatment Human Experimental Research (MOTHER) project is the most current and comprehensive research study that investigates the safety and efficacy of maternal and prenatal exposure to methadone and buprenorphine [115, 119, 131, 156]. According to the study, buprenorphine exposed neonates required 89 % less morphine to treat NAS and spent 43 % less time in the hospital compared to methadone exposed neonates. However, there was a higher compliance in the methadone group compared to buprenorphine [125]. Recent studies also suggest a lower incidence of NAS with buprenorphine compared to methadone [5, 119, 157]. Unlike methadone, buprenorphine is not a highly regulated drug, so it can be used on addicts on an outpatient basis thereby removing the stigma associated with addiction treatment.

Pain management in the perinatal period: Opioid dependence is associated with heightened sensitivity to pain, chronic hyperalgesia, and tolerance to opioid pain medication, making peripartum pain management particularly challenging [158, 159]. Multimodal pain therapy is the best option for opioid addicted patients [159]. Patients maintained on buprenorphine typically require higher doses of opioid agonists throughout the postoperative course to achieve adequate pain relief. Buprenorphine and methadone should be continued into the postpartum period [156].

Recommendations for the treatment of acute pain in these patients include the following: [160]

1. Use shorter acting opioid analgesics in addition to the maintenance dose of buprenorphine and titrate to achieve effective pain control.
2. Divide the total buprenorphine maintenance dose over the course of 24 h and rely solely on the analgesic properties of buprenorphine.
3. Replace the buprenorphine with methadone and then add another short acting opioid analgesic for breakthrough pain.
4. Replace buprenorphine with another opioid analgesic (e.g., intravenous fentanyl or morphine).
5. Add regional anesthetic blockade where possible.

Substance abuse rehabilitation programs with either methadone or buprenorphine should be continued in the postpartum period [161]. These patients should have easy access to psychosocial support groups, contraceptive counseling, drug rehabilitation services, and relapse prevention programs [119].

Cannabis

Cannabis, also known as marijuana, is a genus of flowering plants that include *Cannabis indica*, *Cannabis sativa*, and *Cannabis ruderalis*. It is used for its fiber (hemp) to produce rope, seeds, and oil for medicinal and recreational purposes. The main ingredient is delta-9-tetrahydrocannabinol (THC). Cannabis is one of the most commonly abused drugs in the world after tobacco and alcohol. There is a reported incidence of 3–16 % in pregnant patients. Medical marijuana has been used in glaucoma, AIDS related anorexia and wasting, neuropathic pain, treatment of spasticity associated with multiple sclerosis, chemotherapy-induced nausea, epilepsy, Tourette's syndrome, and agitation in Alzheimer's disease [162].

Pharmacology: Cannabis plants contain a set of unique compounds, collectively called phytocannabinoids, which produce a "state of high" after consumption [163]. Endocannabinoids (eCB) are endogenously produced cannabinoid-like substances that produce psychiatric effects [164]. Anandamide is an endocannabinoid also known as N-arachidonoylethanolamine. CB1 receptors [163] are found in the brain and peripheral tissues whereas CB2 receptors are only present in the periphery. Cannabis produces its psychotropic effects by increasing dopamine levels [165]. Cannabis also potentiates glycine receptors [166]. Cannabis can be smoked or ingested. The effects it produces are similar, irrespective of the route of administration. Cannabis is often consumed for its psychoactive and physiological effects, which include heightened mood or euphoria, relaxation, perceptual alterations, time distortion, exaggeration of sensory experiences and increase in appetite. The unwanted side-effects include a decrease in short-term memory, dry mouth, impaired motor skills, reddening of the eyes, and feelings of paranoia or anxiety.

Maternal effects: Mothers who smoke or ingest cannabis also smoke cigarettes and abuse other substances including alcohol. Long-term use of cannabis leads to mood disorders and exacerbation of psychotic disorders in people prone for neurocognitive disorders. Cannabis can cause bronchitis and emphysema like cigarette smoking. Chronic use can cause hormonal issues and interfere with fertility and ovulation [167].

Fetal effects: Use of cannabis in pregnancy is associated with an increased risk of negative outcomes to the fetus. Cannabis readily crosses the placenta. The increased neonatal morbidity is mainly due to a shortening of the gestation period which leads to prematurity and small for gestational age and low birth weight babies. The active ingredient is excreted in breast milk, and lactating mothers should be advised not to use marijuana [168]. Behavioral abnormalities have been observed in the neonates and infants who are later prone to develop neuropsychiatric and cognitive disorders [169] and problems with drug addiction [170].

Three popular studies have looked at fetal and neonatal effects of marijuana. These include Ottawa Prenatal Prospective Study (OPPS) [171], Maternal Health Practices and Child development Study (MHCPD) [172], and Generation R Study [168]. The OPPS and MHPCD studies both showed increased behavioral problems and decreased performance on language comprehension, sustained attention, memory, and visual perceptual tasks in children after 4 years of age. Generation R is an ongoing study looking at growth and physical development, behavioral and cognitive development, diseases in childhood and health care for pregnant women and children. This study will also help in developing strategies for treating pregnant women abusing marijuana and their children [168].

Functional MRI was used in studying the effects of prenatal exposure of marijuana and was a part of the longitudinal study from the OPPS cohort. They found a direct relationship between the amount of marijuana used and the abnormal neural activity in the left inferior and middle frontal gyri, left parahippocampal gyrus, left middle occipital gyrus, and left cerebellum. There was also significantly less activity in right inferior and middle frontal gyri. These results suggest that prenatal marijuana exposure alters neural functioning during visuospatial working memory processing in young adulthood [173].

Prenatal use of cannabis produces effects on the kids in the neonatal period that continue into adulthood. Neonatal behavior was assessed using the Brazelton Neonatal Behavior Assessment Scale (NBAS) in the OPPS and MHPCD study. There was some amount of irritability resulting in tremors and startles with different sleep patterns observed on EEG [174].

Perinatal management: Pregnant mothers abusing marijuana should be closely monitored for intrauterine growth problems with frequent ultrasound scans between 24 and 36 weeks gestation.

Pharmacotherapy: Current drugs available for treating cannabis dependence cannot be used routinely in pregnant women due to concerns about teratogenicity. The treatment modalities are limited in this population. Pharmacotherapy can be tried by substituting with an agonist like dronabinol or by using rimonabant [175], an antagonist/

inverse agonist. Neuromodulation techniques using drugs that centrally alter the neurotransmitters like dopamine, glutamate norepinephrine, and 5 hydroxy trypt-amine can help treat the addiction. Several drugs have been used, such as entocapone, *N*-acetyl cysteine, atamoxetine, buspirone, and divalproex. Increasing the levels of endocannabinoids in the brain can also help with cannabis dependence [176]. Fatty acid amide hydrolase (FAAH), also known as anandamide amidohydrolase, is a member of the serine hydrolase family of enzymes shown to break down anandamide. Inhibitors of FAAH will increase the endogenous cannabinoids and prevent with-drawal and craving. Psychotherapy in the form of motivational enhancement therapy and cognitive-behavioral therapy is also effective and may be more useful in pregnant women. Cannabis causes withdrawal symptoms when stopped abruptly [177]. The features of cannabis withdrawal are mood disturbances, decreased appetite, sleep disturbances, and gastrointestinal problems. Withdrawal symptoms start within a week and last for a few weeks [178]. There are no approved medications for treat-ment of withdrawal symptoms. Substitution of cannabis with an agonist for the CB1 receptor like dronabinol or marinol has been effective. Other drugs such as lithium, divalproex [179], nefazodone, and lofexidene have been used to treat symptoms of withdrawal. Combination therapy with lofexidene and oral THC has been proven to be more promising than any drug given alone.

Solvents

Inhalants are a broad class of agents: they include volatile solvents, anesthetics, and alkyl nitrites. Volatile solvents such as toluene and 1,1,1-trichloroethane (TCE) are ubiquitous and present in most household cleaners, paints, glues and chemicals, and are most commonly abused in the young, including the pregnant population [180, 181]. Volatile agents such as halothane and methoxyflurane and nitrous oxide have been abused as well. Currently, 22 million people in the United States have used inhalants, with 13 % of high school children admitting to use. The use among women in their reproductive years is increasing [182]. Inhalation abuse occurs more commonly in the poor, mentally ill, and youth involved with crimes. Abuse is com-mon, primarily due to low cost and easy access to these agents. Over half of abusers are women of reproductive age [183], which raises concern about their effects on pregnancy and newborn.

Pharmacology: Inhalants can produce systemic effects within 1–3 min of inhalation due to their lipophilicity. The different methods of inhalation include sniffing, spraying, bagging, cuffing, and huffing. They cause euphoria and disinhibition, which progresses to stupor, loss of consciousness and respiratory depression with higher doses. Mechanisms by which inhalants cause behavioral effects are not well understood, though glutamatergic, GABAergic, dopaminergic, and opioidergic neurotransmission have been implicated [184, 185]. The dopaminergic pathways in the prefrontal cortex and nucleus accumbens specifically are involved in the rein-forcement and reward behaviors in solvent abuse. Inhalants also interact with other cellular targets such as glycine, serotonergic, and nicotine acetylcholine receptors [186]. Medications which target these transmitters and receptors form the crux of treatment rationale in acute and chronic inhalation use.

Systemic effects: The CNS effects of acute solvent inhalation are very similar to that of alcohol intoxication, such as altered perception of sensory stimuli, dizziness, slurred speech, blurry vision, loss of coordination, and headache. Acute use has been associated with burns and fatal accidents [187]. Solvent abuse can cause cognitive impairment in the form of memory loss, learning and attention deficits. Chronic use of toluene can cause diffuse brain atrophy, encephalopathy, parkinsonism, and cerebellar degeneration [188]. It can also cause cardiac dysfunction, ventricular fibrillation, and myocardial infarction. Respiratory problems such as pulmonary hypertension and adult respiratory distress syndrome have been reported. Chronic inhalation can cause renal tubular acidosis affecting both distal and proximal renal tubules leading to electrolyte abnormalities such as hypokalemia, hypophosphatemia, and hypomagnesaemia. Renal tubular acidosis is thought to occur due to accumulation of hippuric acid, a toxic metabolite of toluene. Sudden sniffing death syndrome occurs due to cardiac arrhythmias, hypoxia, suffocation, aspiration, and electrolyte abnormalities [189].

Ethylene glycol causes more severe systemic effects in pregnant women. Toxic metabolites such glycolic acid causes severe CNS depression and seizures followed by cardiopulmonary instability and renal failure. Induced emesis, gastric lavage, antidotes such as fomepizole or ethanol (which prevents the conversion of ethylene glycol to toxic metabolites) and hemodialysis could increase survival after acute ingestion of ethylene glycol.

Effects on pregnancy and fetus: Most of the evidence on fetal effects caused by solvents comes from case reports and animal studies. Volatile agents readily cross the placenta due to their lipophilicity and affect the fetus. Intrauterine growth restriction, preterm delivery, and high fetal mortality have been reported with toluene exposure [190, 191]. Several studies have shown an association between high solvent exposure during pregnancy and oral cleft malformations, renal-urinary and cardiac defects and CNS abnormalities [192, 193]. Toluene exposed infants have specific facial characteristics such as microcephaly, deep set eyes, micrognathia, and body dysmorphology, such as blunted finger tips, small nails, and abnormal palmar creases [180]. The constellations of these signs and symptoms were classified as fetal solvent syndrome, which shares some clinical features with FASD in newborns that have been exposed to alcohol. Long-term effects, such as development delays, language impairment, hyperactivity and postnatal growth retardation, become evident later in life [190]. The newborn can exhibit signs of withdrawal, such as excessive crying, CNS irritability and poor feeding, if the mother has been using these substances constantly before delivery.

Perinatal management: Inhalant abusers are among the sickest of the substance abusers [194] and have comparatively poor treatment outcomes [195].

Providing optimal medical care for any inhalant abuser starts with a high index of suspicion and a keen diagnostic awareness leading to detection, intervention, and then treatment. Inhalants are not detected by routine urine drug screening. When benzene, toluene, or a similar agent has been chronically abused, then specific testing for their major urinary metabolites, phenol and hippuric acid respectively, can be helpful for the treatment-compliance plan [130].

Acute intoxication requires acute medical management starting with the "ABCs" of life support, stabilization of the patient, and further management in a hospital setting. Further management would include hydration and cardiorespiratory monitoring. Myocardial sensitization would preclude the use of pressors and bronchodilators. There is no reversal agent available for acute inhalant intoxication. Decontamination of the patient's clothing and skin may be needed [184].

Chronic toluene abusing parturient may present with renal tubular acidosis. In addition to renal bicarbonate wasting, potassium, phosphate, and magnesium are also lost in the urine and may result in severe deficiencies of each [191]. These electrolyte abnormalities can cause severe muscle weakness, quadriparesis and cardiac arrhythmias, and require aggressive correction. Management of pregnancies in which abuse is recognized should be aimed at early detection of renal tubular acidosis, preterm labor, and fetal growth retardation. Renal tubular acidosis at the time of delivery is associated with significant newborn acidosis and a longer newborn hospitalization. The infants should be followed up for postnatal growth retardation, microcephaly, and developmental delay.

Pharmacotherapy: Pharmacotherapies have not been evaluated in the pregnant solvent-abusing women or their children [181]. Some of the pharmacological therapies that have been tried in the nonpregnant solvent abuser are discussed below.

Pharmacotherapies may be used at multiple stages of the risk chain. First, agents may be used to decrease the addictive drive for inhalants and thereby promote abstinence. The anticonvulsant lamotrigine has been used to promote abstinence for 6 months [196]. Similarly, the dopamine D2 receptor partial receptor agonist aripiprazole resulted in reduced inhalant use [197]. This drug, a partial agonist at serotonin 5-HT_{1A} receptors and an antagonist at 5-HT_{2A} blocks addictive behavior mediated by the mesolimbic dopamine system.

Second, pharmacotherapy can be used to reduce withdrawal symptoms among inhalant dependent individuals. Baclofen at 50 mg/day produced a significant reduction of withdrawal symptoms within 48 h of treatment [198]. This effect may be the result of the action of baclofen at GABA receptors in the ventral tegmental area. Treatment with benzodiazepines, barbiturates, or anti-seizure medications like diphenylhydantoin may also help with withdrawal symptoms [199]. Newborns exhibiting withdrawal signs, which included high-pitched crying, sleeplessness, hyperactive Moro reflex, tremor and hypotonia and difficulty in feeding, responded to phenobarbital treatment [200].

Third, pharmacotherapy might address the neuropsychiatric consequences of inhalant use. Antipsychotic medications carbamazepine and haloperidol caused significant reductions in psychiatric symptoms by reducing dopaminergic activity and neuronal hyperexcitability.

Fourth, pharmacotherapies may reduce behavioral symptoms linked with acute and chronic solvent abuse. The GABA analog vigabatrin attenuates conditioned response through dopamine release inhibition [201]. Finally, pharmacotherapies may be useful in preventing the initiation or relapse to volatile substance abuse by targeting neurocognitive and neuroaffective processes dysregulated in addiction. Drugs like methylphenidate, although not studied in inhalant abuse, have been used in other forms of addiction [202]. In addition, anxiolytics, antidepressants, mood stabilizers and corticotrophin-releasing factor 1 receptor antagonists might be useful in reducing emotional distress and trauma that often drive people with inhalant use disorder to self-medicate.

Solvent abuse tends to occur disproportionately in young adults from impoverished or marginal cultural groups with a wide array of medical, psychiatric and behavioral problems [185]. The most appropriate model of treatment for these patients is an adaptation of a mental health, social rehabilitation model structured as a day or partial hospital program. This is a long-term process requiring extensive resources. Staff involved in their management should be trained in mental health-oriented approaches including behavior therapy and be knowledgeable of various rehabilitative approaches as well.

Conclusions

Problematic substance abuse in pregnancy is prevalent in the US population. There are many challenges in the diagnosis and management of pregnant women with substance abuse disorders. Early identification of certain substance-dependencies in pregnant women improves maternal and fetal outcomes. Pregnancy in the substance-dependent women should be co-managed by the obstetrician–gynecologist and addiction medicine specialist. Healthcare providers, including those outside obstetrics and gynecology, can make a significant impact on improving pregnancy outcomes by providing compassionate, non-judgmental, supportive care to these women with complex physical, emotional, social, and environmental characteristics of addiction. Infants born to women who used substances during pregnancy should be closely monitored by a pediatric healthcare provider for neonatal abstinence syndrome and other effects of maternal substance use.

References

1. Wong S, Ordean A, Kahan M. Substance use in pregnancy. J Obstet Gynaecol Can. 2011;33(4):367–84.
2. Harwell TS, Spence MR, Sands A, Iguchi MY. Substance use in an inner-city family planning population. J Reprod Med. 1996;41(9):704–10.
3. Ostrea Jr EM, Knapp DK, Tannenbaum L, Ostrea AR, Romero A, Salari V, et al. Estimates of illicit drug use during pregnancy by maternal interview, hair analysis, and meconium analysis. J Pediatr. 2001;138(3):344–8.

4. Behnke M, Smith VC. Prenatal substance abuse: short- and long-term effects on the exposed fetus. Pediatrics. 2013;131(3):e1009–24.
5. Jones HE, Finnegan LP, Kaltenbach K. Methadone and buprenorphine for the management of opioid dependence in pregnancy. Drugs. 2012;72(6):747–57.
6. Wendell AD. Overview and epidemiology of substance abuse in pregnancy. Clin Obstet Gynecol. 2013;56(1):91–6.
7. Substance Abuse and Mental Health Services Administration. Results from the 2010 national survey on drug use and health: summary of national findings. HHS Publication No. (SMA) 11-4658. Rockville: Substance Abuse and Mental Health Services Administration; 2011.
8. Keegan J, Parva M, Finnegan M, Gerson A, Belden M. Addiction in pregnancy. J Addict Dis. 2010;29(2):175–91.
9. Arria AM, Derauf C, Lagasse LL, Grant P, Shah R, Smith L, et al. Methamphetamine and other substance use during pregnancy: preliminary estimates from the Infant Development, Environment, and Lifestyle (IDEAL) study. Matern Child Health J. 2006;10(3):293–302.
10. Landau R, Cahana A, Smiley RM, Antonarakis SE, Blouin JL. Genetic variability of mu-opioid receptor in an obstetric population. Anesthesiology. 2004;100(4):1030–3.
11. Calhoun F, Attilia ML, Spagnolo PA, Rotondo C, Mancinelli R, Ceccanti M. National Institute on Alcohol Abuse and Alcoholism and the study of fetal alcohol spectrum disorders. The International Consortium. Ann Ist Super Sanita. 2006;42(1):4–7.
12. Schempf AH, Strobino DM. Illicit drug use and adverse birth outcomes: is it drugs or context? J Urban Health. 2008;85(6):858–73.
13. Ludlow JP, Evans SF, Hulse G. Obstetric and perinatal outcomes in pregnancies associated with illicit substance abuse. Aust N Z J Obstet Gynaecol. 2004;44(4):302–6.
14. American Psychiatric Association. Diagnostic and Statistical Manual of Mental Disorders (DSM-V). 5th ed. Arlington: American Psychiatric Publishing; 2013.
15. Birnbach DJ, Browne IM, Kim A, Stein DJ, Thys DM. Identification of polysubstance abuse in the parturient. Br J Anaesth. 2001;87(3):488–90.
16. Morse B, Gehshan S, Hutchins E. Screening for substance abuse during pregnancy: improving care, improving health. Arlington: National Center for Education in Maternal and Child Health; 1997.
17. Washington State Department of Health. Substance abuse during pregnancy: guidelines for screening. Tumwater: Washington State Department of Health; 2013.
18. Howell EM, Heiser N, Harrington M. A review of recent findings on substance abuse treatment for pregnant women. J Subst Abuse Treat. 1999;16(3):195–219.
19. Chang G, Wilkins-Haug L, Berman S, Goetz MA. The TWEAK: application in a prenatal setting. J Stud Alcohol. 1999;60(3):306–9.
20. Carroll JC, Reid AJ, Biringer A, Midmer D, Glazier RH, Wilson L, et al. Effectiveness of the Antenatal Psychosocial Health Assessment (ALPHA) form in detecting psychosocial concerns: a randomized controlled trial. CMAJ. 2005;173(3):253–9.
21. Ewing JA. Detecting alcoholism. The CAGE questionnaire. JAMA. 1984;252(14):1905–7.
22. Chasnoff IJ, Neuman K, Thornton C, Callaghan MA. Screening for substance use in pregnancy: a practical approach for the primary care physician. Am J Obstet Gynecol. 2001;184(4):752–8.
23. Chasnoff IJ, McGourty RF, Bailey GW, Hutchins E, Lightfoot SO, Pawson LL, et al. The 4P's Plus screen for substance use in pregnancy: clinical application and outcomes. J Perinatol. 2005;25(6):368–74.
24. Chasnoff IJ, Wells AM, McGourty RF, Bailey LK. Validation of the 4P's Plus screen for substance use in pregnancy validation of the 4P's Plus. J Perinatol. 2007;27(12):744–8.
25. Yonkers KA, Gotman N, Kershaw T, Forray A, Howell HB, Rounsaville BJ. Screening for prenatal substance use: development of the Substance Use Risk Profile-Pregnancy scale. Obstet Gynecol. 2010;116(4):827–33.
26. Harrison PA, Sidebottom AC. Systematic prenatal screening for psychosocial risks. J Health Care Poor Underserved. 2008;19(1):258–76.

27. Harrison PA, Godecker A, Sidebottom A. Validity of the prenatal risk overview for detecting drug use disorders in pregnancy. Public Health Nurs. 2012;29(6):563–73.
28. Fleming MF, Barry KL, MacDonald R. The alcohol use disorders identification test (AUDIT) in a college sample. Int J Addict. 1991;26(11):1173–85.
29. Hays RD, Merz JF, Nicholas R. Response burden, reliability, and validity of the CAGE, Short MAST, and AUDIT alcohol screening measures. Behav Res Methods Instrum Comput. 1995;27:277–80.
30. Veloso LU, de Souza MCF. Prevalence and factors associated with alcohol use among pregnant adolescents. Rev Lat Am Enfermagem. 2013;21(1):433–41.
31. Miller GA. The Substance Abuse Subtle Screening Inventory (SASSI) manual. 2nd ed. Springville: SASSI Institute; 1999.
32. Horrigan TJ, Piazza NJ, Weinstein L. The substance abuse subtle screening inventory is more cost effective and has better selectivity than urine toxicology for the detection of substance abuse in pregnancy. J Perinatol. 1996;16(5):326–30.
33. Horrigan TJ, Piazza N. The substance abuse subtle screening inventory minimizes the need for toxicology screening of prenatal patients. J Subst Abuse Treat. 1999;17(3):243–7.
34. Lozano J, Garcia-Algar O, Vall O, de la Torre R, Scaravelli G, Pichini S. Biological matrices for the evaluation of in utero exposure to drugs of abuse. Ther Drug Monit. 2007;29(6):711–34.
35. Garcia-Algar O, Vall O, Alameda F, Puig C, Pellegrini M, Pacifici R, et al. Prenatal exposure to arecoline (areca nut alkaloid) and birth outcomes. Arch Dis Child Fetal Neonatal Ed. 2005;90(3):F276–7.
36. Pichini S, Altieri I, Zuccaro P, Pacifici R. Drug monitoring in nonconventional biological fluids and matrices. Clin Pharmacokinet. 1996;30(3):211–28.
37. Klein J, Karaskov T, Koren G. Clinical applications of hair testing for drugs of abuse—the Canadian experience. Forensic Sci Int. 2000;107(1–3):281–8.
38. Montgomery D, Plate C, Alder SC, Jones M, Jones J, Christensen RD. Testing for fetal exposure to illicit drugs using umbilical cord tissue vs meconium. J Perinatol. 2006;26(1):11–4.
39. Cirimele V, Kintz P, Mangin P. Drug concentrations in human hair after bleaching. J Anal Toxicol. 1995;19(5):331–2.
40. Land DB, Kushner R. Drug abuse during pregnancy in an inner-city hospital: prevalence and patterns. J Am Osteopath Assoc. 1990;90(5):421–6.
41. Halstead AC, Godolphin W, Lockitch G, Segal S. Timing of specimen collection is crucial in urine screening of drug dependent mothers and newborns. Clin Biochem. 1988;21(1):59–61.
42. Caplan YH, Goldberger BA. Alternative specimens for workplace drug testing. J Anal Toxicol. 2001;25(5):396–9.
43. Oei JL, Kingsbury A, Dhawan A, Burns L, Feller JM, Clews S, et al. Amphetamines, the pregnant woman and her children: a review. J Perinatol. 2012;32(10):737–47.
44. Ladhani NN, Shah PS, Murphy KE. Prenatal amphetamine exposure and birth outcomes: a systematic review and metaanalysis. Am J Obstet Gynecol. 2011;205(3):219–7.
45. Kuczkowski KM. The effects of drug abuse on pregnancy. Curr Opin Obstet Gynecol. 2007;19(6):578–85.
46. Ganapathy V. Drugs of abuse and human placenta. Life Sci. 2011;88(21–22):926–30.
47. Jones HE, O'Grady KE, Tuten M. Reinforcement-based treatment improves the maternal treatment and neonatal outcomes of pregnant patients enrolled in comprehensive care treatment. Am J Addict. 2011;20(3):196–204.
48. Nawrot P, Jordan S, Eastwood J, Rotstein J, Hugenholtz A, Feeley M. Effects of caffeine on human health. Food Addit Contam. 2003;20(1):1–30.
49. Browne ML. Maternal exposure to caffeine and risk of congenital anomalies: a systematic review. Epidemiology. 2006;17(3):324–31.
50. Weng X, Odouli R, Li DK. Maternal caffeine consumption during pregnancy and the risk of miscarriage: a prospective cohort study. Am J Obstet Gynecol. 2008;198(3):279–8.

51. Back SA, Craig A, Luo NL, Ren J, Akundi RS, Ribeiro I, et al. Protective effects of caffeine on chronic hypoxia-induced perinatal white matter injury. Ann Neurol. 2006;60(6):696–705.
52. Centers for Disease Control and Prevention (CDC). Alcohol use and binge drinking among women of childbearing age—United States, 2006-2010. MMWR Morb Mortal Wkly Rep. 2012;61(28):534–8. 7-20-2012.
53. Pruett D, Waterman EH, Caughey AB. Fetal alcohol exposure: consequences, diagnosis, and treatment. Obstet Gynecol Surv. 2013;68(1):62–9.
54. Abel EL, Sokol RJ. A revised conservative estimate of the incidence of FAS and its economic impact. Alcohol Clin Exp Res. 1991;15(3):514–24.
55. Serdula M, Williamson DF, Kendrick JS, Anda RF, Byers T. Trends in alcohol consumption by pregnant women. 1985 through 1988. JAMA. 1991;265(7):876–9.
56. Hoyme HE, May PA, Kalberg WO, Kodituwakku P, Gossage JP, Trujillo PM, et al. A practical clinical approach to diagnosis of fetal alcohol spectrum disorders: clarification of the 1996 institute of medicine criteria. Pediatrics. 2005;115(1):39–47.
57. Heberlein A, Leggio L, Stichtenoth D, Hillemacher T. The treatment of alcohol and opioid dependence in pregnant women. Curr Opin Psychiatry. 2012;25(6):559–64.
58. Grant TM, Brown NN, Dubovsky D, Sparrow J, Ries R. The impact of prenatal alcohol exposure on addiction treatment. J Addict Med. 2013;7(2):87–95.
59. Ghuran A, Nolan J. Recreational drug misuse: issues for the cardiologist. Heart. 2000;83(6):627–33.
60. Sajo E. Pharmacology of substance abuse. Lippincotts Prim Care Pract. 2000;4(3):319–35.
61. Reynolds EW, Bada HS. Pharmacology of drugs of abuse. Obstet Gynecol Clin North Am. 2003;30(3):501–22.
62. Warner DO. Perioperative abstinence from cigarettes: physiologic and clinical consequences. Anesthesiology. 2006;104(2):356–67.
63. U.S. Department of Health and Human Services. The health consequences of smoking: a report of the Surgeon General. Washington, DC: Department of Health and Human Services; 2004.
64. American College of Obstetricians and Gynecologists. Smoking cessation during pregnancy. Obstet Gynecol. 2010;116:1241–4.
65. Hegaard HK, Kjaergaard H, Moller LF, Wachmann H, Ottesen B. The effect of environmental tobacco smoke during pregnancy on birth weight. Acta Obstet Gynecol Scand. 2006;85(6):675–81.
66. England LJ, Kendrick JS, Wilson HG, Merritt RK, Gargiullo PM, Zahniser SC. Effects of smoking reduction during pregnancy on the birth weight of term infants. Am J Epidemiol. 2001;154(8):694–701.
67. Public Health Service. Treating tobacco use and dependence. 2008. http://www.surgeongeneral.gov/tobacco/treating_tobacco_use08.pdf
68. Colman GJ, Joyce T. Trends in smoking before, during, and after pregnancy in ten states. Am J Prev Med. 2003;24(1):29–35.
69. Preventive Services US. Task Force. Counseling and interventions to prevent tobacco use and tobacco-caused disease in adults and pregnant women: U.S. Preventive Services Task Force reaffirmation recommendation statement. Ann Intern Med. 2009;150:551–5.
70. Windsor R, Oncken C, Henningfield J, Hartmann K, Edwards N. Behavioral and pharmacological treatment methods for pregnant smokers: issues for clinical practice. J Am Med Womens Assoc. 2000;55(5):304–10.
71. Swamy GK, Roelands JJ, Peterson BL, Fish LJ, Oncken CA, Pletsch PK, et al. Predictors of adverse events among pregnant smokers exposed in a nicotine replacement therapy trial. Am J Obstet Gynecol. 2009;201(4):354–7.
72. Pfizer Labs. Chantix® (varenicline) tablets: highlights of prescribing information. New York: Pfizer Labs; 2010. Ref Type: Pamphlet.
73. American College of Obstetricians and Gynecologists. Use of psychiatric medications during pregnancy and lactation. ACOG Practice Bulletin No. 92. Obstet Gynecol. 2008;111:1001–20.
74. U.S. Food Drug Administration. Information for healthcare professionals: varenicline (marketed as Chantix) and bupropion (marketed as Zyban, Wellbutrin, and generics). Rockville: U.S. Food and Drug Administration; 2010.

75. Porter LS, Porter BO. A blended infant massage—parenting enhancement program for recovering substance-abusing mothers. Pediatr Nurs. 2004;30(5):363–72. 401.
76. Kuczkowski KM. The cocaine abusing parturient: a review of anesthetic considerations. Can J Anaesth. 2004;51(2):145–54.
77. Keegan A. Cocaine plus alcohol, a deadly mix. NIDA Notes. 1991;6:18.
78. Om A, Ellahham S, DiSciascio G. Management of cocaine-induced cardiovascular complications. Am Heart J. 1993;125(2 Pt 1):469–75.
79. Chao CR. Cardiovascular effects of cocaine during pregnancy. Semin Perinatol. 1996;20(2):107–14.
80. Nahas GG, Trouve R, Manger WM. Cocaine, catecholamines and cardiac toxicity. Acta Anaesthesiol Scand Suppl. 1990;94:77–81.
81. Nanda A, Vannemreddy P, Willis B, Kelley R. Stroke in the young: relationship of active cocaine use with stroke mechanism and outcome. Acta Neurochir Suppl. 2006;96:91–6.
82. Blaho K, Winbery S, Park L, Logan B, Karch SB, Barker LA. Cocaine metabolism in hyperthermic patients with excited delirium. J Clin Forensic Med. 2000;7(2):71–6.
83. Woods Jr JR, Plessinger MA. Pregnancy increases cardiovascular toxicity to cocaine. Am J Obstet Gynecol. 1990;162(2):529–33.
84. Kuczkowski KM. Cardiovascular complications of recreational cocaine use in pregnancy: myth or reality? Acta Obstet Gynecol Scand. 2005;84(1):100–1.
85. Buehler BA. Cocaine: how dangerous is it during pregnancy? Nebr Med J. 1995;80(5):116–7.
86. Bhuvaneswar CG, Chang G, Epstein LA, Stern TA. Cocaine and opioid use during pregnancy: prevalence and management. Prim Care Companion J Clin Psychiatry. 2008;10(1):59–65.
87. Bateman DA, Chiriboga CA. Dose-response effect of cocaine on newborn head circumference. Pediatrics. 2000;106(3):E33.
88. Kuczkowski KM. Peripartum care of the cocaine-abusing parturient: are we ready? Acta Obstet Gynecol Scand. 2005;84(2):108–16.
89. Bae S, Zhang L. Prenatal cocaine exposure increases apoptosis of neonatal rat heart and heart susceptibility to ischemia-reperfusion injury in 1-month-old rat. Br J Pharmacol. 2005;144(7): 900–7.
90. Chaplin TM, Freiburger MB, Mayes LC, Sinha R. Prenatal cocaine exposure, gender, and adolescent stress response: a prospective longitudinal study. Neurotoxicol Teratol. 2010;32(6):595–604.
91. Bingol N, Fuchs M, Diaz V, Stone RK, Gromisch DS. Teratogenicity of cocaine in humans. J Pediatr. 1987;110(1):93–6.
92. Handler A, Kistin N, Davis F, Ferre C. Cocaine use during pregnancy: perinatal outcomes. Am J Epidemiol. 1991;133(8):818–25.
93. Chasnoff IJ, Chisum GM, Kaplan WE. Maternal cocaine use and genitourinary tract malformations. Teratology. 1988;37(3):201–4.
94. Williams JH, Ross L. Consequences of prenatal toxin exposure for mental health in children and adolescents: a systematic review. Eur Child Adolesc Psychiatry. 2007;16(4):243–53.
95. Bauer CR, Langer JC, Shankaran S, Bada HS, Lester B, Wright LL, et al. Acute neonatal effects of cocaine exposure during pregnancy. Arch Pediatr Adolesc Med. 2005;159(9): 824–34.
96. Paine TA, Jackman SL, Olmstead MC. Cocaine-induced anxiety: alleviation by diazepam, but not buspirone, dimenhydrinate or diphenhydramine. Behav Pharmacol. 2002;13(7):511–23.
97. Vidaeff AC, Mastrobattista JM. In utero cocaine exposure: a thorny mix of science and mythology. Am J Perinatol. 2003;20(4):165–72.
98. Higgins ST, Delaney DD, Budney AJ, Bickel WK, Hughes JR, Foerg F, et al. A behavioral approach to achieving initial cocaine abstinence. Am J Psychiatry. 1991;148(9):1218–24.
99. Hull L, May J, Farrell-Moore D, Svikis DS. Treatment of cocaine abuse during pregnancy: translating research to clinical practice. Curr Psychiatry Rep. 2010;12(5):454–61.
100. Kleber HD. Pharmacologic treatments for heroin and cocaine dependence. Am J Addict. 2003;12 Suppl 2:S5–18.
101. Bagasra O, Forman LJ, Howeedy A, Whittle P. A potential vaccine for cocaine abuse prophylaxis. Immunopharmacology. 1992;23(3):173–9.

102. Fox BS, Kantak KM, Edwards MA, Black KM, Bollinger BK, Botka AJ, et al. Efficacy of a therapeutic cocaine vaccine in rodent models. Nat Med. 1996;2(10):1129–32.

103. Kosten TR, Rosen M, Bond J, Settles M, Roberts JS, Shields J, et al. Human therapeutic cocaine vaccine: safety and immunogenicity. Vaccine. 2002;20(7–8):1196–204.

104. Hicks MJ, De BP, Rosenberg JB, Davidson JT, Moreno AY, Janda KD, et al. Cocaine analog coupled to disrupted adenovirus: a vaccine strategy to evoke high-titer immunity against addictive drugs. Mol Ther. 2011;19(3):612–9.

105. Martell BA, Arnsten JH, Krantz MJ, Gourevitch MN. Impact of methadone treatment on cardiac repolarization and conduction in opioid users. Am J Cardiol. 2005;95(7):915–8.

106. Paula S, Tabet MR, Farr CD, Norman AB, Ball Jr WJ. Three-dimensional quantitative structure-activity relationship modeling of cocaine binding by a novel human monoclonal antibody. J Med Chem. 2004;47(1):133–42.

107. Norman AB, Norman MK, Buesing WR, Tabet MR, Tsibulsky VL, Ball WJ. The effect of a chimeric human/murine anti-cocaine monoclonal antibody on cocaine self-administration in rats. J Pharmacol Exp Ther. 2009;328(3):873–81.

108. Rosenberg JB, Hicks MJ, De BP, Pagovich O, Frenk E, Janda KD, et al. AAVrh.10-mediated expression of an anti-cocaine antibody mediates persistent passive immunization that suppresses cocaine-induced behavior. Hum Gene Ther. 2012;23(5):451–9.

109. Danger Y, Devys A, Gadjou C, Galons H, Blanchard D, Follea G. Development of monoclonal antibodies directed against cocaine and cocaethylene: potential new tools for immunotherapy. Hybrid Hybridomics. 2004;23(4):212–8.

110. National Institute on Drug Abuse. NIDA survey provides first national data on drug use during pregnancy. 1995. http://archives.drugabuse.gov/NIDA_Notes/NNVol10N1/NIDASurvey.html. Accessed 1 July 2012.

111. Azadi A, Dildy III GA. Universal screening for substance abuse at the time of parturition. Am J Obstet Gynecol. 2008;198(5):e30–2.

112. Velez M, Jansson LM. The Opioid dependent mother and newborn dyad: non-pharmacologic care. J Addict Med. 2008;2(3):113–20.

113. Fitzsimons HE, Tuten M, Vaidya V, Jones HE. Mood disorders affect drug treatment success of drug-dependent pregnant women. J Subst Abuse Treat. 2007;32(1):19–25.

114. Martin JA, Campbell A, Killip T, Kotz M, Krantz MJ, Kreek MJ, et al. QT interval screening in methadone maintenance treatment: report of a SAMHSA expert panel. J Addict Dis. 2011;30(4):283–306.

115. Heil SH, Jones HE, Arria A, Kaltenbach K, Coyle M, Fischer G, et al. Unintended pregnancy in opioid-abusing women. J Subst Abuse Treat. 2011;40(2):199–202.

116. Stoelting RK, Hillier S. Pharmacology and physiology in anesthetic practice. 4th ed. Philadelphia: Lippincott Williams and Wilkins; 2006.

117. Mello NK, Mendelson JH. Buprenorphine suppresses heroin use by heroin addicts. Science. 1980;207(4431):657–9.

118. Davis MP, Pasternak GW. Opioid receptors and opioid pharmaxodynamics. Oxford: Oxford University Press; 2013.

119. Johnson RE, Jones HE, Fischer G. Use of buprenorphine in pregnancy: patient management and effects on the neonate. Drug Alcohol Depend. 2003;70(2 Suppl):S87–101.

120. Volkow ND, Wang GJ, Fowler JS, Tomasi D, Telang F. Addiction: beyond dopamine reward circuitry. Proc Natl Acad Sci USA. 2011;108(37):15037–42.

121. Pickens CL, Airavaara M, Theberge F, Fanous S, Hope BT, Shaham Y. Neurobiology of the incubation of drug craving. Trends Neurosci. 2011;34(8):411–20.

122. Trescot AM, Datta S, Lee M, Hansen H. Opioid pharmacology. Pain Physician. 2008;11(2 Suppl):S133–53.

123. National Institute on Drug Abuse. Commonly abused prescription drugs. Bethesda: National Institute on Drug Abuse; 2011.

124. Bart G. Maintenance medication for opiate addiction: the foundation of recovery. J Addict Dis. 2012;31(3):207–25.

125. Center for Abuse Center for Substance Abuse Treatment. Medication assisted treatment for opioid addiction during pregnancy. ASHMSA/CSAT treatment improvement protocols. Rockville: Substance Abuse and Mental Health Services Administration (US); 2013.

126. Rothman JK. Causes. Am J Epidemiol. 1976;104:587–92.

127. Zierler S, Rothman KJ. Congenital heart disease in relation to maternal use of Bendectin and other drugs in early pregnancy. N Engl J Med. 1985;313(6):347–52.

128. Bracken MB. Drug use in pregnancy and congenital heart disease in offspring. N Engl J Med. 1986;314(17):1120.

129. Shaw GM, Malcoe LH, Swan SH, Cummins SK, Schulman J. Congenital cardiac anomalies relative to selected maternal exposures and conditions during early pregnancy. Eur J Epidemiol. 1992;8(5):757–60.

130. Broussard CS, Rasmussen SA, Reefhuis J, Friedman JM, Jann MW, Riehle-Colarusso T, et al. Maternal treatment with opioid analgesics and risk for birth defects. Am J Obstet Gynecol. 2011;204(4):314–11.

131. Kaltenbach K, Berghella V, Finnegan L. Opioid dependence during pregnancy. Effects and management. Obstet Gynecol Clin North Am. 1998;25(1):139–51.

132. Osborn DA, Jeffery HE, Cole MJ. Opiate treatment for opiate withdrawal in newborn infants. Cochrane Database Syst Rev. 2010;(10):CD002059.

133. Coghlan D, Milner M, Clarke T, Lambert I, McDermott C, McNally M, et al. Neonatal abstinence syndrome. Ir Med J. 1999;92(1):232–3. 236.

134. Johnson RE, Chutuape MA, Strain EC, Walsh SL, Stitzer ML, Bigelow GE. A comparison of levomethadyl acetate, buprenorphine, and methadone for opioid dependence. N Engl J Med. 2000;343(18):1290–7.

135. Drozdick III J, Berghella V, Hill M, Kaltenbach K. Methadone trough levels in pregnancy. Am J Obstet Gynecol. 2002;187(5):1184–8.

136. Kreek MJ. Medical safety and side effects of methadone in tolerant individuals. JAMA. 1973;223(6):665–8.

137. Strang J, Hall W, Hickman M, Bird SM. Impact of supervision of methadone consumption on deaths related to methadone overdose (1993-2008): analyses using OD4 index in England and Scotland. BMJ. 2010;341:c4851.

138. Cornish R, Macleod J, Strang J, Vickerman P, Hickman M. Risk of death during and after opiate substitution treatment in primary care: prospective observational study in UK General Practice Research Database. BMJ. 2010;341:c5475.

139. Bart G. CSAT's QT, interval screening in methadone report: outrageous fortune or sea of troubles? J Addict Dis. 2011;30(4):313–7.

140. Kaltenbach K, Finnegan LP. Perinatal and developmental outcome of infants exposed to methadone in-utero. Neurotoxicol Teratol. 1987;9(4):311–3.

141. Ling W, Casadonte P, Bigelow G, Kampman KM, Patkar A, Bailey GL, et al. Buprenorphine implants for treatment of opioid dependence: a randomized controlled trial. JAMA. 2010;304(14):1576–83.

142. Picard N, Cresteil T, Djebli N, Marquet P. In vitro metabolism study of buprenorphine: evidence for new metabolic pathways. Drug Metab Dispos. 2005;33(5):689–95.

143. Fudala PJ, Bridge TP, Herbert S, Williford WO, Chiang CN, Jones K, et al. Office-based treatment of opiate addiction with a sublingual-tablet formulation of buprenorphine and naloxone. N Engl J Med. 2003;349(10):949–58.

144. Walsh SL, Preston KL, Stitzer ML, Cone EJ, Bigelow GE. Clinical pharmacology of buprenorphine: ceiling effects at high doses. Clin Pharmacol Ther. 1994;55(5):569–80.

145. Martin WR. Realistic goals for antagonist therapy. Am J Drug Alcohol Abuse. 1975;2(3–4):353–6.

146. Comer SD, Sullivan MA, Vosburg SK, Manubay J, Amass L, Cooper ZD, et al. Abuse liability of intravenous buprenorphine/naloxone and buprenorphine alone in buprenorphine-maintained intravenous heroin abusers. Addiction. 2010;105(4):709–18.

147. Jasinski DR, Pevnick JS, Griffith JD. Human pharmacology and abuse potential of the analgesic buprenorphine: a potential agent for treating narcotic addiction. Arch Gen Psychiatry. 1978;35(4):501–16.

148. Reisinger M. Buprenorphine as new treatment for heroin dependence. Drug Alcohol Depend. 1985;16(3):257–62.

149. Tiong GK, Olley JE. Effects of exposure in utero to methadone and buprenorphine on enkephalin levels in the developing rat brain. Neurosci Lett. 1988;93(1):101–6.

150. van Baar A, de Graaff BM. Cognitive development at preschool-age of infants of drug-dependent mothers. Dev Med Child Neurol. 1994;36(12):1063–75.
151. van Baar AL, Soepatmi S, Gunning WB, Akkerhuis GW. Development after prenatal exposure to cocaine, heroin and methadone. Acta Paediatr Suppl. 1994;404:40–6.
152. Messinger DS, Bauer CR, Das A, Seifer R, Lester BM, Lagasse LL, et al. The maternal life-style study: cognitive, motor, and behavioral outcomes of cocaine-exposed and opiate-exposed infants through three years of age. Pediatrics. 2004;113(6):1677–85.
153. Abdel-Latif ME, Pinner J, Clews S, Cooke F, Lui K, Oei J. Effects of breast milk on the severity and outcome of neonatal abstinence syndrome among infants of drug-dependent mothers. Pediatrics. 2006;117(6):e1163–9.
154. Liu AJ, Nanan R. Methadone maintenance and breastfeeding in the neonatal period. Pediatrics. 2008;121(4):869–70.
155. Geraghty B, Graham EA, Logan B, Weiss EL. Methadone levels in breast milk. J Hum Lact. 1997;13(3):227–30.
156. Jones HE, Kaltenbach K, Heil SH, Stine SM, Coyle MG, Arria AM, et al. Neonatal absti-nence syndrome after methadone or buprenorphine exposure. N Engl J Med. 2010;363(24):2320–31.
157. Ebner N, Rohrmeister K, Winklbaur B, Baewert A, Jagsch R, Peternell A, et al. Management of neonatal abstinence syndrome in neonates born to opioid maintained women. Drug Alcohol Depend. 2007;87(2–3):131–8.
158. Hoflich AS, Langer M, Jagsch R, Bawert A, Winklbaur B, Fischer G, et al. Peripartum pain management in opioid dependent women. Eur J Pain. 2012;16(4):574–84.
159. Jones HE, O'Grady K, Dahne J, Johnson R, Lemoine L, Milio L, et al. Management of acute postpartum pain in patients maintained on methadone or buprenorphine during pregnancy. Am J Drug Alcohol Abuse. 2009;35(3):151–6.
160. Alford DP, Compton P, Samet JH. Acute pain management for patients receiving mainte-nance methadone or buprenorphine therapy. Ann Intern Med. 2006;144(2):127–34.
161. Dryden C, Young D, Hepburn M, Mactier H. Maternal methadone use in pregnancy: factors associated with the development of neonatal abstinence syndrome and implications for healthcare resources. BJOG. 2009;116(5):665–71.
162. Muller-Vahl KR, Schneider U, Kolbe H, Emrich HM. Treatment of Tourette's syndrome with delta-9-tetrahydrocannabinol. Am J Psychiatry. 1999;156(3):495.
163. Russo EB. Cannabis and cannabinoids: pharmacology, toxicology, and therapeutic potential. London: Routledge; 2002.
164. Mechoulam R, Gaoni Y. A total synthesis of DL-Delta-1-tetrahydrocannabinol, the active constituent of hashish. J Am Chem Soc. 1965;87:3273–5.
165. Kathmann M, Flau K, Redmer A, Trankle C, Schlicker E. Cannabidiol is an allosteric modu-lator at mu- and delta-opioid receptors. Naunyn Schmiedebergs Arch Pharmacol. 2006;372(5):354–61.
166. Hejazi N, Zhou C, Oz M, Sun H, Ye JH, Zhang L. Delta9-tetrahydrocannabinol and endoge-nous cannabinoid anandamide directly potentiate the function of glycine receptors. Mol Pharmacol. 2006;69(3):991–7.
167. Huizink AC, Ferdinand RF, Ormel J, Verhulst FC. Hypothalamic-pituitary-adrenal axis activ-ity and early onset of cannabis use. Addiction. 2006;101(11):1581–8.
168. El MH, Tiemeier H, Steegers EA, Jaddoe VW, Hofman A, Verhulst FC, et al. Intrauterine cannabis exposure affects fetal growth trajectories: the Generation R Study. J Am Acad Child Adolesc Psychiatry. 2009;48(12):1173–81.
169. de Moraes Barros MC, Guinsburg R, de Araujo PC, Mitsuhiro S, Chalem E, Laranjeira RR. Exposure to marijuana during pregnancy alters neurobehavior in the early neonatal period. J Pediatr. 2006;149(6):781–7.
170. Huizink AC. Prenatal cannabis exposure and infant outcomes: overview of studies. Prog Neuropsychopharmacol Biol Psychiatry. 2014;52:45–52.
171. Fried PA. Marihuana use by pregnant women: neurobehavioral effects in neonates. Drug Alcohol Depend. 1980;6(6):415–24.

172. Richardson GA, Day NL, Taylor PM. Effect of prenatal alcohol, marijuana, and tobacco exposure on neonatal behavior. Infant Behav Dev. 1989;12(2):199–209.

173. Smith AM, Fried PA, Hogan MJ, Cameron I. Effects of prenatal marijuana on visuospatial working memory: an fMRI study in young adults. Neurotoxicol Teratol. 2006;28(2): 286–95.

174. Richardson GA, Day NL, Goldschmidt L. Prenatal alcohol, marijuana, and tobacco use: infant mental and motor development. Neurotoxicol Teratol. 1995;17(4):479–87.

175. Fernandez JR, Allison DB. Rimonabant Sanofi-Synthelabo. Curr Opin Investig Drugs. 2004;5(4):430–5.

176. Clapper JR, Mangieri RA, Piomelli D. The endocannabinoid system as a target for the treatment of cannabis dependence. Neuropharmacology. 2009;56 Suppl 1:235–43.

177. Budney AJ, Hughes JR, Moore BA, Vandrey R. Review of the validity and significance of cannabis withdrawal syndrome. Am J Psychiatry. 2004;161(11):1967–77.

178. Budney AJ, Moore BA, Sigmon SC, Higgins ST. Contingency-management interventions for cannabis dependence, in cannabis dependence; its nature, consequences, and treatment. In: Roffman RA, Stephens RS, editors. Cannabis dependence; its nature, consequences, and treatment. New York: Cambridge; 2006. p. 155–79.

179. Haney M, Hart CL, Vosburg SK, Nasser J, Bennett A, Zubaran C, et al. Marijuana withdrawal in humans: effects of oral THC or divalproex. Neuropsychopharmacology. 2004;29(1): 158–70.

180. Hannigan JH, Bowen SE. Reproductive toxicology and teratology of abused toluene. Syst Biol Reprod Med. 2010;56(2):184–200.

181. Jones HE, Balster RL. Inhalant abuse in pregnancy. Obstet Gynecol Clin North Am. 1998;25(1):153–67.

182. Medina-Mora ME, Real T. Epidemiology of inhalant use. Curr Opin Psychiatry. 2008;21(3): 247–51.

183. Pearson MA, Hoyme HE, Seaver LH, Rimsza ME. Toluene embryopathy: delineation of the phenotype and comparison with fetal alcohol syndrome. Pediatrics. 1994;93(2):211–5.

184. Williams JF, Storck M. Inhalant abuse. Pediatrics. 2007;119(5):1009–17.

185. Howard MO, Bowen SE, Garland EL, Perron BE, Vaughn MG. Inhalant use and inhalant use disorders in the United States. Addict Sci Clin Pract. 2011;6(1):18–31.

186. Garland EL, Howard MO. Volatile substance misuse: clinical considerations, neuropsychopharmacology and potential role of pharmacotherapy in management. CNS Drugs. 2012;26(11):927–35.

187. Bowen SE, Daniel J, Balster RL. Deaths associated with inhalant abuse in Virginia from 1987 to 1996. Drug Alcohol Depend. 1999;53(3):239–45.

188. Gautschi OP, Cadosch D, Zellweger R. Postural tremor induced by paint sniffing. Neurol India. 2007;55(4):393–5.

189. Hall MT, Edwards JD, Howard MO. Accidental deaths due to inhalant misuse in North Carolina: 2000-2008. Subst Use Misuse. 2010;45(9):1330–9.

190. Arnold GL, Kirby RS, Langendoerfer S, Wilkins-Haug L. Toluene embryopathy: clinical delineation and developmental follow-up. Pediatrics. 1994;93(2):216–20.

191. Wilkins-Haug L, Gabow PA. Toluene abuse during pregnancy: obstetric complications and perinatal outcomes. Obstet Gynecol. 1991;77(4):504–9.

192. Cordier S, Ha MC, Ayme S, Goujard J. Maternal occupational exposure and congenital malformations. Scand J Work Environ Health. 1992;18(1):11–7.

193. Bowen SE, Hannigan JH. Developmental toxicity of prenatal exposure to toluene. AAPS J. 2006;8(2):E419–24.

194. Beauvais F, Jumper-Thurman P, Plested B, Helm H. A survey of attitudes among drug user treatment providers toward the treatment of inhalant users. Subst Use Misuse. 2002;37(11): 1391–410.

195. Sakai JT, Mikulich-Gilbertson SK, Crowley TJ. Adolescent inhalant use among male patients in treatment for substance and behavior problems: two-year outcome. Am J Drug Alcohol Abuse. 2006;32(1):29–40.

196. Shen YC. Treatment of inhalant dependence with lamotrigine. Prog Neuropsychopharmacol Biol Psychiatry. 2007;31(3):769–71.
197. Erdogan A, Yurteri N. Aripiprazole treatment in the adolescent patients with inhalants use disorders and conduct disorder: a retrospective case analysis. Yeni Symposium. eni Symposium; 2010. p. 229–33.
198. Muralidharan K, Rajkumar RP, Mulla U, Nayak RB, Benegal V. Baclofen in the management of inhalant withdrawal: a case series. Prim Care Companion J Clin Psychiatry. 2008;10(1): 48–51.
199. Westermeyer J. The psychiatrist and solvent-inhalant abuse: recognition, assessment, and treatment. Am J Psychiatry. 1987;144(7):903–7.
200. Tenenbein M, Casiro OG, Seshia MM, Debooy VD. Neonatal withdrawal from maternal volatile substance abuse. Arch Dis Child Fetal Neonatal Ed. 1996;74(3):F204–7.
201. Lee DE, Schiffer WK, Dewey SL. Gamma-vinyl GABA (vigabatrin) blocks the expression of toluene-induced conditioned place preference (CPP). Synapse. 2004;54(3):183–5.
202. Goldstein RZ, Woicik PA, Maloney T, Tomasi D, ia-Klein N, Shan J, et al. Oral methylphenidate normalizes cingulate activity in cocaine addiction during a salient cognitive task. Proc Natl Acad Sci USA. 2010;107(38):16667–72.

Chapter 36
Substance Abuse in the Elderly

Danie Babypaul, Michal Czernicki, and Sreekumar Kunnumpurath

Key Points

- Definition
- The problem
- Risk factors
- The patterns
- Screening
- Diagnosis
- Treatment
- The future

Definition

According to *DSM-IV-TR* criteria, the diagnosis of substance abuse requires a "maladaptive pattern of substance use leading to clinically significant impairment or distress, requiring (1) failure to fulfil major role obligations, (2) recurrent use in

D. Babypaul, M.B.B.S., D.A., M.D. (Anaesthesiology) (✉)
Department of Anesthetics, Royal Glamorgan Hospital, Ynysmaerdy, Llantrisant,
Rhondda Cynon Taf CF72 8XR, UK
e-mail: daniebp@yahoo.com

M. Czernicki, F.R.C.A., F.F.P.M.R.C.A., M.D.
Department of Anesthesia and Pain Management, Nottingham University Hospital
United Kingdom, 3 Melrose Gardens, Nottingham, Nottinghamshire, UK
e-mail: mczernicki@yahoo.com

S. Kunnumpurath, M.B.B.S., M.D., F.F.P.M.R.C.A., F.R.C.A., F.C.A.R.C.S.I
Department of Anesthetics and Pain Management, Epsom and St. Helier University Hospitals
NHS Trust, Wryth Lane, Carshalton SM5 1AA, UK
e-mail: skunnumpurath@gmail.com

© Springer Science+Business Media New York 2015
A.D. Kaye et al. (eds.), *Substance Abuse*, DOI 10.1007/978-1-4939-1951-2_36

physically hazardous situations, (3) related legal problems, or (4) continued use despite social or interpersonal problems as a consequence of substance effects. The diagnosis also requires that an individual does not meet the criteria for substance dependence [1, 2].

The Problem

Substance abuse among the elderly is one of the rapidly growing health problems. More people are living longer and more of them are abusing drugs and alcohol in their later years. Recent census data estimates that nearly 35 million people in the United States are 65 years or older. Substance abuse among those 60 years and older (including misuse of prescription drugs) currently affects about 17 % of this population. The number of Americans aged 50+ years with a substance use disorder is projected to double from 2.8 million in 2002–2006 to 5.7 million in 2020 [3].

There are approximately 78 million baby boomers in the United States and estimates are that a boomer turns 50 every 7 s. And many of these boomers are taking the abuse of cocaine, heroin, marijuana, and other illicit drugs into their "golden years." Although alcohol remains the top substance of choice among older adults, the aging baby boom cohort has resulted in illicit drugs accounting for a growing proportion of users and admissions to treatment facilities [4].

Elderly substance abuse is a tricky subject. Not only can the signs be mistaken for other problems such as dementia or depression but the abuse can sometimes be unintentional. Substance abuse in the elderly is most often seen in the form of alcoholism but can also be abuse of illicit drugs (heroin, cocaine, marijuana etc.), nicotine, over-the-counter medications, and prescription medications.

Alcohol remained the most common primary substance of abuse among older adults admitted for treatment, but the proportion of admissions reporting alcohol as the primary substance of abuse dropped from 84.6 % in 1992 to 59.9 % in 2008 [5].

In comparison, the proportion of older adult admissions reporting heroin as the primary substance of abuse more than doubled, from 7.2 % in 1992 to 16 % in 2008, and the proportion reporting cocaine as the primary substance of abuse quadrupled from 2.8 to 11.4 %. The proportion of older adult admissions reporting prescription pain relievers, marijuana, or amphetamines as primary substances of abuse also increased but remained small compared with admissions related to alcohol, heroin, and cocaine [6].

Data from the U.S. Drug Abuse Warning Network (DAWN) indicate that there were more than a half million visits to emergency departments involving nonmedical use of pharmaceuticals in 2004. Opioids and benzodiazepines were the two most cited medications among all visits (32 % and 27 %, respectively) and among adults aged 55+ years (33 % and 21 %, respectively). Most of the visits involved use of other substances (mainly alcohol): 65 % of visits for opioids and 76 % of visits for benzodiazepines [7].

   Prescription opioid abuse is an epidemic in the United States. In 2010, there were reportedly as many as 2.4 million opioid abusers in this country, and the number of new abusers had increased by 225 % between 1992 and 2000. Sixty percent of the opioids that are abused are obtained directly or indirectly through a physician's prescription [8].

Risk Factors

- Death of separation from a family member
- Retirement
- Reduced income
- Sleep impairment
- Family conflict
- "Young" elder, unmarried, male
- Previous illicit substance abuse
- Current methadone maintenance
- Licit drug or alcohol use
- Comorbid mental illness, especially depression and/or anxiety
- Substance abuse among close contacts
- Involvement in crime, especially drug crime
- Social isolation/poor social support
- Inmate status
- Short-term memory loss

The Patterns

Early Onset

In early-onset abusers, substance abuse develops before age 65. In these individuals, the incidence of psychiatric and physical problems tends to be higher than that in their late-onset counterparts. It is estimated that early-onset substance abusers make up two-thirds of the geriatric alcoholic population [9].

   Admission data from TEDS have revealed that the vast majority of older admissions (aged 55+ years) indicate first substance use before age 30 years (90 % in men; 70 % in women). Using national data from adults aged 50 to 59 years, researchers have estimated that approximately 90 % of drug users initiated illicit drug use by age 30 years and about 72 % initiated nonmedical use of prescription drugs by that age. Around 3 % initiated illicit drug use and 9 % initiated nonmedical prescription drug use at age 50 years or older. Hence, a comparatively large proportion of early-onset drug users will be more likely than late-onset users to have a wide range of medical, psychiatric, or social problems that will require more intensive or integrated treatments and monitoring. Older early-onset drug users not only may differ from older late-onset drug users in demographic characteristics (men vs. women) but also in risk factors and health status. Screening or assessments for drug use problems among older adults should include age of first drug use. Early onset users require a more comprehensive assessment of substance use and psychiatric histories than late-onset users [10].

Late Onset

In late-onset substance abusers, these behaviors are often thought to develop subsequent to stressful life situations that include losses that commonly occur with aging (e.g., death of a partner, changes in living situation, retirement, and social isolation). These individuals typically experience fewer physical and mental health problems than early-onset abusers.

Women are more likely than men to initiate substance use in late life. Less problematic groups of late life onset users may benefit from more timely brief or low-intensity interventions. Late-onset users may need a more thorough evaluation of recent changes in personal health status and environmental factors that could trigger the onset of drug use.

Screening

Substance abuse among older adults has been described as an "invisible epidemic" because problematic substance use and disorders tend to be under recognized, under diagnosed, or under treated [11].

Several screening instruments are usually accurate in identifying alcohol misuse. Screening tools effective in detecting older adults who may have an alcohol problem are the Cut down, Annoyed, Guilty, Eye-opener (CAGE); the Short Michigan Alcoholism Screening Test—Geriatric version (SMAST-G); and the Alcohol Use Disorder Identification Test (AUDIT). Selecting a screening tool depends on its purpose. While screening is important, it should but does not always effectively lead to treatment [12]. Inappropriate use of other psychotropic medications requires careful clinical assessment and questioning of spouse or family caregiver.

The Florida BRITE Project was the state's first attempt to establish a multisite, older adult-specific substance abuse and misuse screening and service program. In addition, the BRITE Project also established depression and suicide screening services [13].

The Drug and Alcohol Problem Assessment for Primary Care (DAPA-PC), developed under a contract from the National Institute on Drug Abuse, is a comprehensive screening system developed for quickly identifying and addressing substance abuse and related problems in a primary care setting. The DAPA-PC system includes a two-level screening instrument, resources for scoring and reporting results, motivational messages, treatment referrals, and informative links, which together address the multifaceted needs of patients dealing with addiction problems and their providers.

Diagnosis

Compared to younger adults, substance abuse disorders present more often as medical or psychiatric conditions in older individuals. Therefore, criteria for substance abuse in younger individuals may not be appropriate for older populations [14]. Both clinicians and researchers have most often relied on the DSM criteria, which were developed and validated in young or middle-aged samples, to diagnose substance abuse. Though it could be another health condition, substance abuse should be considered as well if there is memory loss, depression, repetitive falls and injuries, legal problems, chronic diarrhea, fluctuating moods, malnutrition, and recent isolation. Elderly substance abuse will not present with the normal red flags of addiction such as change in employment, absenteeism, and withdrawal from society as they usually are retired and engage in fewer activities socially.

The following signs may indicate an elderly substance abuse related problem:

1. Changes in sleeping habits
2. Unexplained bruises
3. Lack of interest in usual activities
4. Sadness, irritability, depression
5. Unexplained chronic pain
6. Changes in eating habits
7. Desire to be alone most of the time
8. Having trouble concentrating
9. Difficulty staying in touch with family or friends
10. Difficulty with memory after having a drink or taking a medication
11. Decreased coordination: frequent falls or walking unsteadily
12. Failing to bathe or to keep clean
13. Chronic diarrhea
14. Legal problems

A comprehensive evaluation should include a thorough physical examination along with laboratory analysis and psychiatric, neurological, and social evaluation. An increased focus on successful identification and subsequent treatment is warranted because research indicates that elderly patients reduce substance use when encouraged by their physician.

Treatment

Substance abuse disorders in older adults, as in younger adults, are frequently comorbid with other psychiatric disorders, including depression, anxiety disorders, adjustment disorders, and bereavement. There is a general lack of evidence-based treatment approaches for substance abuse in the elderly. As a result, much of what is recommended is based on interventions that have been validated in younger populations. It is important to understand specific ways to engage the elderly patient. In general, the choice of treatment depends on the severity of the condition and the level of functional impairment and varies from hospitalization to outpatient care.

Brief intervention is the recommended first step, followed, if necessary, by intervention, motivational interviewing, or specialized treatment; intervention strategies need to be non-confrontational and supportive. Elder-specific strategies that address age-specific psychological, social, and health concerns and contexts are recommended to incorporate into treatment plans for older substance abusers. Specifically, the following general approaches are recommended for treatment of older substance abusers

- Cognitive-behavioral approaches
- Group-based approaches
- Individual counselling
- Medical/psychiatric approaches
- Marital and family involvement/family therapy
- Case management/community-linked services and outreach

Peer self-help approaches, such as Alcoholics Anonymous, are often better when they are comprised exclusively of older adults. It is critical to understand that there is no one-size-fits-all approach. Treatment and other interventions must be tailored to the needs of the individual.

There is good evidence that older adults do as well as young people when it comes to treating substance abuse and that they may even do somewhat better. There are often direct health benefits, improved cognition, more independent living, more and better social connectedness, and new hobbies.

The Future

The greatest limitation to a modern understanding of illicit substance abuse among the elderly is the lack of data. In the future, as awareness of this phenomenon grows and clinicians begin to consider it as a possibility, hopefully studies of illicit drug use will expand their populations to include a greater number of older adults, and more studies will appear focusing particularly on the elderly. There is a continued need to monitor trends (especially nonmedical use and abuse of prescription opioids), key demographic characteristics, and health conditions associated with drug use among older adults. To improve early identification and treatment for the older population, there is a clear need to develop and test screening instruments specifically for this population. Studies are needed to identify the best ways to integrate screening into general medical settings as well as to understand the neurobiology of substance use disorders in the older adult with medical and cognitive comorbidities and to determine which specific treatment interventions are safe and effective.

It is of utmost importance to mobilize resources and prepare for the significant impact that the growth of the aging population will have on our mental health and substance abuse delivery systems. To adequately address the need, our supporting systems need to join forces now to advocate for appropriate planning and funding.

Summary

Substance abuse is a complex problem in the elderly population. Substance misuse among the older population is largely overlooked and underreported. Many factors contribute to this, not least the fact that presentation may be atypical and hence easily missed by the medical practitioner. There may be many clues to its existence, provided the physician remains alert to these. Despite this it is quite comforting to know that once identified, the evidence to date suggests that older people may respond at least as well as younger people to treatment [15].

References

1. Taylor MH, Grossberg GT. The growing problem of illicit substance abuse in the elderly: a review. Prim Care Companion CNS Disord. 2012;14(4):PCC.11r01320.
2. American Psychiatric Association. Diagnostic and statistical manual of mental disorders. 4th ed. Text revision. Washington, DC: American Psychiatric Publishing; 2000.
3. Wu LT, Blazer DG. Illicit and nonmedical drug use among older adults: a review. J Aging Health. 2011;23(3):481–504.
4. Colliver JD, Compton WM, Gfroerer JC, Condon T. Projecting drug use among aging baby boomers in 2020. Ann Epidemiol. 2006;16:257–65.
5. Brennan PL, Moos RH. Late-life drinking behaviour: the influence of personal characteristics, life context, and treatment. Alcohol Health Res World. 1996;20:197–204.
6. Reardon C. The changing face of older adult substance abuse. Soc Work Today. 2012;12(1):8.
7. Substance Abuse and Mental Health Administration. Office of applied studies. The DAWN Report: emergency department visits involving illicit drug use by older adults. 2008. http://www.samhsa.gov/data/2k10/DAWN015/015IllicitAbuse.pdf
8. Lembke A. Why doctors prescribe opioids to known opioid abusers. N Engl J Med. 2012;17:1580–1.
9. Bogunovic O. Substance abuse in aging and elderly adults. Psychiatric Times. 2012;29(8):39–40. http://www.psychiatrictimes.com/geriatric-psychiatry/substance-abuse-aging-and-elderly-adults.
10. Patterson TL, Jeste DV. The potential impact of the baby-boom generation on substance abuse among elderly persons. Psychiatr Serv. 1999;50:1184–8.
11. Moore AA, Seeman T, Morgenstern H, et al. Are there differences between older persons who screen positive on the CAGE questionnaire and the Short Michigan Alcoholism Screening Test-Geriatric Version? J Am Geriatr Soc. 2002;50:858–86.
12. Steinhagen KA, Friedman MB. Substance abuse and misuse in older adults. Aging Well. 2001;3:20.
13. Schonfeld L, King-Kallimanis BL, Duchene DM, et al. screening and brief intervention for substance misuse among older adults: the Florida BRITE project. Am J Public Health. 2010;100(1):108–14.
14. Patterson TL, Lacro JP, Jeste DV. Abuse and misuse of medications in the elderly. Psychiatric Times. 1999;16(4):54–7.
15. McGrath A, Crome P, Crome IB. Substance misuse in the older population. Postgrad Med J. 2005;81:228–31.

Chapter 37
Substance Abuse Among Healthcare Professionals

Natacha Telusca, Kingsuk Ganguly, Chrystina Jeter, and Jordan L. Newmark

Key Points

- Risk factors and causes of substance abuse
- Physical pain
- Emotional and psychiatric difficulties
- Stress associated with work/life
- Recreational use
- Avoidance of withdrawal symptoms
- Evaluation and treatment
- Consequence of physician abuse and barriers
- Considerations in special populations
- Risk factors for relapse
- Education and prevention
- Long-term follow up and monitoring

Introduction and Background

Substance-related impairment of healthcare professionals places the patient, provider, and general public at risk for harm. Although the information contained in this chapter can apply to any number of healthcare providers, the focus of this particular chapter will be on substance abuse among physicians.

N. Telusca M.D. (✉) • K. Ganguly, M.D. • C. Jeter, M.D. • J.L. Newmark, M.D.
Department of Anesthesiology, Perioperative and Pain Medicine, Stanford University
School of Medicine, 450 Broadway Street, Pav C, 4th Floor, Redwood City, CA 9406, USA
e-mail: ntelusca@gmail.com; kingganguly@gmail.com;
Chrystina.jeter@gmail.com; jnewmark@stanford.edu

© Springer Science+Business Media New York 2015   503
A.D. Kaye et al. (eds.), *Substance Abuse*, DOI 10.1007/978-1-4939-1951-2_37

504 N. Telusca et al.

The currently accepted definition of physician impairment, which includes substance-related disorders, is defined by the American Medical Association as "any physical, mental, or behavioral disorder that interferes with ability to engage safely in professional activities," [1]. Rates of substance abuse among physicians are estimated to mirror that of the general population, between 10 and 12 % [1, 2]. Rates of prescription drug abuse and dependence, however, are thought to be much higher among physicians than other non-healthcare professionals [2]. Prescription medication abuse in physicians is estimated to be 5–10 times that of the general population [3]. Though physicians in residency generally have lower rates of substance abuse, emergency medicine and psychiatry had the highest rates among residents in one study conducted in the 1990s [4]. The literature is inconsistent regarding specific abuse patterns among medical students, nurses, and pharmacists. However, there is limited data that suggests misuse and abuse of substances tends to begin before matriculation into professional schools [3].

Risk Factors and Causes of Substance Abuse

Risk Factors

Risk factors for addiction include: personal and family history of substance abuse, history of depression or other psychiatric illnesses, age 16–45 years, and history pre-adolescent sexual abuse specifically in female victims [5]. Healthcare providers have easy access to potent drugs, which is an additional risk factor for substance abuse.

Causes of Substance Abuse

The reasons for abusing prescription medications (and any substances) are broad but are generally confined to five major areas: (1) managing physical pain, (2) emotional and/or psychiatric difficulties, (3) management of stressful work/life, (4) recreational use, and (5) avoidance of withdrawal symptoms [2]. Each will be discussed below.

Physical Pain

Many providers report an inciting medical event, which initiates their substance use. Injuries, illness, and chronic pain have frequently been identified as reasons for opioid use. With continued use of substances, physical and/or psychological dependence can occur. As providers become more psychologically and physically dependent, they may begin "doctor shopping" and/or self-prescribing in an effort to maintain their dependencies [3].

Emotional and Psychiatric Difficulties

Providers have reported abusing anti-depressants, anxiolytics, and opioids in an effort to deal with their own anxieties or depression [3].

Stress Associated with Work/Life

Misuse and abuse of sedatives and/or opioids in an effort to cope with work- and life-related stress and burnout is common. Providers may initially take substances to deal with a physical ailment, such as back pain, but then achieve a secondary benefit of stress reduction, which encourages them to continue misusing [3].

Recreational Use

Frequently, the goal of abusing prescription medications is to experience euphoria, or get "high". A mixture of benzodiazepines and/or opioids with alcohol exaggerates the effect of both without having to take additional doses to achieve euphoria [3].

Avoidance of Withdrawal Symptoms

Providers may wish to stop their misuse of a substance, but cannot, secondary to the discomfort associated with physical or psychological withdrawal. The literature also notes the use of prescription drugs to "detox" from another substance. For example, utilizing Xanax, a benzodiazepine, to mask the withdrawal effects of alcohol while at work has been cited as the prelude for misuse of benzodiazepines [3].

Evaluation and Treatment

Denial is an important barrier, which prevents early intervention and treatment of impaired providers [6]. Brooke and colleagues reviewed medical data on 144 impaired physicians and found that the average duration of drug or alcohol abuse before receiving treatment is about six and a half years [7]. Early intervention is very important to save the impaired physician's life and protect patients from avoidable harm [6]. Physicians have an ethical duty to intervene when their colleague is suspected of experiencing a substance abuse disorder [1].

All states of the USA have Physician Health Programs (PHPs) designed to help identify impaired physicians and guide their evaluation, treatment, and after-care monitoring [8]. PHPs do not primarily provide treatment; their main goals are early detection of substance abuse disorders. Rather, they participate in assessment and evaluation of potential cases, referral to treatment programs, long-term monitoring, and reporting to licensing agencies [9]. They also provide general addiction education programs for all physicians in their states, and conduct thorough evaluations of addiction treatment programs that serve as referral sites [9].

The majority of PHPs are independent nonprofit entities, while others are part of state medical associations or licensing boards; however they all operate in agreement with their state licensing boards [9]. The majority of the state PHPs refer impaired physicians to the same five to seven treatment programs, allowing for long-term relationships between the programs and the PHPs [9]. These relationships force the PHPs to remain accountable, and establish standards and outcomes [9].

It is preferred that impaired physicians seek treatment voluntarily through a PHP, which can advocate for them before their state medical board [8]. Conversely, if an impaired physician is first reported to his or her state medical board before any involvement of a PHP, his license is at greater risk for suspension and revocation [8].

Initial Evaluation and Intervention

The usual treatment course for the impaired provider entails a progression of three stages: Initial evaluation and intervention, formal treatment, and long-term support and monitoring [8]. A critical step in evaluating the provider is to establish the level of confidentiality that can be assured for him or her, as well as the referring individuals, and then identifying who can access medical records [6]. It is imperative to maintain confidentiality of assessment and treatment to the greatest extent feasible due to the potential implications to the licensing and professional standing of the provider [6].

Knight recommends utilizing the principles of directive intervention when approaching or evaluating a colleague suspected of substance abuse. He summarizes these principles through the mnemonic device, "FRAMER," (Table 37.1). The first phase is to collect the *facts* to include any written or verbal complaints regarding the physician's appearance, behaviors, or performance. Documentation should report specific observations and avoid drawing conclusions. The second phase is for the concerned colleague to determine his legal *responsibility* for reporting the suspected colleague to licensing authorities. The third phase is to arrange for an intervention meeting at a private location, and bring *another person* to witness the conversation.

Table 37.1 Principles of directive interventions

F	Gather all of the FACTS
R	Determine your RESPONSIBILITY for reporting; consult confidentially with medical and legal experts
A	Bring in ANOTHER PERSON
M	Begin the meeting with a MONOLOGUE, in which you present the facts and summarize your responsibility
E	Insist on a comprehensive EVALUATION. Refrain from giving a diagnosis
R	Insist on a REPORT BACK and signed releases allowing all parties to communicate freely

Adapted from [10]

The person should preferably be a professional from the state PHP. The beginning of the meeting should be a short *monologue* listing the specific reports from others and observations by the concerned colleague. A referral for a comprehensive *evaluation* to assess the underlying problem and need for treatment should be made, and a *report back is* required from the evaluator as well as a signed release that permits open communication among all involved parties [10].

Once the diagnosis is established, a thorough comprehensive history and physical exam should be collected to include a complete medical and psychosocial history, a physical examination, and appropriate diagnostic tests [1, 6]. The medical interview should include questions regarding the negative impact on performance at work and home; the use of substances in dangerous situations; legal, social, or relationship problems secondary to substance abuse; tolerance or withdrawal symptoms; craving and effort to quit; and other substance-related physical or psychological problems [6]. Information regarding the source of the substance should also be gathered. The impaired physician may have obtained the substances from various sources, including stealing hospital or office supplies, diverting from patients, conspiring with patients to share prescriptions, fraudulent prescriptions, and/or ordering directly from drug companies [6]. The ability to obtain medications and substances online via the internet provides an additional level of complexity which should be explored. Obtaining collateral information from professional colleagues, coworkers, and employers is very useful. However, it is important to protect the privacy of the provider, so confidentiality agreements should be obtained from those sources. Collateral history from family members can be conflicting and inaccurate; therefore it is recommended to avoid asking these individuals about the provider in question [6].

The impaired physician should be screened for psychiatric illness and treated appropriately [11, 12]. Comorbid psychiatric illnesses, particularly depression, are common in addicted patients [13, 14]. It is therefore reasonable to expect that these symptoms would be common in physicians as well. Wijesinghe and colleagues reviewed data on 157 impaired providers and found 61 % had comorbid psychiatric disorders, including bipolar depression, schizophrenia, and major depression being the most common. The investigator must also determine the level of care that matches the needs of the impaired physician, which can include an outpatient or inpatient residential setting [15]. Many impaired physicians are treated in an inpatient setting because of the severity of their substance abuse disorder [8].

Treatment

The results of the evaluation should guide the next steps in management, which include treatment modalities such as medications, referral to treatment centers, a formal relationship with the PHP, and a monitoring contract. [9]. Comprehensive rehabilitation has been shown to be very effective [16]. McLellan reports that most impaired American physicians who received treatment from the PHPs had very good outcomes at 5 years. During long-term monitoring, 81 % had negative urine test results, and about 95 % who completed monitoring were still licensed and working 5 years after treatment commenced [17].

It is essential that impaired physicians undergo longer and more aggressive treatment than the general population because of the potential public health consequences [1]. The length of time for rehabilitation in the general population is usually about 28 days. Providers, on the other hand, require 3- to 6-month structured intensive treatment programs, followed by 5 years of outpatient treatment and monitoring [1]. For identifying effective treatments centers, PHPs can provide assistance. About 70 % of impaired physicians receive treatment in a residential treatment center for about 90 days, and the other 30 % are admitted to an intensive day treatment setting [9]. Smith and colleagues analyzed data on 120 impaired physicians who underwent treatment for various types of chemical dependency treatments, and they found that residential long-term (3–4 months) treatment tailored to healthcare professionals is very successful [18].

During the first few days of treatment, the impaired physician is observed closely for any signs and symptoms of acute drug withdrawal and comorbid medical conditions [10]. When the provider is stabilized, a period of intensive residential rehabilitation is begun. This usually includes individual and group therapy, educational sessions, and attendance at Alcoholics Anonymous (AA), Narcotics Anonymous (NA), and other meetings [9, 10]. The physician may require additional evaluation, such as neuropsychological tests, and/or psychopharmacological evaluation and treatment [10].

Pharmacotherapy is rarely used as part of the treatment of substance abuse. A small number of the treatment programs utilize maintenance or antagonist medications [9]. Reports from PHPs revealed that about one third of the participating physicians received antidepressant and non-benzodiazepine anti-anxiety medications as part of their treatments [9].

Consequence of Physician Abuse and Barriers

Although the prevalence of substance abuse disorders among providers is similar to that of the general population, the consequences are perilous to the physician, patients, and general public [19]. It is impractical and dangerous for physicians to work while seeking treatment. Furthermore, treatment is expensive, costing upwards of $20,000, which is rarely covered by insurance companies [10]. The net effect of lost income plus expenses of treatment can put physicians in significant financial distress [1]. Other dire consequences can include suicide or accidental drug overdose. Other than putting their patients in harm's way, substance abuse can harm others, such as accidents secondary to DUI or domestic violence at home [1]. These events adversely impact a physician's home life, not to mention opening up a plethora of legal implications for the physician. A physician's high level of executive thinking, which serves them well as a healthcare provider, can actually cloud their own personal problems. Physicians can be more skillful in hiding their addictive patterns from others and can attempt to rationalize their addiction as a form of self-treatment. Even if a family member were to find out, the financial and social implications may cause them not to act either. The fear of reprimand from medical boards further hinders a physician's desire to seek help. Fortunately, the developments of PHPs have allowed physicians to seek help outside of the purview of state medical boards [1]. PHPs offer education, rehabilitation, and surveillance without the threat of punitive action. These programs can work with groups such as AA while also performing routine drug screening exams to ensure that physicians remain in compliance [1].

During the acute treatment period, physicians must be excused from providing care. This can be for an unspecified amount of time. These providers must undergo a history and physical examination, followed by extensive laboratory testing that is performed under standards of high scrutiny. A 3–4 month treatment period has been shown to be more successful [10]. Many ethical dilemmas arise during this time, such as when, and if, a physician should return to practice, what to tell the physician's patients during their absence, and whether they can return to the same practice. Fortunately, most physicians who remain in monitoring programs where they are routinely evaluated and required to submit to laboratory testing, are successful in transitioning back to practice [10]. It is best to tell their patients that the physician is on a personal medical leave and any further divulgence of information can potentially harm longstanding doctor patient relationships. However, as a result of any illegal actions, it is not uncommon for physicians not to be allowed back into their original practice. The prospects of moving to another practice can prove to be daunting. Employers frequently ask for referrals from previous jobs. When and if a physician should divulge his history of substance abuse to a new potential employer must be carefully planned. It is best for the physician to first make amends with his former employer, as future employers will likely contact his or her last place of work. The physician should continue to work with his or her PHP and have them provide documentation to his former and potential employers to prove his ongoing commitment to abstinence [10]. The ability to show earnest reform is the best possible way for a provider to avoid future problems. It is also wise for the physician to have these documentations reviewed by his or her attorney [10]. The legal implications of substance abuse, especially if they involve prescription drugs, are far reaching. A physician may have been diverting drug samples to himself or writing prescriptions under pseudonyms. These violations will come with sanctions from the medical board, and the physician thus must obtain legal counsel [10].

Physician abuse can begin rather benignly, with physicians believing that they are self-medicating, rather than abusing, due to stress, anxiety, or depression. This can further snowball as they will eventually require higher dosages to achieve the same effect secondary to tolerance. This escalation can cloud a physician's judgment—they may still believe they are capable of taking care of patients, when in fact, acute intoxication or withdrawal symptoms can pose a danger to patient care. Substance abuse eventually leads to higher stress and anxiety, which too compromises physician performance. The rigors of establishing medical licensure and the risk of losing it pose the greatest barrier for physicians to seek help. Impaired providers spend an average of 6–7 years of substance abuse before finally seeking treatment [10]. Furthermore, when they are seeking help, it is usually not due to self-referral, but from an intervention. With appropriate confidentiality measures, there are many avenues the impaired physician can take to seek help. It can begin by seeing their primary care physician, who can then provide referral to an addiction medicine specialist and/or psychiatrist [10].

Both the American Medical Association (AMA) and the Joint Commission on the Accreditation of Healthcare Organizations (JCAHO) urge the reporting impaired physicians [19]. It is indeed the fiduciary responsibility of physicians to report a colleague, whether it is a peer or a superior. The Federation of State Physician Health Programs (FSPHP), a national nonprofit organization that oversees most PHPs, offers information on its website on how to ethically identify and assist impaired physicians (www.fsphp.org).

Considerations in Special Populations

Anesthesiologists represent a special clinical population among impaired physicians, given that they have an increased, readily available access to parenteral opioids. There are a number of observable behaviors that are seen in anesthesiologists who are addicted to opioids (see Table 37.2) [20]. They have a higher representation in treatment programs, and also a threefold higher risk of drug related deaths compared to their internal medicine colleagues [21]. Anesthesiologists who returned to their practice have a higher rate of relapse compared to those who switched specialties [21]. Psychiatrists and emergency medicine physicians are the highest self-reporters of substance abuse [10].

Table 37.2 What to Look for Inside the Hospital. Addicts sign out ever-increasing quantities of narcotics

1.	Addicts frequently have unusual changes in behavior such as wide mood swings, periods of depression, anger and irritability alternating with periods of euphoria.
2.	Charting becomes increasingly sloppy and unreadable.
3.	Addicts often sign out narcotics in inappropriately high doses for the operation being performed.
4.	They refuse lunch and coffee relief.
5.	Addicts like to work alone in order to use anesthetic techniques without narcotics, falsify records, and divert drugs for personal use.
6.	They volunteer for extra cases, often where large amounts of narcotics are available (e.g., cardiac cases).
7.	They frequently relieve others.
8.	They are often at the hospital when off duty, staying close to their drug supply to prevent withdrawal.
9.	They volunteer frequently for extra call.
10.	They are often difficult to find between cases, taking short naps after using.
11.	Addicted anesthesia personnel may insist on personally administering narcotics in the recovery room.
12.	Addicts make frequent requests for bathroom relief. This is usually where they use drugs.
13.	Addicts may wear long-sleeved gowns to hide needle tracks and also to combat the subjective feeling of cold they experience when using narcotics.
14.	Narcotic addicts often have pinpoint pupils.
15.	An addict's patients may come into the recovery room complaining of pain out of proportion to the amount of narcotic charted on the anesthesia record.
16.	Weight loss and pale skin are also common signs of addiction.
17.	Addicts may be seen injecting drugs.
18.	Untreated addicts are found comatose.
19.	Undetected addicts are found dead.

Adapted from [20]

Risk Factors for Relapse

Evidence based studies have shown 1 in 4 monitored physicians relapse at least once [19]. A family history of substance abuse is one of the strongest risk factors for relapse [21]. Nearly 75 % of surveyed physicians who reported substance abuse had a family history of this, which further increased the risk of relapse [21]. The use of a major opioid, such as parenteral fentanyl, has also been associated with relapse [21]. Physicians with a concomitant psychiatric disorder are also more likely to reengage in substance abuse [21]. The triumvirate of opioid abuse, family history, and coexisting psychiatric illness, increases the risk of relapse by 13-fold [21]. This warrants the need for impaired physicians to undergo extensive mental health evaluation during their monitoring period. It is not surprising then that during this period, one may be diagnosed with an additional psychiatric disease. Having a relapse increases the likelihood of future relapses, emphasizing the need for continuing education for reformed physicians [21]. Aggressive and continued monitoring appears to be the most effective way for physicians to overcome the barrier of substance abuse.

Education and Prevention

Education at an early age is the best way to prevent addiction from even happening [1]. As many providers who present with substance abuse have a concomitant complex medical history of other psychological disorders and a positive family history, prevention is key. Substance abuse education should begin as early as possible, in elementary school and continuing throughout one's educational career. The Higher Education Act of 1965 required medical schools to establish programs on substance abuse education [1]. Other medical schools have taken this one step further, by creating clerkships dedicated to addiction medicine, exposing medical students not only to the knowledge of substance abuse education but also to its clinical applications [1]. Residency programs, particularly those at high risk, such as anesthesiology and emergency medicine, should provide education on the topic beginning in orientation and frequently do so. Prevention is ideal, but education to physicians with a history of substance abuse should be broader to reduce the risk of relapse. Recommending changes to the work environment, such as avoiding overnight calls or reducing work hours, can potentially reduce the stressors that can cause a physician to relapse [1].

Long-term Follow up and Monitoring

Once the impaired provider completes substance abuse treatment, a continued care contract is established by the PHP [9]. The details of the contract include support, counseling, and monitoring, usually for 5 years [9]. The majority of the PHPs obligate impaired physicians to participate frequently in AA, NA, or other self-help groups, and provide verification of attendance to personal counseling [9]. Random drug testing is performed during the monitoring period. The physicians are also required to attend meetings with the PHP for continued medical care and evaluation [9]. Urine is the most often obtained sample for drug screening [9]. Hair, blood, saliva, and breath samples can also be used. Physicians are usually tested about four times per month during the first year for an average of 48 tests, and as the end of the monitoring period approaches, the number of tests tapers to about 20 per year [9].

Conclusion

Substance abuse among healthcare professionals carries a great risk of harm to patients, providers, and society. Physicians have an ethical duty to intervene when a colleague is suspected of substance abuse. Early intervention is crucial to protect the impaired physicians, as well as maintain patient safety and protect the public at large. Treatment options do exist—with the appropriate assessment, therapy, and long-term follow up with monitoring, and other resources as outlined in this chapter, providers may return to direct patient care and practice high quality medicine.

References

1. Merlo L, Gold M. Prescription opioid abuse and dependence among physicians: hypotheses and treatment. Harv Rev Psychiatry. 2008;16(3):181–94.
2. Merlo L, Supachoke S, et al. Reasons for misuse of prescription medication among physicians undergoing monitoring by a physician health program. J Addict Med. 2013;7(5):349–53.
3. Merlo L, et al. Patterns of substance use initiation among healthcare professionals in recovery. Am J Addict. 2013;22(6):605–12.
4. Conrad S, Storr CL, et al. Resident physician substance use, by specialty. Am J Psychiatry. 1992;149:1348–54.
5. Webster LR. Predicting aberrant behaviors in opioid-treated patients: preliminary validation of the opioid risk tool. Pain Med. 2005;6(6):432–42.
6. Galanter M, Kleber HD. Textbook of substance abuse treatment. 4th ed. Washington, DC: American Psychiatric Publishing; 2008.
7. Brooke D, Edwards G, Taylor C. Addiction as an occupational hazard: 144 doctors with drug and alcohol problems. Br J Addict. 1991;86:1011–6.
8. Ross S. Clinical pearl: identifying an impaired physician. In: Ross S, editor. Ethics journal of the American Medical Association. Chicago: American Medical Association; 2003.
9. DuPont RL, Skipper GL, Carr G, Gendel M, McLellan AT. The structure and function of physician health programs in the United States. J Subst Abuse Treat. 2009;37(1):1–7.
10. Knight JR. A 35-year-old physician with opioid dependence. JAMA. 2004;292(11):1351–7.
11. Bovasso G. The long-term treatment outcomes of depression and anxiety comorbid with substance abuse. J Behav Health Serv Res. 2001;28:42–57.
12. Charney DA, Paraherakis AM, Gill KJ. Integrated treatment of comorbid depression and substance use disorders. J Clin Psychiatry. 2001;62:672–7.
13. Havassy BE, Alvidrez J, Owen KK. Comparisons of patients with comorbid psychiatric and substance use disorders: implications for treatment and service delivery. Am J Psychiatry. 2004;161:139–45.
14. Mertens JR, Lu YW, Parthasarathy S, Moore C, Weisner CM. Medical and psychiatric conditions of alcohol and drug treatment patients in an HMO: comparison with matched controls. Arch Intern Med. 2003;163:2511–7.
15. Wijesinghe CP, Dunne F. Substance use and other psychiatric disorders in impaired practitioners. Psychiatr Q. 2001;72:181–9.
16. Shore JH. The Oregon experience with impaired physicians on probation: an eight-year follow-up. JAMA. 1987;257(21):2931–4.
17. McLellan AT, Skipper GS, Campbell M, DuPont RL. Five year outcomes in a cohort study of physicians treated for substance use disorders in the United States. BMJ. 2008;337:a2038.
18. Smith PC, Smith JD. Treatment outcomes of impaired physicians in Oklahoma. J Okla State Med Assoc. 1991;84:599–603.
19. Gastfriend DR. Physician substance abuse and recovery. what does it mean for physicians-and everyone. JAMA. 2005;293(12):1513–5.
20. Berry AJ. Chemical dependence in anesthesiologists: what you need to know when you need to know it. ASA Task Force on Chemical Dependence of the ASA Committee on Occupational Health of Operating Room Personnel; 1998.
21. Domino KB, Hornbein TF, Polissar NL, Renner G, Johnson J, Alberti S, Hankes L. Risk factors for relapse in health care professionals with substance use disorders. JAMA. 2005;293(12):1453–60.

Chapter 38
Podiatric Problems and Management in Patients with Substance Abuse

Gabriel V. Gambardella, Chioma N. Odukwe Enu, Brian M. Schmidt, and Peter A. Blume

Key Points

- Postoperative pain in podiatric surgery
- General overview of the acute pain pathway
- The role of local anesthesia in podiatric surgery
- Preemptive analgesia
- Patient-controlled analgesia and indwelling peripheral nerve catheters
- A multimodal approach to analgesia
- Presentations of patient with substance abuse in podiatric medicine

Introduction

Postoperative pain is not uncommon following foot and ankle surgery, particularly in cases of major reconstruction or trauma surgery. Perioperative pain control is crucial to the overall outcome of surgery and achieving patient satisfaction.

G.V. Gambardella, D.P.M. (✉)
Department of Podiatric Medicine and Surgery, Yale New Haven Hospital, New Haven, CT, USA
e-mail: gvg5@caa.columbia.edu

C.N.O. Enu, D.P.M. • B.M. Schmidt, D.P.M.
Department of Podiatric Medicine and Surgery, Yale New Haven Hospital/
VA Healthcare System, New Haven, CT, USA
e-mail: chiomaoduk@yahoo.com; bmcsch85@gmail.com

P.A. Blume, D.P.M.
Department of Podiatric Medicine and Surgery, Yale New Haven Hospital/
VA Healthcare System, New Haven, CT, USA

Department of Surgery, Anesthesia and Orthopedics and Rehabilitation Medicine,
Yale University School of Medicine, Yale New Haven Hospital, New Haven, CT, USA
e-mail: peterb@esnet.net

© Springer Science+Business Media New York 2015
A.D. Kaye et al. (eds.), *Substance Abuse*, DOI 10.1007/978-1-4939-1951-2_38

Management of acute postsurgical pain becomes a more challenging task in patients with a history of substance abuse, particularly that of opioid dependence. This chapter aims to discuss postoperative pain in podiatric surgery, as well as the acute pain pathway and different therapeutic modalities of achieving pain control. Furthermore, we highlight the various clinical presentations made to the podiatric surgeon that may indicate substance abuse and the subsequent management of the pathology.

Postoperative Pain in Podiatric Surgery

Patients typically seek treatment from a podiatric surgeon to relieve pain, whether acute from a traumatic event or chronic from long-standing or unaddressed pathology, which oftentimes will require surgical intervention. The goal of surgery is to provide each patient with a satisfactory surgical outcome, usually by means of achieving a significant pain reduction from the preoperative state while maximizing long-term function. However, absolute pain relief can never be guaranteed to a patient, and proper patient selection and education is paramount, particularly in cases of elective procedures. Having a comprehensive discussion with the patient preoperatively and setting realistic expectations can help prevent patient dissatisfaction postoperatively. Patients should be educated extensively with regard to postoperative pain, including the anticipated onset, duration, and quality of pain; when pain medication should be initiated; if the pain medication will resolve all or only some of the pain; the amount of pain to be expected; and the difference between normal and abnormal pain [1].

Pain following foot and ankle surgery can be attributed to many factors, including postoperative edema; nerve injury (transection, traction); altering physiologic biomechanics (failure to restore a normal metatarsal parabola); postoperative hematoma (poor intraoperative hemostasis); over- or under-correction of deformity; inappropriate surgical procedure (correcting only one plane of a flatfoot deformity with multi-planar components); failure to address coexisting pathology (performing a total ankle replacement while disregarding significant frontal plane deformity); non-anatomical alignment (fusion of the subtalar joint in inversion); painful scar; hardware failure (poor construct, osteoporotic bone); bone healing complications (secondary to smoking, systemic disease, alcohol abuse, or premature mobilization); joint stiffness (prolonged immobilization); avascular necrosis (poor surgical technique, extensive periosteal stripping); infection (suboptimal aseptic technique, prolonged operative time); failure to recognize coexisting pathology (exacerbation of an arthritic midtarsal joint following subtalar joint arthrodesis); iatrogenic causes (cartilage injury during arthroscopy); anticipated (posttraumatic arthritis following surgical reduction and fixation of a tibial pilon fracture or comminuted calcaneal fracture of the posterior facet); and failure to immediately recognize and treat a postoperative complication. Clearly, treatment should be individualized and directed toward addressing the causative agent.

Even with the aforementioned causes of postoperative pain eliminated, it is normal for patients to experience some degree of pain following surgery, and it is the responsibility of the treating physician to minimize this discomfort without jeopardizing the health of the patient. When surgery is performed on a patient with a history of substance abuse or opioid dependence, control of the acute on chronic pain becomes much more complex and can extend further into the postoperative period.

Acute postoperative pain following podiatric surgery can be attributed to many factors, such as the small compartments of the foot that cannot accommodate significant swelling, the natural dependent position of the foot increasing the propensity for edema, and the trauma-induced pain inherent with osseous surgery and disruption of the highly innervated periosteum. Assessing postoperative pain in 10,008 ambulatory surgical patients, Chung reported the highest incidence of severe pain occurred following orthopedic surgery [2]. With anatomical subdivision, ankle surgery was ranked fifth in terms of postoperative pain severity. Foot surgery was not directly acknowledged in the study.

The most severe pain experienced following foot and ankle surgery has been reported to be at 3 days post-procedure, which can be more severe than preoperative pain levels [3]. Pain experienced has been related to the anticipated severity of postoperative pain by the patient. Following the initial 3-day period, pain is likely to dissipate until the 6-week mark, when the majority of patients report complete pain relief. Patients who experienced a greater intensity of postoperative pain typically demonstrated a greater pain severity preoperatively [2, 3, 4].

There are various tools available for the podiatric surgeon to monitor pain progression postoperatively. Perhaps the most commonly employed tool is the visual analogue scale (VAS)—a 10 cm linear scale ranging from 0 to 10 that is reported subjectively by the patient, where 0 represents no pain and 10 represents unbearable, excruciating pain. The VAS also incorporates specific facial expressions correlating to the numerical pain level, which can certainly be beneficial for the pediatric population, as well as adults. Another frequently used tool is the American Orthopaedic Foot and Ankle Society (AOFAS) scale, which is subdivided by anatomy (Ankle-Hindfoot, Midfoot, and Hallux Metatarsophalangeal-Interphalangeal scales). Using this scale, pain is recorded as none, mild, moderate, or severe. Function and alignment are other documentable categories included in the AOFAS scales that can assist in corresponding pain to other measurable postoperative outcomes. However, the AOFAS scales are typically implemented to ascertain the long-term result of surgery. Therefore, this scale does not monitor pain progression during the acute postoperative period but rather identifies the ultimate change in pain from the preoperative status once the final clinical result has been established.

Consideration of an analgesic regimen should begin prior to surgery. Implementing a multimodal approach that begins with preemptive techniques, continues intraoperatively, and extends into the postoperative period should be a fundamental practice of pain control. When pain is anticipated to be severe in the immediate postoperative period and achieving sufficient pain relief with oral analgesics is unlikely, the patient should be admitted to the hospital for at least 24-h surveillance while receiving patient-controlled analgesia (PCA), nurse-controlled intravenous (IV) analgesics, or indwelling peripheral nerve catheters while being closely monitored for potentially fatal side effects. In some cases, and when available, a portable nerve catheter system can allow a patient to be safely discharged following surgery.

Because of the potential for significant postoperative pain following podiatric surgery, it is important for the surgeon to make attempts to minimize symptoms. One must therefore be knowledgeable of the acute pain pathway to efficiently obstruct the perception of a noxious stimulus.

General Overview of the Acute Pain Pathway

Acute postoperative pain can be associated with significant morbidity and patient dissatisfaction. This is extremely true in podiatric surgery, when patients are often-times restricted from using the operative limb and continued pain prevents the patient from ambulating. A keen understanding of the physiological pathway from a stimulus and local tissue reaction to perception of pain via stimulation-induced activation of various cortical and subcortical regions, including the insula and anterior cingulate cortex [5], is essential.

A simplified yet clinically invaluable model of the acute pain pathway has been reported by Meyr and Steinberg where the process is broken down into four sequential "attack points" [6]. Familiarizing oneself with this knowledge and understanding the mechanism of actin of individual analgesics becomes essential in achieving optimal analgesia.

The first attack point, "stimulus," initiates the pathway, and involves induction of a local tissue response that, in turn, activates afferent nociceptive nerve fibers (A-delta and C) mediated by the interchange of ions leading to cellular depolarization. In podiatric surgery, the initial stimulus is classically that of a surgical blade incising through the epidermal and dermal layers creating a local inflammatory response while also directly injuring microscopic nerve terminals. However, the stimulus can also be chemical (utilization of phenol for a matricectomy), thermal (laser ablation of verrucae or hemangiomas), or mechanical (manual spreading of tissue layers).

The second attack point, termed "transmission," involves the physical propagation of the action potential—the result of neuronal depolarization of the peripheral nerve—to the dorsal horn of the spinal cord where the first synapse occurs.

The activity between the afferent peripheral nerve and second-order neuron in the dorsal horn brought upon by multiple action potentials defines "modulation," or the third attack point. In essence, this stage embodies the "gate control theory." A complex converging network of neuronal input from the peripheral nervous system (PNS) and central nervous system (CNS) transpires, mediated by various proteins and hormones. An imbalance between excitatory and inhibitory factors determines if the signal is transmitted to higher centers of the CNS, or blunted. A detailed account of this process and the involved neuro-stimulators and neuro-inhibitors is beyond the defined scope of this chapter.

"Perception" signifies the fourth and final attack point, much of which "represents taking a quantitative CNS stimulus and translating it into a qualitative physical and emotional response" [3]. If excitation during modulation overwhelms inhibition, the electrical signal will ascend the lateral spinothalamic tracts and terminate in the somatosensory cortex, frontal cortex, and limbic system. Once information is processed, a physical and emotional response to the stimulus is provoked.

The Role of Local Anesthesia in Podiatric Surgery

The role of local anesthesia (LA) cannot be overemphasized in podiatric surgery, as many of our cases can be performed under monitored anesthesia care (MAC) with LA administration. Even when general anesthesia (GA) is utilized, a pre-incisional "block" can help delay pain perception postoperatively. Infiltration of LA acts primarily on the transmission attack point [6], preventing action potential propagation and thwarting peripheral input to the CNS. However, it does not directly inhibit dorsal horn activity or central sensitization. In our practice, bupivacaine and lidocaine are the most commonly utilized LAs.

One must understand the pharmacokinetics and pharmacodynamics of LAs prior to administration to achieve the desired outcome. These agents produce their effects by binding to the sodium channels on the intracellular membranes of the neuron generating a membrane stabilizing effect, decreasing the rate of cellular depolarization, and blocking the initiation of an action potential. The sensations of pain, temperature, and light touch are primarily impeded. Care must be taken to avoid overdose that can trigger life-threatening convulsive seizures, potentiate sedative- and opioid-induced respiratory depression, and affect methemoglobinemia (secondary to prilocaine's metabolite, o-toluidine) [7].

LAs are available in two forms, an amide or ester. Those classified as amides are processed by the liver, and therefore should be avoided, or dose modified, in patients with hepatic dysfunction. The esters are metabolized in the plasma by pseudocholinesterases and pose a greater risk for allergic reaction, specifically to the paraben moiety metabolite. Patients with a history of allergic reaction to a specific LA should be offered an agent from the other class.

Choosing the appropriate agent based on local infection status, lipid solubility and agent ionization will largely influence a block and its efficacy [8]. This becomes critical when confronting a diabetic foot infection that requires incision and drainage or radical tissue debridement. All LAs are weak bases, and exist largely in the ionized form in an alkaline environment. However, the regional pH becomes more acidic in the setting of infection which alters the ionization of the agent determined by its dissociation constant (pKa). In this scenario, the ionized compound dissociates rendering it less capable of traversing the lipid membrane of the cell to exert its effect. Therefore, it may be prudent to perform a more proximal block to achieve satisfactory anesthesia. A buffering agent, such as sodium bicarbonate, can be added to the anesthetic to facilitate transmembranous diffusion in cases of infection and local acidity.

To extend the effective duration and increase allowable dosage of an LA, epinephrine can be added to the solution. For example, 300 mg of lidocaine can safely be administered in adults, which increases to 500 mg with the addition of epinephrine. Similarly, the maximum allowable dosage for bupivacaine increases from 175 to 225 mg with the addition of epinephrine. Contraindications to the use of the vasoactive drug exist, including peripheral vascular disease and Reynaud's phenomenon, which must be considered prior to usage.

The podiatric surgeon implements various blocks depending on the surgical procedure involved. Regional blocks, such as the popliteal sciatic nerve block, are useful in cases involving trauma, such as ankle and calcaneal fractures, and major reconstruction, such as a pantalar arthrodesis, cavus foot reconstruction, Charcot reconstruction, or supramalleolar osteotomy. Local blocks, such as the Mayo block, involve infiltration of local anesthetic in the periphery of the surgical area. They are commonly employed in cases of hallux valgus correction, hammertoe repair, and other various forefoot procedures, as well as cutaneous surgery about the foot. Depending on the LA utilized, effects seldom last long after discharge from the post-anesthesia care unit (PACU).

The ankle block is commonly utilized for global forefoot reconstruction, complex midfoot reconstruction, partial foot amputations, foot trauma, and select tendon procedures. Many reference five nerves to the foot involved in an ankle block. However, this is incorrect and it should be noted that there are six identifiable nerves at the level of the ankle, including, from medial to lateral, the tibial nerve, saphenous nerve, deep peroneal nerve, two terminal branches of the superficial peroneal nerve (medial and intermediate dorsal cutaneous nerves), and sural nerve. The saphenous nerve, sural nerve, and branches of the superficial peroneal nerve lie in the subcutaneous tissue, while the deep peroneal and tibial nerves travel deep to the deep fascia alongside their arterial and venous counterparts. Because of the variability of nervous anatomy about the ankle, we recommend performing a ring block around the ankle by raising a continuous subcutaneous wheel to ensure adequate anesthetization of the four superficial nerves. The deep peroneal nerve can be found between the tendons of extensor hallucis longus and extensor digitorum longus at the level of the ankle joint, lateral to the anterior tibial artery. The tibial nerve is located in the third compartment of the flexor retinaculum posterior to the artery and vein. When anesthetizing the deep peroneal and tibial nerves, aspiration should be performed prior to administration so as not to inadvertently infiltrate a blood vessel.

The "Mayo block" is performed at the level of the first tarso-metatarsal joint and proximal first interspace. It is useful in osseous and soft tissue procedures about the first ray, including metatarsal osteotomies, phalangeal procedures, partial ray amputations, and first metatarso-phalangeal joint arthroplasty and arthrodesis. Targeted nerves include the medial terminal branch of the deep peroneal nerve in the first interspace, the distal extent of the saphenous nerve running along the medial border of the foot, the medial plantar nerve, and the hallucal branch of the medial dorsal cutaneous nerve innervating the dorsal distal aspect of the hallux on its medial side.

A similar injection performed on the lateral aspect of the foot is sometimes referred to as the "reverse Mayo block." The fifth ray and corresponding digit are anesthetized for procedures involving that specific anatomical area, such as Tailor's bunion correction and correction of fifth digit deformities. The sural nerve, lateral plantar nerve, and intermediate dorsal cutaneous nerve and its branches are anesthetized with this block.

Anesthetizing digital nerves is critical for performing some of the most basic podiatric procedures distal to the metatarso-phalangeal joint, such as hammertoe repair and nail surgery. The dorsal and plantar digital nerves on the medial and lateral aspects of the digit are anesthetized.

Benefits of a presurgical LA injection include prolonged anesthesia during the immediate postoperative period, a less required amount of inhalational anesthetic intraoperatively, and a longer time before an analgesic is required postoperatively [9–14]. With reference to podiatric surgery, Murray and co-workers evaluated 40 consecutive patients undergoing bilateral hallux valgus surgery under GA and an ankle block, and discharged with oral analgesics [11]. None of the patients presented to the emergency department for inadequate pain control, and 85 % of the patients reported they would recommend this surgery.

Studies evaluating the effects of a popliteal sciatic nerve block demonstrate anesthesia duration to be 14–20 h when combining 0.5 % bupivacaine with epinephrine [12–14]. These authors pointed out that this block may provide incomplete anesthesia in some patients, however patients exhibiting complete blocks required similar amounts of narcotic analgesics. "Rebound pain" following the diminishing effect of LA has been reported in patients undergoing ankle fracture fixation with a popliteal block [15], indicating a need for a more efficacious approach to central sensitization inhibition.

Needoff, Radford, and Costigan compared the postoperative effects of a pre-incisional ankle block of 0.5 % bupivacaine to normal saline for osseous first ray procedures [16]. Postoperative pain levels were assessed at the 6, 24, 48, and 72 h marks. A significant difference was only confirmed at the 6-h evaluation, with the group receiving bupivacaine exhibiting lower pain levels. The authors reported no difference in total analgesic consumption between the groups, once again implying the need for a more aggressive approach to inhibiting central sensitization.

Migues and colleagues demonstrated that the proximal popliteal block may not offer any advantage over a peripheral foot block for certain procedures [17]. In their study, patients undergoing elective unilateral forefoot surgery demonstrated a non-statistically significant difference between the two approaches in terms of anesthesia duration. Postoperative satisfaction rates of approximately 96 % were achieved. Furthermore, when compared to epidural anesthesia in pediatric patients undergoing surgical correction of clubfoot deformity, a peripheral nerve block was not indicative of a longer lasting analgesic effect, nor did it decrease opioid consumption during the first 24 postoperative hours [18].

Although we consider a preoperative LA injection to be standard practice in podiatric surgery, this alone has shown to be inadequate to maintain optimal analgesia once the effect diminishes [12, 13, 16, 19].

Preemptive Analgesia

It is imperative for any surgeon to be pro-active rather than re-active to pain in order
to provide optimal analgesia. The definition of preemptive analgesia remains somewhat debatable, but for the purpose of this writing we will reference Kissin's
description as "prevention of the establishment of central sensitization caused by
incisional and inflammatory stimuli, covering the perioperative period" [20].

In the absence of preemptive analgesia, the "wind-up" mechanism of pain becomes
pronounced. This entails sensitization of the CNS to a noxious stimulus creating a
hyperalgesic state secondary to central neuroplasticity, rendering pain management a
more difficult feat. *Suppressing* central sensitization after it is already induced may
be more difficult than *preventing* sensitization of the dorsal horn from a noxious
stimulus [21, 22]. Without the use of adjunctive presurgical medications when GA is
utilized, the CNS will receive stimuli input from afferent ascending pathways [23]
that ultimately may lead to sensory amplification postoperatively. Several interventions can be employed by the surgeon to circumvent this phenomenon.

The effects of gabapentin and pregabalin in the preoperative period when added to
a perioperative pain management regimen have been studied extensively. Although
typically prescribed for chronic neurogenic pain states, they have been advocated as a
promising adjunct in the immediate postoperative period in terms of reducing pain
and opioid consumption when administered preemptively [24–26] in non-podiatric
surgery. In a double-blinded randomized study evaluating its efficacy in foot and
ankle surgery, pre- and postoperative consumption of pregabalin was not found to be
beneficial when compared to placebo [27]. The perioperative protocol in the study
included neuraxial anesthesia, sciatic nerve blockade, and orally and intravenously
administered opioids. The authors theorized that their use of spinal anesthesia and a
peripheral nerve block had already prevented central sensitization, creating perhaps a
masked effect of pregabalin. In another study, a single preoperative dose of 300 mg
pregabalin given to patients undergoing minor orthopedic surgery resulted in a significant reduction in anxiety and need for opioid analgesics when compared to placebo,
although postoperative pain scores did not significantly differ [28].

Aside from a decreased amount of consumed opioids, benefits of central sensitization inhibition include shorter hospital stay, earlier mobilization, decreased incidence
of ileus, and a decreased risk of developing a chronic pain syndrome [29].

Patient-Controlled Analgesia and Indwelling Peripheral Nerve Catheters

Patient-controlled analgesia, or PCA, is appropriately utilized following major
reconstructive and trauma surgery about the foot and ankle when pain intensity is
anticipated to be severe. It is particularly beneficial when adequate pain management is expected to be problematic, commonly encountered in patients exhibiting
opioid dependency. This modality bypasses first-pass metabolism and essentially
provides 100 % bioavailability of the medication while offering the benefit of a

rapid onset. By setting parameters, such as defined intervals between medication administration and maximum allowable dosages within a certain timeframe, a patient can safely receive smaller, yet repetitive, on-demand and around-the-clock doses of opioid that can be titrated depending on the amount of perceived pain [30]. In patients with chronic opioid consumption, the "fentanyl challenge" can be utilized to determine postoperative dosing of opioids using PCA [31]. In this study, preoperative consumption of morphine-equivalent doses of fentanyl was calculated, and an IV infusion rate of 2 µg/kg/min was infused until spontaneous respiration was depressed. The duration of infusion was then recorded. Once spontaneous respiration depression was noted, GA was administered. To maintain respiratory safety postoperatively, the basal dose of hourly analgesic requirement was decreased by 50 %, with a lockout interval of 15 min. The basal infusion rate was then titrated at 4-h intervals to achieve a demand dose rate of 2–3 doses per hour. Alternatively, analgesic requirements can be calculated by providing the basic daily requirements of an IV equi-analgesic divided over intervals in a 24-h period. When a heightened pain component is involved with the surgery, one should anticipate providing a 30–50 % increase of the preoperative equivalent [32].

The difficulty in treating opioid-tolerant patients cannot be overstated. These patients tend to exhibit consistently higher postoperative pain scores than opioid-naïve patients [33] undergoing similar operative procedures. It is recommended that patients be given an opioid preoperatively and their daily opioid consumption be converted to an IV equivalent and administered over 24 h as an hourly infusion to avoid withdrawal [34]. If the patient's pain is poorly controlled with this method, or if side effects are experienced, the patient should be rotated onto other opioids while initially reducing the dose by 30–50 % [of the daily equivalent] to allow for incomplete cross-tolerance among the different opioids [34].

Indwelling peripheral nerve catheters also play a vital role in postoperative pain management following major podiatric surgery by providing a continuous therapeutic amount of LA that can continue days after surgery. Following total ankle arthroplasty, a continuous popliteal infusion of bupivacaine decreased pain levels at 6, 12, 18, and 24 h postoperatively, while also lowering opiate consumption and enhancing patient satisfaction [35].

When compared to 0.9 % saline in patients undergoing moderately painful lower extremity surgery, ropivacaine was found to provide significantly better postoperative analgesia when administered through a portable patient-controlled sciatic perineural catheter [19]. Eighty percent of patients did not require an opioid analgesic during the infusion, compared to 7 % of those receiving placebo. On a scale from 0 to 10 (0 being dissatisfied and 10 being very satisfied), the ropivacaine group scored 9.7 ± 0.9, while the patients receiving placebo scored much lower, 5.5 ± 3. A continuous parasacral sciatic nerve block can also be beneficial in providing long-term analgesia in surgery about the foot and leg, such as triple arthrodesis and below-knee amputation (BKA) [36].

Following major foot and ankle surgery, 0.2 % ropivacaine infused continuously in a lateral sciatic nerve block decreased morphine requirements by 29 % and 62 % during the first and second postsurgical days, respectively [37]. Following open repair of intra-articular calcaneal fractures, ambulatory patients receiving a continuous peripheral nerve block through an infusion pump demonstrated a reduction in orally and intravenously administered narcotics during the first postoperative day [38].

Furthermore, the efficacy of using stimulating nerve catheters when compared to other methods has been studied [39]. Following hallux valgus surgery, patients were provided with a portable self-controlled infusion system of 0.2 % ropivacaine anesthetizing the sciatic nerve in the popliteal fossa. In this study, the authors found that the use of a stimulating catheter resulted in less consumption of local anesthetic in the first 48 h post-surgery and only 25 % of the patients required rescue opioid analgesia.

A Multimodal Approach to Analgesia

While we always advocate the implementation of a multimodal approach to pain control, this practice becomes especially important when addressing pain in the substance abuse patient, particularly those who are opioid tolerant and on methadone maintenance therapy. Thus far, we have highlighted the benefits and limitations of local anesthesia in podiatric surgery.

The concept of multimodal analgesia aims to provide superior pain relief by administering analgesics from various classes with contrasting pharmacokinetic profiles, such as opioids, non-steroidal anti-inflammatory drugs (NSAIDs), and other non-opioids analgesics. Although prescribed much more in the United States than in other countries [40], opioids remain the mainstay of treating acute, moderate to severe, postoperative pain in both the opioid-tolerant and opioid-naïve patient, although the former will likely require a significantly greater amount and for an increased duration postoperatively.

Subjectively reported postoperative pain scores are likely to be more severe and dissipate at a slower rate in opioid-dependent individuals when compared to their opioid-naïve counterparts [41, 42]. Therefore, it is important to maintain the patient on his or her baseline narcotic requirement in the perioperative period and provide additional opioid as necessary postoperatively. Balancing the need for effective pain relief and minimizing the risk of overdose while achieving dose-reduction and preventing withdrawal symptoms is challenging and a primary concern, oftentimes warranting an interdisciplinary and collaborative approach [43, 44].

Perioperative administration of NSAIDs and non-opioid analgesics should always be considered as an option in the multimodal analgesic regimen. Inflammatory-mediated prostaglandins contribute significantly to postoperative pain, and the value of NSAIDs is demonstrated in their ability to block prostaglandin synthesis [45]. Selective inhibitors of the cyclo-oxygenase (COX)-2 pathway have proven to lessen mechanical allodynia postoperatively in rat models [46] and attenuate the adverse cardiovascular side effects encountered with conventional NSAIDs, although both selective and nonselective COX inhibitors have been shown to decrease opioid use in the postoperative setting in opioid-naïve patients [47]. Turan et al. evaluated 110 consecutive patients having elective hallux valgus surgery under GA [48]. Pain management began immediately following surgery with a selective COX-2 inhibitor and paracetamol. Postoperatively, the patients were instructed to take the COX-2 inhibitor daily, and the paracetamol as a rescue agent. An opioid analgesic was prescribed as a second rescue medication. During the follow-up period, the researchers reported that 34 % of the patients only required the coxib medication taken as directed; 41 % required paracetamol, and only 25 % required paracetamol and the opioid. Seventy-five percent of the patients did not require opioid analgesia, and only 9 % of patients experienced severe pain.

A combination of oral dexamethasone and paracetamol has also proven to decrease consumption of oxycodone following repair of hallux valgus deformity [49]. Adding tramadol (a narcotic-like centrally acting analgesic) to paracetamol has been shown to significantly decrease analgesic requirements in the acute postoperative setting following hand and foot surgery when compared to paracetamol monotherapy [50].

Because podiatric surgery frequently necessitates the healing of osteotomies, fractures, and arthrodeses for surgical success, NSAIDs should be used with discretion as they depress the inflammatory phase of healing. The clinical relevance of NSAID capability to affect bone turnover and healing is largely under debate [51–55].

Ketamine, an N-methyl-D-aspartate receptor antagonist, has proven to be beneficial in reducing the postoperative opioid requirement when administered intraoperatively in opiate-dependent individuals [56]. Loftus and co-workers demonstrated a 37 % reduction in opiate requirement in the acute postoperative period when ketamine was administered [56]. Furthermore, in their randomized, prospective, double-blinded, and placebo-controlled trial, the researchers reported total morphine consumption to be significantly reduced at the 6-week mark with ketamine utilization intraoperatively when compared to placebo, and also noted a significant reduction in reported pain. When administered preemptively, ketamine produces opioid-sparing effects in opioid abusers [57]. However, not everyone is a candidate for ketamine, and it should be reserved for select patients.

Transcutaneous electrical nerve stimulation (TENS) is a non-pharmacological, noninvasive, electro-analgesic modality that elicits a segmental analgesic effect by stimulating A-beta afferent nerve fibers and inhibiting second-order neurons [58, 59]. This modality proved to reduce analgesic medication consumption by 74.9 % in one study following foot surgery [60]. Similarly, Hamza and colleagues demonstrated a reduction in opioid requirements and consequently, opioid-related side effects, when utilized in combination with PCA postoperatively following major gynecological procedures. However, its use as an isolated treatment for acute pain remains questionable [61]. Following total knee arthroplasty, the authors found no reduction in the amount of PCA utilized when TENS was added as an adjunctive therapy [62].

To the authors' knowledge, no clear benefit of tricyclic antidepressants has been published for acute pain in the postoperative setting following foot and ankle surgery. However, when compared to placebo, low dose amitriptyline did not produce an opioid-sparing effect nor an improvement in general well-being when used as a co-analgesic following orthopedic surgery [63], although the preoperative oral administration of mirtazapine has been shown to reduce preoperative anxiety as well as the onset and severity of postoperative nausea and vomiting following spinal anesthesia [64].

As previously discussed, the podiatric surgeon must be vigilant of each patient's condition, and preoperative planning of postoperative pain control is crucial. Preoperatively medicating patients to minimize central sensitization, administering pre-incisional regional or local nerve blocks, and continuing analgesia with a PCA, indwelling peripheral nerve catheter, and adjuvant medications can assist in reducing opioid requirements and increase pain tolerability postoperatively.

Presentations of Patient with Substance Abuse in Podiatric Medicine

Identification of drug abuse in podiatric medicine requires a comprehensive examination with high index of suspicion, as signs and symptoms of drug abuse can mimic other commonly encountered podiatric pathologies. Local physical findings can be seen acutely or may present in a delayed manner depending on the type of drug being used and duration of use.

The skin is always the first site examined, and may demonstrate stigmata, or "track marks," discoloration, and signs of infection [21]. Injection marks at the site of administration are present in all intravenous drug users (IVDU) and may be the most common presentation of drug abuse [65, 66]. The most common pedal sites demonstrating these marks include the interdigital spaces, which offer discretion, and the medial plantar arch for the accessibility of larger, superficial veins. With repeated use, "shooting tattoos" may appear, representing that the user is following the vein proximally. Because many times drugs are prepared with the use of flames and needles, soot deposition may be visualized on the skin [67]. Swelling is also common and is determined to be secondary to lymphatic obstruction [68–70].

Cutaneous infections are also a common presentation representing IV drug administration. Abscesses and cellulitis have been reported in 11–65 % of IVDUs [68, 69, 71–73]. However, this is viewed from an entire body perspective and the incidence of cutaneous infections to the foot may vary. Risk factors for developing infections include intradermal injection, absence of aseptic technique, improperly sterilized or unsterile equipment, poor hygiene of the drug user, adulterants acting as irritant substances and foreign bodies, and injecting a combination of heroin and cocaine [67, 74, 75]. Tuazon et al. found that 68 % of street heroin samples and 89 % of paraphernalia were contaminated with various pathogens, including coagulase-negative Staphylococcus, Clostridium species, Gram-negative bacteria, and/or fungi [76]. Similarly, Moustoukas and co-workers observed contamination in 61 % of heroin samples [77]. Infection with Human Immunodeficiency Virus (HIV), female gender, foreign nationality, combined heroin/cocaine injection, prostitution, injection frequency, and obtaining syringes through a needle exchange program have been associated with abscess formation [73].

In addition, the pharmacological properties of the drugs, such as the vasoconstrictive effect of cocaine, may potentiate an infectious process [78] by allowing the agent to remain in a localized area for a prolonged period of time, thus increasing the host susceptibility to potentially infectious organisms. A wide range of pathogens have been isolated in these infections, with Gram-positive cocci being the most frequent. Anaerobes, particularly of the Clostridium species are the second most common, while Gram-negative bacteria are isolated less frequently. The source of the pathogens is variable, although most originate from the skin and oropharyngeal flora. Indeed, some IVDUs lick needles and use their saliva to "cleanse" the skin, moisten the cotton wool, or dilute the drug [74, 75, 78].

While the overall incidence of necrotizing fasciitis cases is low, it remains a limb- and potentially life-threatening consequence of IV drug abuse and has been associated with the use of black tar heroin [79–81]. Other local manifestations seen in this population include lymphangitis, thrombophlebitis, pyoderma, ecthyma gangrenosum, pseudoaneurysm, ischemia and tissue necrosis, and myonecrosis, or gas gangrene (Fig. 38.1) [82–84].

When infection results from substance abuse, treatment should be directed toward eradicating the causative organism with antibiotic therapy, orally or intravenously administered depending on infection severity and bone involvement. Abscesses must be addressed through surgical incision and drainage, and excisional debridement of necrotic and infected tissue. In cases of extensive infection, tissue necrosis, and gangrene that require radical tissue debridement, it may not be possible, or recommended, to perform primary wound closure. Patients may require periodic wound evaluations postoperatively and local wound care with regular debridements for an undefined amount of time until a healthy, granular wound bed is obtained.

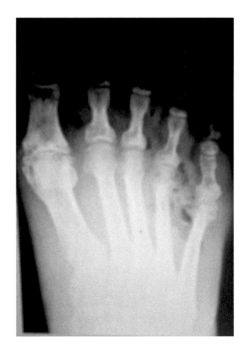

Fig. 38.1 Radiograph demonstrating gas gangrene. Note the radiolucencies about the fourth interspace. A finding of subcutaneous emphysema in the foot is a surgical emergency, and mandates immediate surgical incision and drainage with debridement of all infected tissue. The patient is at risk for partial foot, or major lower extremity, amputation

Fig. 38.2 Closure of a
posterior lower leg wound
following radical
debridement of a severe foot
infection using a reverse sural
artery flap. A split thickness
skin graft was harvested from
the ipsilateral extremity to
cover the donor site

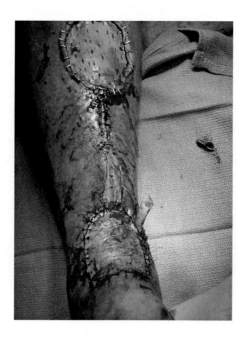

Once it is clinically established that all infected and devitalized tissue has been excised, advanced wound reconstruction techniques to obtain wound closure can be considered. This may ultimately require skin grafting or local, or free, flap closure (Fig. 38.2).

Aside from infection, osteo-articular disease of the foot and ankle can manifest in patients with substance abuse. Neuropathic osteoarthropathy, or Charcot foot, presents as a warm, edematous foot in the acute stage, somewhat resembling a cellulitis. Radiographically, the pathology is hallmarked by osteolysis and fragmentation of involved osseous structures, as well as joint subluxation with marked instability noted clinically (Fig. 38.3). Although it is most commonly encountered in the United States in patients with peripheral neuropathy secondary to diabetes mellitus, it can be attributed to virtually any disease or pathological process predisposing to peripheral neuropathy, including chronic alcoholism [85, 86].

First-line treatment of the disease in the acute phase includes immobilization, usually by means of total-contact casting, in an attempt to maintain or restore anatomical alignment of the foot prior to osseous consolidation. If this fails, significant deformity may result, which may include the classic rocker-bottom foot type (Fig. 38.4). The foot is then predisposed to significantly increased plantar pressures during gait, increasing the propensity for callus formation, tissue breakdown, ulceration, and ultimately infection.

When the diagnosis of Charcot arthropathy is made or suspected, it is imperative to obtain consultation from a podiatric foot and ankle surgeon who is well trained in the conservative management of the disease as well as Charcot reconstruction,

Fig. 38.3 Dorso-plantar (DP) radiograph of a right foot with Charcot arthropathy. Note the osteolysis and dislocation of the tarso-metatarsal joint

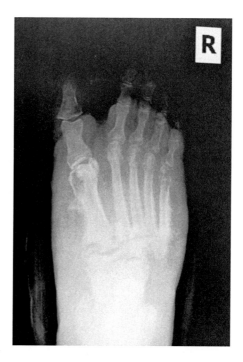

Fig. 38.4 Lateral radiograph of a right foot with Charcot arthropathy. Note the significant collapse of the midtarsal joint and negative calcaneal inclination angle creating a rocker-bottom foot type. Soft tissue volume is significantly increased

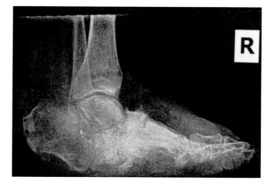

should surgical intervention become necessary. Limb salvage surgery may require correctional osteotomies and multiple joint arthrodeses using various forms of fixation, including screws, plates, intramedullary nails, and external fixation devices. Bone grafting can be used to negate the shortening of the foot or leg inherent with the surgery. The ultimate goal of reconstructive surgery is to prevent a major lower extremity amputation by constructing a stable, plantigrade foot capable of ambulation while minimizing the risk for tissue breakdown in the future. Although successful limb salvage has been reported in over 90 % of patients [87–89], complications

Fig. 38.5 Lateral radiograph demonstrating osteonecrosis of the talus. Note the increased radiodensity of the talar body as well as flattening of the talar dome signifying early subchondral collapse

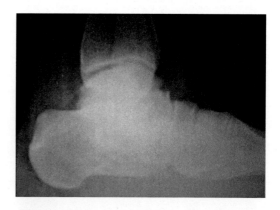

Fig. 38.6 MRI, T-2 weighted image, of a foot with osteonecrosis of the talus secondary to chronic steroid use. Note the increased signal throughout the talar body extending to the head of the talus

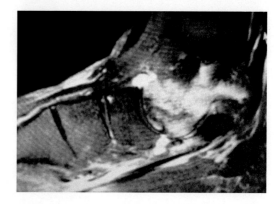

are common and include pin tract infections, malunions, nonunions, impaired wound healing, hematomas, superficial and deep infections, osteomyelitis, hardware failure, need for revision, and lower extremity amputation [90–93].

Although typically attributed to vascular disruption following trauma, pedal osteonecrosis can also be an indicator of substance abuse, and has been described in patients with cocaine, alcohol, and steroid abuse [94–98]. This condition can be debilitating, and manifests clinically as significant pain that can likely be attributed to vascular compromise resulting in osseous ischemia and bone marrow infarction [97, 98]. Furthermore, range of motion can be restricted due to accompanying pain. When a history of trauma is not related, the physician must investigate other possible etiologic factors of the pathology. Radiographically, one may note an increased radiodensity, or osseous sclerosis, as well as subchondral collapse and fragmentation depending on the stage of the disease (Fig. 38.5). Magnetic resonance imaging is a valuable imaging modality to aid in the diagnosis of osteonecrosis (Figs. 38.6 and 38.7), and may demonstrate the "double-line" sign, signifying a region of hyperemic granulation tissue surrounded by sclerotic bone (Fig. 38.7) [99]. Treatment is determined by the stage of the disease, location, and the amount of bone affected, in

Fig. 38.7 MRI, T-1 weighted image, of a foot with talar osteonecrosis. Note the "double-line" sign about the talar dome

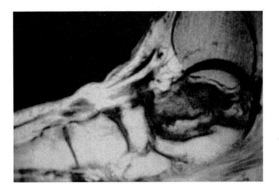

addition to dismissing the causative toxin. Conservatively, the podiatric surgeon prescribes NSAIDs to achieve pain reduction, modifies the patient's weight-bearing status to the respective extremity to promote healing, and encourages physical therapy to maintain joint mobility. In severe cases of osteonecrosis, or when conservative treatment fails, surgery becomes necessary, and includes core decompression, partial or complete ostectomy, bone grafting, joint arthrodesis, and arthroplasty, or joint replacement surgery [100–105].

Conclusion

Postoperative pain management following foot and ankle surgery can be challenging, particularly in substance abuse patients. Implementing a multimodal approach utilizing the described techniques and medications can significantly improve postoperative subjective pain levels and overall patient satisfaction and surgical success. Treatment methods should be customized to meet the specific requirements of each patient. Furthermore, various presentations of substance abuse about the foot and ankle have been described, and should prompt further investigation when suspicion is high.

References

1. Meyr AJ, Steinberg JS. Clinical pain management peri-operative scenarios. Clin Podiatr Med Surg. 2008;25(3):517–35.
2. Chung F, Ritchie E, Su J. Postoperative pain in ambulatory surgery. Anesth Analg. 1997;85(4): 808–16.
3. Chou LB, Wagner D, Witten DM, Martinez-Diaz GJ, Brook NS, Toussaint M, Carroll IR. Postoperative pain following foot and ankle surgery: a prospective study. Foot Ankle Int. 2008;29(11):1063–8.
4. Aida S, Fujihara H, Taga K, Fukuda S, Shimoji K. Involvement of presurgical pain in preemptive analgesia for orthopedic surgery: a randomized double blinded study. Pain. 2000;84(2–3):169–73.

5. Tracey I, Mantyh PW. The cerebral signature for pain perception and its modulation. Neuron. 2007;55(3):377–91.
6. Meyr AJ, Steinberg JS. The physiology of the acute pain pathway. Clin Podiatr Med Surg. 2008;25(3):305–26.
7. Becker DE, Reed KL. Essentials of local anesthetic pharmacology. Anesth Prog. 2006;53(3):98–108.
8. Robertson GS, Ristic CD, Bullen BR. The incidence of congenitally absent foot pulses. Ann R Coll Surg Engl. 1990;72(2):99–100.
9. Ke RW, Portera SG, Lincoln SR. A randomized blinded trial of preemptive local anesthesia in laparoscopy. Prim Care Update Ob Gyns. 1998;5(4):197–8.
10. Altintas F, Bozkurt P, Ipek N, Yucel A, Kaya G. The efficacy of pre-versus postsurgical axillary block on postoperative pain in paediatric patients. Paediatr Anaesth. 2000;10(1):23–8.
11. Murray O, Holt G, McGrory R, Kay M, Crombie A, Kumar CS. Efficacy of outpatient bilateral simultaneous hallux valgus surgery. Orthopedics. 2010;33(6):394.
12. Herr MJ, Keyarash AB, Muir JJ, Kile TA, Claridge RJ. Lateral trans-biceps popliteal block for elective foot and ankle surgery performed after induction of general anesthesia. Foot Ankle Int. 2006;27(9):667–71.
13. Grosser DM, Herr MJ, Claridge RJ, Barker LG. Preoperative lateral popliteal nerve block for intraoperative and postoperative pain control in foot and ankle surgery: a prospective analysis. Foot Ankle Int. 2007;28(12):1271–5.
14. Rongstad K, Mann RA, Prieskorn D, Nichelson S, Horton G. Popliteal sciatic nerve block for postoperative analgesia. Foot Ankle Int. 1996;17(7):378–82.
15. Goldstein RY, Montero N, Jain SK, Egol KA, Tejwani NC. Efficacy of popliteal block in postoperative pain control after ankle fracture fixation: a prospective randomized study. J Orthop Trauma. 2012;26(10):557–61.
16. Needoff M, Radford P, Costigan P. Local anesthesia for postoperative pain relief after foot surgery: a prospective clinical trial. Foot Ankle Int. 1995;16(1):11–3.
17. Migues A, Slullitel G, Vescovo A, Droblas F, Carrasco M, Perrin Turenne H. Peripheral foot blockade cersus popliteal fossa nerve block: a prospective randomized trial in 51 patients. J Foot Ankle Surg. 2005;44(5):354–7.
18. Rodrigues MR, Paes FC, Duarte LT, Nunes LG, Costa VV, Saraiva RA. Postoperative analgesia for the surgical correction of congenital clubfoot: comparison between peripheral nerve block and caudal epidural block. Rev Bras Anestesiol. 2009;59(6):684–93.
19. Ilfield BM, Morey TE, Wang RD, Enneking FK. Continuous popliteal sciatic nerve block for postoperative pain control at home: a randomized, double-blinded placebo-controlled study. Anesthesiology. 2002;97(4):959–65.
20. Kissin I. Preemptive analgesia. Anesthesiology. 2000;93(4):1138–43.
21. Woolf CJ, Wall PD. Morphine sensitive and morphine-insensitive actions of C-fiber input on the rat spinal cord. Neurosci Lett. 1986;64(2):221–5.
22. Dickenson AH, Sullivan AF. Electrophysiological studies on the effect of intrathecal morphine on nociceptive neurons in the rat dorsal horn. Pain. 1986;24(2):211–22.
23. Frerichs JA, Janis LR. Preemptive analgesia in foot and ankle surgery. Clin Podiatr Med Surg. 2003;20(2):237–56.
24. Behdad S, Ayatollahi V, Bafghi AT, Tezerjani MD, Abrishamkar M. Effect of gabapentin on postoperative pain and operation complications: a randomized placebo controlled trial. West Indian Med J. 2012;61(2):128–33.
25. Balaban F, Yagar S, Ozgok A, Koc M, Gullapoglu H. A randomized, placebo-controlled study of pregabalin for postoperative pain intensity after laparoscopic cholecystectomy. J Clin Anesth. 2012;24(3):175–8.
26. Bornemann-Cimenti H, Lederer AJ, Wejbora M, et al. Preoperative pregabalin administration significantly reduces postoperative opioid consumption and mechanical hyperalgesia after transperitoneal nephrectomy. Br J Anaesth. 2012;108(5):845–9.
27. Yadeau JT, Paroli L, Kahn RL, Jules-Elysee KM, et al. Addition of pregabalin to multimodal analgesic therapy following ankle surgery: a randomized double-blind, placebo-controlled trial. Reg Anesth Pain Med. 2012;37(3):302–7.

28. Gonano C, Latzke D, Sabeti-Aschraf M, Kettner SC, Chiari A, Gustorff B. The anxiolytic effect of pregabalin in outpatients undergoing minor orthopaedic surgery. J Psychopharmacol. 2011;25(2):249–53.
29. Seeman P. The membrane actions of anesthetics and tranquilizers. Pharmacol Rev. 1972;24:583–655.
30. Ferrante FM, Orav EJ, Rocco AG, Gallo J. A statistical model for pain in patient-controlled analgesia and conventional intramuscular opioid regimens. Anesth Analg. 1988;67(5):457–61.
31. Davis JJ, Swenson JD, Hall RH, Dillon JD, Johnson KB, Egan TD, Pace NL, Niu SY. Preoperative "fentanyl challenge" as a tool to estimate postoperative opioid dosing in chronic opioid-consuming patients. Anesth Analg. 2005;101(2):389–95.
32. Richebe P, Beaulieu P. Perioperative pain management in the patient treated with opioids: continuing professional development. Can J Anaesth. 2009;56(12):969–81.
33. Costa JR, Coleman R. Post-operative pain management using patient-controlled analgesia. Clin Podiatr Med Surg. 2008;25(3):465–75.
34. Marshall S, Jackson M. Acute pain management for opioid tolerant patients. Update Anaesthesia. 2011;35–9. http://e-safe-anaesthesia.org/e_library/10/Acute_pain_management_for_opioid_tolerant_patients_Update_20.pdf.
35. Gallardo J, Lagos L, Bastias C, Henriquez H, Carcuro G, Paleo M. Continuous popliteal block for postoperative analgesia in total ankle arthroplasty. Foot Ankle Int. 2012;33(3):208–12.
36. Morris GF, Lang SA. Continuous parasacral sciatic nerve block: two case reports. Reg Anesth. 1997;22(5):469–72.
37. Chelly JE, Greger J, Casati A, Al-Samsam T, McGarvey W, Clanton T. Continuous lateral sciatic blocks for acute postoperative pain management. Foot Ankle Int. 2002;23(8):749–52.
38. Hunt KJ, Higgins TF, Carlston CV, Swenson JR, McEachern JE, Beals TC. Continuous peripheral nerve blockade as postoperative analgesia for open treatment of calcaneal fractures. J Orthop Trauma. 2010;24(3):148–55.
39. Casati A, Fanelli G, Koscielniak-Nielsen Z, Cappelleri G, et al. Using stimulating catheters for continuous sciatic nerve block shortens onset time of surgical block and minimizes postoperative consumption of pain medication after hallux valgus repair as compared with conventional nonstimulating catheters. Anesth Analg. 2005;101(4):1192–7.
40. Lindenhovius AL, Helmerhrst GT, Schnellen AC, Vrahas M, Ring D, Kloen P. Differences in prescription of narcotic pain medication after operative treatment of hip and ankle fractures in the United States and the Netherlands. J Trauma. 2009;67(1):160–4.
41. Rapp SE, Ready LB, Nessly ML. Acute pain management in patients with prior opioid consumption: a case-controlled retrospective review. Pain. 1995;61:195–201.
42. Chapman CR, Donaldon G, Davis J, Ericson D, Billharz J. Postoperative pain patterns in chronic pain patients: a pilot study. Pain Med. 2009;10:481–7.
43. Huxtable CA, Roberts LJ, Somogyi AA, MacIntyre PE. Acute pain management in opioid-tolerant patients: a growing challenge. Anaesth Intensive Care. 2011;39(5):804–23.
44. Alford DP, Compton P, Samet JH. Acute pain management for patients receiving maintenance methadone or buprenorphine therapy. Ann Intern Med. 2006;144(2):127–34.
45. DiPrima JG, Keating SE, DeVincentis AF. The use of naproxen in controlling postoperative pain in podiatric surgery. J Foot Surg. 1986;25(4):273–7.
46. Yamamoto T, Sakashita Y, Nozaki-Taguchi N. Anti-allodynic effects of oral COX-2 selective inhibitor on post-operative pain in the rat. Can J Anaesth. 2000;47(4):354–60.
47. Maund E, McDaid C, Rice S, Wright K, Jenkins B, Woolacott N. Paracetamol and selective and non-selective non-steroidal anti-inflammatory drugs for the reduction in morphine-related side effects after major surgery: a systematic review. Br J Anaesth. 2011;106:292–7.
48. Turan I, Assareh H, Rolf C, Jakobsson JG. Etoricoxib, paracetamol, and dextropropoxyphene for postoperative pain management: a questionnaire survey of consumption of take-home medication after elective hallux valgus surgery. Foot Ankle Spec. 2008;1(2):88–92.

49. Mattila, Kontinen VK, Kalso E, Hynynen MJ. Dexamethasone decreases oxycodone consumption following osteotomy of the first metatarsal bone: a randomized controlled trial in day surgery. Acta Anaesthesiol Scand. 2010;54(3):268–76.

50. Spagnoli AM, Rizzo MI, Palmieri A, Sorvillo V, Quadrini L, Scuderi N. A single blind controlled comparison of tramadol/paracetamol combination and paracetamol in hand and foot surgery. A prospective study. In Vivo. 2011;25(2):291–5.

51. Konstantinidis I, Papageorgiou SN, Kyrgidis A, Tzellos TG, Kouvelas D. Effect of nonsteroidal anti-inflammatory drugs on bone turnover: an evidence based review. Rev Recent Clin Trials. 2013;8(1):48–60.

52. Hernandez RK, Do TP, Critchlow CW, Dent RE, Jick SS. Patient-related risk factors for fracture-healing complications in the United Kingdom General Practice Research Database. Acta Orthop. 2012;83(6):653–60.

53. Kidd LJ, Cowling NR, Wu AC, Kelly WL, Forwood MR. Selective and non-selective cyclooxygenase inhibitors delay stress fracture healing in the rat ulna. J Orthop Res. 2013;31(2): 235–42.

54. Kurmis AP, Kurmis TP, O'Brien JX, Dalen T. The effect of nonsteroidal anti-inflammatory drug administration on acute phase fracture-healing: a review. J Bone Joint Surg Am. 2012;94(4):815–23.

55. Welting TJ, Caron MM, Emans PJ, Janssen MP, et al. Inhibition of cyclooxygenase-2 impacts chondrocyte hypertrophic differentiation during endochondral ossification. Eur Cell Mater. 2011;22:420–36.

56. Loftus RW, Yeager MP, Clark JA, Brown JR, Abdu WA, Sengupta DK, Beach ML. Intraoperative ketamine reduces perioperative opiate consumption in opiate-dependent patients with chronic bak pain undergoing back surgery. Anesthesiology. 2010;113(3):639–46.

57. Gharaei B, Jafari A, Aghamohammadi H, Kamranmanesh M, et al. Opioid-sparing effect of preemptive bious low-dose ketamine for moderate sedation in opioid abusers undergoing extracorporeal shock wave lithotripsy: a randomized clinical trial. Anesth Analg. 2012;116(1):75–80.

58. Mulvey MR, Bagnall AM, Johnson MI, Marchant PR. Transcutaneous nerve stimulation (TENS) for phantom pain and stump pain following amputation in adults. Cochrane Database Syst Rev. 2010;(5):CD007264.

59. Claydon LS, Chesterton LS, Barlas P, Sim J. Dose-specific effects of transcutaneous electrical nerve stimulation (TENS) on experimental pain: a systematic review. Clin J Pain. 2011;27(7):635–47.

60. Chen CC, Lin CS, Ko YP, Hung YC, Lao HC, Hsu YW. Premedication with mirtazapine reduces preoperative anxiety and postoperative nausea and vomiting. Anesth Analg. 2008;106(1):109–13.

61. Walsh DM, Howe TE, Johnson MI, Sluka KA. Transcutaneous electrical nerve stimulation for acute pain. Cochrane Database Syst Rev. 2009;(2):CD006142.

62. Berit R, Van der Wall H. Transcutaneous electrical nerve stimulation for postoperative pain relief after total knee arthroplasty. J Arthroplasty. 2004;19(1):45–8.

63. Kerrick JM, Fine PG, Lipman AG, Love G. Low-dose amitriptyline as an adjunct to opioids for postoperative orthopedic pain: a placebo-controlled trial. Pain. 1993;52(3):325–30.

64. Chang FL, Ho ST, Sheen MJ. Efficacy of mirtazapine in preventing intrathecal morthine-induced nausea and vomiting after orthopaedic surgery. Anaesthesia. 2012;65(12):1206–11.

65. Kringsholm B, Christoffersen P. Morphological findings in fatal drug addiction. An investigation of injection marks, endocrine organs and kidneys. Forensic Sci Int. 1989;40(1):15–24.

66. Rathod NH, De Alarcon R, Thomson IG. Signs of heroin usage detected by drug users and their parents. Lancet. 1967;2(7531):1411–4.

67. Shuster MM, Lewin ML. Needle tracks in narcotic addicts. N Y State J Med. 1968;68(24):3129–34.

68. Stone MH, Stone DH, MacGregor H. Anatomical distribution of soft tissue sepsis sites in intravenous drug misusers attending an accident and emergency department. Br J Addict. 1990;85(11):1495–6.

69. Hussey HH, Katz S. Infections resulting from narcotic addiction: report of 102 cases. Am J Med. 1950;9(2):186–93.
70. Vollum DI. Skin lesions in drug addicts. Br Med J. 1970;2(5710):647–50.
71. Beaufoy A. Infections in intravenous drug users: a two-year review. Can J Infect Control. 1993;8(1):7–9.
72. Vishov D, Sullivan M, Astemborski J, Nelson KE. Bacterial infections and skin cleaning prior to infection among intravenous drug users. Public Health Rep. 1992;107(5):595–8.
73. Spijkerman IJ, Ameijden EJ, Mientjes GH, Coutinho RA, van den Hoek A. Human immuno-deficiency virus infection and other risk factors for skin abscesses and endocarditis among injection drug users. J Clin Epidemiol. 1996;49(10):1149–54.
74. Murphy EL, DeVita D, Liu H, Vittinghoff E, Leung P, Ciccarone DH, Edlin BR. Risk factors for skin and soft-tissue abscesses among injection drug users: a case-control study. Clin Infect Dis. 2001;33(1):35–40.
75. Binswanger IA, Kral AH, Bluthenthal RN, Rybold DH, Edlin BR. High prevalence of abscesses and cellulitis among community-recruited injection drug users in San Francisco. Clin Infect Dis. 2000;30(3):579–81.
76. Tuazon CU, Hill R, Sheagren JN. Microbiologic study of street heroin and injection paraphernalia. J Infect Dis. 1974;129(3):327–9.
77. Moustoukas NM, Nichols RL, Smith JW, Garey RE, Egan RR. Contaminated street heroin. Relationship to clinical infections. Arch Surg. 1983;118(6):746–9.
78. Bergstein JM, Baker IV EJ, Aprahamian C, Schein M, Wittmann DH. Soft tissue abscesses associated with parenteral drug abuse: presentation, microbiology and treatment. Am Surg. 1995;61(2):1105–8.
79. Bosshardt TL, Henderson VJ, Organ CH. Necrotizing soft-tissue infections. Arch Surg. 1996;131(8):846–52; discussion 852–54.
80. Chen JL, Fullerton KE, Flynn NM. Necrotizing fasciitis associated with injection drug use. Clin Infect Dis. 2001;33(1):6–15.
81. Callahan TE, Schecter WP, Horn JK. Necrotizing soft tissue infection masquerading as cutaneous abscess following illicit drug injection. Arch Surg. 1998;133(8):812–7.
82. Haiart DC, Andrade B, Murie JA. Gas gangrene following intra-arterial injection of oral medication in a drug abuser. Eur J Vasc Surg. 1992;6(5):565–6.
83. Conrad C, Steffen T, Gutzwiller F. Development of skin diseases in intravenous drug dependent patients treated with heroin substitution. Praxis (Bern 1994). 2000;89(46):1899–906.
84. Woodburn KR, Murie JA. Vascular complications of injecting drug misuse. Br J Surg. 1996;83(10):1329–34.
85. Shibuya N, La Fontaine J, Frania SJ. Alcohol-induced neuroarthropathy in the foot: a case series and review of the literature. J Foot Ankle Surg. 2008;47(2):118–24.
86. Arapostathi C, Tentolouris N, Jude EB. Charcot foot associated with chronic alcohol abuse. BMJ Case Rep. 2013;5:2013.
87. Pinzur MS, Gil J, Belmares J. Treatment of osteomyelitis in charcot foot with single-stage resection of infection, correction of deformity, and maintenance with ring fixation. Foot Ankle Int. 2012;33(12):1069–74.
88. Dalla Paola L, Volpe A, Varotto D, Postorino A, Brocco E, Senesi A, Merico M, De Vido D, Da Ros R, Assaloni R. Use of a retrograde nail for ankle arthrodesis in Charcot neuroar-thropathy: a limb salvage procedure. Foot Ankle Int. 2007;28(9):967–70.
89. Grant WP, Garcia-Levin SE, Sabo RT, Tam HS, Jerlin E. A retrospective analysis of 50 consecutive Charcot diabetic salvage reconstructions. J Foot Ankle Surg. 2009;48(1):30–8.
90. Herscovici D, Sammarco GJ, Sammarco VJ, Scaduto JM. Pantalar arthrodesis for post-traumatic arthritis and diabetic neuroarthropathy of the ankle and hindfoot. Foot Ankle Int. 2011;32(6):581–8.
91. Mittlmeier T, Klaue K, Haar P, Beck M. Should one consider primary surgical reconstruction in charcot arthropathy of the feet? Clin Orthop Relat Res. 2010;468(4):1002–11.
92. Zarutsky E, Rush SM, Schuberth JM. The use of circular wire external fixation in the treatment of salvage ankle arthrodesis. J Foot Ankle Surg. 2005;44(1):22–31.

93. Mendicino RW, Catanzariti AR, Saltrick KR, Dombek MF, Tullis BL, Statler TK, Johnson BM. Tibiotalocalcaneal arthrodesis with retrograde intramedullary nailing. J Foot Ankle Surg. 2004;43(2):82–6.
94. Assouline-Dayan Y, Chang C, Greenspan A, Shoenfeld Y, Gershwin ME. Pathogenesis and natural history of osteonecrosis. Semin Arthritis Rheum. 2002;32(2):94–124.
95. Ziraldo L, O'Connor MB, Blake SP, Phelan MJ. Osteonecrosis following alcohol, cocaine, and steroid use. Subst Abus. 2011;32(3):170–3.
96. Panchbhavi VK, Leontaritis NM. A case report of atypical magnetic resonance images of the hindfoot following cocaine injection in the foot and a review of osteonecrosis in calcaneus. Foot Ankle Surg. 2008;14(4):215–50.
97. McCarthy I. The physiology of bone blood flow: a review. J Bone Joint Surg Am. 2006;88 Suppl 3:4–9.
98. DiGiovanni CW, Patel A, Calfe R, Nickisch F. Osteonecrosis in the foot. J Am Acad Orthop Surg. 2007;15(4):208–18.
99. Zurlo JV. The double-line sign. Radiology. 1999;212(2):541–2.
100. Grice J, Cannon L. Percutaneous core decompression: a successful method of treatment of Stage I avascular necrosis of the talus. Foot Ankle Surg. 2011;17(4):317–8.
101. Ross JS, Rush SM, Rodd NW, Jennings MM. Modified Blair tibiotalar arthrodesis for post-traumatic avascular necrosis of the talus: a case report. J Foot Ankle Surg. 2013;52(6):776–80.
102. Stapleton JJ, Zgonis T. Concomitant osteomyelitis and avascular necrosis of the talus treated with talectomy and tibiiocalcaneal arthrodesis. Clin Podiatr Med Surg. 2013;30(2):251–6.
103. Yu G, Zhao Y, Zhou J, Zhang M. Fusion of talonavicular and naviculocuneiform joints for the treatment of Muller-Weiss disease. J Foot Ankle Surg. 2012;51(4):415–9.
104. Nicolo M, Paolo R, Francesco C, Andrea M, Longo UG, Vincenzo D. Hemiarthroplasty in a patient affected by osteonecrosis of the first metatarsal head following chevron osteotomy: a case report. Foot (Edinb). 2010;20(1):32–4.
105. Brosky II TA, Menke CR, Xenos D. Reconstruction of the first metatarsophalangeal joint following post-cheilectomy avascular necrosis of the first metatarsal head: a case report. J Foot Ankle Surg. 2009;48(1):61–9.

Chapter 39
Substance Abuse and Respiratory Disease

Martin D. Knolle, Sumit Chatterji, and Thomas B. Pulimood

Key Points

- Smoking is a popular way to ingest recreational drugs
- Nicotine addiction is a widespread problem
- Effective therapies to manage nicotine addiction exist
- Smoking of drugs causes structural lung damage and predisposes to infections

Introduction

Drug abuse is a growing problem, with estimates that the total healthcare burden of drug abuse is in the order of $137 billion/year and overall costs reaching $621 billion/year. Currently, the highest percentage of healthcare costs is attributable to tobacco ($97 billion/year) [1]. However, drug abuse patterns are constantly changing. Current monitoring by the National Institute for Drug Abuse shows that most drug abuse currently appears to be in decline. However, there are some notable exceptions. Marijuana use appears to be on the rise in adolescents [2].

M.D. Knolle, M.A., M.B., B.Chir., Ph.D., M.R.C.P.
Addenbrooke's Hospital, Cambridge University Hospital NHS Foundation Trust,
Cambridge, UK
e-mail: martinknolle@gmail.com

S. Chatterji, M.A., M.B., B.Chir., F.R.C.P
Respiratory Department, Peterborough & Stamford Hospitals, Cambridge, UK
e-mail: Sumit.chatterji@nhs.net

T.B. Pulimood, F.R.C.P., F.H.E.A. (✉)
West Suffolk Hospital, A University of Cambridge Teaching Hospital, Bury St. Edmunds, UK
e-mail: tpulimood@nhs.net

© Springer Science+Business Media New York 2015
A.D. Kaye et al. (eds.), *Substance Abuse*, DOI 10.1007/978-1-4939-1951-2_39

This chapter focuses on the effects of drug abuse on the lung. Perhaps unsurprisingly, we will focus on the effects of smoking and possible strategies to reduce smoking. In addition, we will examine ways in which other drugs can affect the lung. Broadly, substance abuse can either affect the lung directly (mainly through smoke inhalation), or indirectly by depressing the respiratory drive or by lowering immune defenses resulting in infection. Furthermore, substance abuse often goes hand in hand with other psychosocial problems, which can pose additional challenges in treatment.

Smoking is a popular form of drug consumption for a number of physiological reasons. The large surface area of the lung means that inhaled drugs can be rapidly absorbed into the blood stream. Once absorbed, they travel directly via the systemic circulation to the brain, where their effects set in within a few (around 10) seconds. This is a more rapid way to achieve an effect than even intravenous injection of drugs. As opposed to ingestion of drugs, there is no first pass metabolism by the liver after gut absorption. The lungs' larger surface area means that a larger dose of drug can be absorbed immediately (compared to nasal ingestion of drugs). The biggest drug problem facing respiratory physicians in quantitative terms is of course tobacco, and its addictive component nicotine.

Tobacco and the Lung: Introduction

Tobacco can be consumed in other forms than smoking, such as sniffing or chewing, however, for reasons outlined above tobacco smoking is by far the most common. The devastating effects of tobacco smoke are seen across a number of organ systems, not just the lung. Cigarette smoking accounts for 430,000 deaths annually in the United States. As such, it is one of the most easily modifiable risk factors for morbidity [3].

The percentage of the US population smoking tobacco is currently around 20 %. Despite the well-publicized risks of smoking, people continue to smoke and also commence smoking. The reasons for this are mainly psychosocial. For example, smoking is perceived as something grown up or a statement of toughness. Following starting to smoke, the addictive properties of nicotine maintain the smoking habit [4].

Tobacco and the Lung: Mechanisms of Addiction

Nicotine activates nicotinic acetylcholine receptors in the central nervous system, which induce dopamine release [5]. The dopamine release is widespread in the central nervous system, including dopamine release in the nucleus accumbens. This is similar to the effects of other addictive drugs, such as cocaine. In addition, nicotine also facilitates the release of dopamine via its release of other neurotransmitters, including glutamate. Other substances inhaled in cigarette smoke may contribute to its addictive effects. The half-life of nicotine is 15–20 min, and the terminal half-life around 2 h. These pharmacokinetics necessitate smokers to regularly replenish their nicotine to maintain concentrations. After smoking throughout the day, nicotine levels fall slowly overnight.

Nicotine ingestion has several positive effects. It leads to reduced stress, anxiety, improved concentration, and reaction time. However, the opposite effects take hold during nicotine withdrawal. Nicotine withdrawal leads to increased levels of corticotrophin-releasing factor, resulting in a stress response. Smokers will feel anxious, irritable, and have low mood. These symptoms of withdrawal ensure that regular smoking is maintained.

Regular cigarette smoking leads to saturation of nicotinic receptors. This results in desensitization of receptors, and a need to maintain high plasma levels of nicotine to avoid withdrawal. The need to "top up" nicotine levels results in conditioned behaviors, which in turn strengthen nicotine addiction. Ritualistic smoking associated with certain activities (after a meal, while drinking in a bar, or during a break, for example) maintains addiction beyond the merely pharmacological levels of addiction.

Tobacco and the Lung: Lung Pathologies

The devastating effects of tobacco smoking on the lung are well-documented and widely known. Lung cancer is the most frequently diagnosed cancer worldwide (and among the top three in the United States), and causes the highest number of deaths of all cancers. Ninety percent of lung cancers occur in smokers.

Lung cancer may present insidiously and is often only detected at a late stage, making curative treatment impossible. Presenting signs include weight loss, cough, shortness of breath, and hemoptysis. Physical signs can include fingernail clubbing, tracheal deviation (in case of a cancer causing endobronchial narrowing and collapse), bronchial breathing or stridor. Lung cancer may also have extrapulmonary manifestations such as symptom of inappropriate antidiuretic hormone secretion (SIADH), hypercalcaemia either due to bone metastasis or secretion of parathyroid hormone-related protein or paraneoplastic effects such as Lambert Eaton Myasthenic Syndrome.

Should a smoker present with a cough persisting more than 3 weeks, a referral to a chest physician should be made. The patient should subsequently be investigated appropriately. Of particular importance is to ascertain performance status, for example using the ECOG/WHO performance scale. Performance status is important in treatment options, as only patients with good performance status are likely to benefit from radical treatment. Investigations should include imaging (chest X-ray, contrast staging CT of the chest and abdomen and positron emission tomography if appropriate), blood tests and tests of respiratory function (spirometry).

The other main associations of cigarette smoking and lung disease is chronic obstructive pulmonary disease (COPD). Smoking destroys elastic lung tissue, resulting in emphysema. The reduced elastic recoil leads to hyperexpansion of the lung. In addition, smoking causes small airways disease with ensuing airflow obstruction.

The majority of cases of COPD are caused by cigarette smoking, however, in some patients, particularly young patient with lower lobe predominant emphysema it is important to consider other causes such as α1-antitrypsin deficiency. However, cigarette smoking causes the majority (80–90 %) of cases of COPD.

Patients with COPD may present with cough, wheeze, and shortness of breath. Patients should be investigated as appropriately with imaging and lung function testing. Treatment of COPD should be undertaken by physicians with expertise in this field. The mainstay of treatment comprises bronchodilator therapy (short- or long-acting β2 adrenoreceptor agonists or long-acting antimuscarinic agents) with or without inhaled or systemic corticosteroids. However, further treatments are emerging ranging from lung volume reduction surgery, endobronchial valves, and new generations of anti-inflammatory agents.

Tobacco: Other Pathologies

Tobacco smoking is a risk factor for a wide number of extrapulmonary diseases. Cigarette smoking is a major risk factor for cardiovascular disease, contributing to up to a third of coronary heart disease deaths. In addition, smoking significantly increases the risk of ischemic stroke [3]. Cigarette smoking is also associated with numerous other cancers.

Tobacco and the Lung: Smoking Cessation Therapies

Smoking cessation has substantial health benefits. Not only does stop smoking modify long-term risk factors for diseases outlined above, it also has immediate health benefits. Within a month, lung function and blood pressure may improve. Long-term risks for developing smoking related disease reduces. The risk of developing heart disease is halved within a year of stopping to smoke; within 15 years the risk is similar to that of a never smoker. The risk of developing lung cancer falls by 30–50 % over 10 years, but remains elevated compared to never smokers even after 20 years. All these benefits result in former smokers living longer than patients who continue to smoke [6].

Smoking cessation can either be promoted on an individual or population levels. While we will not review population level efforts in detail, these include public health campaigns to draw attention to the dangers of smoking, banning of tobacco advertising (for example at sports events) or plain cigarette packaging recently adopted by some countries.

Interestingly, most smokers would like to give up smoking. However, breaking the smoking habit due is difficult due to its addictive nature, consisting of both a physical addiction and conditioned behavior. Thus, before embarking on therapy it is useful to assess the patients' nicotine dependence and their motivation to stop. This helps to tailor therapy as patients with little dependence and high motivation to stop may well do so with minimal support, while other patients will require more support. There are questionnaires available to quantify nicotine addiction (for example the Fagerstrom questionnaire) to aid quantify levels of nicotine addiction [7].

Smoking cessation therapy can consist of advice, psychological support, or pharmacological treatment, alone or in combination (for the Department of Health Guidelines see Table 39.1). There is data to suggest that simple advice to stop smoking has a 1:40 success rate. While this is low, it still is a very cost-effective method.

Table 39.1 Key recommendations for tobacco replacement (US Department of Health and Human Services) [9]

1.	Tobacco dependence is a chronic disease that often requires repeated intervention and multiple attempts to quit. Effective treatments exist, however, that can significantly increase rates of long-term abstinence
2.	It is essential that clinicians and healthcare delivery systems consistently identify and document tobacco use status and treat every tobacco user seen in a healthcare setting
3.	Tobacco dependence treatments are effective across a broad range of populations. Clinicians should encourage every patient willing to make a quit attempt to use the counseling treatments and medications recommended in this Guideline
4.	Brief tobacco dependence treatment is effective. Clinicians should offer every patient who uses tobacco at least the brief treatments shown to be effective in this Guideline
5.	Individual, group, and telephone counseling are effective, and their effectiveness increases with treatment intensity. Two components of counseling are especially effective, and clinicians should use these when counseling patients make a quit attempt
	Practical counseling (problem solving/skill training)
	Social support delivery as part of treatment
6.	Numerous effective medications are available for tobacco dependence, and clinicians should encourage their use by all patients attempting to quit smoking—except when medically contraindicated or with specific populations for which there is insufficient evidence of effectiveness (i.e., pregnant women, smokeless tobacco users, light smokers, and adolescents)
	Seven first-line medications (five nicotine and two non-nicotine) reliably increase long-term smoking abstinence rates
	Bupropion
	Nicotine (gum/inhaler/lozenge/nasal spray/patch)
	Varenicline
	Clinicians also should consider the use of certain combinations of medications identified as effective in this Guideline
7.	Counseling and medication are effective when used by themselves for treating tobacco dependence. The combination of counseling and medication, however, is more effective than either alone. Thus, clinicians should encourage all individuals making a quit attempt to use both counseling and medication
8.	Telephone quit line counseling is effective with diverse populations and has a broad reach. Therefore, clinicians and healthcare delivery systems should both ensure patient access to quit lines and promote quit line use
9.	If a tobacco user currently is unwilling to make a quit attempt, clinicians should use the motivational treatment shown in this Guideline to be effective in increasing future quit attempts
10.	Tobacco dependence treatments are both clinically effective and highly cost-effective relative to interventions for other clinical disorders. Providing coverage for these treatments increases quit rates. Insurers and purchasers should ensure that all insurance plans include the counseling and medication identified as effective in this Guideline as covered benefits

This success rate can be increased almost fourfold by behavioral support therapy. This therapy should be aimed at understanding the patient's nicotine addiction providing appropriate advice on how to avoid succumbing to conditioned smoking behavior. The difference between the physical addiction and conditioned behavior needs to be clearly explained to the patient [8]. Combination of psychological therapy with pharmacological therapy increases quit rates over and above single strand therapy.

In combination with psychological therapy, pharmacological therapy can effect around a 30 % quit rate. Pharmacological therapy can be broadly subdivided into nicotine replacement therapy (NRT) and non-nicotine replacement therapy [9].

NRT aims to reduce physical addiction by providing an alternative source of nicotine. NRT can take different forms, including lozenges, nasal spray, gum, inhaler, and patches. Lozenges are available over the counter in two strengths, 2 mg for less dependent smokers and 4 mg for more dependent smokers. Nasal spray provides faster relief from symptoms than other forms of NRT. It should be used for approximately 2 months and then slowly withdrawn. Gum similarly comes in 2 and 4 mg strength for lighter and heavy smokers, respectively. The maximum recommended dose is 15×4 mg gums/day. The physical act of chewing may also help to alleviate some of the conditioned behavioral addiction to nicotine. Nicotine inhalers provide the addition of the conditioned movement and smoking actions to nicotine replacement. Nicotine inhalers should be used for around 2–3 months, and then gradually reduced. Nicotine patches again come in different strengths, which should be prescribed according to number of cigarettes smoked. Patches should be worn during the day for 8 weeks and then weaned to lower strength patches. Patches should not be worn overnight as this may result in nightmares.

Bupropion is a non-nicotine replacement smoking cessation agent. It is an antidepressant that reduces desire to smoke by inhibiting dopamine, serotonin, and noradrenaline reuptake. As these are key mediators of nicotine dependence, increasing their brain levels helps overcome physical addiction. Burpropion achieves up to 30 % quit rates in smokers smoking over 10 cigarettes/day [10]. Smokers should start taking it 2 weeks before their anticipated quit date, and then continue it for a further 8 weeks. Bupropion is contraindicated in patients with epilepsy, a central nervous system tumor, eating disorders, and those taking monoamine oxidase inhibitors.

Varenicline is an $\alpha 4\beta 2$-nicotinic receptor partial agonist. It should be slowly titrated in over a couple of weeks and then continued for 3 months. It may increase quit rates by up to 38 %.

Second-line pharmacological pharmacy includes clonidine and nortriptyline. Some combinations of medications may also be considered. Nicotine patches can be effective in combination with NRT gum, spray, inhaler, or bupropion.

Marijuana and the Lung

Dissecting the specific effects of marijuana on the lung can be complicated by the fact that marijuana abuse often coexists with tobacco smoking. In addition, the well-documented effects of marijuana on memory make self-reported studies of marijuana exposure more difficult to interpret. A further difficulty in studying how marijuana affects the lung is the variety of ways of smoking marijuana. In Europe, the smoking of cannabis resin (hash) is more widespread, while in the United States smoking of dried leaves and the tops of the plants tends to be more prevalent. Also methods of smoking vary from unfiltered cigarettes (joint) to pipes to smoking cannabis through water pipes. For purposes of this chapter, we will not distinguish between different forms of smoking and refer to marijuana smoking for all of them. Perhaps because of the different formulations and ways to smoke marijuana the precise effects of marijuana smoking on the lung remain controversial.

Regardless of formulation and way of inhalation, it is common for marijuana smokers to share their drug. This can either occur by sharing smoking implements or exhaling smoke into another person's mouth. Unsurprisingly, these practices can lead to a spread of respiratory infections. In particular, spread of TB has been associated with marijuana smoking in some patients [11].

Interestingly, some effects of marijuana appear different from those of tobacco smoke while others are very similar. Cannabis smoke contains cannabinoids (including Δ9-tetrahydrocannabinol), while tobacco smoke contains nicotine. Other than these, the smoke composition of marijuana and tobacco is similar in many components including carcinogens (carbon monoxide, cyanide, acrolein, benzene, vinyl chlorides, phenols, nitrosamines, reactive oxygen species, and polycyclic aromatic hydrocarbons). Given that many of the carcinogens are shared between tobacco smoke and marijuana smoke, it is perhaps not surprising that several reports link marijuana smoking with an increased risk of lung cancer [12].

As alluded above, the precise effects of cannabis smoke on the lung remain controversial, in particular with regard to lung function. Marijuana on its own, or in conjunction with tobacco smoke has been shown to induce airway inflammation in otherwise healthy subjects [13]. Long-term use of marijuana is associated with symptoms of chronic obstructive pulmonary disease [14, 15]. This includes symptoms of cough, wheeze, and sputum production. Stopping marijuana smoking leads to symptomatic improvement (if tobacco smoking is stopped as well) [16].

In terms of lung function, a recent cohort study suggests that low levels of marijuana smoking did not appear to adversely affect lung function [17]. This is supported by systemic reviews, which appear to support the view that short-term marijuana use does not have a detrimental effect on lung function [15], albeit causing symptoms of chronic bronchitis. However, other studies suggest that marijuana is detrimental to lung function. It has been estimated that a single marijuana joint is equivalent to up to 5 tobacco cigarettes in terms of causing airflow obstruction. Cannabis smoking reduces lung density (as assessed by CT scanning) and causes lung hyperinflation [18]. When assessing lung function, some report a dose-dependent relationship between marijuana smoking and airway obstruction [19].

In addition, there is a well-documented relationship between marijuana smoking and the development of bullae in the lung [20]. In particular large, apical bullous disease may exist and may result in the development of pneumothoraces in marijuana smokers [21]. It is particularly interesting to note that despite the bullous disease, many patients do not display deterioration in lung function. In patients with large bullous disease care has to be taken in environments where transpulmonary pressures are elevated. Pneumothoraces in bullous disease may be more likely when for example diving or flying. The management of these pathological effects on the lung are no different to those advocated above for tobacco smoke-related lung disease.

In summary, marijuana has several effects on the lung. While the effect on lung function remains unclear, marijuana is associated with airway inflammation, symptoms of chronic bronchitis, spread of pulmonary infections, lung cancer, and bullous lung disease with increased risk of secondary spontaneous pneumothorax.

Cocaine and the Lung

In its pure form, cocaine is often administered intranasally by sniffing of "lines". There are many case reports that link this behavior to the occurrence of pneumothoraces, possibly due to a Valsalva maneuver being performed during the sniffing of cocaine. Similar effects have also been reported to occur with nasal amphetamine abuse.

Crack cocaine is the freebase form of cocaine. Crack cocaine is prepared from normal cocaine by "cooking" it with a weak base, such as bicarbonate of soda (common baking salt) and is consumed by inhalation. Due to the large surface area of the lungs, rapid absorption of the smoked cracked cocaine (compared to "intranasal" cocaine), results in an effect (a "high") within seconds. The rapid, intense onset of euphoria is caused by a release of dopamine in the brain. As the high is more rapid and intense compared to intranasal cocaine, crack cocaine is thought to be more addictive [22]. Following the high, dopamine levels drop, resulting in low mood.

Clinically, crack cocaine smokers may present with a wide variety of symptoms. These can be attributable to the drug itself or often due to contaminants present accidently or deliberately [23]. Symptoms may include a productive cough (with sputum which may be discolored black), wheeze, dyspnea, and chest pain.

The most widely recognized condition caused by smoking crack cocaine is "Crack Lung" [24]. Patients with crack lung present acutely with fever, hypoxia, hemoptysis, and respiratory failure. Histologically, crack lung may demonstrate diffuse inflammatory alveolar infiltrates and alveolar hemorrhage [25]. The inflammatory infiltrate may be rich in eosinophils. Other damage caused to the lung by smoking crack cocaine includes thermal airway injury, pneumothorax, and pneumomediastinum [26]. Long-term smoking of crack cocaine may result in interstitial pneumonitis [27]. In addition, crack cocaine has been associated with pulmonary arterial hypertension [28], as have other stimulants such as amphetamine.

Management of acute presentations of crack cocaine smoking is largely supportive. The patient's respiratory status should be assessed using oxygen saturations and arterial blood gases and oxygen supplemented or respiratory support given as indicated. Imaging with chest radiograph or CT will a) confirm the extent of damage caused by the smoking of crack cocaine and b) rule out other pathologies (such as a pneumothorax).

Some reports suggest corticosteroids have been used with good effect in acute presentations of crack cocaine-induced lung injury [24].

Long-term sequelae such as fibrosis and pulmonary hypertension should be fully assessed and be managed by physicians with specialist interest in these areas. Assessment should include full pulmonary function testing, appropriate imaging such as high-resolution CT chest, CT pulmonary angiogram and echocardiography. Treatment will depend on the predominant pathology and severity of symptoms. Some cases may be severe enough to be referred for lung or heart/lung transplant assessment but only if drug rehabilitation and complete abstinence from drug use for at least 6 months can be demonstrated.

Alcohol and the Lung

Alcohol can have acute and chronic effects on the lung. Acutely, alcohol is a respiratory depressant. Patients may present with a reduced consciousness, low respiratory rate, and acute respiratory failure. The priority in these patients is airway protection, as emesis combined with the reduced consciousness may result in aspiration of gastric contents. Should aspiration of solids or semisolids have occurred, these may have to be removed acutely if causing respiratory compromise. Once a safe airway is established, other aspects of alcohol poisoning also need to be addressed. This includes administration of thiamine to prevent Wernicke's encephalopathy. Rarely, alcohol levels reach blood concentrations high enough to require management with hemodialysis.

As mentioned above, aspiration is a frequently encountered problem in patients with alcohol addiction. Aspiration can lead to a sterile pneumonitis or induce bacterial aspiration pneumonia. Thus, patients with acute alcohol intoxication and clinico-radiological suggestion of aspiration pneumonitis should be covered with broad-spectrum antibiotics with cover for gram-negative and anaerobic bacteria.

Alcohol abuse in the absence of acute intoxication is also a risk factor for developing pneumonia. In addition to the risk of aspiration, other lung defense mechanisms are impaired by alcohol. This includes poor oral hygiene, impaired gag reflexes, impaired mucociliary clearance, and direct effects on leukocytes [29]. Furthermore, malnourishment secondary to chronic alcohol abuse contributes to the risk of developing pneumonia due to impaired immune responses. Due to the impaired lung defenses atypical pulmonary infections, for example those caused by gram-negative bacteria such as Klebsiella, or mycobacterium tuberculosis, are more common. Pneumonia is often more severe in patients with chronic alcohol dependency. Other factors to note are that alcohol abuse is an independent risk factor for the development of acute respiratory distress syndrome. Furthermore, it is also a risk factor for the development of chronic obstructive pulmonary disease, possibly through oxidative stress [30].

Benzodiazepines and the Lung

Benzodiazepines are sometimes used, often in conjunction with opioids, to palliate patients suffering from dyspnea. However, acute benzodiazepine abuse may present with a clinical presentation similar to that of acute alcohol intoxication. Benzodiazepine abuse frequently presents in the setting of deliberate self-harm with the taking of a deliberate overdose. An overdose of benzodiazepines may result in reduced conscious level and respiratory depression. Thus, airway protection and adequate respiratory support are paramount. Aspiration pneumonia should be covered with broad-spectrum antibiotics. As opposed to alcohol, excess benzodiazepine may be countered by specific antidote. Flumazenil is a benzodiazepine receptor antagonist. Flumazenil does however have a number of side effects of its own that restrict its use. For example, it lowers the seizure threshold and may result in cardiac arrhythmias. In addition, its relatively short half-life (compared to benzodiazepines) requires repeat doses or an intravenous infusion to prevent recurrence of sedation. Thus, it may be considered safer in some patients to prioritize airway protection and ventilatory support over the reversal of the benzodiazepines.

Heroin and the Lung

Heroin smoking ("chasing the dragon") may have similar consequences to crack cocaine smoking. The study of the effects of heroin smoking is complicated by the fact that the vast majority of heroin smokers also smoke tobacco. Patients who smoke heroin may develop bronchiectasis, eosinophilic pneumonia, emphysema, bullous lung disease, pneumothoraces, and pulmonary hypertension. Chronic heroin smoking results in impaired lung function and shortness of breath [31]. In addition, cases of acute pulmonary edema secondary to heroin smoking have been reported. Furthermore, the respiratory depressant effects of heroin (see below) may also occur after inhalational use. Treatment is supportive and should focus on helping patients overcome heroin addiction.

Injecting heroin (or indeed any recreational drug taken intravenously) may also have effects on the lung. Acutely, heroin injection can reduce respiratory drive and consciousness. In these circumstances airway protection is the key priority. Intravenous naloxone can be administered as an effective antidote to a heroin overdose. Care needs to be taken because the half-life of naloxone is shorter than that of heroin and repeat administration may be required.

Non-sterile injection may result in infection that embolizes via the blood stream to the lung. On radiography multifocal nodular or cavitating lesions may be seen. This may occur in the presence or absence of right-heart infective endocarditis.

In addition, intravenous drug users are at higher risk of developing human immunodeficiency virus (HIV) infection. Individuals with HIV are more prone to pneumonia and infection with less commonly seen bacteria. This includes gram-negative bacteria, *Mycobacterium tuberculosis*, atypical mycobacteria, viral pneumonias, or fungal pneumonias (for example pneumocystis jiroveci).

TB Treatment in Drug Users

As alluded in a number of chapters above, drug abuse frequently increases the risk of respiratory infections. Few of these are as challenging to manage as mycobacterium tuberculosis, which occurs with increased frequency as the result of drug abuse. In addition drug abuse and the social situation of many patients abusing drugs increases the risk of multidrug resistant or extensively drug resistant mycobacterium tuberculosis infection. Thus, it is important that cases of mycobacterium tuberculosis in this population are adequately treated. However, this can often be challenging, in particular due to poor adherence to a drug regime requiring the regular taking of a number of different tablets over a period of months to years. This may be improved by directly observed therapy where patients take their medications in the presence of a healthcare worker. Due to logistical problems, some of these patients are managed on a thrice weekly rather than daily dosing. Yet this improves adherence and adequate treatment of mycobacterium tuberculosis in this hard-to-reach population.

Summary

Smoking of recreational drugs is a popular method of drug consumption. The respiratory consequences are myriad and are primarily through direct insult caused by chemicals or heat. Opportunistic pulmonary infections are more common and often more severe, with the drug-associated social behaviors often serving as risk factors for transmission of infection. Finally, some drugs of abuse cause respiratory depression and may compromise the airway if taken in overdose or as a severe idiosyncratic reaction. Reducing tobacco smoking and nicotine dependence remain a primary healthcare priority in most developed countries with lung cancer and COPD causing significant morbidity and mortality as well as burden on health economics. All healthcare practitioners should encourage smokers to enrol with smoking cessation programs and be vigilant to early symptoms of lung cancer and COPD.

References

1. http://www.drugabuse.gov/related-topics/trends-statistics. Accessed 1 Sept 2013.
2. Substance Abuse and Mental Health Services Administration. Results from the 2010 National Survey on Drug Use and Health: summary of National Findings, NSDUH series H-41, HHS publication no. (SMA) 11-4658. Rockville: Substance Abuse and Mental Health Services Administration; 2011.
3. Ockene IS, Houst Miller N, For the American Heart Association Task Force on Risk Reduction. Cigarette smoking, cardiovascular disease, and stroke. Circulation. 1997;96:3243–7.
4. Jarvis MJ. Why do people smoke. BMJ. 2004;328(7433):277–9.
5. Benowitz NL. Nicotine addiction. N Engl J Med. 2010;362(24):2295–303.
6. Edwards R. The problem of tobacco smoking. BMJ. 2004;328(7433):217–9.

7. West R. Assessment of dependence and motivation to stop smoking. BMJ. 2004;328(7433):338–9.
8. Coleman T. Use of simple advice and behavioural support. BMJ. 2004;328(7433):397–9.
9. Fiore MC, Jaen CR, Baker TB, Bailey WC, et al. Treating tobacco use and dependence: 2008 update. Rockville: US Department of Health and Human Services, Public Health Service; 2008.
10. Hurt RD, Sachs DPL, Glover ED, Offord KP, et al. A comparison of sustained-release bupropion and placebo for smoking cessation. N Engl J Med. 1997;337:1195–202.
11. Oeltmann JE, Oren E, Haddad MB, Lake LK, Harrington TA, Ijaz K, Narita M. Tuberculosis outbreak in marijuana users, Seattle, Washington, 2004. Emerg Infect Dis. 2006;12(7):1156–9.
12. Aldington S, Harwood M, Cox B, Weatherall M, Beckert L, Hansell A, Pritchard A, Robinson G, Beasley R. Cannabis and the risk of lung cancer: a case-control study. Eur Respir J. 2008;31(2):280–6.
13. Roth MD, Arora A, Barsky SK, Kleerup EC, Simmons M, Tashkin DP. Airway inflammation in young marijuana and tobacco. Am J Respir Crit Care Med. 1998;157(3):928–37.
14. Tashkin DP, Coulson AH, Clark VA, Simmons M, Bourque LB, Duann S, Spivey GH, Gong H. Respiratory symptoms and lung function in habitual heavy smokers or marijuana alone, smoker of marijuana and tobacco, smoker of tobacco alone, and nonsmokers. Am Rev Respir Dis. 1987;135(1):209–16.
15. Tetrault JM, Crothers K, Moore BA, Mehra R, Concato J, Fiellin DA. Effects of marijuana smoking on pulmonary function and respiratory complications: a systematic review. Arch Intern Med. 2008;167(3):221–8.
16. Tashkin DP, Simmons MS, Tseng CH. Impact of changes in regular use of marijuana and or/ tobacco on chronic bronchitis. COPD. 2012;9(4):367–74.
17. Pletcher MJ, Vittinghoff E, Kalhan R, Richman J, Safford M, Sidney S, Ling F, Keresz S. Association between marijuana exposure and pulmonary function tests over 20 years. JAMA. 2012;307(2):173–81.
18. Aldington S, Williams M, Nowitz M, Weatherall M, Pritchard A, McNaughton A, Robinson G, Beasley R. Effects of cannabis on pulmonary structure, function and symptoms. Thorax. 2007;62(12):1058–63.
19. Taylor DR, Fergusson DM, Milne BJ, Horwood LJ, Moffitt TE, Sears MR, Poulton R. A longitudinal study of the effects of tobacco and cannabis exposure on lung function in young adults. Addiction. 2002;97(8):1055–61.
20. Johnson MK, Smith RP, Morrison D, Laszlo G, White RJ. Thorax. 2000;55(4):340–2.
21. Beshay M, Kaiser H, Niedhart D, Remond MA, Smid RA. Emphysema and secondary pneumothorax in young adults smoking cannabis. Eur J Cardiothorac Surg. 2007;32:834–8.
22. Hatsukami DK, Fischman MW. Crack cocaine and cocaine hydrochloride. Are the differences myth or reality. JAMA. 1996;276(19):1580–8.
23. Kon OM, Redhead JB, Gillen D, Fothergill J, Henry JA, Mitchell DM. Crack lung caused by an impure preparation. Thorax. 1996;51:959–60.
24. Forrest JM, Steele AW, Waldron JA, Parsons PE. Crack lung: an acute pulmonary syndrome with a spectrum of clinical and histopathological findings. Am Rev Respir Dis. 1990;142(2):462–7.
25. Restrepo CS, Carrillo JA, Martines S, Ojeda P, Rivera AL, Hatta A. Pulmonary complications from cocaine and cocaine-based substances: imaging manifestations. Radiographics. 2007;27:941–56.
26. Haim DY, Lippman ML, Goldberg SK, Walkenstein MD. The pulmonary complications of crack cocaine. A comprehensive review. Chest. 1995;107(1):233–40.
27. O'Donnell AE, Mappin FG, Sebo TJ, Tazelaar H. Interstitial pneumonitis associated with "crack" cocaine abuse. Chest. 1991;100(4):1155–7.
28. Abenheim L, Moride Y, Brenot F, Rich S, Benichou J, Kurz X, Higenbottam T, Oakley C, Wouters E, Aubier M, Simonneau G, Begaud B. Appetite-suppressant drugs and the risk of primary pulmonary hypertension. N Engl J Med. 1996;335:609–16.
29. Kershaw CD, Guidot DM. Alcoholic lung disease. NIAAA Publications. http://pubs.niaaa.nih.gov/publications/arh311/66-75.htm.
30. Kaphalia L, Calhoun WJ. Alcoholic lung injury: metabolic, biochemical and immunological aspects. Toxicol Lett. 2013;222(2):171–9.
31. Buster MCA, Rook L, Van BRussel GHA, van Ree J. Chasing the dragon, related to the impaired lung function among heroin users. Drug Alcohol Depend. 2002;68(2):221–8.

Chapter 40
Medically Supervised Withdrawal for Opioid Dependence

Sanford M. Silverman

Key Points

- Overuse and abuse of prescription opioids
- Opioid dependence
- Medical treatment of opioid withdrawal
- Opioid withdrawal neurochemistry: noradrenergic (autonomic)
- Opioid withdrawal neurochemistry: dopaminergic (affective)
- Clonidine
- Naltrexone
- Ultra rapid opioid withdrawal
- Opioid agonist therapy (OAT)
- Buprenorphine and precipitated withdrawal
- Patient selection
- Stages of change
- Initial assessment
- Induction
- Maintenance
- Withdrawal without maintenance
- Use in pregnancy

Opium from the poppy has been cultivated for thousands of years. Many ancient civilizations utilized opium for pain relief and to allow surgeons to treat patients. Opium was utilized in ancient Sumeria in 3400 BC and by the Egyptians in 1300 BC. Hippocrates documented the pain killing narcotic in 460 BC. The word "narcotic" is derived from ancient Greek "to benumb." Opium was widely utilized in its

S.M. Silverman, M.D. (✉)
Comprehensive Pain Medicine, Florida Society of Interventional Pain Physicians (FSIPP),
100 East Sample Rd., Ste 200, Pompano Beach, FL 33064, USA
e-mail: sanfordsilverman@cpmedicine.com

© Springer Science+Business Media New York 2015
A.D. Kaye et al. (eds.), *Substance Abuse*, DOI 10.1007/978-1-4939-1951-2_40

unprocessed form through the mid-nineteenth century, until morphine was isolated. This led to a variety of semisynthetic and synthetic derivatives which are used today.

In the nineteenth century, Britain suppressed China to allow the continued widespread distribution of opium throughout that country. This led to two opium wars in 1839 and 1858. After 1860, opium use continued to increase with widespread domestic production in China, until more than 25 % of the male population was regular consumers by 1905. Recreational or addictive opium use in other nations however remained rare into the late nineteenth century. Opium was very popular among nineteenth century authors such as John Keats and Elizabeth Barrett Browning.

Opium was prohibited in many countries during the early twentieth century. This led to the modern pattern of opium production, which also was a precursor for tightly regulated legal prescription drugs and illegal recreational drug use.

Afghanistan is the principal site for the illicit production of opium. This was decimated in 2000 when the ruling Taliban banned its use. Its production has steadily increased since the USA led war in Afghanistan resulted in the fall of the Taliban in 2001.

Historically, opioid dependence in the USA has been a public health problem for most of the twentieth century. Before the Harrison Narcotic Act of 1914 was enacted, physicians could prescribe opioids for any condition, including opioid dependence. In 1919, the US Supreme Court ruled that the Harrison Act disallowed prescription of opioids for maintenance purposes (opioid dependence), which effectively ended opioid-based treatment for addiction.

After World War I, many cities established maintenance clinics for opioid addiction in response to a huge wave of heroin addicts. New York City pioneered efforts to engage the treatment of more than 8,000 addicts through its health department.

Unfortunately, these clinics were forced to close with the passage of the Harrison Act. From the 1920s forward, physicians were discouraged from treating opioid addiction, and it was reconceptualized as a criminal rather than a medical problem.

Interestingly enough, a parallel epidemic of cocaine abuse occurred within the USA in the late 1800s. Cocaine was originally synthesized in 1860, followed by amphetamine in 1887. In 1909 the International Opium Commission was established to regulate narcotics. In 1919 methamphetamine was synthesized and in the 1930s, the Benzedrine inhaler became available and was quickly abused. It was ultimately banned in the 1950s.

It was not until the 1970s when opioid addiction was addressed at the federal level with methadone regulations (21 CFR Part 291) in 1972 and the Narcotic Addict Treatment Act of 1974, which created federal and state licensed methadone clinics.

A physician who wishes to treat opioid addiction with methadone must obtain additional registration from the Drug Enforcement Administration (DEA) and the Department of Health and Human Services, with additional approval from state authorities, thus creating an intimidating beaurocratic gauntlet that few physicians are willing to negotiate.

The Drug Addiction Treatment Act (DATA) of 2000, an amendment to the Controlled Substances Act, allows certified physicians to prescribe and dispense Schedule III, IV, and V narcotic drugs that have been approved by the Food and Drug Administration (FDA) for use in addiction treatment (i.e., maintenance or medical withdrawal/detoxification). In October 2002, the FDA approved Schedule III sublingual buprenorphine tablets for the treatment of opioid dependence.

Prior to the use of buprenorphine for the treatment of opioid dependence, only methadone or Levo-alpha-acetylmethanol (LAAM) where approved for in the USA. Eventually LAAM was replaced solely by methadone, and outpatient treatment clinics were restricted to methadone as the sole opioid agonist for the treatment of dependence.

The USA is suffering again from an opioid epidemic; prescription drug abuse. As it is said, history repeats itself.

Overuse and Abuse of Prescription Opioids

The global epidemic of chronic pain and disability led to the explosion of prescription opioid use and abuse [1]. The sales of opioid analgesics quadrupled between 1999 and 2010. Hydrocodone sales increased by 280 % from 1997 to 2007, while methadone usage increased 1,293 %, and oxycodone usage increased by 866 % [2]. The estimated number of prescriptions filled for opioids exceeded 256 million in the USA in 2009 [3, 4].

Hydrocodone with acetaminophen was the number one prescription in the USA from 2006 through 2011 [5]. In addition, a UN report illustrated that the US population, constituting 4.6 % of the world's population consumed 83 % of the world's oxycodone and 99 % of hydrocodone in 2007 [6]. In the state of Florida, over 9.2 million units of oxycodone were dispensed from physician's offices in the 6 months between the months of October 2008 and March 2009. During the same time period, of the top 50 US physicians *dispensing* oxycodone from their offices, 49 were in Florida [7]. In a nationwide comparison of oxycodone purchases by practitioners between January and June 2010, Florida saw over 41 million units purchased compared to 1.1 million units for the remaining states [8].

Opioid Dependence

Opioid dependence is often preceded by opioid abuse, the former being a more serious condition. The DSM IV criteria for both are as follows:

Opioid Abuse

- One or more of the following in a 12-month period
  - Failure to fulfill major role obligations at work, school, or home
  - Recurrent substance use in situations in which it is physically hazardous

- Current substance-related legal problems (e.g., arrests for substance-related disorderly conduct)
- Continued substance use despite having persistent or recurrent social or interpersonal problems caused or exacerbated by the effects of the substance

Opioid Dependence

- More than three of the following during last 12 months:

  - Tolerance
  - Withdrawal syndrome
  - Larger amounts/longer period intended
  - Inability to/persistent desire to cut down or control
  - Increased amount of time spent in activities necessary to obtain opioids
  - Social, occupational, and recreational activities given up or reduced
  - Opioid use is continued despite adverse consequences

The disease of addiction is a complex interaction between genetic, biological, environmental, and psychosocial factors. It is defined (abridged version) as follows [9]:

- Addiction is a primary, chronic disease of brain reward, motivation, memory, and related circuitry.
- Dysfunction in these circuits leads to characteristic biological, psychological, social, and spiritual manifestations.
- This is reflected in an individual pathologically pursuing reward and/or relief by substance use and other behaviors.
- Addiction is characterized by the inability to consistently abstain, impairment in behavioral control, craving, diminished recognition of significant problems with one's behaviors and interpersonal relationships, and a dysfunctional emotional response.
- Like other chronic diseases, addiction often involves cycles of relapse and remission.
- Without treatment or engagement in recovery activities, addiction is progressive and can result in disability or premature death.

Medical Treatment of Opioid Withdrawal

Opioid withdrawal or abstinence syndrome is a normal physiologic effect which occurs with abrupt cessation, usually after prolonged administration. It is variable in its presentation, with some patients exhibiting little to no symptoms. Withdrawal implies physical dependence, which is natural physiologic response to many pharmacologic agents. Many people experience headache and lethargy upon cessation of caffeinated beverages (coffee, etc.). Serious withdrawal can also occur to selective serotonin reuptake inhibitors (paroxetine).

The signs and symptoms of opioid withdrawal are:

- Dysphoric mood
- Nausea and vomiting
- Muscle aches
- Lacrimation or rhinorrhea
- Pupillary dilation, piloerection, or sweating
- Diarrhea
- Yawning
- Fever
- Insomnia

The symptoms of dysphoria and anhedonia truly drive the disease of addiction. In addition, environmental, genetic, and psychosocial factors play major roles.

Opioid Withdrawal Neurochemistry: Noradrenergic (Autonomic)

Opioids acutely depress norepinephrine activity in Locus Coeruleus. Tolerance develops with chronic use and up regulation of central noradrenergic activity occurs. There is also decreased efficacy (less analgesia) at mu receptor via uncoupling and protein kinase inhibition.

Withdrawal results in increased in adrenergic (autonomic) activity with elevations in blood pressure, heart rate, peristalsis, diaphoresis, myalgias, sweating, piloerection, and increased CNS irritability.

Opioid Withdrawal Neurochemistry: Dopaminergic (Affective)

Opioids acutely raise dopamine levels in mesolimbic pathway. Tolerance develops with chronic use and dopamine levels and transmission decrease over time. Dopamine is the neurotransmitter which mediates pleasure and hedonic tone.

Withdrawal (affective) results in low levels of dopamine transmission leading to anhedonia, dysphoria, and depression.

The pharmacologic treatment of opioid withdrawal involves use of medications which target different areas of the nervous system to modulate both be autonomic and affective symptoms. These medications include:

- Opioids which are less euphorigenic that are substituted for the abused drug; Opioid Agonist Therapy; OAT (methadone, buprenorphine)
- Benzodiazepines as adjunctive agents to reduce the anxiety component of withdrawal (diazepam, lorazepam, alprazolam, etc.)

- Agents which reduce the central hyperadrenergic response mediated through Locus Coeruleus (clonidine)
- Opioid antagonists to treat craving and maintain abstinence (naloxone, naltrexone)
- Antidiarrheals and antiemetics for associated symptoms

Clonidine

Clonidine is an alpha-2 adrenergic agonist which binds to presynaptic receptors on adrenergic neurons. Specifically, these are located in the Locus Coeruleus and possibly in the A1 and A2 cell groups of the medulla that project to the extended amygdala. Clonidine is FDA approved for the treatment of hypertension. Its major limiting side effect is hypotension.

Clonidine has been shown to significantly reduce the autonomic symptoms of opioid withdrawal and to be significantly better than placebo and nearly comparable to a slow methadone taper [10]. It has been the most commonly used approach over the past 20 years and does not require a physician to meet specific legal requirements, as does methadone and buprenorphine.

The dosing of clonidine starts at 0.1–0.4 mg every 4–6 h as needed for withdrawal symptoms. Typically the dose is increased until the patient experiences orthostatic hypotension or diastolic blood pressure below 60 mm. Antiemetics and antidiarrheals may also be utilized to treat associated withdrawal symptoms.

Naltrexone

The concept of using a pure opioid mu receptor antagonist is that all clinical effects of the mu receptor are blocked. In other words, the patient will not experience euphoria or elevation of hedonic tone. Once the patient is detoxified from the opioid (5–7 days for short-acting opioids, 7–10 days for long-acting agents), a challenge dose of antagonist is given to determine if withdrawal occurs. If not, the patient is then maintained on naltrexone to suppress cravings and other signs and symptoms of opioid dependence.

In general this technique demonstrates poor patient compliance but may be effective in certain selected patient populations, such as professionals (physicians, attorneys, etc.) where the consequences of relapse are quite high. In these groups it may represent the best method of maintenance therapy.

Dosing of naltrexone starts at 25 mg per day and may be increased a maximum of 100 mg daily. An intramuscular formulation of naltrexone approved in 2010 (Vivitrol® Alkermes, Inc.) may be administered on a monthly basis.

Ultra Rapid Opioid Withdrawal

This technique involves administering opioid antagonists intravenously (naloxone) to provoke withdrawal, usually under anesthesia. The emergent symptoms are treated with other medications such as clonidine, benzodiazepines, antiemetics, and antidiarrheals. Withdrawal essentially resolves in 2–3 days with the patient on a full dose of antagonist (naltrexone). This technique remains controversial as there are few well-designed clinical studies to support its use. However, it may be justifiable in certain healthy patients who cannot undergo long-term detoxification based on logistical concerns. It may facilitate rapid conversion to naltrexone for maintenance but is not without.

Opioid Agonist Therapy

Methadone

Methadone is given in liquid form once or twice daily, either observed or with take-home doses. The goal is to suppress withdrawal and cravings. Maintenance dosing can be performed on an indefinite basis.

Methadone is very inexpensive. It is metabolized primarily by the 3A4 and secondarily by the 2D6 cytochrome P450 system in the liver. The L-isomer provides analgesic and sedative effects. The D-isomer is an NMDA receptor antagonist and may provide a certain niche treatment for difficult to treat chronic pain conditions, such as neuropathic pain.

Liquid methadone has a slow onset of action but is rapidly absorbed orally. The half-life of methadone is quite variable and ranges from 24 to 150 h depending on the dose. The average daily dose of liquid methadone in the USA for the treatment of opioid dependence is 80–120 mg.

The metabolism of methadone may be affected by certain inhibitors and inducers of the CYP3A4 system (Table 40.1).

A potentially lethal side effect of methadone has been reported involving prolongation of the QT interval. Specifically, this is a dose-dependent phenomenon and severe ventricular arrhythmias such as Torsades de Pointes have been reported. Since methadone has a long plasma half-life, it may accumulate. Furthermore, the use of a CYP 3A4 inhibitors increase the risk of this arrhythmia. Potential factors that may predispose patients to Torsades de Pointes include preexisting bradycardia, congenital QT prolongation, hypokalemia, and concomitant use of medications inducing QT prolongation.

Clinical experience demonstrates that methadone requires multiple doses throughout the day to treat chronic pain. The analgesic half-life (approximately 6–8 h) appears to be much less than the plasma half-life. When using methadone for chronic pain control, one must also recognize that it demonstrates incomplete cross-tolerance with other opioids. Specifically, the dose of methadone (with respect to morphine equivalents) is not constant and varies with dose (Table 40.2).

Table 40.1 Substrates, inhibitors and inducers of the CYP 2D6 and 3A4 enzymes

Enzyme	Substrates	Inhibitors	Inducers
CYP2D6	Amitriptyline, buproprion, clomipramine, clozapine, clonazepam, codeine, clonazepam, codeine, desipramine, dextromethorphan, doxepin, fluoxetine, haloperidol, hydrocodone, imipramine, methadone, modafinil, morphine, nortriptyline, olanzapine, oxycodone, paroxetine, sertraline, tiagabine, tramadol, venlafaxine	Citalopram (weak), desipramine, fluoxetine, olanzapine (weak), paroxetine, sertraline, venlafaxine (weak)	Carbamazepine, phenobarbital, phenytoin
CYP3A4	Alfentanil, alprazolam, amitriptyline, buproprion, citalopram, clozapine, cyclosporine, dexamethasone, dextromethorphan, etoposide, fentanyl, fluoxetine, ifosfamide, imipramine, ketamine, lidocaine, meperidine, modafinil, paclitaxel, prednisone, sertraline, tamoxifen, tiagabine, venlafaxine, vincristine	Dexamethasone, dextromethorphan, fluoxetine, paroxetine (weak), sertraline, venlafaxine	Carbamazepine, dexamethasone, erythromycin, modafinil, phenobarbital, phenytoin

Table 40.2 Incomplete cross tolerance of methadone in pain medicine

Initial dose of morphine (mg)	Ratio morphine/methadone
30–90	4:1
91–300	8:1
>300	12:1

Modified from Ripamonti C, Zecca E, Bruera E.An update on the clinical use of methadone for cancer pain. Pain. 1997 Apr;70(2–3):109–15 [22]

30 mg MSO_4 ~ 7 mg methadone
300 mg MSO_4 ~ 40 mg methadone
400 mg MSO_4 ~ 30 mg methadone

Buprenorphine

Naturally occurring opiates from the poppy include morphine, codeine, and thebaine. Buprenorphine is a thebaine derivative. It is a synthetic opioid which has certain unique properties which make it ideal for the treatment of opioid dependency. Specifically buprenorphine:

- Is highly potent
- Is an antagonist at the kappa opioid receptor
- Is a partial agonist at the mu opioid receptor
- Has an extremely high affinity for the mu receptor, binding more tightly than other opioids or opioid antagonists
- Slowly dissociates from the mu receptor with milder withdrawal symptoms

Buprenorphine is poorly absorbed orally with an extensive first pass effect. However, buprenorphine has excellent sublingual and transdermal absorption, and thus better bioavailability (refer to Fig. 23.1).

Since buprenorphine has *less* activity at the mu receptor, it is referred to as a partial agonist. Specifically, buprenorphine has a ceiling effect with respect to analgesia, respiratory depression, and other opioid side effects. This accounts for its milder withdrawal symptoms.

Buprenorphine is also an antagonist at the kappa opioid receptor, which may provide a unique role in treating opioid induced hyperalgesia and significant opioid tolerance [11]. Buprenorphine is FDA approved for the treatment of opioid dependence in its sublingual form (generic, and Subutex® [Reckitt Benckiser Group]) and in a 4:1 ratio to naloxone (Suboxone® [Reckitt Benckiser Group]). Zubsolv® (Orexo AB) tablets are a naloxone combination product available in September 2013.

Buprenorphine is commercially available to treat pain as parenteral formulation (Buprenex® [Reckitt Benckiser Group]) and as a transdermal formulation (Butrans® [Purdue Pharma L.P.]). It should be noted that the only legally approved form of buprenorphine for the treatment of opioid dependence is the sublingual form.

In 2000 the US Congress passed the DATA which permits qualified physicians to obtain a waiver from the separate registration requirements of the Narcotic Addict Treatment Act of 1974 to treat opioid addiction with Schedule III, IV, and V opioid medications or combinations of such medications. These medications have been specifically approved by the FDA for such indication.

For the treatment of opioid dependence, both the medication and the practitioner must meet certain requirements. Requirements for the practitioner are listed below:

1. The physician holds a subspecialty board certification in addiction psychiatry from the American Board of Medical Specialties.
2. The physician holds an addiction certification from the American Society of Addiction Medicine.
3. The physician holds a subspecialty board certification in addiction medicine from the American Osteopathic Association.
4. The physician has completed not less than 8 h of training with respect to the treatment and management of opioid-addicted patients. This training can be provided through classroom situations, seminars at professional society meetings, electronic communications, or otherwise. The training must be sponsored by one of five organizations authorized in the DATA 2000 legislation to sponsor such training, or by any other organization that the Secretary of the Department of Health and Human Services (the Secretary) determines to be appropriate.
5. The physician has participated as an investigator in one or more clinical trials leading to the approval of a narcotic drug in Schedule III, IV, or V for maintenance or detoxification treatment, as demonstrated by a statement submitted to the Secretary by the sponsor of such approved drug.
6. The physician has other training or experience, considered by the State medical licensing board (of the State in which the physician will provide maintenance or detoxification treatment) to demonstrate the ability of the physician to treat and manage opioid-addicted patients.

7. The physician has other training or experience the Secretary considers demonstrates the ability of the physician to treat and manage opioid-addicted patients.

Once these criteria are met, the physician may apply to obtain a waiver from the DEA and SAMHSA/CSAT (Substance Abuse and Mental Health Services Administration/Center for Substance Abuse Treatment). Upon submission (Notification of intent to use Schedule III, IV, or V Drugs For Maintenance And Detoxification Treatment Of Opiate Addiction; Under 21 USC 823(g)(2)) SAMHSA/CSAT has 45 days to determine if the physician meets the requirements. The DEA then assigns an "X number" to the physician, in addition to their standard DEA number, which allows them to prescribe controlled substances for the treatment of opioid dependence established by DATA 2000. Physicians may treat up to 30 patients for opioid dependence with sublingual buprenorphine. As of 2007, a physician can treat up to 100 patients with secondary notification to SAMHSA/CSAT.

Only specific formulations of buprenorphine can be utilized under DATA 2000. It is illegal to use Buprenex® to treat opioid dependence. Sublingual buprenorphine is the *only* schedule III drug currently approved by the FDA to treat opioid dependence established by law under DATA 2000.

Prior to its use in the USA, buprenorphine in its sublingual form was used very successfully in Europe for the treatment of opioid addiction. Unfortunately, the single component formulation was also illicitly abused in Europe, in particular Great Britain, which prompted the combined formulation, (which deters abuse) widely utilized in the USA.

Over 10 years of clinical research have supported the use of buprenorphine and its combination with naloxone as an alternative to methadone. It is also quite safe exhibiting a ceiling effect on respiratory depression. The therapeutic index of buprenorphine is relatively high (refer to Table 23.2).

Buprenorphine and Precipitated Withdrawal

Buprenorphine has a very high affinity for the mu receptor. It competes and subsequently displaces full opioid agonists from the mu receptor. Buprenorphine also has a lower intrinsic activity than a full agonist. When administered to a patient physically dependent on a full agonist, this reduced mu receptor activity is experienced by the patient as withdrawal. Therefore, if a patient is currently using a full mu agonist and is *not* in withdrawal, the administration of buprenorphine will *precipitate* withdrawal. Hence, patients must be in some degree opioid withdrawal in order to be treated with buprenorphine (refer to Fig. 23.2).

Patient Selection

Not all patients are appropriate for office-based medically supervised withdrawal using sublingual buprenorphine. Relative contraindications to its use in this setting include poly-substance abuse, history of multiple relapses, poor compliance, poor psychosocial functioning, and medical instability. Absolute contraindications to the use of buprenorphine include severe side effects from previous exposure or hypersensitivity to naloxone.

In addition, the patient must present in the preparation or action phase in the *stages of change*.

Stages of Change

The Stages of Change Model was originally developed in the late 1970s and early 1980s by James Prochaska and Carlo DiClemente at the University of Rhode Island [12]. They were studying how smokers were able to cope with their nicotine dependence.

This model involves six stages that take a person from the beginning, learning to identify a problem, and to the end, living without that problem (Fig. 40.1). The model provides a behavioral road map for addiction, and assists these patients to recognize their place in the change process.

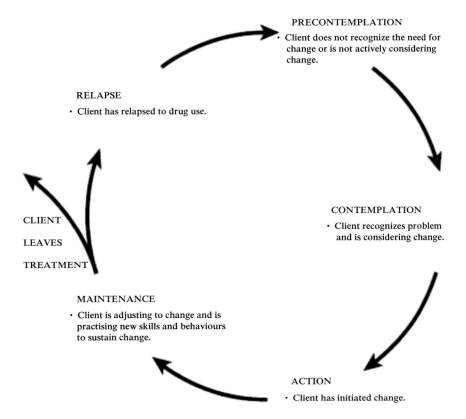

Fig. 40.1 Overview of the stages of change. Modified from Prochaska, J.O. and DiClemente, C.C. Transtheoretical therapy: Toward a more integrative model of change. Modified from *Psychotherapy: Theory, Research and Practice 1982; 19 (3); 276–288* [13]

The Stages of Change are:

1. Pre-contemplation
2. Contemplation
3. Determination
4. Action
5. Maintenance, relapse, recycle
6. Termination

Pre-contemplation

In this stage, an individual may not even recognize that he or she has a problem. Patients are not yet thinking about changing their behavior directly, and may believe that other people are overreacting to them and their behaviors. Patients can be in this stage for decades.

Contemplation

The patient is open to consider that a problem exists, and that there may be a need to change. However a commitment to change has *not* yet been made; there is not yet direct action although one may undertake to learn more about the nature of their addiction.

Determination/Preparation

The patient makes a decision to stop using, to make a change.

Action

The patient recognizes and admits that a problem exists, and has developed a plan to make changes. They modify their behaviors, environment, relationships, and experiences to overcome the problem. They put the plan they made in the determination stage into action, such as enrolling in treatment.

Maintenance, Relapse, and Recycling

Change has been achieved—a pattern of addictive behaviors has been replaced with sobriety and strides into recovery. The patient recognizes the benefits of successful change. However, relapse is still a risk and the patient must continue in therapy.

Termination

At some point in the maintenance stage, the threat of relapse is reduced. When triggers arise, such as personal crisis or financial hardship, the person has a support system. Substances no longer emerge as a response to crisis.

Initial Assessment

A complete psychiatric and mental status examination should be done prior to treatment. A referral to the appropriate specialist/psychiatrist should be considered for any patient with a significant coexisting psychiatric disorder. The medical history should be carefully evaluated to include intravenous drug abuse, alcoholism, HIV and appropriate laboratory evaluation ordered.

Induction

Induction is the process by which the patient presents for administration of buprenorphine for medically supervised withdrawal. A determination must be made as to how the patient should discontinue their opioids so as to present in moderate withdrawal. This depends on whether the patient is using short-acting versus long-acting opioids. In general, long-acting opioids should be discontinued 24 h prior to induction and short-acting opioids approximately 12 h. The physician should also ascertain whether the patient has experienced withdrawal in the past and how soon these symptoms occur after stopping opioids. The Clinical Opiate Withdrawal Scale (COWS) [13] can be utilized to objectively quantify withdrawal status. The induction should not proceed until the patient is an adequate withdrawal (COWS = 8–11, Table 40.3).

The patient is instructed on proper sublingual administration. The dosing should begin at 2–4 mg, and a repeat assessment of COWS should be done approximately 1 h later. The dose may then be repeated and titrated to the severity of withdrawal symptoms. Most patients will respond to a maximum of 16 mg of sublingual buprenorphine during induction. At 16 mg, 75–95 % of the mu receptors are blocked by buprenorphine [14]. If precipitated withdrawal should occur, repeated doses of buprenorphine should be given until withdrawal symptoms abate (up to 32 mg).

Table 40.3 The Clinical Opioid Withdrawal Scale

Patient's Name:_____	Date: _____			
Buprenorphine induction:				
Enter scores at time zero, 30 min after first dose, 2 h after first dose, etc.				
Times:	_____	_____	_____	_____
Resting Pulse Rate: (record beats per minute)				
Measured after patient is sitting or lying for one minute				
0 pulse rate 80 or below				
1 pulse rate 81–100				
2 pulse rate 101–120				
4 pulse rate greater than 120				
Sweating: *over past ½ hour not accounted for by room temperature or patient activity.*				
0 no report of chills or flushing				
1 subjective report of chills or flushing				
2 flushed or observable moistness on face				
3 beads of sweat on brow or face				
4 sweat streaming off face				
Restlessness *Observation during assessment*				
0 able to sit still				
1 reports difficulty sitting still, but is able to do so				
3 frequent shifting or extraneous movements of legs/arms				
5 Unable to sit still for more than a few seconds				
Pupil size				
0 pupils pinned or normal size for room light				
1 pupils possibly larger than normal for room light				
2 pupils moderately dilated				
5 pupils so dilated that only the rim of the iris is visible				
Bone or Joint aches *If patient was having pain previously, only the additional component attributed to opiates withdrawal is scored*				
0 not present				
1 mild diffuse discomfort				
2 patient reports severe diffuse aching of joints/ muscles				
4 patient is rubbing joints or muscles and is unable to sit still because of discomfort				
Runny nose or tearing *Not accounted for by cold symptoms or allergies*				
0 not present				
1 nasal stuffiness or unusually moist eyes				
2 nose running or tearing				
4 nose constantly running or tears streaming down cheeks				

(continued)

Table 40.3 (continued)

GI Upset: *over last ½ hour*				
0 no GI symptoms				
1 stomach cramps				
2 nausea or loose stool				
3 vomiting or diarrhea				
5 Multiple episodes of diarrhea or vomiting				
Tremor *observation of outstretched hands*				
0 No tremor				
1 tremor can be felt, but not observed				
2 slight tremor observable				
4 gross tremor or muscle twitching				
Yawning *Observation during assessment*				
0 no yawning				
1 yawning once or twice during assessment				
2 yawning three or more times during assessment				
4 yawning several times/min				
Anxiety or Irritability				
0 none				
1 patient reports increasing irritability or anxiousness				
2 patient obviously irritable anxious				
4 patient so irritable or anxious that participation in the assessment is difficult				
Gooseflesh skin				
0 skin is smooth				
3 piloerection of skin can be felt or hairs standing up on arms				
5 prominent piloerection				
Total scores				
Score: 5–12 = mild				
13–24 = moderate				
25–36 = moderately severe				
More than 36 = severe withdrawal				

From: Wesson DR, Ling W; The Clinical Opiate Withdrawal Scale (COWS); J Psychoactive Drugs 2003; 35: 253–259 [13]

Maintenance

Ideally most patients can be stabilized on once daily sublingual dosing with average doses quite variable (8–16 mg). As the patient is weaned down from the initial induction dose, dosing may shift to every other day to facilitate complete discontinuation of buprenorphine. The dosing may also be given 2–3 times daily, which is often effective in patients experiencing chronic pain, since the analgesic half-life of buprenorphine, like methadone is relatively short, approximately 6–8 h.

Maintenance follow-up visits should include assessment for intoxication, adverse events, cravings, concomitant use of other illicit/prescription drugs, and withdrawal symptoms. The use of urine drug testing can be very informative in this setting. Counseling and behavioral therapy are necessary integral components of any chemical dependency treatment program.

The objectives of maintenance treatment are to reduce the mortality from overdose and infection from needle use. The overall harm reduction provided by maintenance treatment includes the reduction of illicit/prescription drug use, HIV, HBV, HCV transmission, and drug-related crime. Overall, the goal is to improve the patient's general health and well-being, social functioning, and the ability to work.

Withdrawal Without Maintenance

In general, withdrawal without maintenance using OAT has poor clinical outcomes as opposed to a maintenance protocol with a gradual withdrawal program [15]. Patients will do better with a comprehensive psychosocial, vocational, and medical program.

Use in Pregnancy

The gold standard during pregnancy has always been methadone maintenance therapy, and then treatment of newborn for neonatal withdrawal. Medical detoxification during pregnancy may cause irreparable harm to the fetus and/or miscarriage. Sublingual buprenorphine without naloxone can be utilized for maintenance therapy during pregnancy. Due to the unknown effects of naloxone on the fetus, the combination formulation is a class C teratogen. Buprenorphine was compared to methadone for the treatment of opioid dependence during pregnancy with similar outcomes. However the newborns in the buprenorphine group displayed less required less morphine to treat neonatal abstinence syndrome, displaying less withdrawal symptoms [16].

Conclusion

Physicians treating opioid dependency must be familiar with the basic pharmacology of opioids and physiologic manifestations of withdrawal. This patient population is complex, and requires a comprehensive evaluation prior to treatment. There is a significant overlap of this population with those who have chronic pain [17]. These patients present a tremendous challenge to the health care system. Evidence-based studies have shown that OAT with methadone, and now with buprenorphine, combined with behavioral therapy can improve the success in the treatment of opioid dependence [18–21].

As prescription opioid abuse is addressed through legislative means and the availability of opioids is reduced, the treatment for these patients who are dependent becomes increasingly important for them. Society will benefit from the reductions in crime, infectious disease, and overutilization of health care costs.

References

1. Manchikanti L, et al. American Society of Interventional Pain Physicians (ASIPP) guidelines for responsible opioid prescribing in chronic non-cancer pain: part I—evidence assessment. Pain Physician. 2012;15:S1–66.
2. Manchikanti L, Fellows B, Ailinani H, Pampati V. Therapeutic use, abuse, and nonmedical use of opioids: a ten year perspective. Pain Physician. 2010;13:401–35.
3. Volkow ND, McLellan TA, Cotto JH. Characteristics of opioid prescriptions in 2009. JAMA. 2011;305:1299–301.
4. Governale L. Outpatient prescription opioid utilization in the U.S., years 2000–2009. Drug Utilization Data Analysis Team Leader, Division of Epidemiology, Office of Surveillance and Epidemiology. Presentation for U.S. Food and Drug Administration, 22 July 2010.
5. IMS Institute for Healthcare Informatics. The use of medicines in the United States: Review of 2011; April 2012.
6. Report of the International Narcotics Control Board 2008. New York: United Nations. 2009.www.incb.org/pdf/annual-report/2008/en/AR_08_English.pdf
7. Broward County Commission on Substance Abuse. Based on data from the Broward County Appraisal Office and Automation of Reports and Consolidated Orders System (ARCOS); 2009.
8. Automation of Reports and Consolidated Orders System (ARCOS). US Drug Enforcement Agency; 2010.
9. Adopted by the American Society of Addiction Medicine Board of Directors; 4/12/2011.
10. Gold M, Redmond DE, Kleber HD. Clonidine blocks acute opioid withdrawal symptoms. Lancet. 1978;1:929–30.
11. Silverman SM. Opioid induced hyperalgesia: clinical implications for the pain practitioner. Pain Physician. 2009;12:679–84.
12. Prochaska JO, DiClemente CC. Transtheoretical therapy: toward a more integrative model of change. Psychother Theory Res Pract. 1982;19(3):276–88.
13. Wesson DR, Ling W. The Clinical Opioid Withdrawal Scale. J Psychoactive Drugs. 2003;35:253–9.
14. Zubieta JK, et al. Buprenorphine-induced changes in mu-opioid receptor availability in male heroin-dependent volunteers: a preliminary study. Neuropsychopharmacology. 2000;23(3):326–34.
15. Kakko J, et al. Buprenorphine improved treatment retention in patients with heroin dependence. Lancet. 2003;361:662–8.
16. Jones HE, et al. Neonatal abstinence syndrome after methadone or buprenorphine exposure. N Engl J Med. 2010;363:2320–31.
17. Webster LR, Webster RM. Predicting aberrant behaviors in opioid-treated patients: preliminary validation of the opioid risk tool. Pain Med. 2005;6(6):432–42.
18. Mattick RP, Ali R, White JM, O'Brien S, Wolk S, Danz C. Buprenorphine versus methadone maintenance therapy: a randomized double-blind trial with 405 opioid-dependent patients. Addiction. 2003;98:441–52.
19. Ling W, et al. A multi-center randomized trial of buprenorphine-naloxone versus clonidine for opioid detoxification: findings from the National Institute on Drug Abuse Clinical Trials Network. Addiction. 2005;100:1090–100.
20. Ahmadi J, Ahmadi K, Ohaeri J. Controlled, randomized trial in maintenance treatment of intravenous buprenorphine dependence with naltrexone, methadone or buprenorphine: a novel study. Eur J Clin Invest. 2003;33:824–9.

21. Ling W, et al. Buprenorphine maintenance treatment of opiate dependence: a multicenter, randomized clinical trial. Addiction. 1998;93:475–86.
22. Ripamonti C, Zecca E, Bruera E. An update on the clinical use of methadone for cancer pain. Pain. 1997;70(2–3):109–15.

Chapter 41
Pain, Addiction, Depression (PAD): Assessment of Pain and Addiction, the Neurobiology of Pain

Hans C. Hansen

Key Points

- Where we are going and what is new
- Assumptions, chronic pain
- Assessment of pain and addiction, the neurobiology of pain
- Principles of pharmacology, PAD
- Pain, addiction, and depression, the sick neuron
- Assessment of pain, addiction, and depression
- Treatment of pain depression and addiction

Medicine requires observation to develop a diagnostic conclusion. Trending from the traditional concept of "stand by your diagnosis," physicians and providers are finding themselves much better suited to maintain a large differential diagnosis, and keep that differential diagnosis dynamic and fluid. We cannot see, touch, feel, or measure pain, and observation many times verifies reality. As pain is a subject of interpretation and a very personal experience, nowhere else in medicine will we be challenged with the assumption that what the patient is telling us is correct, and we have little opportunity to follow the timeline, or "the story," to a true point of validation. In other words, many times pain is just going to have to be assumed to be present, and the patient is telling you the correct information that the clinician needs to have to treat them effectively, in a safe and controlled environment. When controlled substances are used, however, the assumption that pain is present has to be weighed against the risk/reward benefit of a chosen therapy. We hope that that risk/reward benefit remains in both the provider's favor, as well as the patient's, but as is often the case, there is no perfect world. More often, the provider of care and the patient experience peaks and valleys of success and frustration [1].

H.C. Hansen, M.D. (✉)
The Pain Relief Center, Conover, NC, USA
e-mail: hhansen@painreliefcenters.com

© Springer Science+Business Media New York 2015
A.D. Kaye et al. (eds.), *Substance Abuse*, DOI 10.1007/978-1-4939-1951-2_41

To best plan for a patient's care, we look to the complex relationship that the brain has with the description of the patient reporting pain is present. Pain rarely stands alone. It is never "I hurt here, therefore my diagnosis is clear." The source of pathology is rarely treated by either special procedure or a pharmaceutical with a cure at hand. Pain is more complex than most maladies. The neurobiology of pain is becoming increasingly important to achieve a good outcome, with minimal risk, and positive reward. As we better understand fine points of the brain's intricacies and the interrelationships of its action, pain, and its neurobiological siblings, addiction and depression, behaviors and motivations of those in pain become a little easier to tolerate [2].

Where We Are Going and What Is New

What We Are

What we are is a complex interrelationship with our environment and genetics. We are all not alike, but we are not dissimilar either. We can learn from the old, and we can understand from the new. A sagittal section of the primitive brain of the rat looks actually very similar to the sagittal primitive human brain (Fig. 41.1). Pain is either acute or chronic, and when pain becomes the disease itself, it will become chronic. Acute pain occurs chronically, much as we see in those who suffer intermittent bouts of impairing back pain, and chronic pain occurs acutely.

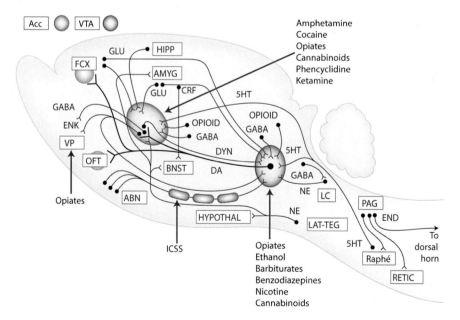

Fig. 41.1 A sagittal section of the primitive brain of the rat looks actually very similar to the sagittal primitive human brain. Adopted from ASAM Review 2014

As chronic pain becomes a part of the person's life, the complex interrelationships with the primitive brain structures divulge common denominators. The lines begin to blur. Pain interrelates to the sections in the brain that are associated with depression, and as the medications used to desperately treat this pain are exposed to certain brain structures, habituation and dependence turns into addiction. Addiction and pain share many of the common threads and pathways in the primitive brain. It is not common sense anymore. When the brain is hijacked, and chronic pain has evolved into the neurobiology of an individual seeking medications for relief, only to find that it isn't the medications anymore, it's the anxiety, the situational depression, and the need for a release from a torment stimulating the reward pathway is soothing and reinforcing. This is the point where pain, addiction, and depression (PAD) finds its common points of relevance.

Assumptions, Chronic Pain

To treat chronic pain a number of assumptions are made. First the physician understands the risk in management of chronic pain, and understands the interrelationships of PAD. Persistent failure of the physician to treat PAD is a poor medical practice, and conversely, failure to prescribe medications to treat these maladies when indicated is also poor medical practice. As common as chronic pain is to the general population, being the most frequent complaint to a physician's office, it is ironic that physicians and providers traditionally receive little or no education about management of PAD [3–5]. This leaves pain undertreated, depression and anxiety interfering with even normal activities of daily living, and the resultant potential for addiction. Failure to treat pain results from the fear of patient harm, and to the fear of regulatory legal or licensing penalties. Treating the pain also stirs up fears of supporting addiction, or allowing an individual to divert or misuse medication [6]. When PAD is undertreated, this fallacy of false generalization leads to invalid diagnostic assumptions such as pseudoaddiction. Pseudoaddiction is really a pseudoreality and antiquated terminology still used today [7, 8]. The feeling that the patient needs more pain medication because they are undertreated, the basis of this concept, pseudoaddiction leads the physician down a rabbit hole, where the drug is now the addicts tool. The original assumptions of pseudoaddiction, when examined, were not based on evidence, or a true expression of reality, but more of an "I think it therefore it is" conclusion. Unfortunately, the patient suffers. By the tip of the pen, the physician has introduced a drug with risk, to a patient population that is vulnerable, fostered by little training, even less evidence, and the drug with risk now, yielding no reward. The patient is walked up the stairs to iatrogenic addiction, and the clinician has given him the keys to the kingdom. It isn't just opioids; it is also central nervous system depressants, stimulants, and the ever present benzodiazepine, that is as much of a drug of crisis as opioids. 6.4 million use psychotherapeutic drugs nonmedically, 4.7 use pain relievers, 1.8 million use tranquilizers, 1.1 million use stimulants, and rising, and 272,000 use sedatives. These numbers vary widely through different reporting and tracking entities, but facts are facts (Box 41.1) [9–11]. Toxic drug exposure is now an epidemic.

Box 41.1: Chronic Pain: Most Abused Prescription Drugs

Most abused prescription drugs

- Opioids
- Central nervous system depressants
- Stimulants

Prescription drug use is on the rise, and the problems that go with prescription drug use, including death, is tracking right with them. It behooves the treating physician who is holding the tip of the pen, to understand that chronic pain isn't just a process where a part of something hurts from the outside in, but is a process that actually "rewires" the nervous system to continue sending signals after the original cause has been healed or removed. The resultant anxiety, depression, insomnia, that make this pain unbearable, is an expected comorbidity [12, 13]. It isn't undertreatment, in many cases, it is mistreatment, with good intent intact. Physicians are charged with treating the patient, but first do no harm. If the latter has been introduced into the community of standard of care, we must treat pain. A physician is often pressured, even bullied into a prescription. The clinician feels painted into a corner. Damned if I do, damned if I don't. Therefore, the physician is best suited by following rules, procedure, protocol, whatever it needs to be called. Here are five.

1. Pain is a description, not an entity
   Pain is an unpleasant sensory/emotional experience based on actual or potential tissue damage. (Merskey: Classification of pain).
   Pain is a very subjective interpretation of an event, or an occurrence, that is interpreted in some part of the brain as pain. It is variable to humans at all levels, and at all ages. There is no good way to measure it, and we do not have reliable tools to do so. Functional indices help, but pain is really biopsychosocial. We can also add the religious influence in certain communities. The Venn Diagram is mind numbing (Fig. 41.2). Within the psychological capacity there are genetic factors, somatoform disorders, personality disorders, and atypical stress responses. Depression cannot be separated from the anxiety, much like it can't be separated from pain and addiction, neurobiologically and by life experience. The associated environmental circumstances of drug use are also associated with poverty, child abuse, unemployment, and peer pressure. The genetic vulnerability is punctuated by family history of addiction, personality disorders, and gene variants associated with risk taking and impulsivity (called the initiation phase). Atypical stress responses lead to poor drug disposition, and the pharmacokinetic genes affecting drug metabolism and transport are also interrelated. Pharmacodynamic genes affecting pain and analgesic responses, as well as the potential for dependence and addiction that follows, are now measured to some degree, but an understanding of how they relate to the relevance of our clinical practice is still evolving. When we initiate drug therapy, we stimulate reward circuitry in the mesocorticolimbic system. The method we give these drugs also plays an important role. Is it IV, is it

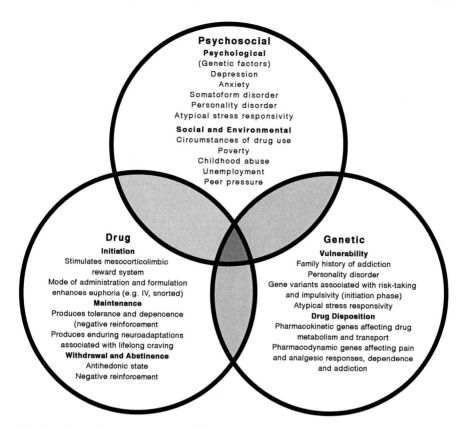

Psychosocial
Psychological
(Genetic factors)
Depression
Anxiety
Somatoform disorder
Personality disorder
Atypical stress responsivity
Social and Environmental
Circumstances of drug use
Poverty
Childhood abuse
Unemployment
Peer pressure

Drug
Initiation
Stimulates mesocorticolimbic
reward system
Mode of administration and formulation
enhances euphoria (e.g. IV, snorted)
Maintenance
Produces tolerance and depencence
(negative reinforcement
Produces enduring neuroadaptations
associated with lifelong craving
Withdrawal and Abstinence
Antihedonic state
Negative reinforcement

Genetic
Vulnerability
Family history of addiction
Personality disorder
Gene variants associated with risk-taking
and impulsivity (initiation phase)
Atypical stress responsivity
Drug Disposition
Pharmacokinetic genes affecting drug
metabolism and transport
Pharmacodynamic genes affecting pain
and analgesic responses, dependence
and addiction

Fig. 41.2 Venn diagram of psychological, environmental, and genetic factors associated with pain. Adopted from ASAM Review 2014

transmucosal, or a pill. Each is important in risk to misuse or abuse stratification. Once a drug is regularly used, the concept of tolerance, dependence, and addiction are followed by neuroadaptive changes in the brain, "rewiring," that can follow an individual for life. There is no cure for addiction, alcoholism, or drug abuse. It is merely managed. Pain is managed, as is depression, and the pathways associated with PAD close this loop. These biological pathways either enforce a positive state, or promote negative reinforcement, always avoiding the anhedonic state. Ultimately, the physician is pressured into the position of "prescribe change this to a period." PAD is not a traditional disease, we heal, but we do not cure.

2. You must have a diagnosis

The treatment of any disease state follows a diagnostic pathway that often leads to conclusion. Traditional medicine relies on the laboratory, imaging, physical exam, and the natural history of disease as it unveils itself to the practitioner. Pain is different. Pain is more of a process. There are no specific tests, and often the practitioner relies on clinical instinct, and weighs heavily on judgment. This is the exact reason that so many practitioners damage themselves and their practice by making bad decisions, most often with good intent. PAD requires well-developed judgment skills. The diagnosis of a painful entity is a complex interaction between the patient's historical elements, physical findings, and any other pieces that can be put together for the best assumptions of a cause and effect. This might include imaging, laboratory tests, and traditional strategies, but more than likely the personality of the patient will be the heaviest component of the diagnostic conclusion, one way or the other. We cannot see, touch, feel, or measure pain, and often the patient's self-descriptors are the best process we have. Variable treatment and the number of types of pain practitioners have flourished because of pain's elusive and subjective pathway. From massage therapists claiming to enhance blood flow and wash away toxins, to the chiropractic community that sees the malpositioning of the spine as a cause of maladies from ear infections, to chronic pain. Naturopaths claim pain within their scope of care.

All Specialties have an opinion. A naturopath will provide a patient with a completely inactive compound that is claimed to invoke a physiologic process, aimed at improving the well-being of the patient. Zero evidence-based documentation can be claimed, but ironically, positive results are occasionally obtained. The same holds true with acupuncture that is used in a variety of clinical settings and cannot be supported by evidence. This invokes the concept of "personality of pain." The process of pain, it's translation by the organism, and the effector processes, have a direct link to the limbic system. These interconnections, that play an important role in the diagnosis and treatment of virtually any painful condition. The personality of pain is defined by the individual that is stricken with the disease of question. The many responses to both personal impairment, and response to treatment, are interrelated with these complex neural pathways.

The greatest challenge any provider has that treats pain is finding a diagnosis. Pain is rarely a singular problem, but more of a confusing, often waxing and waning production of the central nervous system that is alive, and subject to neuroplastic changes. This is why pain is best treated "inside out" as opposed to "outside in". Peripheral manifestations of painful trigger points, the neuropathies, even neurohormonally driven pain states are commonly linked to the central nervous system. The flawed construct of managing a peripheral trigger point is more likely seen as aggravating a peripheral manifestation of a central nervous system event. Even referral patterns. For example, patients often believe that thoracic discomfort in the parascapular region is related to some type of thoracic problem when in fact, more likely a referred pattern from a lower cervical facet. The assumption is further supported by blocking that facet at the medial branch, alleviating some of the patient's pain [14]. This is how a pain practitioner is best suited to determine the diagnosis. Not by specific laboratory tests, per say, imaging, or a historical complaint, but embracing a pragmatic and thoughtful merging of judgment, experience, knowledge, and evidence based support. A strong diagnosis is necessary to treat any disease state, underscored by the personality of pain. Due to the central nervous influences, most pain is never stagnant. The previously expressed mantra, acute pain occurs chronically and chronic pain occurs acutely, expects pain to be unpredictable. With the central nervous system involved, it is not surprising that pain is often migratory, and never clearly defines its position.

Another problem with the diagnosis of the individual in pain is the necessity for regulatory and reimbursement institutions to understand medical decision-making. The mere act of writing a controlled substance requires a diagnosis, supported by the medical record, and which in turn displays historical and physical findings [6, 15]. When these are elusive, the diagnosis might come into question, adding an element of risk to the practitioner rendering care. Enhanced scrutiny comes to bear if the actions taken by the practitioner have little if any consistent clinical findings. Diagnosis such as fibromyalgia, interstitial cystitis, myofascial pain, and abdominal pain are a few examples of pain states that have virtually no consistent clinical findings. There will be reluctance to accept the judgment by the practitioner when the patient looks normal, and psychiatric overtones are assumed. The practitioner's judgment and compassion are unnecessarily scrutinized and dismissed. Evidence based guidelines, which are very important to make the right decisions in most cases, will be used against providers increasing the risk of audits, and the punishing regulatory influences that are mandated at the State and Federal level. Each provider is increasingly required to demonstrate a higher level of evidence for medical decision-making. Tender points, perceived radiculopathies, neuropathies with poor sensory documentation will start to feel pushback, and access to care for many painful entities will be reduced or denied. This by no means implies that these diagnoses don't exist, but are considered "unimportant" because they aren't maiming or killing people. Therein lies the pain provider's paradox. Clear, concise documentation, to support a position that can only be vaguely described by the less informed, presented to uninterested or financially pressured institutions, to effect what is right for the patient, and avoid what is wrong for the physician and patient, denial of service.

Over the next few years, documentation will also require the provider to be digitally secured. The medical record once told a story, the presentation of the disease and its course. The electronic health record is unlikely to do that. Pain providers will not have the opportunity to support their judgment and their diagnosis in the electronic health record unless care is exercised to ensure the proper information is introduced to the digital environment. Most health information systems are finding their way and are becoming more friendly. Likened to the early age of aviation, a great deal of standardization, cross talk, and cooperation will need to be introduced to the medical communities by the health record vendors. That is not taking place at this time. Although the will is there, and the mandates are evolving, it will be many years before EHR's look the same and provide the type of information over a standardized medical landscape. What is clear is that the pain provider's most important tool, a strong diagnosis, backed by valid information and good judgment is going to be more difficult to present, and support in the early transition to the digital landscape.

3. The Referral rule

Simply put, if you don't believe in a disease, or a diagnosis, you cannot treat it effectively. The complex and vague nature of pain requires a new way of presenting information, often bundled with neurobiological assumptions. Some believe fibromyalgia does exist. Possibly interstitial cystitis is not a bladder problem, but a peripheral manifestation of a central nervous system disease, much the way CRPS is. Inside out not outside in. Common features of situational anxiety and depression, mixed depressive disorder (MDD), and the resistance to treatment are common denominators, PAD. The lack of clear diagnostic criteria, and the confusion by practitioners across many specialties attributes to delayed diagnosis and treatment. In the case of interstitial cystitis, Hunner's ulcers may be present, or not, and fibromyalgia may meet criteria of the American Rheumatology Association, but it might not. If a provider needs to see, touch, feel, and measure the disease state, and does not render judgment as the most important diagnostic pathway in a pain practitioner's armamentarium, often these disease diagnoses will be brushed aside. When a pain practitioner uses terminology to describe their patient's personality, rather than structuring a diagnosis with the disease, treatment will be chaotic and without focus for example. Discounting an individual who has widespread pain, and is fatigued, demonstrating pelvic pain, frequent headaches, will miss the foundation of a diagnosis such as fibromyalgia. Fibromyalgia is a syndrome, it is not a disease, and this can be said about many of our pain diagnosis. A syndrome is a collection of problems, not a specific entity. We might find great success at treating headache, and muscle pain, less so abdominal pain, irritable bowel, or the pelvic pain comorbidities often accompanying fibromyalgia (The Fibro 5). Successful treatment of each of these states could greatly improve a person's quality of life. Furthermore, most pain problems are accompanied with situational depression and anxiety. Treating the depression and isolation of an individual suffering from CRPS will improve their peripheral manifestation of disease. A pain practitioner that does not assess the idiosyncrasies of his or her diagnosis, or cherry picks, does their patients no favor. It is easy to be lured into a practice of spine injections, no meds, and no complex chronic patients. Pain is too broad based. If the provider cannot recognize the need to offer diversified care, they need to refer that patient out.

4. Know Thy Meds. Pick five classes, pick five drugs

Thankfully, pain practitioners are being influenced less and less by pharma, and responsible prescribing is rarely motivated by industry association. Unfortunately, that is just part of the story. The specialty of pain medicine is often accused unjustly of initiating the opioid epidemic. Most controlled substances come out of the primary care field, and often by the time the pain practitioner absorbs the patient, opioids are either problematic, or on their way to being a focus in the patient's perceived required pain regimen. Opioids, benzodiazepines, and barbiturates are items of significant risk to a patient, and this risk poorly perceived by the medical community. The epidemic is by the tip of a pen, connected to an individual that believes a diagnosis is present, and driven by good judgment. In fact based on the root word, epidemic, judgment was lacking at the tip of that pen. Rarely is ill will the driving mechanism to poor prescriptive practice. Practitioners that are untrained in the management of pain often do not know about adjunctive medications which reduce the opioid load. A rich grasp of pharmacologic knowledge is imperative to sound treatment, and the pain practitioner is best suited to be the clinical pharmacologist. Understanding how medications work within their classes, and the expectations of treatment, is imperative, particularly when controlled substances are being used. Even noncontrolled medications have consequences attached to them. More people die from NSAID related causes than from HIV. Controlled substances add more risk. More people die from opioid related deaths in the USA than from motor vehicle accidents.

Principles of Pharmacology, PAD

The reaction of an agent at the cellular level is measured in time. This may range from milliseconds to hours. Channeled linked receptors which are ionotropic, hyperpolarize or depolarize a cell resulting in cellular effect. On the time scale this is measured in milliseconds. This would be typically a nicotinic acetylcholine receptor for example. Another rapid response occurs at the G protein coupled receptor, which is metabotropic, resulting in a second messenger protein phosphorylation. The resultant calcium release results in cellular effects, and is measured in minutes. Typically this would be muscarinic acetylcholine receptor. Kinase linked receptors such as an insulin receptor, phosphorylate protein, which then follows to cellular effect. Finally receptors to gene transcription (nuclear receptors) and messenger RNA synthesis, ultimately synthesize proteins, which can take hours and then result in cellular effect. An example would be an estrogen receptor (Fig. 41.3).

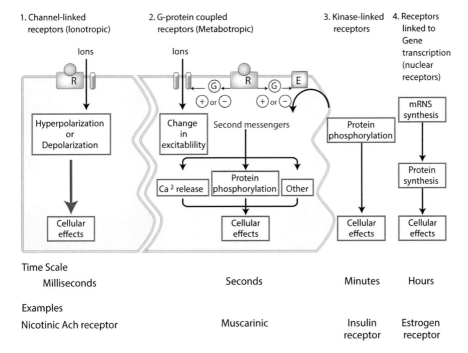

Fig. 41.3 Receptors to gene transcription and messenger RNA synthesis ultimately synthesize proteins, which can take hours to result in cellular effect; for example: estrogen receptor. From Ries RK, Fiellin DA, Miller SC, Saitz R, eds. Principles of Addiction Medicine, 4th ed. Philadelphia: Lippincott Williams & Wilking, 2009

Metabolism

The metabolism of drug is best understood by breaking down nomenclature in genes and pseudogenes. Termed CYP, the enzyme is first followed with the family letter, a subfamily letter, and then a form number. For example, CYP3a designates a metabolic pathway that results in metabolism of about 50 % of known drugs. There are 50 known cytochrome CYPP450 enzyme systems (Fig. 41.4). The enzymes are exposed to oxidation, or polarization, that may results in elimination (Fig. 41.5). Dissected, NADPH reduction to NADP by P450 reductase drives metabolism at P450 enzyme metabolizing drugs combining to hydrogen atoms with oxygen, and results in a water molecule. The most efficient system is in the liver, followed by lungs, GI, skin, and kidney (Fig. 41.6).

Elimination/Excretion

Elimination is a process of excretion of apparent drug/metabolite. Excretion results in removal of the drug or agent without changing the drug. Clearance on the other hand is a rate at which this occurs, with $T\frac{1}{2}$, being the half-life with 50 % change, in time, to or from a steady state. A steady state typically takes five half lives for a drug to obtain, and is a relatively level state (Box 41.2).

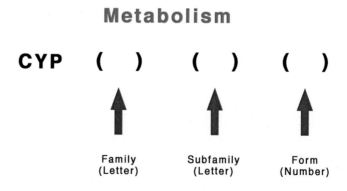

Fig. 41.4 The metabolism of drug is best understood by breaking down nomenclature in genes and pseudogenes. Termed CYP, the enzyme is first followed with the family letter, a subfamily letter, and then a form number. Adopted from ASAM Review 2014

Metabolism

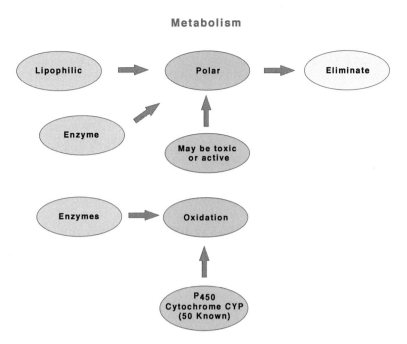

Fig. 41.5 The enzymes are exposed to oxidation, or polarization, that may results in elimination. Adopted from ASAM Review 2014

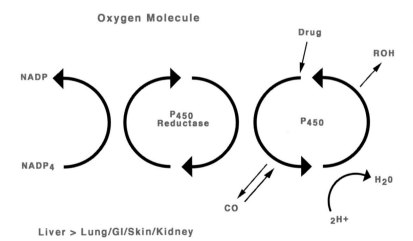

Fig. 41.6 Dissected, NADPH reduction to NADP by P450 reductase drives metabolism at P450 enzyme metabolizing drugs combining to hydrogen atoms with oxygen, and results in a water molecule. The most efficient system is in the liver, followed by lungs, GI, skin, and kidney. From Ries RK, Fiellin DA, Miller SC, Saitz R, eds. Principles of Addiction Medicine, 4th ed. Philadelphia: Lippincott Williams & Wilking, 2009

> **Box 41.2: Elimination/Secretion**
>
> *Elimination*—Metabolism or excretion of parent drug/metabolite
> *Excretion*—Removal without changing the drug
> *Clearance*—Rate that this occurs
> $t\frac{1}{2}$—half life, 50% change, in time, to or from steady state

Tolerance/Dependence (Fig. 41.7)

The concept of tolerance/dependence is important for the practitioner to understand if the drug chosen is useful, and if a response is normal to the drug. The concept of tolerance is a resultant effect of repeated use of an agent, which reduces its response. This is illustrated in a dose response curve. Normal response is left on the X axis, a tolerant individual, shifts the curve to the right. Movement of that curve one way or the other can result in either an adverse event or mortality, or in the case of dependence, shifting the curve to the left might result in withdrawal (Fig. 41.8). So a normal response to a drug does not necessarily result in tolerance or dependence, but this concept explains

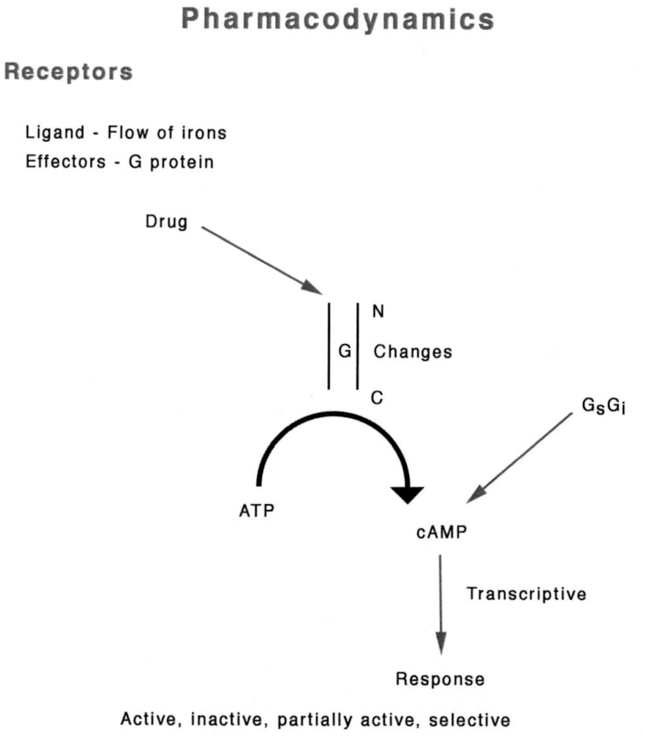

Fig. 41.7 Tolerance/dependence: pharmacodynamics. From Ries RK, Fiellin DA, Miller SC, Saitz R, eds. Principles of Addiction Medicine, 4th ed. Philadelphia: Lippincott Williams & Wilking, 2009

Tolerance/Dependence

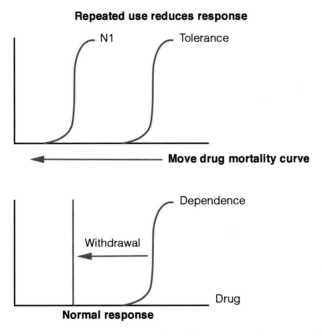

Fig. 41.8 The concept of tolerance is a resultant effect of repeated use of an agent, which reduces its response. This is illustrated in a dose response curve. Normal response is *left* on the X axis, a tolerant individual, shifts the curve to the *right*. Movement of that curve one way or the other can result in either an adverse event or mortality, or in the case of dependence, shifting the curve to the *left* might result in withdrawal. Adopted from ASAM Review 2014

with more clarity is it pain or is it tolerance/dependence. Furthermore, this illustrates the drive toward addiction. Tolerance and dependence are not addiction, but the development of tolerance in humans over time to obtain the same effect requires an increased amount of drug. If an inexperienced or younger user is mapped on a timeline, and opioid use is constant, its diminished effect, which is usually for anxiolysis, is not achieved over time, and tolerance is developed. This requires the individual to increase the dose in the experienced user. The drug level increases to obtain the same euphoria or anxiolysis effect. This is termed resetting the *hedonic set point* and is dopamine driven. The Y axis reveals an increase in drug dose, where the X axis, representing time pushes the drug to the right, and is a real life application of tolerance/dependence dose response curves. The user, addict or not, is taking more drug, and will eventually lead to adverse consequence if not identified, responded to, and intervened. This concept of tolerance is necessarily applied to any strategy of drug utilization. Some drugs develop tolerance very quickly, others not so much. Knowing different classes of drugs, and being clear within those classes allows the use of cotherapeutics as opposed to the pure drug, resulting in a probable improved outcome. Tolerance can be delayed, diminished, or even avoided if drugs are used in combination therapy, or with other modalities, such as interventions. Extending the concept of tolerance to the PAD model, the practitioner better manages the risk, reward benefit that pharmacologic agents and controlled substances impose. Although not always possible, in most cases, an exit strategy for controlled substances may be obtained. The controlled substance crisis that is evident in today's society is in direct relation to the fact that practitioners began treatment, without a plan, and without viable benchmarks. Where are we now, 3 months from now, 6 months from now, and have we improved, is measured by true functional and realistic parameters. Employ the diagnosis, the belief in that diagnosis to a treatment strategy, good judgment and then picking the correct pharmacologic management substantially reduces the controlled substance load, and reduces the likelihood that abuse evolves.

Addiction

The patient is an "addict." Commonly employed terminology and commonly misused. Addiction is rewarding, reinforcing, is pleasurable, and it activates brain circuitry. The neurobiology of addiction is complex, and the degree of activation correlates with an addiction tendency. This may be genetic, or environmental, and most likely a combination of both. Addiction correlates to a number of behaviors [16]. In more simple ways of characterizing those is by four C's.

- Impairment control over drug use
- Compulsive use of the drug
- Continued use of the drug despite harm
- Craving for the drug (Kanter, Manchikanti)

This pleasure and reward circuitry in the brain is driven by the reward neurotransmitter Dopamine (DA) (Fig. 41.9). Dopamine is considered the mother of all addictive things, and reinforces its activity at multiple points in this brain reward circuitry. Key structures include the nucleus accumbens, ventral tegmental area, amygdala, locus coeruleus, and various dynamic outflow circuitry. The nucleus (NUACC) receives dopamine (DA) and shares this dopaminergic reward relationship (Fig. 41.10). The nucleus accumbens encodes receipt as a reward, and responds to a varying degree, including anticipation, prediction, expectancy, and disappointment (Box 41.3). Almost all addictive drugs are dopamine activators. Dopamine antagonists are important in this consideration, but problematic. It would seem that dopamine antagonists would diminish the desire, but can increase the drug intake to compensate. This ever-present dopaminergic relationship at various stages of the reward circuitry turns the brain on fire with the drug desire, centering dopamine as an addict's gasoline (accelerant). Addicts have circuitry and reward deficiency. Adding relevance to dopamine's affect on the addict is the observation that decreased dopamine D2 receptors decreases metabolism in the cingulate gyrus. This is a part of the brain that inhibits the drive to use a substance, therefore is unopposed. Conversely, people with increased D2 seem less likely to develop a substance abuse

NH2
R
OH
OH
Dopamine; R=H
Norepinephring; R=OH
NHR
CH3
Amphetamine; R=H
Methamphetamine; R=CH3
Benzphetamine; R=benzyl
H3C
NH2
CH3
Phentermine
NHR
HO
OH
Phenylephrine

Fig. 41.9 Pleasure and reward circuitry in the brain is driven by the reward neurotransmitter Dopamine. From Ries RK, Fiellin DA, Miller SC, Saitz R, eds. Principles of Addiction Medicine, 4th ed. Philadelphia: Lippincott Williams & Wilking, 2009

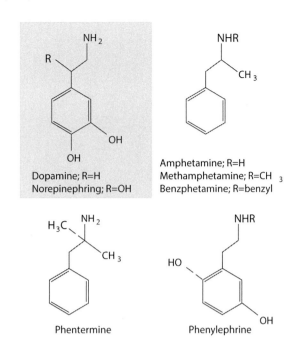

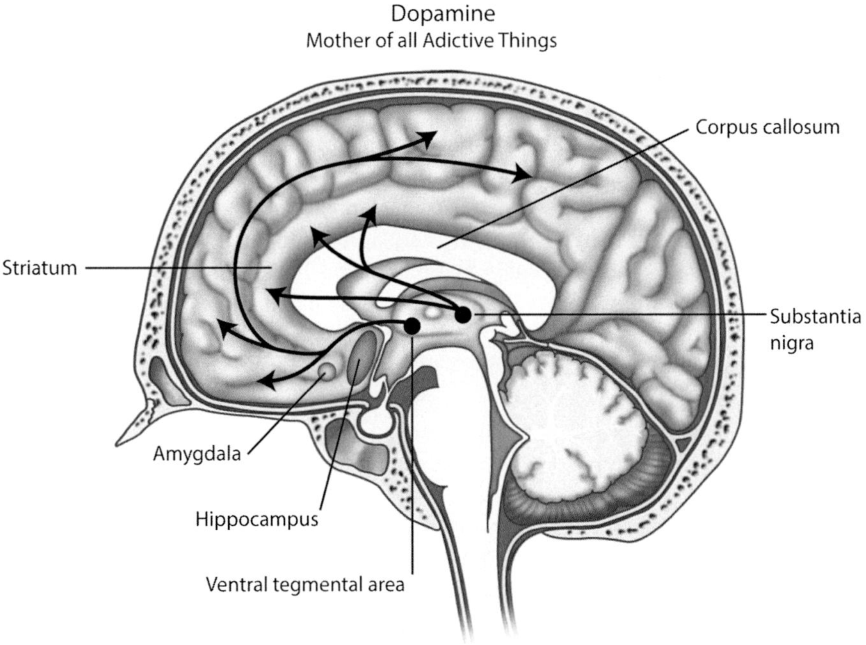

Dopamine
Mother of all Adictive Things
Corpus callosum
Striatum
Substantia nigra
Amygdala
Hippocampus
Ventral tegmental area

Fig. 41.10 The nucleus (NUACC) receives dopamine (DA) and shares this dopaminergic reward relationship. Adopted from ASAM Review 2014

Box 41.3: Addiction: Nucleus Accumbens (NUACC) and Dopamine (DA)

- Dopaminergic reward relationship
- Encodes receipt of reward
- Degree of reward
- Anticipation
- Expectancy
- Prediction
- Disappointment

disorder than those with decreased D2. An additional dopamine receptor, D3, is found only in this pleasure reward circuitry. It seems to be accountable to reward. Where D2 is dysphoric when blocked, addicts that experience a block at D3 diminish drug seeking and drug triggered relapse with queues, triggers, incubation, and craving [17]. This receptor is of interest to pharma as a treatment for addiction [6].

Neurobiology, Pain, Addiction, Depression

The similarities between the sagittal section in the primitive rat brain and the human are striking. Primitive as it is, it is just as important as many higher cognitive functional components of the brain. This primitive region will pull a human being, the highest functioning organism on the planet, and devolve the human into a compulsive illogical, irrational being. It is truly the stupid center. "The seat of an addict's soul lies in the nucleus accumbens"—Griffith Edwards. The intimate relationship between the ventral tegmental area, nucleus accumbens and the prefrontal cortex is influenced by the lateral hypothalamus, and orbital frontal cortex. The nucleus accumbens is the brain reward center, and it mediates motivation to behavior, most notably associated with incentive. This center relies on dopamine transmission, and is irrelevant of the addict's choice of pleasure. Not just opioids, food, sex, gambling, are all well known to enhance activity at the nucleus accumbens. When the addictive drug is exposed, the reward center substrates the brain to behave as do naturally occurring biologically essential rewards such as food, sex, etc. Addictive drugs drive much of their addictive power by activating these reward substrates and centers, with mechanisms more powerful than the naturally biological central reward. There is experimental evidence for this. The anterior cingulate gyrus anticipates the reward, the amygdala adds emotion to the reward, and the nucleus accumbens is the motivation. A well-known experiment is the progressive ratio of self-administration. The rat will press a bar designed to increase the workload on the animal to yield an injection. First attempts may require only two pushes for injection, then 4, 8, 16, and 32. The break point is defined as the ratio when the animal will abruptly stop pushing to get the injection and its subsequent reward. An electrode is placed at the intracranial self-stimulation (ICSS) connection between the hypothalamus, which stimulates the ventral tegmental area, and in turn the nucleus accumbens. The complex interrelationship between the prefrontal cortex, hippocampus, amygdala, locus coeruleus, and other primitive brain regions underlie the intense relationship between these structures and reward (Figs. 41.11 and 41.12). Most drugs of abuse have this relationship to the limbic system. Addictions alter neurochemistry in the

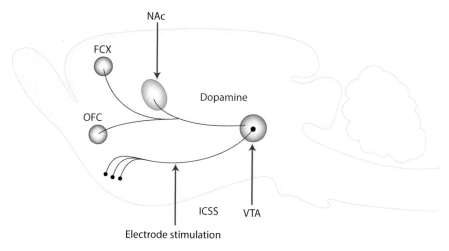

Fig. 41.11 The complex interrelationship between the prefrontal cortex, hippocampus, amygdala, locus coeruleus, and other primitive brain regions underlie the intense relationship between these structures and reward. Adopted from ASAM Review 2014

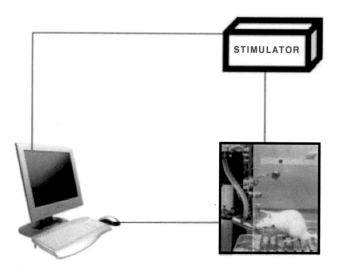

Fig. 41.12 The complex interrelationship between the prefrontal cortex, hippocampus, amygdala, locus coeruleus, and other primitive brain regions underlie the intense relationship between these structures and reward. Adopted from ASAM Review 2014

limbic system, the personality of pain. Addiction and depression, as well as pain direct the individual to actions and reactions that are intimately linked to these processes. Drug seeking behavior, is therefore driven by emotion, not logic. An example of this is relapse. Those with a great deal to lose, financially, emotionally, culturally, familial, and professionally (such as a physician), often relapse. Consequences are usually understood, and a successfully treated individual does not have to relapse. The example of a physician, with lifelong aspirations and training, are put in peril by the addicted brain. The stupid center at work on emotion deep in limbic structures. Relapse is the norm, and is part of the inherent disease of addiction. With so much to lose, it would be an obvious assumption that those successfully treated would not relapse, ultimately putting so much at risk, but not born out in reality. Emotion, not logic, hijacks the addicts brain. It is easy to become judgmental of the addict, but it is far more compassionate to understand the intimate relationship of these mechanisms and the need to apply science to understanding and, again, judgment. The progression of the disease of addiction begins recreationally, occasional use, then steady use. Once the reward driven state is obtained, a habit driven use occurs. No longer is it rewarding, no longer is the euphoric high obtained. Most addicts will relate a feeling of anxiety and dysphoria, and not the party high that they once obtained. The transition from ventral striatum to the dorsal striatum brain turns habit driven use to compulsive use. Eventually the denial, or the bottoming out "crash" occurs, and treatment is initiated. Once the achievement of abstinence is obtained, the addict is persistently vulnerable to craving and relapse. Expect this relapse. The neurobiology of PAD teaches us that humans are not always in command of their fate. Genetics, environment, events, and comorbid disease states are so important to include in the differential diagnosis of PAD for this reason.

Pain, Addiction, and Depression, the Sick Neuron

The interrelationship between the ventral tegmental area and the nucleus accumbens changes over time and exposure to the inciting event [18]. Continued opioid exposure, particularly those that are genetically predisposed to addiction, results in poor connections between the axons, and the interrelating structures in the brain. Long-term substance abuse and drug exposure results in a poorly functioning unhealthy neuron in the ventral tegmental area, which affects function at the nucleus accumbens (Fig. 41.13). These impaired dendritic connections affect PAD, as well as many higher cognitive functions such as learning and memory. A process of neurodegeneration progresses, with atrophy and loss of neurons in glial cells. This is the concept of neurodegeneration, and neurodegeneration disorders are the likely cause of treatment resistant depression. Poor resultant sleep, depression, and a propensity toward a pain state, is a cycle of reinforcement, and often patients look to any type of hope. With depressed mood, the sick neuron, and accompanying situational depression and anxiety, comes the realization that this is not a new problem, but a problem that has just recently been characterized and understood. With the stigma of PAD, also comes the societal segregation that has been seen since

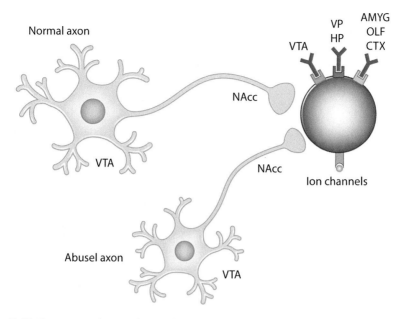

Fig. 41.13 Long-term substance abuse and drug exposure results in a poorly functioning unhealthy neuron in the ventral tegmental area, which affects function at the nucleus accumbens. Adopted from ASAM Review 2014

Table 41.1 Mood, receptors, and depression		
Medieval	Depression and humors (Black Bile)
Seventeenth century	Duelism—mind, body, social environment
Early twentieth century	Sigmund Freud—brain would describe mental illness
Current	Receptor technology

medieval times. Called depression in humors, or black bile, during the seventeenth century, a dualism of mind, body, and environment was postulated. Early in the twentieth century Sigmund Freud demonstrated the brain described mental illness. Today, technology can alter the central brain receptor, PAD states are realizing potent new treatment paradigms (Table 41.1). The concept of neurodegeneration begins in the hippocampus, and involves the primitive brain. The connections to the amygdala and prefrontal cortex are critical to learning and memory. Cognitive emotion is associated with human behavior (Fig. 41.14). Brain drive neurotrophic factor, BDNF, is a key component in learning and memory. BDNF supports brain health. BDNF is a neurotrophin family nerve growth factor which supports neuron survival and synapses. BDNF is also affected by environmental factors and genetics. There is no place in the brain other than the dentate gyrus of the hippocampus where neurons continue to be born. This is a process of neurogenesis where BDNF supports the health of the brain cells, and promotes new neurons (Fig. 41.15). This is termed

Stress and Depression

Neurogenisis — Hippocampus
Rats, Monkeys, Humans

Neurons continue to be born in dentate gyrus of hippocampus

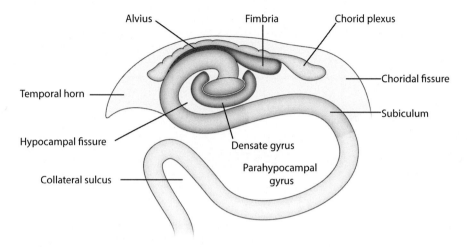

Fig. 41.14 The concept of neurodegeneration begins in the hippocampus, and involves the primitive brain. The connections to the amygdala and prefrontal cortex are critical to learning and memory. Cognitive emotion is associated with human behavior. Adopted from ASAM Review 2014

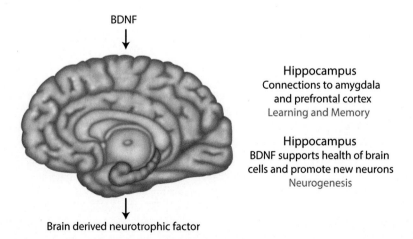

Fig. 41.15 BDNF is also affected by environmental factors and genetics. There is no place in the brain other than the dentate gyrus of the hippocampus where neurons continue to be born. This is a process of neurogenesis where BDNF supports the health of the brain cells, and promotes new neurons. Adopted from ASAM Review 2014

neurogenesis. The dentate gyrus is found in the hippocampal fissure, and approximates, the fimbria. The subiculum follows to the perihippocampal gyrus. These interrelated structures found in rats, monkeys, and even humans within the hippocampus, are the foundation of neurogenesis. Stress and depression intimately affect this area. There is an upregulation of neurogenesis with antidepressants, and reverse atrophy of the sick neurons that are present in PAD. The increased expression of BDNF in an upregulated brain enhances connectivity in the hippocampus, and BDNF protein is supported and encoded by the BDNF gene. This is termed positive metoplasticity. The stem cells are stimulated, BDNF is enhanced, and neurogenesis follows at this basal forebrain. PAD directly influence this positive event. When BDNF is diminished, depression worsens. Stress also is a precursor to mood disorder. Stress decreases BDNF. Stress would be considered an environmental factor, as is genetics. Stress increases glucocorticoids, which downregulate hippocampal synaptic activity, and is termed negative metoplasticity. The organic states of PAD are seen with loss of cognition, enhanced dementia, amyloid formation, obesity, and epilepsy, and all share negative metoplasticity. Memory disturbances and poor learning are also observed. Stress and depression actually improve with increased physical activity. Exercise stimulates neurogenesis. Where glucocorticoids and steroids suppress dentate gyrus neurogenesis (Gould), exercise stimulates neurogenesis. The target receptor is the serotonin receptor. 5 HT1a, serotonin receptors have a high concentration in the dentate gyrus of the hippocampus, and have long been known to be affected by serotonin enhancing agents. BDNF messenger RNA is upregulated in the hippocampus with physical activity and antidepression treatment and the result is a feeling of wellbeing. Could this be runner's high? Stress on the other hand, leads to neuronal atrophy at the cellular level. Decrease BDNF and neurogenesis at the hippocampal level, and the resultant situational depression, anxiety increases. BDNF is actually required for brain survival. There are factors that clinicians can take advantage of that enhance BDNF and brain health. By blocking the NMDA receptor, (N-methyl-D aspartate) eukaryotic elongation factor 2 (EF2) is either diminished or stopped. By decreasing this EF2 kinase, there is an increased translation phosphorylation (inactivated form) of eukaryotic elongation factor 2 and a rapid increase in BDNF. Therefore, to inhibit EF2 kinase, it is possible to obtain a rapid antidepressant effect. The converse is true as well. High concentrations of EF2 kinase suppress BDNF function leading to further situational depression, anxiety, and pain. EF2 is believed to affect background activity and spontaneous nerve firing, or "background noise." Spontaneous nerve firing is important and carries a strong role in plasticity. Electroconvulsive therapy is effective at restoring background noise, and enhancing mood most likely by this effect of the BDNF. Another emerging therapy is ketamine. Ketamine is a NMDA receptor antagonist, and noncompetitive. It decreases the effectiveness of the neurotransmitter, glutamate, which binds to opioid receptors. Ketamine does not block NMDA activity, but it does block the background noise link between spontaneous noise and depression. A single dose of ketamine activates the mammalian target of rapamycin (mTOR) signaling pathway. Ketamine is an on switch to mTOR ketabolism [19–21] (Figs. 41.16 and 41.17).

Synaptogenesis

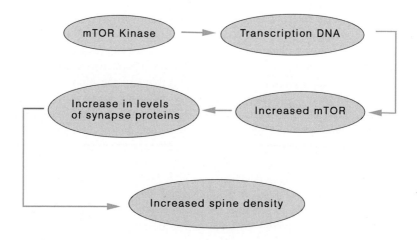

Synapses and spine morphology
necessary for learning and memory

Fig. 41.16 Synaptogenesis. Adopted from ASAM Review 2014

BDNF

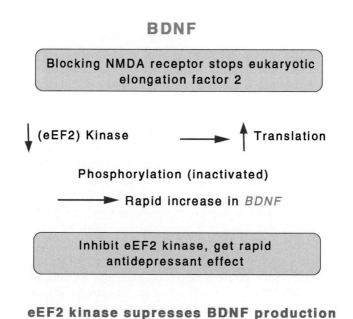

eEF2 kinase supresses BDNF production

Fig. 41.17 BDNF. Adopted from ASAM Review 2014

Concept of Synaptogenesis

Depression results from the brain failure to grow new neurons at key regions, and is receptor regulated. Ketamine activates mTOR, this ubiquitous protein kinase involved in protein synthesis and synaptic plasticity. This process of *synaptogenesis* by mTOR kinase results in transcriptive DNA increasing mTOR, which increases the levels of synapse proteins, resulting in an increased spine density. Spine density enhances activity at the synapse and this spine morphology is necessary for learning and memory. The sick neuron has poor dendritic spine formation, and ketamine has been demonstrated to increase the spine formation, sometimes a matter of hours. Aberrant TOR activities are also seen in diabetes, obesity, heart disease, cancer, pain, and addiction. Dendritic spine density wakes up a drug addicted, drug preferring VTA connection to the nucleus accumbens, and enhances a normal state. Both electroconvulsive therapy and ketamine subsequently reset the background noise/activity, and spontaneous activity. With 2 out of 3 patients who do not respond to common antidepressants, those that are treated with ketamine improved within hours. Those suffering from severe forms of depression, such as MDD, often have failed conventional antidepressant therapy. This treatment resistant depression rapidly responds to ECT and ketamine, suggesting that pain and addiction, which share common pathways, might respond as well [22–24].

The Concept of PAD

Work by Duman describing neurotrophic theory and depression in 2011 began with nerve growth factors, influencing serotonin cellular transcriptive events, and the antidepressant effect in the hippocampus. This link between antidepressants and the C AMP pathway (creb-C AMP responsive to element bringing protein) regulates change in the hippocampus to produce this antidepressant effect (Fig. 41.18). With drugs such as ketamine being so effective with the rapid onset timeline, can other ketamine like agents be developed to allow traditional antidepressants and emerging drugs with similar characteristics to ketamine in development to catch up with the depression and comorbidities. Ketamine and antidepressant medications then may restore cell density and regular higher order synaptic plasticity in the hippocampus. With so many painful disease states poorly defined and understood, it makes sense that fibromyalgia and CRPS would be one of the first diagnoses to be positively affected by ketamine [25–29].

Assessment of Pain, Addiction, and Depression

As we have seen with the neurodynamics and biology of pain and depression, it is a brain disease, and not a purely psychiatric disorder. Therefore, psychodynamics is always a part of the diagnosis. PAD is behavioral, so we would expect behavioral

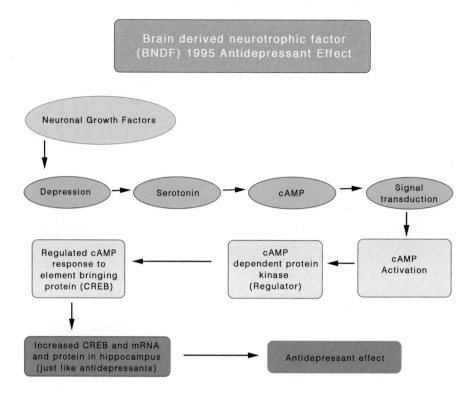

Fig. 41.18 Duman's neurotrophic theory of depression [20]

abnormalities, including relapse, psychiatric comorbidities, and anxiety and depression to be relatively common in these states. With loss, the self is first to go, followed by loss of image, respect, reliance, reliability, coping, interpersonal relationships, developed compulsiveness, and aggression, are often seen with PAD. Also these patients experience significant financial, legal, and employment stressors that complicate the treatment paradigm. To assess these first we understand the disease state and the consequences of the different stages of these diseases. They range in severity from mild to severe, therefore a range of different specialties treat these conditions. Specialty sensitive, it can be years before the proper clinician finally evaluates and manages a complex pain, addiction, or depression.

Treatment of Pain, Depression, and Addiction

Rule #5, Putting It All Together

From a professional standpoint we all want to improve your pain, but from a realistic standpoint we want to improve an individual's function. PAD are best treated with good judgment, compassion, and care, a sound understanding of the science behind the behaviors, and realizing that people can be helped, even by nontraditional means [20]. The provider understands the purpose of obtaining benchmarks, 3, 6, 9, and 12 months, to better place the foundation of these improvements. It might be as simple as going to the grocery, riding in a car longer, or taking less medicine. The patient should document these improvements with realistic expectations that PAD are managed, and not necessarily cured. The light at the end of the tunnel will never be a truck, and that there are options available, and progressive understanding of the science behind PAD, which enhances outcome. At the end of the day, the risk/reward of treatment falls in the patient and practitioner's favor, and the course of care is clearly understood and justified, with a support system in place. Even an exit strategy for opioids can be entertained with understanding advanced pharmacologic management, brain neurobiology, and adjunctive medical care. This mixed modality approach may include interventional techniques, and psychological and behavioral techniques. The point of understanding the neurobiology of PAD is to choose pathways, and not develop obstructions to care. There is not one pathway for any particular patient that is firm, and adjustments are usually made along the way. Developing this understanding removes barriers to communication, and ultimately improves quality of life.

References

1. Rasor J, et al. Using opioids for patients with moderate to severe pain. J Am Osteopath Assoc. 2007;107(9 Suppl 5):ES4–10.
2. Trescot AM, et al. Opioids and the management of chronic non-cancer pain: an update of American Society of Interventional Pain Physicians (ASIPP) guidelines. Pain Physician. 2008;11:S5–62.
3. Woolfert MZ. Opiod analgesics for pain control: Wisconsin physicians knowledge, beliefs, attitudes, and prescribing practices. Pain Med. 2010;11(3):425–33.
4. Spitz A, et al. Primary care provider's perspective on prescribing opioids to older adults with chronic non-cancer pain: a qualitative study. BMC Geriatr. 2010;11:35.
5. Joranson DE. Pain management, controlled substances, and state medical board policy: a decade of change. J Pain Symptom Manage. 2002;23(2):138–47.
6. Rannazzisi JT. The DEAs daunting act to ensure public health and safety. Clin Pharmacol Ther. 2007;81(6):805–6.
7. Weissman DE, Haddox JD. Opioid pseudoaddiction-an iatrogenic syndrome. Pain. 1989; 36(3):363–6.
8. Schultz TF. Medical review officer handbook. 8th ed. London: Quadrangle Research; 2002.
9. Substance Abuse and Mental Health Services Administration (US). Report no: (US); 2012 (SMA) 12-4681. 2012. www.samhsa.gov/data/NSDUH/zk10NSDUH/zkResults.pdf

10. Centers for Disease Control and Prevention. Unintentional drug poisoning in the United States. 2010. p. 190. http://www.cdc.gov/home-andrecreactionalsafety/pdf/poison-issue-brief.pdf
11. Substance Abuse and Mental Health Services Administration. Results from 2010 National Survey on Drug Use and Health: Mental Health Findings. NSDUH series H-42 HHS publication number (SMA) 11-4667. Rockville: Substance Abuse and Mental Health Services Administration; 2012. www.samhsa.gov/data/nsduh/2k10mh_findings/2k10mhresults.pdf
12. Laxmaiah Manchikanti MD. Opioid epidemic in the United States. Pain Physician. 2012;15: ES9–38.
13. Laxmaiah Manchikanti MD, et al. American Society of Interventional Pain Physicians (ASIPP) guidelines for responsible opioid prescribing and chronic non-cancer pain: part 1—evidence assessment. Pain Physician. 2012;15:S1–66.
14. Laxmaiah Manchikanti MD, et al. American Society of Interventional Pain Physicians (ASIPP) guidelines for responsible opioid prescribing and chronic non-cancer pain: part 2—guidance. Pain Physician. 2012;15(3 Suppl):ES 67–92.
15. Controlled Substance Act [21 USC 829; 21 C.F.R, 1306.04(a)].
16. Reis RK. Basic science and core concepts. In: Principles of medicine. 4th ed. Philadelphia: Lippincott Williams and Wilkins; 2009. p. 1–11.
17. Reis RK. The anatomy of addiction. In: Principles of medicine. 4th ed. Philadelphia: Lippincott Williams and Wilkins; 2009. p. 27–35.
18. Heidbreder C. Selective antagonism of dopamine D3 receptors as a target for drug addiction pharmacotherapy: a review of pre-clinical evidence. CNS Neurol Disord Drug Targets. 2008;7(5):410–21.
19. Reis RK. Neurobiology of addiction from a developmental perspective. In: Principles of medicine. 4th ed. Philadelphia: Lippincott Williams and Wilkins; 2009. p. 1391–1406.
20. Duman RS. Signaling pathways underlying rapid antidepressant actions of ketamine. Neuropharmacology. 2012;62(1):35–41.
21. Schoenfeld TJ, et al. Stress, stress hormones, and adult neurogenesis. Exp Neurol. 2012;233(1): 12–21.
22. Manchikanti L, Boswell MV, Singh V, Benyamin RM, Fellows B, Abdi S, Buenaventura RM, Conn A, Datta S, Derby R, Falco FJE, Erhart S, Diwan S, Hayek SM, Helm S, Parr AT, Schultz DM, Smith HS, Wolfer LR, Hirsch JA. Comprehensive evidence-based guidelines in the management of chronic spinal pain. Pain Physician. 2009;12:699–802.
23. WormBook: The online review of C elegans biology synaptogenesis. Santa Cruz: Department of Molecular Cell and Developmental Biology; 2005.
24. Machado-Viera R. Brain derived neurotrophic factor and initial antidepressant response to an N-methyl-D-aspartate antagonist. J Clin Psychiatry. 2009;70(12):1662.
25. DiazGranados N, et al. Rapid resolution of suicidal ideation after single infusion of an N-methyl-D-aspartate antagonist in patients with treatment-resistant major depressive disorder. J Clin Psychiatry. 2010;71(12):1605–11.
26. Murrough JW. Antidepressant efficacy of ketamine in treatment-resistant major depression: to site randomized control trial. Mol J Psychiatry. 2013;170(10):134–42.
27. Keifer RT, et al. Complete recovery from intractable complex regional pain syndrome, CRPS type 1, following anesthetic, ketamine, and midazolam. Pain Pract. 2007;7(2):147–50.
28. Schwartzman RJ, et al. Outpatient intravenous ketamine for the treatment of complex regional pain syndrome: double blind placebo controlled study. Pain. 2009;147(1–3):107–15.
29. Haley S, et al. Neuroplasticity and the next wave of antidepressant strategies. Front Cell Neurosci. 2013;7:218.

Chapter 42
Between Social Welfare and Public Health: Substance Abuse and Co-occurring Disability

Song Kim and Alan David Kaye

Key Points

- Terms and definitions
- Social security disability claims
- Drug abuse and alcoholism in social disability programs: a brief history
- Drug abuse and addiction category today
- Coping with the disease of having a disease
- Treatments for co-occurring disorders

Through the decades, disability was defined along a number of dimensions. From the purview of labor and law, the US Social Security disability programs introduced in 1945 [1] framed a disabled individual as one unable to fully participate in civic and economic activities, requiring financial assistance from the state. Americans with Disability Act of 1990 operates on a sociopolitical model, in which a disabled person is entitled to reasonable accommodation in order to function in society without discrimination [2]. Both reflect what scholar Brucker deems a "positive" social construction of disability [3], that of equality and nondiscrimination.

Introduction of substance abuse as a disability does not neatly fit into this discourse of charity and integration. Some states like Louisiana and Michigan have considered and imposed laws to require drug testing for welfare recipients, barring those who test positive from food stamps, and other aids [4]. Chicago Housing

S. Kim, B.S. (✉)
Tulane University School of Medicine,
1430 Tulane Avenue, New Orleans, LA 70112, USA
e-mail: skim17@tulane.edu

A.D. Kaye, M.D., Ph.D.
Departments of Anesthesiology and Pharmacology, Louisiana State University
Health Sciences Center, Louisiana State University Interim Hospital,
and Ochsner Kenner Hospital, New Orleans, LA, USA

© Springer Science+Business Media New York 2015
A.D. Kaye et al. (eds.), *Substance Abuse*, DOI 10.1007/978-1-4939-1951-2_42

Authority, for example, has a policy requiring random drug testing of residents without grounds for suspicion [5]. Along the same lines, ADA excludes active users of illicit substances from employment and to give tests for illegal use of drugs, a "punitive" model [3] consistent with the above.

The medical and public health community has come to a scientific consensus on addiction and substance dependence as a neurobiological disorder, deserving of treatment and insurance like other disorders [6].

Edward and colleagues' seminal dimensional theory on alcohol dependence described substance abuse as occurring on a continuum of biological drives and problems, paving the way for a preventative and holistic approaches to substance abuse in practice today [7]. Accordingly, in 1980 American Psychiatric Association Diagnostic and Statistical Manual of Mental disorders (DSM) included substance abuse as its own category, in a break way from earlier editions that categorized substance abuse as a manifestation of personality disorders [8].

The above purviews of medicine and law paint an ambiguous picture of substance abuse that spans a spectrum between irresponsible personal choice and disability. The chapter further elaborates on this biaxial model of substance abuse in the historical context of Social security disability programs and current public health guidelines.

Terms and Definitions

Disability is defined using a number of different models. Americans with Disability Act, for example, has a threefold definition for an individual disability, who (1) has a physical or mental impairment that substantially limits one or more major life activities; or (2) has a record of such an impairment; or (3) is regarded as having such an impairment [2]. Social Security programs, the focus of this chapter, subscribes to the first part the definition, the major life activity being gainful work.

The term "substance abuse" used throughout the chapter refers to both substance abuse and substance dependence, as suggested in the latest edition of DSM [9]. It encompasses the use of both alcohol and other psychoactive substances.

Social Security Disability Claims

There are two public assistance programs operated by the Social Security Administration for the disabled: Disability Insurance (DI) and Supplemental Security Income (SSI) programs. Disability Insurance is an insurance program, in which tax deductions taken out of a healthy worker's payroll over time determines the benefits should he/she become disabled. By contrast, the Supplemental Security Income (SSI) is a welfare program for those determined to be disabled and with few, minimal financial resources [10].

To qualify for disability benefits, a potential claimant fills out documents required for disability determination process: the Social Security application, and documents of medical records from physicians, psychiatrists, and other treatment centers [11]. Nonmedical sources such as non-clinical social workers, licensed chemical dependency practitioners, or other medical-sources such as nurse practitioners, physicians' assistants and therapists, must be reviewed together with findings from a medical physician [12].

A field office first verifies nonmedical eligibility such as marital status, employment, and SS coverage. A federally funded agency known as the Disability Determination Service, consisting of a physician (or psychologist) and disability examiner, then reviews the submitted reports and determines eligibility for benefits [11]. This is the same agency that conducts Continuing Disability Review (CDR) every 3 years or more depending on the severity of the claimant's conditions, to determine whether the benefits should continue in light of any medical improvements relating to ability to work [13].

The application process is a lengthy one, perhaps taking several months or years after submission until receiving a decision. If denied, the claimant may request appeal by self-representing, or selecting a relative or a legal representative for hearing [14].

Drug Abuse and Alcoholism in Social Disability Programs: A Brief History

Drug Abuse and Alcoholism (DA&A) category in the SSI programs was a controversial addition that introduced a complex psychosocial dimension to the understanding of the disabled. In the earlier years of the program, low-income individuals whose primary diagnosis was substance abuse could claim their condition as worthy of receiving benefits. In the years since its implementation, the legitimacy of DA&A as a disability would continue to be questioned and scrutinized.

1972

Social Security Act Amendments first introduced the DA&A to its disability programs. The provisions specified that claimants applying for assistance would be required to undergo treatment, and select a representative payee (a third party managing benefit checks on behalf of the recipient). To administer the treatment mandate, Referral and Monitoring Agencies were to be established in every state in order to direct the SSI beneficiaries to necessary services [15].

By this time, DA&A appeared in the Listing of Impairments as a "functional nonpsychotic disorder." It seemed to imply that some physical and functional deficit would have to accompany the addictive behaviors, but there were no such specifications, confounding the evaluation process [16].

1994

Due to an unforeseen increase in DA&A status applicants qualifying for benefits since the passage of Social Security Act Amendments, the *Social Security Independence and Program Improvements Act* sought to tighten the disability programs [15]. The push for change likely came from incredulous politicians, who were concerned that the tax dollars financed people who were responsible for their own problems and possibly using the check to obtain more illicit substance [17]. Concomitantly, legal sanctions against fraudulent claims were expanded during this time [18].

The act thus mandated a stricter supervision over the recipients whose primary impairment was drug addiction and alcoholism. It would place a 3-year restriction on both SSI and DI benefits to these "material" individuals, who must demonstrate compliance to treatment to the investigating RMA, or face payment suspension. Those who suffered from non drug-related primary disorder were exempt from the 3-year limit [15] As Hogan et al. conclude, it implied that addiction was not taken to be a permanent disorder [17].

1996

Underlying these previous provisions was a "presumption of culpability" toward DA&A claimants; no other specific disability categories explicitly required a third-party representative payee or an ongoing state surveillance over the course of their treatments [16]. However daunting the said requirements, they proved difficult in management; Hunt notes from the retrospective 1997 Department of Health and Human services report that in a 18-month period between 1994 and 1995, RMAs referred 2,182 cases to the SSA for a CDR following successful completion of a substance abuse treatment program. Only 32 cases were terminated [16].

Under *Contract with America Advancement Act*, SSA terminated benefits for over 120,000 of 160,000 SSI beneficiaries, whose primary impairment was drug addiction, alcoholism, or both, as of January 1, 1997 [15].

Drug Abuse and Addiction Category Today

Through a history wrought with administrative challenges and political climate of the time, no longer can individuals with a diagnosis of substance abuse qualify for disability if their condition is "material," that is, if the individual would not be disabled physically and mentally in *absence of the addictive behaviors*. Addiction occurring secondary to another irreversible disorder, or physical and mental conditions resulting from a lifelong addiction passes the "materiality" criterion.

Table 42.1 Drug Abuse and Alcoholism (DAA) evaluation process

1. Does the claimant have DAA?	a. No—No DAA materiality determination necessary
	b. Yes—Go to step 2
2. Is the claimant disabled considering all impairments, including DAA?	a. No—Do not determine DAA materiality (Denial)
	b. Yes—Go to step 3
3. Is DAA the only impairment?	a. Yes—DAA material (Denial)
	b. No—Go to step 4
4. Is the other impairment(s) disabling by itself while the claimant is dependent upon or abusing drugs or alcohol?	a. No—DAA material (Denial)
	b. Yes—Go to step 5
5. Does the DAA cause or affect the claimant's medically determinable impairment(s)?	a. No—DAA not material (Allowance)
	b. Yes, but the other impairment(s) is irreversible or could not improve to the point of nondisability—DAA not material (Allowance)
	c. Yes, and DAA could be material—Go to step
6. Would the other impairment(s) improve to the point of non-disability in the absence of DAA?	a. Yes—DAA material (Denial)
	b. No—DAA not material (Allowance)

Adapted from [12]

Table 42.1 is the algorithm outlined by SSA, which effectively excludes claimants with a primary diagnosis of drug abuse and addiction. However, if a person qualifies under another diagnosis, secondary substance use disorder diagnoses are acceptable. The Social Security Administration has developed a lengthy list of mental and physical disorders deemed to interfere with gainful activities. Known as the Listing of Impairments, it describes disabling conditions under each physiological system, with ongoing treatments to be documented, and recommended methods of examination.

Substance abuse disorder category is defined to be "behavioral changes or physical changes associated with the regular use of substances that affect the central nervous system." The required level of severity for the disorder is met with requirements for the following mental/organ disorders:

1. Organic mental disorders
2. Depressive syndrome
3. Anxiety disorders
4. Personality disorders
5. Peripheral neuropathies
6. Liver damage
7. Gastritis
8. Pancreatitis
9. Seizures [19]

Physicians provide a letter on behalf of the SS disability applicant, to include behavioral observations and other symptoms consistent with the Listing of Impairment guidelines. Thus for a patient with a substance abuse disorder, evidence of the above *independent of substance use* must be provided in order to meet "materiality" criterion. The National Health Care for the Homeless recommend that physicians document: (1) claimant's physical and mental status during abstinence, (2) whether the drug use may be owing to the patient attempting to manage symptoms of underlying illnesses, and (3) irreversible damage resulting from substance use that may fall under the eligible impairments listed in the Listing of Impairments, such as cirrhosis that would not improve even after the patient has ceased drug use [20]. Regardless of the primary diagnosis specified in the SSI/DI application, the office develops further evidence on DA&A with allegation such as multiple emergency department visits due to the effects of substance abuse, or current treatment for substance dependence. This is excluding the cases in which the disablement by another impairment is unrelated to and is not exacerbated by DA&A, or irreversible [12].

"Coping with the Disease of Having a Disease"

Even though the current SSA definition of disability permits little room for substance abuse, the reciprocal relationship between substance abuse and non-drug induced disability is well documented. The Department of Health and Human Services estimates that in persons with disabilities, substance abuse rate is 2–4 times higher than in the general population [21]; severe mental illness, traumatic spinal cord, and brain injuries have the highest prevalence rate approaching 50 % [22]. Hearing impairments, learning disability, blindness and visual impairments, and burn victims are other disabilities with high incidence of substance abuse [23]. Quite likely, personal difficulties such as social isolation and management of severe symptoms lend themselves to the disabled persons succumbing to substance abuse, turning to alcohol and drugs as a defensive mechanism to "cope with the disease of having a disease" [24].

The current status of DA&A is such that a disability recipient with a substance abuse problem continues to receive funding, without having to follow a prescribed treatment for the latter [12]. It remains up to the individual to seek treatment, and the primary physician or other care-giving worker to address the issue. Some may believe that granting disability benefits to active substance abusers will only hamper the patient's rehabilitative efforts, increase his or her drug use. Timely enough, investigations on the matter in 1995 served to bolstered the argument of DA&A opponents. The NEJM paper showed that cocaine use, psychiatric symptoms, and hospital admissions increased each month around the time of disability check receipt for schizophrenic patients with cocaine dependence [25]. In spite of the limitations of the study, it affirmed the popular belief that public dollars were enabling recipients' addictive habits [16]. Other authors since then have reported that disability beneficiaries with substance addiction are no more likely than an average person in the workforce to increase substance use, and that SSI/SSDI benefits can significantly improve their quality of life [26]. Brucker's meta-analysis of

National Survey on Drug Use and Health across general populations and benefit recipients bears mixed findings. The author discovered that compared to the rate in the overall general population, alcohol abuse was more common among DI and SSI recipients. Encouragingly, the results showed that disability beneficiaries were more likely to participate in treatment than persons with substance use not enrolled in the assistance programs [3].

Treatments for Co-occurring Disorders

Substance abuse treatment services are covered by public and private health insurances, and out-of-pocket expenditure in different proportions: According to SAMHSA, public expenditures for substance use was 76 % while only 45 % of all health care was publicly funded [27]. The data nevertheless bodes well for disability beneficiaries, most of whom receive national health insurance coverage. DI recipients become automatically eligible for Medicare after 2 years, entitling them to a disability check along with medical coverage for substance abuse treatment. Most SSI recipients also qualify for Medicaid, with SSI receipt being an eligibility category in many states [28]. However, because substance abuse treatment and rehabilitation are optional Medicaid benefits left to the discretion of the states, coverage may vary substantially; 40 out of 50 states covered inpatient hospitalization for substance abuse, most often acute admissions for detoxification, 25 states extensive outpatient services for substance abuse such as daytime treatment centers, 15 states residential substance abuse services, and 13 states case management services for substance users [29]. Out-of-pocket payment per substance use visit has been steadily increasing from 2007 to 2011, and remains far greater than those per mental health, medical, or surgical admission [30].

Tackling addiction in a clinical population especially at risk for unhealthy substance use is not an easy task. On the demand side, people with cognitive and mental disorder are already less likely than their healthy counterparts to seek treatment for substance abuse [31]. On the supply side, existing substance abuse programs are found to be insufficiently responsive or accessible to the needs of the disabled, in spite of the Americans with Disabilities Act mandate.

Complicating access to treatment in particular is the lack of facilities equipped to serve particular disabled groups [32]. In New York State, for example, of 12 state-sponsored addiction treatment centers only one offers specialized services for the deaf and hard of hearing, and another one for traumatic brain injury cases [33]. The fiscal difficulties of ADA compliances shift the principal focus of managing co-occurring disorders to mental health provider trainings for substance abuse.

Because healthcare professionals may address only the patient's disability rather than the full range of his or her health, they may not anticipate substance abuse as a problem. Encouragingly, providers in rehabilitative medicine are beginning to increasingly recognize substance abuse as a prevalent issue in their clientele.

As a survey of TBI and TCI treatment centers have discovered, more centers are using institutionalized approaches such as regular screening and written guidelines than 30 years ago [34, 35]. More screening tools are now available. The New York State Office of Mental Health (OMH) and the Office of Alcoholism and Substance Abuse Services (OASAS) have since 2008 recommended licensed mental health and chemical dependency clinics statewide to screen all patients for the presence of a co-occurring mental health and substance use disorder, with specific tools recommended for each setting [36].

Beyond the screening and assessment steps, the traditional therapies used to ameliorate substance abuse symptoms is likely not amenable to persons with social, cognitive, emotional constraints. The 12-step program used by Alcoholics Anonymous, for example, emphasizes spirituality as a principal component of a successful treatment outcome, to which patients with various cognitive disorders may not be receptive [37]. To address the gap in treatment of co-occurring disorders, treatment and research communities have spearheaded efforts to design integrative co-treatment plans, each unique to a known mental disorder combined with substance abuse such as schizophrenia and borderline disorders [38]. While supporting further development of the unified approach, SAMHSA research panel acknowledges the difficulties of systems integration [38], revealing the disparate historical growth of the fields in spite of the inextricable link between substance abuse and mental health.

Conclusion

The demise of the DA&A disability program to target substance abusers was perhaps inevitable, due to the complex structure and requirements evolving from the paternalistic nature of the program. Regardless of its shortcomings, SSI/DI benefits secured financing for the large constituent of disabled population suffering from the dual conditions. Perhaps a greater cooperation with other social service agencies is needed to balance the goals of financial support and treatment, a large gap left behind by the DA&A termination. For example, SAMHSA launched the SSI/DI Outreach, Access and Recovery (SOAR) initiative to bridge local mental health services to public assistance programs, training providers to help enroll identified outpatients in SSI/DI [39]. A federal agency with a vested interest in public health and human services, SAMHSA is right to focus on the twofold aim of rehabilitation and access to benefits. In the meanwhile, those at risk for substance use may greatly benefit from the recent advancements in holistic and preventative approaches that delve deeper into the human psyche and well-being.

Disclosure The authors have no relationships with pharmaceutical companies or products to disclose, nor do they discuss off-label or investigative products in this chapter.

References

1. Kearney, JR. Social security and the "D" in OASDI: the history of a federal program insuring earners against disability. Washington, DC: Social Security Bulletin, 2006;66(3).
2. Americans with Disability Act of 1990, s. 12182 (a).
3. Brucker, D. Disability, substance abuse and public disability benefits [PhD thesis]. New Brunswick: Rutgers State University of New Jersey; 2007. Available from ProQuest Dissertations & Theses Database [cited 29 Jun 2013].
4. American Civil Liberty Union. Drug testing of public assistance recipients as a condition of eligibility[Internet].2008.http://www.aclu.org/drug-law-reform/drug-testing-public-assistance-recipients-coition-eligibility [updated 8 Apr 2008; cited 18 Aug 2013].
5. American Civil Liberty Union of Illinois. Long-time resident challenges Chicago' Housing Authority's "stigmatizing" drug testing program [Internet]. 2013. http://www.aclu-il.org/long-time-resident-challenges-chicago-housing-authoritys-stigmatizing-drug-testing-program/ [updated 15 Aug 2013; cited 18 Aug 2013].
6. American Society of Addiction Medicine. Public policy statement: definition of addiction [Internet]. 2011. http://www.asam.org/for-the-public/definition-of-addiction [updated 11 Apr 2011; cited 15 Jul 2013].
7. Li TK, Hewitt BG, Grant BF. The Alcohol Dependence Syndrome, 30 years later: a commentary. Addiction [serial online]. 2007;102(10):1522–30. Available from PubMed [cited 20 Jun 2013].
8. Babor TF. Substance-related problems in the context of international classificatory systems. In: Lader M, Edwards G, Drummond D, editors. The nature of alcohol and drug related problems. New York: Oxford University Press; 1992.
9. American Psychiatric Publishing. Substance-related and addictive disorders [Internet]. 2013. http://www.dsm5.org/Documents/Substance%20Use%20Disorder%20Fact%20Sheet.pdf [cited 15 Jul 2013].
10. Social Security Administration. Benefits for people with disabilities [Internet]. 2013. http://www.ssa.gov/disability/ [updated 26 Jun 2013; cited 15 Jul 2013].
11. Social Security Administration. Disability determination process. 2013. http://www.ssa.gov/disability/index.htm [updated 26 Jun 2013; cited 15 Jul 2013].
12. Social Security Administration. Social Security Ruling, SSR 13-2p; Titles II and XVI: evaluating cases involving drug addiction and alcoholism. Washington, DC: Social Security Administration (US); 2013 February. Federal Register 78(34).
13. Social Security Administration. Continuing disability review, Understanding supplemental security income. Washington, DC: Social Security Administration (US); 2013.
14. van Vleet R, McAlpine K. How to apply for disability benefits. In: Kaye AD, Urman R, editors. Understanding pain: what you need to know to take control. Santa Barbara: Praeger; 2011.
15. Waid MD, Barber SL. Follow-up of former drug addict and alcoholic beneficiaries. Washington, DC: Research and Statistics Note; 2001. October. Report No: 2001-02.
16. Hunt SR, Baumohol J. Drink, drugs and disability: an introduction to the controversy. Contemp Drug Probl. 2003;30(1/2):9–76.
17. Hogan SR, Unick GJ, Speiglman R, Norris JC. Social welfare policy and public assistance for low-income substance abusers: the impact of 1996 welfare reform legislation on the economic security of former supplemental security income drug addiction and alcoholism beneficiaries. J Sociol Social Welfare. 2008;35(1):221–45.
18. Social Security Administration. Social Security Administration Created as an Independent Agency: Public Law 1-3-296. Washington, DC: Social Security Administration (US); 1995. Social Security Bulletin 58(1): p. 57–65.
19. Social Security Administration. Section 12.10 Substance abuse disorders. Disability evaluation under social security part iii—listing of impairments. http://www.ssa.gov/disability/professionals/bluebook/12.00-MentalDisorders-Adult.htm [cited 15 May 2013].

20. Post P, Perret Y, Ander S, Dalton M, Zevin B. Documenting disability for persons with substance use disorders and co-occurring impairments; a guide for clinicians. Nashville: National Health Care for the Homeless Council, Inc.; 2007.
21. Department of Health and Human Services. Substance abuse and disability. http://www.hhs.gov/od/about/fact_sheets/substanceabuse.html [cited 30 May 2013].
22. Stinson FS, Grant BF, Dawson DA, Ruan WJ, Huang B, Saha T. Comorbidity between DSM-IV alcohol and specific drug use disorders in the United States. Results from the national Epidemiologic survey on alcohol related conditions. Drug Alcohol Depend. 2005;80:105–16.
23. Rehabilitation Research and Training Center on Drugs and Disability. Alcohol and other drug abuse statistics among persons with disabilities. In: Wolkstein E, Moore D, editors. Substance abuse, disability, and vocational rehabilitation. Dayton: Rehabilitation Research and Training on Drugs and Disability, Wright State University; 1996.
24. Sharoff LJ. Coping with the disease of having a disease: a holistic perspective. J Psychosoc Nurs Ment Health Serv. 1998;35:43–5.
25. Shaner A, Eckman TA, Roberts LJ, Wilkins JN, Tucker DC, Tsuang JW, Mintz J. Disability income, cocaine use, and repeated hospitalization among schizophrenic cocaine abusers: a government-sponsored revolving door? New Engl J Med. 1995;333(12):777–83.
26. Rosen MI, McMahon TJ, Lin H, Rosenheck RA. Effect of social security payments on substance abuse in a homeless mentally ill cohort. Health Serv Res. 2006;41(1):171–91.
27. Mark TL, Coffey RM, Vandivort-Warren R, Harwood HJ, King EC, and MHSA Spending Estimates Team. U.S. spending for mental health and substance abuse treatment, 1991–2001. Health Affairs. 2005;133–42.
28. Social Security Administration. Trends in the social security and supplemental security income disability programs. Washington, DC: Social Security Administration (US); 2006 August. No. 13-11831.
29. Robinson G, Kaye N, Bergman D, Moreaux M, Baxter K. State profiles of mental health and substance abuse services in medicaid. Rockville: Substance Abuse and Mental Health Services Administration (US); 2005 January. Pub ID: NMH05-0202.
30. Carolina-Nicole H, Hargraves J, Stanton G. Issue brief #5: the impact of Mental Health Parity and Addiction Equity act on inpatient admissions. Washington, DC: Health Care Cost Institute; 2003.
31. Slayter EM. Disparities in access to substance abuse treatment among people with intellectual disabilities and serious mental illness. Health Soc Work. 2010;35(1):49–59.
32. Capps CF, Luck RS, West SL. Physical inaccessibility negatively impacts the treatment participation of persons with disabilities. Addict Behav. 2007;32(7):1494–7.
33. New York State Office of Alcoholism and Substance Abuse services. OASAS Addiction Treatment Center Directory. http://www.oasas.ny.gov/atc/directory.cfm [cited 30 May 2013].
34. Basford JR, Rohe DE, Barnes CP, DePompolo RW. Substance abuse attitudes and policies in US rehabilitation training programs: a comparison of 1985 and 2000. Arch Phys Med Rehabil. 2002;83(4):517–22.
35. Bombardier CH, Turner AP. Alcohol and other drug use in traumatic disability. In: Frank RG, Rosenthal M, Caplan B, editors. Handbook of rehabilitation psychology. 2nd ed. Washington, DC: American Psychological Association; 2010.
36. New York State Office of Mental Health. Screening for Co-occurring Disorders OMH and OASAS Guidance Document [Internet]. 2008 [updated 31 Jul 2008; cited 10 Jul 2013]. http://www.omh.ny.gov/omhweb/resources/providers/co_occurring/adult_services/screening.html.
37. Timko T. Outcomes of AA for special populations. In: Galanter M, Kaskutas LA, editors. Alcoholism research: alcoholics anonymous and spirituality in addiction recovery, Recent developments in alcoholism, vol. XVIII. New York: Springer; 2008.
38. Center for Substance Abuse Treatment. Substance abuse treatment for persons with co-occurring disorders. Treatment Improvement Protocol (TIP) Series 42. Rockville: Substance Abuse and Mental Health Services; 2005. DHHS Publication No. SMA05-3992.
39. Substance Abuse and Mental Health Services (SAMHSA) SSI/SSDI Outreach, Access and Recovery (SOAR) Technical Assistance Center. 2011 SOAR outcomes. Rockville: Substance Abuse and Mental Health Services; 2012 February.

Chapter 43
Effects of Substance Abuse on the Cardiovascular System and Its Management

Adnan Khan Malik, Ann Marie Melookaran, Gnana S. Simon, and Qingbing Zhu

Key Points

- Alcohol
- Cocaine
- Opioids
- Barbiturates
- Amphetamines
- Benzodiazepines
- Marijuana
- Tricyclic Antidepressants
- Salicylic Acid
- Acetaminophen
- Steroids
- Nicotine
- Ketamine (Ketamine hydrochloride)
- Methamphetamine
- Caffeine
- Dextromethorphan
- Organic Solvents
- MDMA
- Hallucinogens (LSD)

A.K. Malik, M.D. • A.M. Melookaran, M.D. • G.S. Simon, M.D., M.B.A.
Department of Anesthesiology, Yale-New Haven Hospital, 20 York Street, New Haven, CT 06511, USA
e-mail: adnan.malik@yale.edu; ann.melookaran@yale.edu; Simon.gnana@gmail.com

Q. Zhu, M.D., Ph.D. (✉)
Department of Anesthesiology, Yale University, School of Medicine, 333 Cedar street, New Haven, CT 06510-8051, USA
e-mail: qingbing.zhu@yale.edu

© Springer Science+Business Media New York 2015
A.D. Kaye et al. (eds.), *Substance Abuse*, DOI 10.1007/978-1-4939-1951-2_43

Alcohol

Alcohol has been demonstrated to have specific neuronal targets and believed to be more complex than previously thought. There are multiple target receptors in the body including ligand-gated ion channels such as GABA, glycine, NMDA, nicotinic acetylcholine receptors, AMPA receptors, Kainate receptor systems, 5-HT3 receptors, dopamine, adenosine receptors, and voltage-gated ion channels. When ingested acutely, the initial effects include mood elevation followed shortly by alcohol's sedative and anxiolytic effects. Chronic ingestion of alcohol can manifest as liver disease (fatty liver and liver cirrhosis), peripheral neuropathy (secondary to malabsorption with vitamin B deficiencies), and Wernicke-Korsakoff syndrome due to thiamine deficiency [1]. Heavy alcohol consumption results in damage to the heart when ingestion dosages exceed 90–100 g/day. Continuous heavy alcohol consumption results in alcoholic cardiomyopathy which is preceded by an increased ventricular wall thickness to diameter ratio [2]. Excessive consumption of alcohol can result in arrhythmias, particularly supraventricular tachyarrhythmia due to its damaging effects on cardiac tissue. Atrial fibrillation was reported to be the most common arrhythmia followed by ventricular arrhythmias. Chronic alcohol consumption was associated with an increased incidence of conduction disturbances, i.e., RBBB, LBBB [3]. While there has been an associated risk of hypertension with heavy alcohol consumption, the link between light and moderate consumption is much less established. Some researches indicated that moderate alcohol intake may have a protective effect on ischemia coronary disease and stroke [4]. Treatment can be supportive via self-help programs such as alcoholics anonymous [5] and more effective when combined with professional psychotherapy [6]. The withdrawal period has been associated with significant ventricular arrhythmias and management should take into consideration this serious complication [7]. Pharmacotherapy with disulfiram has been classically utilized to promote alcohol abstinence. Disulfiram prevents the conversion of acetaldehyde to acetate by alcohol dehydrogenase. The resulting accumulation of acetaldehyde results in an unpleasant sensation, which serves as a deterrent for future consumption [8]. Acamprosate has been shown to result in abstinence from usage for up to 1 year when compared to psychosocial treatment alone [9]. Naltrexone has also been utilized for the treatment by presumably preventing cravings; however, the exact mechanism is unknown [4]. Other non-conventional treatment options have found ondansetron, when combined with psychotherapy, to result in abstinence for a longer period in individuals who are categorized as "early-onset alcoholics" (heavy drinkers prior to the age of 25) [10] while sertraline has been shown to reduce drinking in late-onset alcoholics [11].

Cocaine

Cocaine, while notorious for its euphoric effects, is often forgotten that it was one of the first local anesthetics that was discovered and served as a template for future local anesthetics. The mechanism of action involved inhibiting nerve impulse by blocking Na voltage-gated channels. In the CNS, cocaine acts as a stimulant by increasing norepinephrine and epinephrine levels in addition to preventing reuptake of norepinephrine, serotonin, and dopamine [1]. Cocaine usage results in a dose-dependent increase in heart rate and blood pressure. Further effects on the cardiovascular system include myocardial ischemia and infarction. The increased sympathetic activity results in an increase of myocardial contractility, hypertension, tachycardia, and myocardial oxygen consumption while concurrently causing myocardial vasoconstriction which can decrease oxygen supply to the heart. The most common symptom is chest pain and the most common cardiac disorder is acute coronary syndrome. As such, there is noted to be a 24-fold increase in the likelihood of developing an acute myocardial infarction shortly after cocaine use. In individuals with normal coronary arteries, focal vasospasm and diffuse coronary vasoconstriction can result in a myocardial infarction. Individuals with atherosclerosis are at an increased risk as the endothelial dysfunction present results in hypersensitivity to the cardiac effects of cocaine. Cocaine can also result in enhanced platelet aggregation by potentiating thromboxane production [12]. Even in the absence of myocardial ischemia, there can be depression of left ventricular function. This can result in transient toxic cardiomyopathy. Cocaine has multiple effects on the rhythm of the heart as it causes sodium channel blockade acting as a class I antiarrhythmic agent. It can result in QT interval prolongation, ventricular arrhythmias including ventricular fibrillation [12]. In addition, the direct effects of cocaine on the endothelium can predispose one to endocarditis. The shearing effects from increased systemic arterial pressure can induce acute aortic dissection [12]. The prevention in reuptake of dopamine results in mood elevation and arousal. When ingested, the acute effects mimic those of other stimulants such as amphetamines. Physiologically, the release of norepinephrine, epinephrine, and dopamine results in intense CNS stimulation which can lower the seizure threshold, hyperpyrexia, tachycardia, hypertension, and diaphoresis. With chronic use, tolerance and dependence can develop in addition to presentation of depression, psychosis, personality disorders, and eating disorders [1]. The need to reduplicate the initial sense of euphoria despite developing tolerance results in altered motivational behavior where the individual will often be highly determined to obtain cocaine regardless of what deeds may be required. Currently there are no other effective treatments aside from abstinence with life support and as such, patients can be treated as outpatients with minimal withdrawal symptoms short of cravings. The recovery of PR intervals to normal range of ECG was found to be correlated well with the length of cocaine abstinence [1].

Opioids

Opioids are a class of medications that were traditionally extracted from the plant Papaver Somniferum; however, they are now able to be derived synthetically. They exert their action by binding to a number of opioid receptors of which four subtypes have been identified including the mu (μ), kappa (κ), delta (δ), and sigma (σ) receptors. The vast majority of opioids that are used clinically have high specificity for the μ-opioid receptors [13]. Most opioids depend on hepatic metabolism for clearance which in turn is dependent on liver blood flow. Of the clinically utilized opioids, morphine and meperidine have the most active metabolites while the by-products of fentanyl, sufentanil, and alfentanil are inactive. Meperidine undergoes metabolism to form normeperidine which when accumulated in high levels can result in seizures. Morphine undergoes conjugation with glucuronic acid to form morphine 3-glucuronide and morphine 6-glucuronide. The end metabolites of both meperidine and morphine require renal elimination. In situations of renal failure, the metabolites accumulate resulting in prolonged ventilator depression and narcosis in the case of morphine, and normeperidine in the case of meperidine resulting in seizures and myoclonic activity. Opioids effects on the cardiovascular system typically are evident by a vagal mediated bradycardia with the exception of meperidine where tachycardia is more likely given its anticholinergic properties. The hypotension resulting from opioid administration is typically due to bradycardia rather than any myocardial depression. Where morphine and meperidine are involved, histamine release can result in venodilation resulting in hypotension. Acute intoxication with opioids often manifests as signs of severe respiratory depression, mitosis, and varying levels of consciousness. The severe respiratory depression can at times also result in pulmonary edema. Acute treatment of opioid toxicity often involves establishing adequate ventilation and the administration of an opioid antagonist (i.e., naloxone) intravenously. Proper administration involves titration with 40 mcg increments in order to minimize opioid withdrawal with typical response seen with less than 0.5 mg of naloxone. If after 5–10 mg of naloxone administration, there is no significant reversal in symptoms, then it is very unlikely that the CNS depression and respiratory depression are primarily due to opioids. Overdose with buprenorphine however can require Naloxone doses as high as 10 mg to reverse its effects due to the strong affinity of buprenorphine to opioid receptors. If a longer acting opioid was the triggering agent for the overdose, then careful attention must be paid to prevent relapse as the duration of naloxone may be shorter than the inciting drug [1]. Methadone regimes are the favorable choice for treatment of opioid withdrawal, while alpha-2 adrenergic agonist may help to reduce the withdrawal symptoms in both in-patient and out-patient settings.

Barbiturates

Barbiturates act by depressing the reticular activating system by suppressing the transmission of excitatory neurotransmitters and mimicking the actions of GABA on chloride channels with inhibitory effects on the CNS. When given intravenously, barbiturates result in hypotension and tachycardia, vasodilation. Cardiac output is minimally affected as the hypotension is offset by increasing heart rate. If the baroreceptor response is blunted, the vasodilation and hypotension can dramatically cause a decrease in cardiac output. The respiratory effects include ventilatory depression, bronchospasm, and laryngospasm and hiccupping are also noted. When examining the effects on the central nervous system, there is a dramatic decrease in cerebral blood flow and intracranial pressure [14]. Treatment involves slow tapering as the withdrawal symptoms can have deleterious effects. Behavioral therapy is a mainstay in managing dependence.

Amphetamines

Amphetamines exert their effects by acting as an indirect catecholamine agonist by causing release of norepinephrine and dopamine from presynaptic neurons while preventing their reuptake and in high doses can have serotonergic effects by release of 5-hydroxytryptamine. Administration can be taken orally or intravenously. The main effects are exerted on the CNS system resulting in stimulatory effects. Psychiatric behavior associates with aggression, anorexia, hyperactivity, psychotic ideation, and high risk behavior. The acute effects involve cardiac conduction, ventricular irritability, hyperpyrexia, hypertension, and seizures [1]. More specific cardiac effects include chest pain, dyspnea, and palpitations. Myocardial infarctions have also been associated with amphetamine use due to thrombus formation. Both acute and chronic amphetamine use has been associated with the development of cardiomyopathy both from direct cardiotoxicity and indirect actions of amphetamines inducing hypertension and ischemia. While most incidences of cardiomyopathy have been linked to oral and intravenous usage, inhalation of methamphetamines can also result in cardiac toxicity [15]. Chronic usage has been shown to result in neurotransmitter depletion, neuronal destruction, cerebrovascular damage, and psychosis. Treatment of amphetamine abuse includes blocking the reinforcing effects and to reduce the urges that result in use. This is accomplished primarily by dopamine agonists by preventing the cravings and dysphoria that is associated with amphetamine use. Tricyclic antidepressants have also been effective in treatment for preventing the depressive symptoms and urges that are associated with withdrawal. Lastly, behavioral therapy is equally as important to prevent relapse [1].

Benzodiazepines

Benzodiazepines are in a class of sedative agents that bind to $GABA_A$ receptors and increased conductance via chloride channels. Metabolism is dependent on hepatic metabolism with oxidation and conjugation to metabolites. As such, liver disease can significantly prolong the duration of action of benzodiazepines. Common effects involve sedation, hypnosis, anterograde amnesia, dose-dependent respiratory depression, and anti-convulsion properties. The hemodynamic effects of benzodiazepine usage involved potent peripheral vasodilation and hypotension [16]. The decrease in systemic vascular resistance and subsequent hypotension along with myocardial depressive effects are masked under general anesthesia secondary to laryngoscopy and intubation [13]. Despite the ability of benzodiazepines to cause vasodilation and mild depression of myocardial contractility, the sympathetic reflexes remain intact. In fact, after administration, catecholamine release tends to stabilize both cardiac output and blood pressure [17]. Acute intoxication with benzodiazepines can be treated with flumazenil which has a high affinity for the benzodiazepine receptor and acts as a competitive antagonist. Its short half-life necessitates repeat dosing or initiation of a continuous infusion due to longer lasting effects of benzodiazepines [13].

Marijuana

Marijuana is a substance that has a psychoactive component called delta-9-tetrahydrocannabinol (THC). It is part of the cannabinoid drugs, which are from the dried hemp plant [18–20]. The most common prescription use of this drug is as an antiemetic [19]. Effects of THC are due to binding to cannabinoid receptors in the central and peripheral nervous system. Acute effects include euphoria, activation of the sympathetic nervous system [18]. Inhalation provides greater euphoria than oral ingestion. THC may cause a decrease in parasympathetic nervous system. Most common objective changes are dose-dependent tachycardia and a mild increase of blood pressure. Occasionally orthostatic hypotension may happen as a result of decreased peripheral vascular resistance [19]. Vasodilation causes conjunctival congestion as well. Acute effect of marijuana may decrease the time of the onset of chest pain in patients with ongoing MI. Due to the result of increase of heart rate, blood pressure, increase of catecholamine levels and carboxyl hemoglobin, smoking of marijuana may increase the risk of the cardiovascular disease [20]. Chronic users may develop tolerance to the psychoactive components of THC. THC effects last about 2 h with a peak onset time of about 1 h and there is no reversal at this time for acute intoxication [18, 19]. Treatment is supportive.

Tricyclic Antidepressants

Tricyclic antidepressants (TCA) are serotonin, norepinephrine reuptake inhibitors. In overdose they can cause significant anticholinergic effects. Acute ingestion may present as intense anticholinergic effects, peripheral alpha adrenergic blockade, and membrane depressant effects [18]. Anticholinergic effects present with cardiovascular effects such as tachycardia, genitourinary effects such as ileus and urinary retention, peripheral effects such as dry skin and flushing as well as other presentations with delirium, fever, and mydriasis. Cardiovascular toxicity, sinus tachycardia, and dysrhythmias with prolongations of the PR, QRS, and QT intervals can also be seen with acute TCA ingestion [18]. In overdose, cardiac dysrhythmias can be fatal and the risk may persist for days after ingestion. Cardiotoxicity from TCA overdose is the most common cause of death, usually associated with hypotension and reduced contractility as well as dysrhythmias [18, 21]. Sodium channel blockade in the myocardium prolongs action potentials which prolongs the refractory period and delays conduction thus widening the QRS complexes. Treatment after acute ingestion can be activated charcoal and gastric lavage initially to eliminate the drug though endotracheal intubation and supportive care may be required if the patient cannot protect their airway [21]. Decreasing free drug by increasing the protein bound drug with alkalization can be done with sodium bicarbonate or hyperventilation. Lipid emulsion may potentially help with reversing cardiotoxicity with TCA overdose in addition to supportive therapy [18, 21].

Salicylic Acid

Salicylic acid is a metabolite of acetylsalicylic acid. Toxicity of salicylic acid is primarily by uncoupling oxidative phosphorylation and disruption of the Krebs cycle which causes an increase in lactate and ketoacids. Metabolic acidosis seen with salicylic acid is due to the lactic acid and ketoacids [18]. Respiratory alkalosis due to stimulation of the CNS respiratory center is also seen with salicylic acid use; patients may present with mixed metabolic acidosis and concomitant respiratory alkalosis [18, 22]. Noncardiogenic pulmonary edema can occur in the first 24 h after overdose [18, 23]. Rarely, ventricular ectopic activity or sinus and atrioventricular nodal conduction disturbance and atrial arrhythmias can be seen with toxic serum salicylate concentrations [23]. Treatment initially after overdose is activated charcoal and gastric lavage. Serum salicylate concentrations should be measured at presentation and compared to the levels after treatment. Sodium bicarbonate and glucose can be given to help alkalinize the serum, and subsequently the urine, and prevent cerebrospinal fluid glucose levels from dropping. Hemodialysis is indicated if >100 mg/dL ingestion as well as if there is refractory acidosis or with renal failure or comatose patients [18].

Acetaminophen

Acetaminophen is an over-the-counter nonsteroidal anti-inflammatory analgesic. Although it has no direct effect on cardiovascular system, acetaminophen may increase blood pressure or even increase risk for cardiovascular risk in human [24, 25]. Acute overdose presents with gastrointestinal symptoms such as nausea, emesis, and abdominal pain [18, 26]. Toxicity is due to centrilobar hepatic necrosis caused by N-acetyl-p-benzoquinoneimine, which is lethal to hepatocytes. This metabolite is usually inactivated when conjugated with glutathione [18]. In situations such as overdose though, glutathione is depleted allowing for the toxic metabolite to persist. Four hours after ingestion the plasma level can be plotted on a Rumack-Matthew nomogram and risk of hepatotoxicity can be stratified to help determine therapeutic options. Activated charcoal and gastric lavage can be used to remove acetaminophen if less than 4 h after ingestion [18]. Treatment with N-acetylcysteine, which depletes glutathione and allows for conjugation of the toxic metabolite, is the most effective within 8 h of ingestion of acetaminophen [26]. Treatment can be both oral and intravenous, though there was a case report regarding adverse effects of intravenous use of N-acetylcysteine in a patient that developed an anaphylactoid reaction [18, 26, 27].

Steroids

Steroid use has both anabolic and androgenic effects. Anabolic steroids can be classified into 17-alpha-alkylated and 17-esterified steroids [26]. The anabolic effects include muscle mass proliferation which is why this can be abused by athletes. Direct myocardial injury such as myocardial cell hypertrophy is caused by anabolic androgenic steroids [26]. Toxicity or intoxication with anabolic steroids can cause cardiovascular diseases such as myocardial infarction or cerebrovascular accidents [28]. Other associated toxicities include liver disease, hypertension, fluid retention, changes in the immune system, and skin changes. The androgenic effects of steroid use can include masculinization of both males and females [29]. Myocardial hypertrophy, regional fibrosis, and necrosis or even new onset heart failure can all be associated with steroids, which increases associated risk with infarct and sudden cardiac death [29]. Chronic use of steroids can suppress adrenocorticotropic hormone secondary to the negative feedback on the hypothalamus from the exogenous steroids. Withdrawal from steroids, when it is chronically used, can present with insomnia, anorexia, restlessness, and fatigue [29]. There is no specific treatment or pharmacologic needs during detoxification, though patients with severe hypothalamic suppression of the gonadotropins may need hormonal replacement [29].

Nicotine

Nicotine is a substance in tobacco from the plant *Nicotiana Tabacum*. It is most often inhaled, dipped, or chewed as it can be absorbed through the respiratory tract, buccal membranes, and skin [30]. Nicotine acts on the nicotinic acetylcholine receptors. Nicotinic receptors are found at the neuromuscular junction, the autonomic ganglia, and central nerve system. Stimulation of these nicotinic receptors causes alertness, skeletal muscle contraction, and sympathetic nervous system stimulation including tachycardia and diaphoresis [31]. Acutely, nicotine may produce a mild euphoria though the tolerance may develop so quickly that this euphoria does not persist [30, 31]. Tolerance may develop to the effects of nicotine stimulation such as tachycardia, increase of blood pressure as well as nausea and emesis. Since nicotine can cause vasoconstriction, there is concern for decreased placental blood flow an oxygen delivery to the fetus [30]. Treatment for nicotine addiction includes 12-step programs, which are also used for other addictions [20]. Nicotine replacement with gum or patches can help with quitting. Clonidine is also used for treatment of nicotine withdrawal [30].

Ketamine (Ketamine Hydrochloride)

Ketamine hydrochloride (Ketamine) is a phencyclidine derivative developed in the 1960s as an anesthetic alternative to PCP [32]. Ketamine is a noncompetitive NMDA antagonist, which is primarily metabolized by the liver through the CYP450 pathway into norketamine [32]. Current indications for ketamine include induction and maintenance of general anesthesia as well as premedication. Acute cardiovascular effects of ketamine include increased arterial and venous pressures, tachycardia, and an increase in cardiac output. Ketamine acts as direct negative ionotrope but the net effect is one of a central sympathetic stimulant [33]. Studies have found that chronic ketamine abuse leads to myocardial apoptosis with subsequent fibrotic remodeling leading to increased arrhythmias [34]. Recent studies have shown a possible role for ketamine in the treatment of depression. Subanesthetic doses of ketamine produce marked and prolonged antidepressant activity [32]. Recreational use of ketamine saw a surge starting in the 1980s, with users seeking a sense of euphoria, increased social interaction, and hallucinations. Higher doses of ketamine are associated with a dissociative state. Other adverse acute effects include nausea/vomiting, increased secretions, nystagmus, increased intracranial pressure, and increased risk of seizure [32]. Prolonged use of ketamine is associated with decreased cognitive function and psychological health [35]. Ketamine also has a role in chronic pain management due to its ability to both inhibit opiate tolerance and resensitize to opiate analgesia [32]. Ketamine toxicity often manifests as respiratory depression and sedation, requiring supportive therapy. Instances of ketamine psychosis have also been described.

Methamphetamine

Methamphetamine is the N-methyl derivative of amphetamine. It acts as an indirect agonist at dopamine, noradrenalin, and serotonin receptors [36]. Methamphetamine is primarily metabolized in the liver through the cytochrome p450 2D6 pathway and produces several metabolites, including amphetamine, 4-hydroxymethamphetamine, and norephedrine [36]. Metabolites that do not appear have significant clinical effects. The effects of methamphetamine are dose dependent. Cardiovascular effects of methamphetamine include hypertension and tachycardia associated with potentiating arrhythmia, acute coronary events, and cardiac death [36]. Studies show that methamphetamine users have both a high and earlier incidence of coronary artery disease. The risk of cardiomyopathy in this population is also increased up to 3–4 folds [36]. In low-to-moderate doses (5–30 mg), common subjective effects include euphoria, arousal, anxiety, paranoia, and hallucinations [36]. Physiologic effects include anorexia, mydriasis, tachycardia, hypertension, and increased body temperature. Studies on higher doses of methamphetamine (55–640 mg) are limited but appear to be characterized psychotic symptoms [36]. Chronic use of methamphetamines is associated with higher incidence of psychotic symptoms. Methamphetamine psychosis is characterized by a paranoid-hallucinatory state, clinically similar to acute paranoid schizophrenia [36]. Symptoms include auditory hallucinations, delusions, and disordered thinking. Regular exposure to methamphetamines is also associated with neurotoxicity, particularly to serotonergic and dopaminergic neurons [36]. Cognitive deficits especially in memory, impulse control, and executive function are also noted. Withdrawal is associated with sudden termination of chronic methamphetamine use. It is characterized by depression, agitation, insomnia, and cognitive deficits [36].

Caffeine

Caffeine (1,3,7-trimethylxanthine) is the most common stimulant in use across the world. Its mechanism of action is through antagonism of adenosine receptors [37]. Through inhibiting adenosine, caffeine increases circulating levels of catecholamines. Caffeine is metabolized primarily in the liver through the cytochrome-450 system. Due to an inability to demethylate caffeine, neonates rely on renal excretion until 3 months of life [37]. Metabolism of caffeine is affected by multiple drugs. For example, alcohol, estrogen, and cimetidine inhibit metabolism of caffeine while alcohol increases it [37]. Of note, regular use of caffeine results in developing tolerance in the course of days. The peak effect of caffeine is achieved within 30–60 min; half-life ranges from 2 to 12 h in adults [37]. Cardiovascular effects of caffeine include mild hypertension and peripheral vasoconstriction [37]. There is no change in cardiac output as this increase in blood pressure is often compensated with decrease in heart rate. Acute effects include increased arousal, vigilance, and decreased fatigue. At higher doses, adverse side effects include insomnia, tremors, and anxiety. It has also been associated with precipitating panic attacks in patients with underlying psychiatric illness. Caffeine increases the respiratory rate and minute ventilation. It also has mild bronchodilator effects. There is increased water and sodium with caffeine due to increased GFR and inhibition of tubular reabsorption [37]. Caffeine toxicity is characterized by catecholamine release with resultant tachycardia as well as hypotension and vasodilatation [37]. Treatment consists of supportive measures. Chronic and heavy caffeine use is associated with a dose-related increased risk of coronary artery disease. Heavy caffeine consumption is also associated with increased cholesterol levels and arrhythmias [37]. Abrupt cessation of caffeine leads to a withdrawal syndrome. The withdrawal symptoms, which include fatigue, anxiety, and headache, can begin within 12 h of stopping intake and last up to 1 week [37].

Dextromethorphan

Dextromethorphan hydrobromide (DXM) is a common ingredient in cough and cold medicines. It is a popular drug of abuse in adolescents due to its easily availability and price point. Dextromethorphan is a weak sigma-1 opioid agonist, strong

NMDA antagonist, and serotonin agonist [38]. Metabolism of dextromethorphan is through the cytochrome CYP2D6 system. Due to genetic variation, up to 5 % of those with European descent have abnormal metabolism leading to rapid DXM toxicity. DXM produces feelings of euphoria and disassociation, likely due to its similarities to PCP and ketamine [38]. Higher doses can lead to hallucinations and psychosis. Other adverse acute effects include hypertension, tachycardia, and ataxia [39]. Chronic use of dextromethorphan can lead to tolerance and cessation is associated with withdrawal predominated by severe depression. Dextromethorphan is often available in combination with other drugs including guaifenesin and acetaminophen [38]. Toxicity is often attributed to accidently ingesting large amounts of these additive drugs. Dextromethorphan toxicity has been associated with behavior changes including aggression and psychosis [39]. Cases of respiratory failure and ARDS have also been reported. Treatment is primarily supportive.

Organic Solvents

The recreational use of organic solvents is highest in children and adolescents. The most common organic solvent abused is toluene, which is found in spray paint and nail polish. Toluene acts as a CNS depressant through enhancing GABA receptors and inhibiting NMDA receptors [40]. This organic solvent is highly lipophilic and is rapidly absorbed in lipid rich organs like the brain and liver. It is well absorbed both orally and nasally. The half-life of toluene in blood is 3–6 h [40]. Metabolism is primarily through the liver (the cytochrome CYP2E1 system) and less so by direct pulmonary exchange [40]. Acute effects include euphoria and grandiosity. Adverse acute effects are dose dependent. At lower doses, these consist include ataxia, headache, and slowed motor and speech [40]. Higher doses can lead to encephalopathy, seizures, arrhythmias, and respiratory depression [40]. Ventricular arrhythmia is the most common cause of death in toluene misuse. Toluene has direct chronotropic effects on cardiac muscle, usually through sensitizing myocytes to catecholamine [41]. Although tachyarrhythmia is more characteristic of toluene toxicity, bradyarrhythmia, cardiomyopathy, vasospasm, and myocardial infarction have been described. The chronic use of toluene has been associated with neurotoxicity; specifically myelin damage and white matter macrophages. MRI studies show white matter loss as early as 4 years [42]. Neurotoxicity consists of optic damage, hearing loss, cerebellum dysfunction, and cognitive decline [40].

MDMA

3,4 methylenedioxy-methamphetamine (MDMA) is also known as ecstasy and is a common drug of abuse. It increases concentrations of serotonin, dopamine, and norepinephrine, with the highest affinity for serotonin [43]. It is metabolized in the liver through the cytochrome CYP2D6 system with a half-life of 8 h [43]. Acute effects include increased energy, euphoria, increased motor coordination, and desire for socialization. These qualities account for MDMA's high use among young adult in party and rave settings [44]. One of the hallmarks of acute MDMA toxicity is hyperthermia, which is often aggravated by the high surrounding temperatures [44]. Hyperthermia is usually accompanied by a chain effect of rhabdomyolysis, acute renal failure, and DIC. MDMA has also been associated with hypertension, tachycardia, arrhythmias, stroke, and cerebral hemorrhages [43]. As a cardiac stimulant, MDMA leads to tachycardia, hypertension, and increased cardiac output in a dose-dependent manner. Notably, it does not have any inotropic effects, which leads to increased myocardial oxygen consumption but with no compensatory increase in contractility [45]. This may explain the instances of arrhythmias, cardiomyopathy, and myocardial infarction with MDMA use reported. Cases of serotonin syndrome and hyperactivity have also been described. Treatment for MDMA toxicity is primarily supportive such as cool, quiet, non-stimulating environment and hydration [44]. Recent studies have shown MDMA associated with increased oxidative stress, free radical production, and mitochondrial dysfunction [46]. Chronic MDMA use is associated with neurotoxicity through the destruction of serotonergic and dopaminergic neurons [43]. There is also an increased incidence of psychiatric illness in chronic MDMA uses, predominated by anxiety and depression.

Hallucinogens (LSD)

Lysergic acid diethylamide (LSD) is a synthetic hallucinogenic substance that has been used for recreational drug use. It can cause sensory distortions for visual, tactile, and auditory senses [47]. It is known to produce hallucinogenic effects as well as changes in behavior [48]. Proposed mechanism of action includes agonist, partial agonist, and antagonist effects at various serotonin, dopaminergic, and adrenergic receptors [49]. Acute administration is usually through mucosal surfaces and the peak effect is usually seen in 30–60 min. Its effects last for about 8–12 h [47] but can persist for days. It is derived from the ergot alkaloids and is structurally similar to other alkaloids and other drugs that are known to inhibit serotonin. Serious side effects include the acute psychotic reaction and hallucinations and the risk of transient reappearance of the hallucinogenic effects later [48]. Sympathetic stimulation results in mydriasis, hypertension, tachycardia, and hyperreflexia. Rarely, ingestion of LSD can result in supraventricular arrhythmias and precipitation of myocardial infarction. This effect is postulated to be secondary to serotonin-induced platelet aggregation and sympathetic arterial vasospasm [49]. Hallucinogen-persisting perception disorder after lysergic acid diethylamide abuse can be a chronic effect of use and is seen as continued spontaneous recurrence of visual hallucinations after use [50, 51]. Treatment methods have included antiepileptics, antidepressants as well as supportive care [50].

Table 43.1 is a summary of the above abuse substances for their effects on the cardiovascular system and treatment.

Table 43.1 The following table is summary of the above abuse substances for their effects on the cardiovascular system and treatment

	CNS	PNS	Acute	Chronic	Withdrawal	Treatment
Alcohol	+	+/−	Tachycardia, Arrhythmia,	BBB, hypertension cardiomyopathy	Ventricular arrhythmia	Supportive, Disulfiram, Self-help+psychotherapy
Cocaine	+	+	Increase HR, HTN, MI, aorta dissection, arrhythmia, vasospasm, vasoconstriction	MI, arrhythmia	Arrhythmia	Supportive
Opioids	+	+	Bradycardia, tachycardia, hypotension	Bradycardia	+	Supportive, naloxone, clonidine
Barbiturate	+	+	Hypotension, tachycardia, vasodilation	+	+	Supportive
Amphetamine	+	+	HTN, arrhythmia, MI,	Cardiomyopathy	+	Supportive, dopamine, TCA, behavioral
Benzodiazepine	+		Vasodilatation, depression of contractility	+	+	Flumazenil
Marijuana	+	+	Tachycardia, hypotension	+	+	Supportive
TCA	+	+	Anticholinergic, hypotension, arrhythmia, death			Gastric lavage, lipid emulsion, charcoal, alkalization, hemodialysis
Salicyclic Acid		+	Arrhythmia			Gastric lavage, charcoal, alkalization, hemodialysis
Acetaminophen	+	+	HTN			N-acetylcysteine
Steroid	+	+	+	Hypertrophy, cardiomyopathy, fibrosis, MI, sudden death	+	Supportive
Nicotine	+	+	Tachycardia, HTN, vasoconstriction		+	Supportive, nicotine, clonidine
Ketamine	+		HTN, tachycardia	Myocardia apoptosis, arrhythmia		Supportive
Methamphetamine	+	+	HTN, arrhythmia, acute coronary events, sudden death	Cardiomyopathy, CAD	+	Supportive
Caffeine	+	+	HTN, tachycardia	Increase risk of CAD, arrhythmia	+	Supportive
Dextromethorphan	+		HTN, tachycardia	+	+	Supportive
Organic solvents	+	+	Ventricular arrhythmia, cardiomyopathy, vasospasm, MI	+		Supportive
MDMA	+	+	HTN, tachycardia, arrhythmia, cardiomyopathy, MI	+		Supportive
Hallucinogens (LSD)	+	+	HTN, tachycardia, arrhythmia, MI			Supportive

+ positive effect, − no effect, *BBB* bundle branch block, *CAD* coronary arterial disease, *CNS* central nerve system, *HR* heart rate, *HTN* hypertension, *MI* myocardial infarction, *PNS* peripheral nerve system

References

1. Lowinson JH, Ruiz P, Millman RB, Langrod JG. Substance abuse: a comprehensive textbook. Philadelphia: Lippincott Williams & Wilkins; 2005.
2. Spies CD, Sander M, Stangl K, Fernandez-Sola J, Preedy VR, Rubin E, et al. Effects of alcohol on the heart. Curr Opin Crit Care. 2001;7(5):337–43.
3. Krasniqi A, Bostaca I, Dima-Cosma C, Crişu D, Aursulesei V. Arrhythmogenic effects of alcohol. Rev Med Chir Soc Med Nat Iasi. 2011;115(4):1052–56.
4. Sesso HD, Cook NR, Buring JE, Manson JE, Gaziano JM. Alcohol consumption and the risk of hypertension in women and men. Hypertension. 2008;51(4):1080–7.
5. Humphreys K, Mankowski ES, Moos RH, Finney JW. Do enhanced friendship networks and active coping mediate the effect of self-help groups on substance abuse? Ann Behav Med. 1999;21(1):54–60.
6. Walsh DC, Hingson RW, Merrigan DM, et al. A randomized trial of treatment options for alcohol-abusing workers. N Engl J Med. 1991;325(11):775–82.
7. Hémery Y, Broustet H, Guiraudet O, Schiano P, Godreuil C, Plotton C, et al. Alcohol and rhythm disorders. Ann Cardiol Angeiol. 2000;49(8):473–9.
8. Martin CR. Identification and treatment of alcohol dependency. Cumbria: M&K publishing; 2008.
9. Swift RM. Drug therapy for alcohol dependence. N Engl J Med. 1999;340(19):1482–90.
10. Johnson BA, Roache JD, Javors MA, et al. Ondansetron for reduction of drinking among biologically predisposed alcoholic patients: a randomized controlled trial. JAMA. 2000;284(8):963–71.
11. Pettinati HM, Volpicelli JR, Kranzler HR, et al. Sertraline treatment for alcohol dependence: Interactive effects of medication and alcohol subtype. Alcohol Clin Exp Res. 2000;24(7):1041–9.
12. Maraj S, Figueredo VM, Morris DL. Cocaine and the heart. Clin Cardiol. 2010;33(5):264–9.
13. Barash PG, Cullen BF, Stoelting RK, Cahalan MK, Stock MC. Clinical anesthesia. Philadelphia: Lippincott Williams & Wilkins; 2009.
14. Morgan G, Mikhail MS, Murrary MJ. Clinical anesthesiology. New York: McGraw-Hill; 2006.
15. Albertson TE, Derlet RW, Van Hoozen BE. Methamphetamine and the expanding complications of amphetamines. West J Med. 1999;170(4):214–9.
16. Hensley FA, Martin DE, Gravlee GP. Cardiac Anesthesia. Philadelphia: Lippincott Williams & Wilkins; 2008.
17. Klein LV, Lide AM. Central alpha-2 adrenergic and benzodiazepine agonists and their antagonists. J Zoo Wildl Med. 1989;20(2):138–53.
18. Stoelting RK, Hines RL, Marschall KE. Psychiatric disease, substance abuse, and drug overdose, Stoelting's anesthesia and co-existing disease. Philadelphia: Churchill Livingstone/Elsevier; 2008. p. 550–6.
19. Andreoli TE, Carpenter CJ, Russell LC. Alcohol and substance abuse, Andreoli and Carpenter's Cecil essentials of medicine. Philadelphia: Saunders; 2010. p. 1230–2.
20. Barash PG. Obstetrical anesthesia clinical anesthesia. Philadelphia: Wolters Kluwer; 2009. p. 1159.
21. Blaber MS, Khan JN, Brebner JA, et al. "Lipid rescue" for tricyclic antidepressant cardiotoxicity. J Emerg Med. 2012;23:465–7.
22. Sabatine MS. Acid-base disturbances, Pocket medicine. Philadelphia: Wolters Kluwer Health/Lippincott Williams & Wilkins; 2011. p. 4–2.
23. Mukerji V, Alpert MA, Flaker GC, Beach CL, Weber RD. Cardiac conduction abnormalities and atrial arrhythmias associated with salicylate toxicity. Pharmacotherapy. 1986;6:41–3.
24. Forman JP, Rimm EB, Curhan GC. Frequency of analgesic use and risk of hypertension among men. Arch Intern Med. 2007;167:394–9.
25. Chan AT, Manson JE, Albert CM, Chae CU, Rexrode KM, Curhan GC, et al. Nonsteroid anti-inflammatory drugs, acetaminophen, and the risk of cardiovascular events. Circulation. 2006;113:1578–87.
26. Andreoli TE, Carpenter CJ, Russell LC. Essentials in critical care medicine, Andreoli and Carpenter's Cecil essentials of medicine. Philadelphia: Saunders; 2010. p. 264–5.

27. Elms AR, Owen KP, Albertson TE, et al. Fatal myocardial infarction associated with intravenous N-acetylcysteine error. Int J Emerg Med. 2011;4:54.
28. Riezzo I, De Carlo D, Neri A, et al. Heart disease induced by AAS abuse, using experimental mice/rats models and the role of exercise induced cardiotoxicity. Mini Rev Med Chem. 2013;11:409–24.
29. Miller NS. The pharmacology of anabolic-androgen steroids, The pharmacology of alcohol and drugs of abuse and addiction. New York: Springer; 1991. p. 125–31.
30. Miller NS. The pharmacology of nicotine, The pharmacology of alcohol and drugs of abuse and addiction. New York: Springer; 1991. p. 241–7.
31. Stoelting RK, Miller RD. Autonomic nervous system, Basics of anesthesia. Philadelphia: Churchill Livingstone; 2007. p. 64–8.
32. Rothman RD, Weiner RB, Pope H, et al. Anabolic androgenic steroid induced myocardial toxicity: an evolving problem in an ageing population. BMJ Case Rep. 2011.
33. Trujillo KA, Smith ML, Sullivan B, Heller CY, Garcia C, Bates M. The neurobehavioral pharmacology of ketamine: implications for drug abuse, addiction and psychiatric disorders. ILAR J. 2011;52:366–78.
34. Pai A, Heining M. Ketamine. Cont Educ Anaesth Crit Care Pain. 2007;7(2):59–63.
35. Li Y, Shi J, Yang BF, Lui L, Han CL, et al. Ketamine-induced ventricular structural, sympathetic and electrophysiological remodelling: pathologic consequences and effects of metoprolol. Br J Pharmacol. 2012;165(6):1748–56.
36. Morgan CA, Muetzelfelt L, Curran HV. Consequences of chronic ketamine self-administration upon neurocognitive and psychological well-being: a 1-year longitudinal study. Addiction. 2010;105(1):121–33.
37. Cruickshank C, Dyer K. A review of the clinical pharmacology of methamphetamine. Addiction. 2009;104:1085–99.
38. Benowitz NL. Clinical pharmacology of caffeine. Annu Rev Med. 1990;41:277–88.
39. Lessenger JE, Feinberg SD. Abuse of prescription and over-the-counter medications. J Am Board Fam Med. 2008;21:45–54.
40. Logan BK, Yaekel JK, Goldfogel G, Frost MP, Sandstrom G, Wickham D. Dextromethorphan abuse leading to assault, suicide and homicide. J Forensic Sci. 2012;57:1388–94.
41. Rosenberg NL, Grigsby J, Dreisbach J, Busenbark D, Grigsby P. Neuropsychologic impairment and MRI abnormalities associated with chronic solvent abuse. Clin Toxicol. 2002;40(1):21–34.
42. Turkoglu C, Aliyev F, Celiker C, Uzunhasan I, Kocas C. Slow heart-slow brain: consequence of short-term occupational exposure to toulene in a young woman: what is the real mechanism. Clin Cardiol. 2009;33(2):68–71.
43. Al-Hajri Z, Del Bigio MR. Brain damage in large cohort of solvent abusers. Acta Neuropathol. 2010;119(4):435–45.
44. Rietjens S, Hondebrink L, Westerink R, Meulenbelt J. Pharmacokinetics and pharmacodynamics of 3,4-methylenedioxymethamphetamine (MDMA): inter individual differences due to polymorphims and drug-drug interactions. Crit Rev Toxicol. 2012;42(10):854–76.
45. Green RA, Cross AJ, Goodwin GM. Review of the pharmocology and clinical pharmacology of 3,4-methylenedioxymethamphetamine (MDMA or "ectasy"). Psychopharmacology (Berl). 1995;119:247–60.
46. Lester SJ, Baggott M, Welm S, Schiller NB, Jones RT, Foster E, et al. Cardiovascular effects of 3,4-Methylenedioxymethamphetamine. A double-blind, placebo-controlled trial. Ann Intern Med. 2000;133:969–73.
47. Nakagawa Y, Suzuki T, Tayama S, Ishil H, Ogata A. Cytotoxic effects of 3,4-Methylenedioxy-N-alkyl amphetamines, MDMA and its analogues, on isolated rat hepatocytes. Arch Toxicol. 2009;83:69–80.
48. Beck F, Bonnet N. The substance experience, a history of LSD. Med Sci. 2013;29:430–3.
49. Jenkins JP. LSD. Encyclopedia Britannica Inc. 2013.
50. Guran A, Nolan J. Recreational drug misuse: issues for the cardiologist. Heart. 2000;83:627–33.
51. Hermle L, Simon M, Ruchsow M, Geppert M. Hallucinogen-persisting perception disorder. Ther Adv Psychopharmacol. 2012;2(5):199–205.

Chapter 44
The Face of Addiction

Debra Short

Key points

- Who is an addict?
- Hydrocodone
- "Hitting bottom"
- Rehab
- Recovery
- Narcotics Anonymous

Who is an addict? I have been a retail pharmacist for almost 15 years, and I learned very quickly how to identify an addict, or, more gently stated, I learned how to recognize patients who struggled with substance abuse issues. I saw the patient recovering from surgery who became dependent on opiates, the tired-looking man coming to the pharmacy to buy needles for his "diabetes", the nervous-looking woman attempting to purchase multiple boxes of pseudoephedrine, the emergency-room-frequenter bringing almost daily prescriptions for painkillers and muscle relaxants. What I failed to realize during all of my years of practice was that the face of addiction would actually be my own.

My story begins innocently enough. The birth of my son in 2010 brought with it the joy and stress of being a new mom, as well as the complications of bursitis in both hips and chronic lower back pain. I received prescriptions from my doctor for hydrocodone and carisoprodol, and I took the medication, even though I felt weak and ashamed that I needed it. My desire to work pain-free outweighed those feelings, and being able to walk and to stand for eight-hour shifts made taking the medication a necessary evil.

D. Short, Pharm.D. (✉)
10192 Creek Trail Circle, Stockton, CA 95209, USA
e-mail: morleybaby@comcast.net

© Springer Science+Business Media New York 2015
A.D. Kaye et al. (eds.), *Substance Abuse*, DOI 10.1007/978-1-4939-1951-2_44

With shocking speed, I developed physical tolerance to the hydrocodone, and the pain in my hips and back rapidly became unmanageable. I recall one of my last appointments with my doctor, where I explained my situation and was told that nothing stronger would be prescribed and that she was concerned about me taking too much medication. I remember feeling panic, but, being a healthcare professional and worrying about appearances, I made vague noises of agreement. I did not want her to know how dire my circumstances actually felt.

I do not remember the exact day or time when the desperation of being in constant pain began to cloud my judgment. At some point, however, I made a series of decisions which would affect my life and my career forever: I started stealing medication from the pharmacy where I worked. Over the course of the next 2 years, I engaged in illegal and immoral behavior, diverting larger and larger quantities of hydrocodone and carisoprodol in an effort to manage an increasingly dangerous addiction. For months, I faced no consequences. My performance at work was not affected. My home life and my relationships did not suffer, and to my detriment, no one at the pharmacy knew what I was doing.

Looking back, I realize that every time I stole medication, I lost a piece of myself. I no longer recognized the woman I had been—the successful college student, the highly productive pharmacist, the caring wife and mother. I had become someone I never thought I would be … an addict.

The phrase "hitting bottom" is often thrown around when addicts talk about their motivation for quitting. In April of 2012, I am pretty sure that the bottom hit me. I was arrested and led out of my store in handcuffs, paraded past my employees and patients. I was officially one of those people I had spent my entire career judging. I was an out-of-control, drug-seeking, law-breaking addict.

I checked myself into rehab and started taking steps to get my life and my career back. I learned there that addiction does not discriminate. Wearing a white coat and calling myself a professional did not protect me from this disease. If anything, being in a position of trust and power kept me from being honest with myself and with those around me. Facing no initial consequences likely perpetuated the drug use that should have killed me many times over.

As I progress in my recovery, I have discovered several important things. First, and foremost, identifying myself as an addict does not carry with it shame. I made bad choices; I am not a bad person. I have also come to understand that I have been given an amazing opportunity for self-discovery and self-improvement. The path my life has taken may not be the one I envisioned for myself, but it is the path I have learned to embrace and to appreciate.

I sit in a meeting of Narcotics Anonymous today, and I can honestly say that I am grateful. Grateful that I am alive and whole. Grateful that I have been given this chance to discover how to live. Grateful that I have the opportunity to share my story with others, in the hope that they might learn from my mistakes. I think, as a healthcare provider, I had forgotten that people who suffer from the disease of addiction are human beings first and addicts second. Ultimately, this experience has made me a better pharmacist and a more empathetic person. Today, I have reclaimed my *own* humanity and have grown to accept myself for who I am. I am Debbie. I am a pharmacist. I am an addict.

Chapter 45
Drug Testing and Adherence Monitoring in Substance Abuse Patients

Steven Michael Lampert, Alan David Kaye, Richard D. Urman, and Laxmaiah Manchikanti

Key Points

- Stratification of risk
- Prescription drug monitoring programs
- Drug testing
- Pill counts
- An algorithmic approach

A Russian proverb was espoused by former president Ronald Regan in the 1980s in negotiations with the Soviet leadership, "Trust, but verify." This same concept [1–3] has been adopted by many physicians working with patients on chronic opioid therapy. Physicians that prescribe chronic opioid therapy have an ethical and legal responsibility to monitor for treatment adherence. One way to enhance the trust between the prescribing physician and the patient is to implement a comprehensive adherence-monitoring program [1–4].

S.M. Lampert, M.D. (✉) • R.D. Urman, M.D., M.B.A., C.P.E.
Department of Anesthesiology, Perioperative and Pain Medicine,
Brigham and Women's Hospital, Harvard Medical School, Boston, MA, USA
e-mail: steven.lampert@alumni.bcm.edu

A.D. Kaye, M.D., Ph.D.
Departments of Anesthesiology and Pharmacology,
Louisiana State University Health Sciences Center Louisiana State University
Interim Hospital, and Ochsner Kenner Hospital, New Orleans, LA, USA
e-mail: alankaye44@hotmail.com

L. Manchikanti, M.D.
Anesthesiology and Perioperative Medicine, University of Louisville, Kentucky,
Paducah, KY, USA
e-mail: drm@asipp.org

© Springer Science+Business Media New York 2015
A.D. Kaye et al. (eds.), *Substance Abuse*, DOI 10.1007/978-1-4939-1951-2_45

Urine drug testing is often part of a standard opioid agreement and one tool used for adherence monitoring. Urine drug testing is done to document compliance with medication management as well as screen for concomitant use of illicit drugs of abuse. Recent well publicized reports have clearly documented the growing prescription opioid epidemic and associated increase in morbidity and mortality including opioid related deaths [1, 5–11]. Hydrocodone with acetaminophen is currently the most prescribed drug in the United States with over 135 million prescriptions filled in 2011 [10]. This is more than triple the number of prescriptions filled for the commonly used anti-cholesterol medication Atorvastatin (Lipitor) [10]. Thus, it is incumbent on the physician prescribing opioids to monitor for compliance and drugs of abuse. Furthermore, published data show that physicians are not able to consistently and accurately determine which patients have problems with compliance or addiction based on behaviors and self-report alone [12, 13].

A busy practitioner is frequently faced with aberrant results of urine drug testing, triggering an in depth discussion with the patient about implications for further continuing care [1, 3, 4]. Ideally, the expectations and consequences of aberrant urine drug testing are thoroughly discussed at the onset of the doctor–patient relationship and clearly spelled out in the opioid agreement before opioid management is initiated [1].

The vast majority of opioids in the United States are prescribed by primary care physicians. 42 % of immediate release opioids and almost 44 % of long acting opioids are prescribed in primary care settings [1]. States have focused efforts on educating physicians on "safe" opioid prescribing practices [14, 15]. These prescribing requirements in multiple states are highly variable, but may include education of pharmacology side effects, complications, fatalities, mandatory inquiry of prescription monitoring program, opioid agreements, multiple screening tests, dose limitations, controlled substance agreement, urine drug testing, and random pill counts with repeat assessments and documentation of physical and functional status improvement and comorbidity [1–4, 14, 15].

Stratification of Risk

Risk stratification in patients on chronic opioid therapy is essentially the process of using demographic and historical information in order to attempt to predict patients at higher risk for opioid misuse [1, 4]. Features commonly described of as risk factors for opioid misuse include socioeconomic factors, chronic pain features, drug-related factors, family history and environmental factors, substance abuse history, and psychiatric history [1, 4]. For example, high risk features include pain in 3 or more body regions, widespread pain without objective signs or diagnostic findings, age less than 45 years, heavy smoking, major or multiple psychological comorbidities including bipolar or personality disorders, family or personal history of substance abuse, unwillingness to participate in multimodal therapy, low level of pain acceptance, and poor coping strategies [1, 3]. On the other hand, low risk features include pain in 3 or less body regions, objective signs, and reliable symptoms confirmed by physical exam or diagnostic studies, age greater than 45 years, non-smokers, little or no psychological co-morbidities, no personal or family history of substance abuse, well-motivated to participate in multimodal therapy, a high level of pain acceptance, and a high level of coping strategies [1, 3].

A number of screening tools have been developed in order to assist the practitioner in screening for risk of abuse and misuse of opioids including aberrant drug related behavior in patients on chronic opioid therapy [16, 17]. Although many of these tools can be time consuming to implement, many have not been validated, and some are even susceptible to deception.

Prescription Drug Monitoring Programs

Prescription Drug Monitoring Programs (PDMP) are state sponsored programs that collect data about prescription drugs and track their flow [1, 18–20]. The data collected include the patient's name, prescribing physician, and the pharmacy that filled the medication. Pharmacies are required by state law to report the data to the database. PDMPs are tools used to identify and prevent drug abuse and diversion. One way they assist prescribers is by helping identify drug-seeking behaviors or "doctor shopping." PDMPs can also used by licensing boards to identify unusual or inappropriate prescribing patterns. The goal of implementing and enhancing prescription monitoring programs is that they could lead to a reduction in emergency room visits, drug overdoses, and deaths due to prescription drug overdose.

Previous studies have shown PDMPs are effective when fully utilized. For example, Baehren and colleagues [15] reported, in an emergency room setting with patients seen for nontraumatic painful conditions but excluding acute injuries, 41 % of physicians altered their prescribing plan after the clinician reviewed PDMP data, with 61 % of patients receiving fewer or no opioid pain medications, whereas 39 % resulted in more opioid medications than previously planned by the physician prior to reviewing the data.

Currently, in all the states with pill mill regulations [14], inquiry of the PDMP database is mandatory, while it is voluntary in other states.

Drug Testing

Drug testing can be implemented using several different methods [1, 3, 21–25]. Breath, blood, oral fluid, urine, sweat, hair, and meconium have been used for toxicology screening. They can all be influenced by the amount and frequency of the substance taken prior to sampling. In clinical ambulatory practice, urine drug screening is most frequently used.

624   S.M. Lampert et al.

Table 45.1 Comparative diagnostic accuracy of immunoassay with liquid chromatography

	Sensitivity/false negative rate	Specificity/false positive rate	Test efficiency (agreement)
Morphine, hydrocodone, codeine, hydromorphone	92.2 %/7.8 %	93.1 %/6.9 %	92.5 %
Oxycodone	75.4 %/24.6 %	92.3 %/7.7 %	90 %
Methadone	96.1 %/3.9 %	98.8 %/1.2 %	98.7 %
Marijuana	90.9 %/9.1 %	98.0 %/2 %	97.8 %
Cocaine	25.0 %/75 %	100 %/0 %	99.4 %
Methamphetamines	40 %/60 %	98.8 %/1.2 %	98.5 %
Amphetamines	47 %/53 %	99.1 %/0.9 %	98.2 %

Adapted with permission from [24]

EIA (enzyme-mediated immunoassay) is often used as an initial screening test. It is a quick, relatively easy and inexpensive test to perform. Although somewhat sensitive, the test is not as sensitive or specific as other methods. For example, the test may be positive for opioids but not detect the specific opioid prescribed, especially synthetic opioids like fentanyl, oxycodone, and hydrocodone [21].

Liquid chromatography/tandem mass spectrometry (LC/MS/MS) and gas chromatography/mass spectrometry (GC/MS) are highly sensitive and specific techniques used to accurately identify and quantify specific drugs and their metabolites. They can be used to confirm an unexpected positive or negative EIA result [21].

Urine drug tests, especially LC/MS/MS and GC/MS can be relatively accurate. However, they are still prone to false positives and false negatives like any diagnostic test. This should be kept in mind when interpreting unexpected results. Analyzing almost 1,000 samples, Manchikanti et al. [24, 25] compared the diagnostic accuracy of immunoassay with liquid chromatography tandem mass spectrometry and found a high degree of agreement (90 % for oxycodone and as much as 99 % for cocaine) between the techniques. Their findings are summarized in Table 45.1. However, these data may not be strictly applied in clinical practice settings as many patients provide the history that they have used different drugs. Consequently, based on the patient history and physical examination, the sensitivity and specificity of an office drug testing protocol may be much higher, requiring very few specimens for ultimate confirmation.

When interpreting urine drug testing results, it is essential to keep in mind how long a given substance can be detected in the urine. For example, opioids like hydrocodone, oxycodone, or morphine may only be detected for 3 or 4 days after the last dose. However, methadone may be detected for 5–10 days after the last dose. Marijuana, on the other hand, can be detected for approximately 3 days after the last use with occasional use but can be detected up to 11 weeks with chronic use as shown in Table 45.2.

Although helpful for drug screening, quantitative urine drug testing by chromatography/mass spectrometry cannot reliably indicate how much actual drug the

Table 45.2 Urine drug testing: typical screening and confirmation cut-off concentrations and detection times for drugs of abuse

Drug	Screening cut-off concentrations ng/mL urine	Confirmation cut-off concentrations ng/mL	Urine detection time	Chromatography (C)
Hydrocodone	300	50	1–2 days	I & C
Oxycodone	100	50	1–3 days	I & C
Morphine	300	50	3–4 days	I & C
Methadone	300	100	5–10 days	I & C
Hydromorphone	300	100	1–2 days	I & C
Meperidine	300	100	1–2 days	I & C
Codeine	300	50	1–3 days	I & C
Benzodiazepines	200	20–50	Up to 30 days	I
Barbiturates	200	100	2–10 days	I & C
Marijuana	50	15	1–3 days for casual use; up to 11 weeks for chronic use	I & C
Cocaine	300	50	1–3 days	I & C
Amphetamine	1,000	100	2–4 days	I & C
Methamphetamine	1,000	100	2–4 days	I & C
Heroin[a]	10	25	1–3 days	I & C
Phencyclidine	25	10	2–8 days	I & C

Adapted with permission from [1]
[a]6-MAM, the specific metabolite is detected only for 6 h

patient is taking. There is significant individual variability in how the body absorbs, distributes, and metabolizes a given drug. As an example, Morphine absorption shows 2.5-fold variability between oral, buccal, and intramuscular routes. Furthermore, first pass metabolism can result in significant variability in the amount of a given drug reaching systemic circulation [21].

As discussed previously, immunoassay techniques are subject to cross reactivity. There are many drugs that can lead to false positive results. When interpreting urine drug test results, an unexpected positive result should be interpreted in the context of the patient's complete medical history and current medication list, including over the counter products and medication prescribed by another physician.

Drugs that may cause a false positive result [1] are listed in Table 45.3.

Combining patient history with urine drug testing is more reliable than either technique alone. In a university based pain clinic study of 122 patients with non-cancer pain treated with opioids, 21 % of patients with no behavioral issues had a positive urine drug screen for either an illicit drug or a non-prescribed controlled substance [12]. Behavioral issues were defined as "lost or stolen prescriptions, consumption in excess of prescribed dosage, visits without appointments, multiple drug intolerances and allergies, and frequent telephone calls" [12].

Table 45.3 Drug cross-reactants

Drug group	Cross reactivity based on product insert	Cross reactivity based on potential cross reaction
Cannabinoids	Dronabinol (Marinol)	NSAIDs
Efavirenz (Sustiva)		
Hemp Seed Oil (Cannabis seed)		
Pantoprazole (Protonix)		
Nexium		
Prilosec		
Opioids	6-Acetylmorphine	
Ethyl morphine		
Oxymorphone		
Oxycodone		
Methadone		
Dextromethorphan	Fluoroquinolones	
Ofloxacin (Floxin)		
Papaverine		
Poppy Seeds		
Rifampicin & Rifampin (Rimactane, Rifadin, Rofact)		
Levofloxacin (Levaquin)		
Amphetamines	Dextroamphetamine + amphetamine (Adderall)	Ephedrine
Methylphenidate		
Trazodone		
Bupropion		
Desipramine		
Amantadine		
Ranitidine		
Phenylpropanolamine		
Vicks Vapor Spray		
Phentermine (Adipex/Obenix/Oby-Trim)		
Pseudoephedrine		
Methamphetamine	d-Methamphetamine	
d-Amphetamine		
Chloroquine (Aralen)		
Desoxyephedrine		
MDMA (Ecstasy)		
Methamphetamine (Desoxyn)	Bupropion (Wellbutrin & Zyban)	
Chloroquine (Aralen)		
Chlorpromazine (Thorazine, Largactil)		
Desipramine (Norpramin)		
Dextroamphetamine (Dexedrine)		
Ephedrine (Ephedra and Ma Huang)		

(continued)

Table 45.3 (continued)

Drug group	Cross reactivity based on product insert	Cross reactivity based on potential cross reaction
Fenfluramine (Fen Phen)		
Labetalol (Labetalol)		
Mexiletine (Mexitil)		
n-acetyl procainamide (Procainamide)		
Phenylephrine (Neo-synephrine)		
Propranolol (Inderal)		
Pseudoephedrine (Claritin-D)		
Quinacrine (Atabrine, Mepacrine)		
Ranitidine (Zantac)		
Selegiline (Selegiline)		
Trazodone (Desyrel, Desyrel Dividose)		
Tyramine (Tyramine)		
PCP	None	Chlorpromazine
Meperidine		
Doxylamine		
Dextromethorphan		
Diphenhydramine (Benadryl)		
Thioridazine (Mellaril)		
Venlafaxine (Effexor)		
Benzodiazepine	Bromazepam (Tenix)	
Clobazam (Mystan)		
Estazolam (ProSom)	Oxaprozin (Daypro)	
Sertraline (Zoloft)		
Some herbal agents		
Cocaine	Benzoylecgonine	
Ecgonine		
Ecgonine Methyl Ester	TAC Solution (TAC Solution)	
ETOH	None	Asthma inhalers (sometimes)
Methadone	None	Propoxyphene
Seroquel		
Barbiturates	Alphenal	Phenytoin (Dilantin)
Primidone (Mysoline)		
Oxycodone	Hydrocodone	
Hydromorphone (Dilaudid)		
Oxymorphone (Numorphan)		
Codeine (Codeine)		

Source: DrugCheck® Cross Reactivity Chart (www.drugcheck.com/_images/DC145_Cross-Reactivity_chart.pdf)
Adapted with permission from [1]

Marijuana is the most common illicit drug found on urine drug testing, followed by cocaine. Opioids are the most common non-prescribed controlled drug found on urine drug testing followed by benzodiazepines, barbiturates, and ethanol.

A study by Michna and colleagues found that "gut instinct" was a poor predictor of an abnormal urine drug test [23]. In a university based pain clinic, retrospective analysis of data from 470 patients found no relationship between urine drug test result and sex, pain site, type of opioid dose or number of opioids prescribed, or prescribing physician [23]. The only correlation found in this population was that younger patients were found to have used illicit substances (mean age 44.1 ± 9.3) and/or additional non-prescribed opioids (mean age 44 ± 10) more often than older patients [23].

Pill Counts

Used in conjunction with interval history, PDMP data, and urine drug testing, pill counting is yet one more tool to monitor for adherence when prescribing chronic opioid therapy. Pill counts can be time consuming and impractical for routine widespread use in a busy ambulatory practice. To be effective, the pill counts should be random. They can be helpful in the event of an unexpected aberrant urine drug screen or when drug-seeking behavior is suspected. For example, a pill count can be helpful when evaluating a patient prescribed daily oxycodone who tests negative for oxycodone or its metabolite. A pill count may help uncover prescription medication diversion or, on the other hand, may support a working hypothesis of laboratory error.

An Algorithmic Approach

An algorithmic approach with risk stratification is shown in Fig. 45.1 and an algorithmic approach for managing a patient with chronic non-cancer pain from the initial visit to the remaining period or until discharged is shown in Fig. 45.2.

Manchikanti et al. [26] described a case of opioid misuse in a patient in an AHRQ publication describing the above algorithmic approach and discussed various issues related in adherence monitoring.

Summary

Physicians that prescribe chronic opioid therapy have an ethical and legal responsibility to monitor for treatment adherence. A comprehensive adherence-monitoring program will include pretreatment and ongoing risk assessment, toxicology

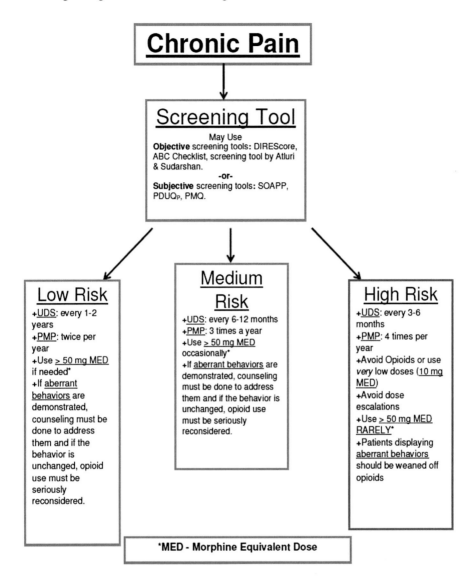

Chronic Pain

Screening Tool

May Use
Objective screening tools: DIREScore,
ABC Checklist, screening tool by Atluri
& Sudarshan.
-or-
Subjective screening tools: SOAPP,
PDUQ_P, PMQ.

Low Risk

+<u>UDS</u>: every 1-2
years
+<u>PMP</u>: twice per
year
+Use ≥ 50 mg MED
if needed*
+If <u>aberrant
behaviors</u> are
demonstrated,
counseling must be
done to address
them and if the
behavior is
unchanged, opioid
use must be
seriously
reconsidered.

Medium Risk

+<u>UDS</u>: every 6-12 months
+<u>PMP</u>: 3 times a year
+Use ≥ 50 mg MED
occasionally*
+If <u>aberrant behaviors</u> are
demonstrated, counseling
must be done to address
them and if the behavior is
unchanged, opioid use
must be seriously
reconsidered.

High Risk

+<u>UDS</u>: every 3-6
months
+<u>PMP</u>: 4 times per
year
+Avoid Opioids or use
very low doses (<u>10 mg
MED</u>)
+Avoid dose
escalations
+Use ≥ 50 mg MED
<u>RARELY</u>*
+Patients displaying
<u>aberrant behaviors</u>
should be weaned off
opioids

*MED - Morphine Equivalent Dose

Fig. 45.1 Risk stratification and adherence monitoring. Adapted with permission from [1]

screening, prescription monitoring program database inquiry, and pill counts. A standard and universally implemented program is the most reliable way to identify potential problems and improve patient safety. It is unwise to use "gut instinct" to decide which patients need monitoring as this method has proven unreliable at best.

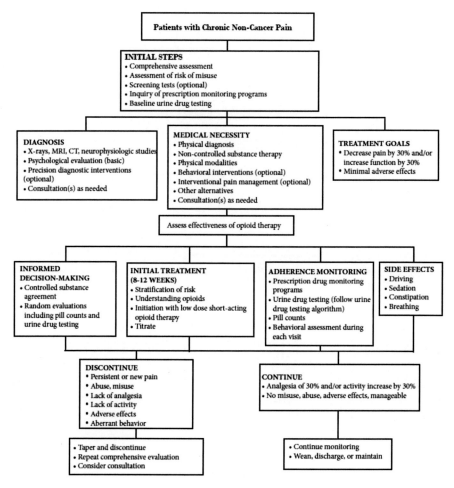

Fig. 45.2 Guidance to opioid therapy. Adapted with permission from [1]

References

1. Manchikanti L, Abdi S, Atluri S, et al. American Society of Interventional Pain Physicians (ASIPP) guidelines for responsible opioid prescribing in chronic non-cancer pain: Part 2—guidance. Pain Physician. 2012;15:S67–116.
2. Manchikanti L, Boswell MV, Hirsch JA. Lessons learned in the abuse of pain-relief medication: a focus on healthcare costs. Expert Rev Neurother. 2013;13:527–43.
3. Christo PJ, Manchikanti L, Ruan X, Bottros M, Hansen H, Solanki D, Jordan AE, Colson J. Urine drug testing in chronic pain. Pain Physician. 2011;14:123–43.
4. Atluri SL, Akbik H, Sudarshan G. Prevention of opioid abuse in chronic non-cancer pain: an algorithmic, evidence-based approach. Pain Physician. 2012;15:ES177–89.
5. Manchikanti L, Helm II S, Fellows B, Janata JW, Pampati V, Grider JS, Boswell MV. Opioid epidemic in the United States. Pain Physician. 2012;15:ES9–38.

6. Centers for Disease Control and Prevention. CDC grand rounds: prescription drug overdoses—a U.S. epidemic. MMWR Morb Mortal Wkly Rep. 2012;61:10–3.
7. Centers for Disease Control and Prevention. Vital signs: overdoses of prescription opioid pain relievers—United States, 1999–2008. MMWR Morb Mortal Wkly Rep. 2011;60:1487–92.
8. Kuehn BM. Prescription drug abuse rises globally. JAMA. 2007;297:1306.
9. Report of the International Narcotics Control Board for 2011. United Nations, New York; 2011. www.unodc.org/documents/southasia/reports/2011_INCB_ANNUAL_REPORT_english_PDF.pdf.
10. The Use of Medicines in the United States: review of 2011. Report by the IMS Institute for Healthcare Informatics. www.imshealth.com.
11. Inocencio TJ, Carroll NV, Read EJ, Holdford DA. The economic burden of opioid-related poisoning in the United States. Pain Med. 2013. doi:10.1111/pme.12183 [Epub ahead of print].
12. Katz NP, Sherburne S, Beach M, et al. Behavioral monitoring and urine toxicology testing in patients receiving long-term opioid therapy. Anesth Analg. 2003;97:1097–102.
13. Chou R, Fanciullo GJ, Fine PG, et al. American Pain Society—American Academy of Pain Medicine Opioids guidelines panel; clinical guidelines for the use of chronic opioid therapy in chronic non-cancer pain. J Pain. 2009;10:113–30.
14. Centers for Disease Control and Prevention. Prescription drug overdose: state law. http://www.cdc.gov/HomeandRecreationalSafety/poisoning/laws/index.html.
15. Baehren DF, Marco CA, Droz DE, et al. A statewide prescription monitoring program affects emergency department prescribing behaviors. Ann Emerg Med. 2010;56:19–23.
16. Solanki DR, Koyyalagunta D, Shah RV, Silverman SM, Manchikanti L. Monitoring opioid adherence in chronic pain patients: assessment of risk of substance misuse. Pain Physician. 2011;14:E119–31.
17. Sehgal N, Manchikanti L, Smith HS. Prescription opioid abuse in chronic pain: a review of opioid abuse predictors and strategies to curb opioid abuse. Pain Physician. 2012;15:ES67–92.
18. Manchikanti L, Whitfield E, Pallone F. Evolution of the National All Schedules Prescription Electronic Reporting Act (NASPER): a public law for balancing treatment of pain and drug abuse and diversion. Pain Physician. 2005;8:335–47.
19. Goodin A, Blumenschein K, Freeman PR, Talbert J. Consumer/patient encounters with prescription drug monitoring programs: evidence from a Medicaid population. Pain Physician. 2012;15:ES169–75.
20. Drug Enforcement Administration and the National Alliance for Model State Drug Laws. A closer look at state prescription monitoring programs. http://www.deadiversion.usdoj.gov/pubs/program/prescription-monitor/summary.htm.
21. Nafziger AN, Bertino Jr JS. Utility and application of urine drug testing in chronic pain management with opioids. Clin J Pain. 2009;25(1):73–9.
22. Standridge JB, Adams SM, Zotos AP. Drug screening: a valuable office procedure. Am Fam Physician. 2010;81:635–40.
23. Michna E, Jamison RN, Pham LD, Ross EL, Janfaza D, Nedeljkovic SS, Narang S, Palombi D, Wasan AD. Toxicology screening among chronic pain patients on opioid therapy: frequency and predictability of abnormal findings. Clin J Pain. 2007;23:173–9.
24. Manchikanti L, Malla Y, Wargo BW, Fellows B. Comparative evaluation of the accuracy of immunoassay with liquid chromatography tandem mass spectrometry (LC/MS/MS) of urine drug testing (UDT) opioids and illicit drugs in chronic pain patients. Pain Physician. 2011;14:175–87.
25. Manchikanti L, Malla Y, Wargo BW, Fellows B. Comparative evaluation of the accuracy of benzodiazepine testing in chronic pain patients utilizing immunoassay with liquid chromatography tandem mass spectrometry (LC/MS/MS) of urine drug testing. Pain Physician. 2011;14:259–70.
26. Manchikanti L, Hirsch JA. The pains of chronic opioid usage [Spotlight]. AHRQ WebM&M [serial online]. September 2013.

Index

© Springer Science+Business Media New York 2015

633

A.D. Kaye et al. (eds.), *Substance Abuse*, DOI 10.1007/978-1-4939-1951-2

Printed in the United States
By Bookmasters